KU-220-283

Advances in the Neurobiology of Anxiety Disorders

Edited by
H. G. M. WESTENBERG
Department of Biological Psychiatry, Academic Hospital Utrecht, The Netherlands

J. A. DEN BOER
Department of Biological Psychiatry, Academic Hospital Groningen, The Netherlands

and

D. L. MURPHY
National Institute of Mental Health, Laboratory of Clinical Sciences, Bethesda, MD, USA

JOHN WILEY & SONS
Chichester · New York · Brisbane · Toronto · Singapore

Copyright © 1996 by John Wiley & Sons Ltd,
            Baffins Lane, Chichester,
            West Sussex PO19 1UD, England

            National   01243 779777
            International   (+44) 1243 779777

All rights reserved.

No part of this book may be reproduced by any means,
or transmitted, or translated into a machine language
without the written permission of the publisher.

Other Wiley Editorial Offices

John Wiley & Sons, Inc., 605 Third Avenue,
New York, NY 10158-0012, USA

Jacaranda Wiley Ltd, 33 Park Road, Milton,
Queensland 4064, Australia

John Wiley & Sons (Canada) Ltd, 22 Worcester Road,
Rexdale, Ontario M9W 1L1, Canada

John Wiley & Sons (Asia) Pte Ltd, 2 Clementi Loop #02-01,
Jin Xing Distripark, Singapore 0512

Library of Congress Cataloging-in-Publication Data

Advances in the neurobiology of anxiety disorders/edited by H. G. M.
    Westenberg, J. A. den Boer and D. L. Murphy.
        p. cm. — (Wiley series on clinical and neurobiological
    advances in psychiatry v. 2)
        ISBN 0 471 96124 8 (alk. paper)
        1. Anxiety—Physiological aspects. 2. Anxiety—Chemotherapy.
    I. Westenberg, Herman Gerrit Marinus. II. Boer, Johan A. den, 1953–.
    III. Murphy, Dennis L. IV. Series.
    [DNLM: 1. Anxiety Disorders—physiopathology. 2. Anxiety
    Disorders—drug therapy.   W1 WI53J v. 2 1996 / WM 172 A2446 1996]
    RC531.A38   1996
    616.85' 223—dc20   96-4645
                                                              CIP

British Library Cataloguing in Publication Data

A catalogue record for this book is available from the British Library

ISBN 0 471 96124 8

Typeset in 10/12pt Times by Saxon Graphics Ltd, Derby
Printed and bound in Great Britain by Bookcraft (Bath) Ltd, Midsomer Norton
This book is printed on acid-free paper responsibly manufactured from sustainable
forestation, for which at least two trees are planted for each one used for paper production.

Advances in the Neurobiology
of Anxiety Disorders

WILEY SERIES ON
CLINICAL AND NEUROBIOLOGICAL PSYCHIATRY

Series Editors: J. A. Den Boer and H. G. M. Westenberg

Volume 1
Advances in the Neurobiology of Schizophrenia
Edited by J. A. Den Boer, H. G. M. Westenberg and H. M. Van Praag

Volume 2
Advances in the Neurobiology of Anxiety Disorders
Edited by H. G. M. Westenberg, J. A. Den Boer and D. L. Murphy

Volume 3
Depression: Neurobiological, Psychopathological and Therapeutic Advances
Edited by A. Honig, M. Ansseau and H. M. Van Praag

Further volumes in preparation

Cover illustration by kind permission of
Andrew W. Goddard, chapter 6, this volume

Contents

Contributors

M. Altemus
NIMH, 9000 Rockville Pike, Bethesda, MD 20892, USA

N. Andrews
Psychopharmacology Research Unit, Guy's Hospital, London SE1 9RT, UK

J. C. Ballenger
Department of Psychiatry, 171 Ashley Avenue, Charleston, SC 29425, USA

R. Balon
University Psychiatric Center, Wayne State University, Suite 200, 2751 Jefferson, Detroit, MI 48207, USA

L. R. Baxter Jr
University of California, Neuropsychiatric Institute, 760 Westwood Plaza, Los Angeles, CA 90024, USA

J. Benjamin
Laboratory of Clinical Science, NIMH, 9000 Rockville Pike, Bethesda, MD 20892, USA

A. L. Brody
University of California, Neuropsychiatric Institute, 760 Westwood Plaza, Los Angeles, CA 90024, USA

D. S. Charney
Veterans Administration Medical Center, 950 Campbell Avenue, West Haven, CT 06516, USA

J. D. Coplan
Columbia University, Department of Psychiatry, 722 West 168th Street, New York, NY 10032, USA

J. A. Den Boer
Department of Psychiatry, University Hospital Utrecht, PO Box 85500, 3500 GA Utrecht, The Netherlands

O. T. Dolberg
Chaim Sheba Medical Center, Department of Psychiatry, Tel Hashomer, 52612 Ramat Gan, Israel

S. E. File
Psychopharmacology Research Unit, Guy's Hospital, London SE1 9RT, UK

D. Foley
Mental Health Research Institute of Victoria, Private Bag 3, Parkville, Victoria 3052, Australia

G. Glas
Department of Psychiatry, Heidelberglaan 100, 3584 CX Utrecht, The Netherlands

D. A. Glitz
Wayne State University, Detroit, MI, USA

A. W. Goddard
Yale University, Department of Psychiatry, New Haven, CT 0619, USA

T. Grady
Duke University Medical Center, Department of Psychiatry, Trent Drive, Durham, NC, USA

B. Greenberg
Laboratory of Clinical Science, NIMH, 9000 Rockville Pike, Bethesda, MD 20892, USA

L. Groenink
Department of Psychopharmacology, Utrecht University, Sorbonne, Laan 16, 3584 CA Utrecht, The Netherlands

S. Hogg
Psychopharmacology Research Unit, Guy's Hospital, London SE1 9RT, UK

R. Joordens
Department of Psychopharmacology, Utrecht University, Sorbonnelaan 16, 3584 CA Utrecht, The Netherlands

R. S. Kahn
Department of Psychiatry, University Hospital Utrecht, PO Box 85500, 350 GA Utrecht, The Netherlands

J. W. Kasckow
Department of Psychiatry, UC College of Medicine, 231 Bethesda Avenue, ML 559, Cincinnati, OH 45267-0559, USA

S. Kindler
Chaim Sheba Medical Center, Department of Psychiatry, Tel Hashomer, 52612 Ramat Gan, Israel

D. F. Klein
Department of Psychiatry, Columbia University, 722 West 168th Street, New York, NY 10032, USA

M. Kotler
Chaim Sheba Medical Center, Department of Psychiatry, Tel Hashomer, 52612 Ramat Gan, Israel

A. Mackinnon
Biostatistics and Psychometrics Unit, Mental Health Research Institute of Victoria, Private Bag 3, Parkville, Victoria 3052, Australia

D. Marazziti
Chaim Sheba Medical Center, Tel Hashomer, 52612 Ramat Gan, Israel

E. Molewijk
CNS Research, Solvay Duphar, PO Box 900, 1380 DA Weesp, The Netherlands

J. Mos
CNS Research, Solvay Duphar BV, PO Box 900, 1380 DA Weesp, The Netherlands

D. L. Murphy
Laboratory of Clinical Science, NIMH, 9000 Rockville Pike, Bethesda, MD 20892, USA

C. B. Nemeroff
Department of Psychiatry and Behavioral Sciences, 1639 Pierce Drive, Suite 4000, Atlanta, GA 30322, USA

B. Olivier
CNS Research, Solvay Duphar BV, C J van Houtenlaan 36, 1381 CP Weesp, The Netherlands

T. Pigott
Department of Psychiatry, Georgetown University Medical Center, 3750 Reservoir Road NW, Washington, DC, USA

Y. Sasson
Chaim Sheba Medical Center, Department of Psychiatry, Tel Hashomer, 52612 Ramat Gan, Israel

S. M. Stahl
Clinical Neuroscience Research Center, 8899 University Center Lane, Suite 130, San Diego, CA 92122, USA

B. A. Van der Kolk
Trauma Center at HRI Hospital, 227 Babcock Street, Brookline, MA 02146, USA

H. J. G. M. Van Megen
Department of Psychiatry, University Hospital Utrecht, PO Box 85500, 350 GA Utrecht, The Netherlands

H. M. Van Praag
Department of Psychiatry, Academisch Psychiatrisch Centrum, P Debijelaan 25, 6229 HA Maastricht, The Netherlands

I. M. Van Vliet
Department of Psychiatry, Academic Hospital, PO Box 85500, 3508 GA Utrecht, The Netherlands

H. G. M. Westenberg Department of Psychiatry, University Hospital Utrecht, PO Box 85500, 3508 GA Utrecht, The Netherlands

S. W. Woods Yale University, Department of Psychiatry, New Haven, CT, USA

T. Zethof CNS Research, Solvay Duphar BV, PO Box 900, 1380 DA Weesp, The Netherlands

J. Zohar Chaim Sheba Medical Center, Tel Hashomer, 52612 Ramat Gan, Israel

Series Preface

In the past twenty years we have witnessed an impressive shift in doctrine, methods of investigation and perspective regarding the relationship between processes in the brain and subjective experience. Parallel to developments in philosophy, where philosophers have become increasingly involved in science, psychiatry has swung towards a more scientific approach as well.

Nowadays, neural systems and certain psychiatric disorders are known to be linked. Major advances in the neurosciences have opened up new research possibilities and have increased our understanding of the relationship between cerebral processes and behavioral, cognitive and emotional disorders. During the last decade our knowledge of different receptors in the brain has expanded with striking speed.

It is without exaggeration that we can state that recent advances in basic molecular biology and related fields will, in the years to come, dramatically increase the possibilities of gaining insight into brain–behavior relationships.

Another major development has been the introduction of imaging techniques in psychiatry. We now have the unprecedented possibility to study brain processes during actual different emotional and cognitive states.

In other areas of psychiatry there is a trend towards a more empirical approach to the investigation of psychiatric disturbance. Major improvements have been made in psychological testing methods and psychometric assessments, as witnessed by the introduction of (semi) standardized interview techniques in areas like axis one diagnoses, as well as in the domain of personality disorders.

The purpose of this series is to focus on major developments in the field of biological psychiatry, particularly those with clinical relevance. Biological factors, important as they are, do not exist in a vacuum and can be affected by environmental, intrapsychic and societal influences which may all have an impact on the biology of the brain.

It is with this conviction in mind that we hope this series will provide the clinical psychiatrist, the experimental psychologist and the neuroscientist with an updated critical overview of advances in our understanding of the biological processes which underpin psychiatric disease.

J. A. Den Boer
H. G. M. Westenberg

Part 1

INTRODUCTION

1 Concepts of Anxiety: A Historical Reflection on Anxiety and Related Disorders

GERRIT GLAS

University Hospital Utrecht and State University of Leiden, The Netherlands

INTRODUCTION

There is perhaps no better way to illustrate the changes in twentieth-century psychiatric thinking, than by delineating the history of the concept of anxiety. One aim of this introductory chapter is to briefly summarize these changes and to sensitize to the social, conceptual and philosophical issues which are involved here.

At the same time, elucidating the historical and conceptual background of our contemporary view of anxiety may also be fruitful for the understanding of anxiety itself, as a conglomerate of concrete phenomena. It may remind us, among others, of the elusive nature of the experience of anxiety, the immense diversity of its (sometimes idiosyncratic) behavioral and physiological manifestations, its mingling with other forms of psychopathology, and, not to mention more, the existential dimension of the experience of anxiety.

In summary, the focus of our historical review will be both on theory and on the phenomenon of anxiety itself. The history of the concept of anxiety can be seen as a reflection of changes in the self-conception of psychiatry. At the same time, these changes show the phenomenon of anxiety from different angles.

ETYMOLOGY

The word anxiety probably derives from the Indo-Germanic root *Angh*, which means to constrict, to narrow, or to strangulate (Lewis, 1967). This root reappears in the Greek word *anchein* which means to strangle, to suffocate, or to press shut. The root *Angh* has survived in Latin, for example in *angor* (suffocation, feeling of entrapment) and *anxietas* (overconcern; shrink back fearfully),

Advances in the Neurobiology of Anxiety Disorders. Edited by H. G. M. Westenberg, J. A. Den Boer and D. L. Murphy
©1996 John Wiley & Sons Ltd

and in some contemporary European languages. In spite of the numerous con-
notations and subtle shifts of meaning, the perception of tightness and constriction of the throat and of the chest can still be recognized as a central element of
meaning in terms derived from the root *Angh* in these modern languages.

 Fear derives from the German stem *freisa* or *frasa*. Phobia and panic on the
other hand have a Greek background. Panic refers to *Pan* or *Panikos*, the Greek
god of the forests and of shepherds, who was thought to have caused panic
among the Persians at Marathon.

FROM ANTIQUITY TO THE MIDDLE OF THE
NINETEENTH CENTURY

First of all, it should be realized that from Antiquity to the middle of the nineteenth-century medicine did not recognize the need for a systematic distinction
between anxiety and depression. This does not mean that the numerous manifestations of anxiety and depression have not been observed and described. On
the contrary, the *Corpus Hippocraticum* and other medical texts, like those of
Galen, Burton and nineteenth-century alienists, contain many lively descriptions of people suffering from conditions which now would be identified as
anxiety or depressive disorder. For centuries, however, these conditions were
encompassed by the broad concept of melancholia.

 This concept, of course, refers to the so-called humoral theory, according to
which disease results from a disturbance in the balance of four bodily fluids:
blood, yellow bile, black bile and phlegm. The earliest formulation of this theory can be discovered in the *Corpus Hippocraticum*, a series of 70 medical texts
dating from the fifth century BC, which are attributed to Hippocrates and his
pupils. Melancholia, or black bile disease, is only briefly mentioned here, with
fear and despondency as its dominant characteristics. The full description of its
effects can be found in the work of Galen (AD 131–201), more than five centuries later. Galen ascribed the anxiety seen in melancholics to a dark-colored
vapor emanating from black bile, as a result of local heating in the hypochon-
drium. This smoky vapor, he thought, rose up into the brain, producing fear and
mental obscuration.

> As external darkness renders almost all persons fearful, with the exception of a
> few naturally audacious ones or those who were specially trained, thus the color
> of the black bile induces fear when its darkness throws a shadow over the area of
> thought [in the brain] (Galenus, p. 93).

According to later writers of the Galenic school, the heating process also
explains the motor restlessness and other behavioral phenomena of this
(hypochondriacal) form of melancholia.

 During the Middle Ages humoral pathology was systematized. One of the
effects was a sharper distinction between melancholia as a result of an excess

(or heating) of natural black bile and melancholia being caused by an excess of unnatural black bile. This unnatural black bile was thought to be produced by combustion, or degeneration, of one of the four bodily fluids. Preoccupation of death, for instance, was associated with combustion or degeneration of black bile, mania with degeneration of yellow bile, apathy with degeneration of phlegm.

Medical literature on melancholia culminates in Robert Burton's *The Anatomy of Melancholy*, published in 1621. Greatly indebted to ancient medicine and philosophy, this peculiar and sometimes rather bizarre work compiles all knowledge of that time on the subject of melancholia. Sorrow and fear are considered to be the major causes of melancholia, sorrow being related to disaster in the present and fear to disaster in the future. In discussing the symptoms of melancholia, Burton shows to be acquainted with many of the forms of anxiety known today: fear of death; fear of losing those who are most important to us; anxiety based on paranoid delusions and delusions of reference; fear associated with depersonalization; delusional depersonalization; hypochondria; anticipatory anxiety; hyperventilation; agoraphobia; and many specific phobias, such as fear of public speaking, fear of heights, and claustrophobia (Burton, 1621, pp. 442–449).

It was ultimately at the end of the eighteenth century that humoral pathology lost its grip on medical thinking. Pathological anatomy had expanded greatly. More emphasis was put on clinical observation and description. It was a time of sensualism and of a fascination with sensibility and sensory perception. Popular notions in medical literature of that time, like irritability and tone, betray a preoccupation with the hypersensitivity of the nervous system and of the senses. The central nervous system gradually replaced the blood, the liver and the spleen, from which, until then, melancholia was thought to originate.

Today, the idea of temperament is all that remains of humoralism, as a metaphorical expression for the experiences of despondent people.

THE TURNING POINT: AGORAPHOBIA AND ANXIETY UNDER CIRCUMSTANCES OF WAR

Flemming's *Über Praecordialangst (On Precordial Pain)*, which dates from 1848, is probably the first medical text devoted to a non-phobic form of anxiety as a more or less specific entity (Schmidt-Degenhard, 1986). It was, however, not this publication which became a turning point in the conceptual history of anxiety and anxiety disorders. For that, we have to wait until 1870, when in a short span of time three articles appeared which would become particularly authoritative. First of these is a short article by Benedikt (1870) entitled *Über Platzschwindel (On Dizziness on Squares)*. It described a patient who, as soon as he entered a street or a square, was overcome by dizziness. Terrified of collapsing mentally and gripped by a tremendous fear he never dared to pass through that place again. Benedikt, thus, believed the anxiety to be secondary to the dizziness of this patient. Two years later, that view was challenged by Westphal (1872), who was the first to use the term agoraphobia in a technical sense. Westphal stated that it was the anxiety that caused the dizziness. He based his hypothesis on clinical observation. Interestingly enough, he was very much aware that the three patients he described were not afraid of streets or squares as such. He stressed the unfounded nature of their anxiety. Theirs was rather a fear of anxiety itself, an anxiety that only much later was linked to particular situations. Westphal's critique on Benedikt anticipates a debate that would reach its climax more than a century later in the controversy about the provocative role of bodily sensations (and their interpretation) in the origin of panic attacks.

In the same period, the American cardiologist Da Costa (1871) wrote another classic on a quite different form of anxiety. Auscultating the cardiac murmurs of more than 300 exhausted soldiers returning from the front, he heard some abnormalities, for which he coined the term "irritable heart". The patients complained of palpitations, pain in the chest and extreme fatigue. Heightened nervous irritability, he believed, was the cause of the condition. The ensuing debate, which became particularly intense during and after the two World Wars, centered around the nature of the intolerance to physical exertion. Thomas Lewis, who studied many such cases among British soldiers in World War I and to whom we owe the term effort syndrome, rejected the one-sided emphasis on the heart and the presumed cardiac origin of the complaints. Although many agreed with this, there still was no unanimity about what actually lay behind the syndrome. Some emphasized the role of psychogenic factors (Culpin, 1920; Wood, 1941), others argued for a multifactorial origin of the condition, pointing to constitution, previous infections, heavy exercise and neurotic mechanisms as precipitating factors (MacKenzie, 1916, 1920; Jones and Lewis, 1941; Jones, 1948).

The debate was settled provisionally by two studies: one by the cardiologist Paul Wood (1941), the other by (Maxwell) Jones (1948), better known as the protagonist of the therapeutic community. According to Wood the symptoms of the "irritable heart" were also prevalent in peacetime and closely resembled those of anxiety neurosis. Especially susceptible were patients who, in childhood, "clung too long to their mothers' skirts" (Wood, 1941, p. 846). Owing to parental overconcern or comments by their physician, these patients would have learned to interpret various normal physiological symptoms as signs of physical danger or heart disease. One should be reminded that this was said long before the formulation of attribution theory (MacKenzie, 1920). Jones concurred with this in his award-winning study. Although he emphasized the reality of the intolerance to physical exertion, he interpreted it as the result of (subconscious) avoidance. His physiological investigations demonstrated namely a slightly smaller increase of the level of lactate in patients compared to normal controls at the subjective maximum of exertion. From this he concluded that the patients stopped exerting themselves before they reached their physiological maximum. The effort syndrome, in fact, was an effort phobia. Jones developed a form of group psychoeducation, using groups of about 100 patients. Experiences with these groups would become important for his later ideas on the therapeutic community.

Wars have contributed greatly to our knowledge of anxiety disorders, in particular the so-called traumatic neuroses. In addition, they direct our attention to the social influences affecting psychiatric diagnosis. The term effort syndrome, for instance, can be seen as a reflection at the diagnostic level of the military importance of the capacity to deliver physical effort.

NEURASTHENIA AND ANXIETY NEUROSIS

In the last decades of the nineteenth century, a new concept, neurasthenia, gained ground. George M. Beard, the American advocate of this idea, considered neurasthenia to be a functional disorder characterized by a deficiency of "nervous energy". This deficiency could express itself in a multitude of symptoms, mainly at the level of the central nervous system, the digestive tract and the reproductive tract (Beard, 1884, 1890). Although not highly prominent among these symptoms, morbid fear and phobias were nevertheless ranked among the most difficult symptoms to cure. The concept of neurasthenia is closely linked to Beard's view of American society, which supposedly generated much more excitation of the nervous system than did European society. "American nervousness", one of Beard's favorite synonyms for neurasthenia, was a typical product of an industrial society in which the upper classes were doomed to a hectic lifestyle.

Beard's contribution to psychopathology has to be sought in his meticulous description of even the most idiosyncratic symptoms and in his attempt to focus psychiatry's attention to patients that could not be found in the hospitals and mental institutions of that time. Neurasthenia was a disease of the street, according to Beard. The idea of nervous energy, with its clearly Romantic and vitalistic background, was abandoned after several decades, as well as the reflex (or irradiation) theory which said that local functional disorders could be transmitted to other organs by the sympathetic nerve.

The history of the classification of anxiety disorders since the time of Beard can be seen as a peeling-away of layers of the concept of neurasthenia. Anxiety neurosis was the first stratum to be laid bare under its surface. Next came all sorts of classificatory subdivisions within anxiety neurosis (Tyrer, 1984).

Hecker initiated the above-mentioned process in a classic article on anxiety states in neurasthenia (Hecker, 1893). He had noticed that the anxiety attacks experienced by many neurasthenia sufferers were not accompanied by any subjective feeling of anxiety. Hecker used the term "larvirt" (larval; larva-like) to denote this absence of a feeling of anxiety. The term "abortiv", on the other hand, indicated the interrupted, incomplete nature of the attacks. These patients did not show the full range of physical symptoms. The picture described by Hecker bears some resemblance to the so-called "limited symptom attacks" in present-day literature on panic disorder.

In 1895, Sigmund Freud, with reference to Hecker, joined the critics of Beard's broad concept of neurasthenia. However, in being more explicit about pathogenesis, Freud went a step further than Hecker (Freud, 1895a, 1895c). He regarded the distinction between neurasthenia and anxiety neurosis to be essential, since anxiety neurosis had a different pathogenesis and required a different treatment. Neurasthenia was a disorder of the way in which the so-called somatic-sexual excitation was released, whereas anxiety neurosis was primarily a disorder in the psychic processing of such excitation.

In the case of anxiety neurosis, Freud imagined that there was a build-up of pressure on the walls of the male seminal vesicles. When this pressure exceeded a given threshold, it was transformed into somatic energy and transmitted, via neural pathways, to the cerebral cortex. Under normal conditions, sexual "fantasy groups" became charged with this energy, leading to sexual excitement (libido) and the pursuit of release. Anxiety neurosis involved a blockage in the psychic processing of this somatic sexual tension. Such a blockage might arise through abstinence, for example, or due to the use of coitus interruptus, or because sexual fantasies had simply failed to take shape. Somatic sexual tension was thus deflected away from the psyche (the cortex) and directed to subcortical paths, finally expressing itself as "inadequate actions". These inadequate actions most characteristically occurred during an anxiety attack.

The pioneering article in which Freud detached anxiety neurosis from neurasthenia includes a description of the symptomatology of the various forms of anxiety which is still valid today (Freud, 1895a). Freud cited anxious expectation as the core symptom of anxiety neurosis. He also distinguished between specific phobias, agoraphobia, free floating anxiety and anxiety attacks. The latter were spontaneous in nature and were described as purely somatic phenomena (Freud, 1895c, pp. 368–369). The aforementioned distinctions anticipated the now generally accepted classification of specific phobias, agoraphobia, generalized anxiety and panic disorder. Freud was not alone in anticipating DSM-III-R. As the authors of DSM-III-R have acknowledged, striking similarities are also to be found in the sixth edition of Emil Kraepelin's handbook of psychiatry (Kraepelin, 1899; Spitzer and Williams, 1985).

Furthermore, it is interesting that Freud considered agoraphobia to be characterized by a fear of panic attacks, and not by fear of streets or squares per se:

> ce que redoute ce malade c'est l'événement d'une telle attaque [what the patient fears is the occurrence of such an attack] (Freud, 1895b, p. 352)

Ultimately however, it was not these interpretations of anxiety neurosis which would survive. Freud's second theory of anxiety, in which anxiety was interpreted as a signal of inner threat, would have much greater influence (Freud, 1926). This second theory had already announced its arrival by around 1895, albeit in a somatic guise. Freud asked why non-processed sexual excitation should express itself specifically in the form of anxiety. In answering this question, a glimpse is afforded of something which much later would become more explicit. Unlike real anxiety, which is based on the perception of external danger, neurotic anxiety is a reaction to inner threat. The core of this inner threat is an inability to process "endogenously" created (sexual) excitation (Freud, 1895a, p. 338). On another occasion Freud put it as follows:

> Anxiety is the sensation of the accumulation of another endogenous stimulus, the stimulus to breathing (Freud, 1894, p. 194)

It is sometimes forgotten that elements of the above hypothesis also appeared in Freud's signal theory. There also the basis of all anxiety is biological helplessness, i.e. the helplessness of the child with respect to its own drive impulses (cf. Freud, 1926, p. 68).

Although the signal theory also concerns the satisfying of needs, it does not relate primarily to sexual needs but rather to those associated with the instinct for self-preservation (cf. Freud, 1933, pp. 100–101). Object loss, the most clear-cut threat recognized by this instinct, becomes the psychological prerequisite for inducing the ego to release a small quantum of anxiety in order to restore a favorable balance of pleasure and pain. The threat of object loss remains linked to the biological state of being at the mercy of one's drive impulses. This linkage is mediated by remembrance symbols which, via separation and birth, ultimately refer to an archaic inheritance of hereditary anxiety responses. In anxious patients, the symptom of gasping for air is no longer seen as a mitigated orgasm but rather as the rudiment of the cry of a newborn child (Freud, 1926, p. 168).

In a negative sense, Freud's second theory of anxiety was of great significance within the classification debate. His view of anxiety as the invariable outcome of all kinds of unresolved neurotic conflict illustrates the nosologically non-specific character he attributed to anxiety. The influence of this view partly explains why the classification of anxiety and anxiety disorders became such a neglected theme in the period between 1930 and 1960.

This is not meant to detract from Freud's merits. In the field of anxiety theory, these merits lay particularly in the concept of anxiety as a reaction to inner threat. This idea, which was without precedent in Freud's days, permanently changed the face of psychiatry. Freud thereby gave a wholly individual treatment to the fundamental distinction between (object-less) anxiety and (object-linked) fear, a theme which for the rest was to find its way into psychiatry via another route (Kierkegaard, Jaspers and existential phenomenology). Moreover, Freud's approach was not limited to the psychoanalytic school. At least one of the contemporary currents in cognitive psychology has built explicitly upon Freud's pioneering concept of anxiety as an inner threat (Beck, 1976; Beck et al., 1985).

PSYCHASTHENIA

One of the most remarkable studies in the history of the classification of anxiety is Pierre Janet's *Les Obsessions et la Psychasthénie* (*The Obsessions and Psychasthenia*), dating from 1903. This work, written in an elegant and still readable style, not only offers an overview of all possible manifestations of pathological anxiety, it also contains numerous vivid descriptions of conditions which today are known as depersonalization, somatoform disorder, hypochondria, stereotyped movement disorder and chronic fatigue syndrome.

Janet argues against the tendency of many of his colleagues to divide the symptom clusters into separate diagnostic entities. Indeed, he presents a classification of his own, by making a distinction between three types of psychasthenia: obsessive thoughts, irresistible movements (compulsions, tics, outbursts of temper as a result of the inability to complete the compulsions) and visceral anxiety (generalized anxiety, panic, phobias and even pain syndromes). These types in their turn are subdivided into various clinical states. Janet nevertheless emphasizes the close ties between these states. In the course of their illness many patients show symptoms of conditions belonging to different types. Moreover, suppression of the target symptoms of one type often leads to the emergence of symptoms belonging to another type of psychasthenia. Blocking of the obsessions, for instance, heightens the anxiety and may induce compulsive behavior. Resisting one's compulsions, on the other hand, often leads to cardiac palpitations and the sensation of suffocation.

The real innovative element of Janet's study, however, is his attempt to fit his numerous observations in a general theory of psychological functioning. Already in the Introduction Janet declares his sympathy with the French psychologist Ribot, who was one of his intellectual fathers and who had made a plea for the close collaboration between medicine and psychology. Common to all patients, says Janet, is a disturbance in psychological functioning, the so-called psychasthenic state or psychasthenia. This state is characterized by three distinctive features, namely:

1. a "sense of incompleteness" ("sentiment d'incomplétude");
2. a diminishing or loss of "the sense (or function) of reality" ("la fonction du réel"); and
3. exhaustion (Janet, 1903, p. 439).

It is not easy to perceive what Janet exactly meant with the first two of these features. Roughly speaking, the sense of incompleteness refers to the subjective feeling that something is missing in one's actions, feelings or intellectual functioning. It is a sense of incapacity and of being unsuccessful. Whatever one does, it seems useless and not to come to an end. Doubt, hesitance, and endless rumination dominate one's activities. Depersonalization, feelings of doubleness and unreality, restlessness, apathy and disgust complete this list of manifestations.

With regard to the second feature, the diminishing of "the sense (or function) of reality", it is at first sight even harder to imagine what Janet had in mind. Citing Spencer, he defines it as "the coefficient of reality of a psychological fact" (Janet, 1903, p. 487). Rephrasing this statement, one could say that certain classes of psychic functioning can be assessed with respect to their degree of reality, i.e. to a certain quality of psychic functioning in relation to actual tasks and circumstances. In sum, the "function of reality" refers to the capacity to be present, spontaneous and effective, particularly in the domain of voluntary action, attention and perception.

Janet, after all, discerns five hierarchical levels of psychological functioning: the function of reality at the upper level; then indifferent activities (routine acts and vague perceptions), the imaging function (memory, imagination, abstract reasoning, and daydreaming) and visceral emotional reactions; and finally, at the lowest level, involuntary muscular movements. The quality of psychological functioning is determined by the so-called psychological tension, the psychic correlate of the nervous energy, which Beard and Freud had alluded to. Lowering of this tension initially leads to a lack of attention, concentration and other synthetic mental functions, in other words, to a loss of "la fonction du réel" and—subsequently—to a disruption of routine activities at the second level. The psychasthenic state is the result of precisely this lowering of psychic tension ("abaissement de la tension psychologique"; Janet, 1903, p. 497).

From this, it will become clear that anxiety is by no means the central symptom in Janet's account of the psychasthenic state. Anxiety occurs when psychic functioning is disturbed from the upper level down to the fourth level, that of the visceral emotional reactions. Anxiety, consequently, belongs to the most elementary of the mental functions:

> Underneath the anger, fear, and love, there is an emotion, that is not specific any more, that is a sum-total of vague respiratory and cardiac complaints, which don't evoke in the mind the idea of any inclination or any particular action. That emotion is called anxiety, the most elementary of the mental functions (Janet, 1903, p. 486; translation by the author)

Clearly, psychasthenia encompasses a broad range of clinical phenomena, including the anxiety disorders of our time. The psychasthenic state, however, is determined by a breakdown of only the highest level of psychic functioning. This implies that even in the case of phobias, obsessive-compulsive disorder and panic attacks, a central role should be assigned to feelings of unreality, incompleteness, ineffectiveness and depersonalization, and not to feelings of fear and anxiety. Emotions and emotion theory play only a secondary role in Janet's description and explanation of these disorders.

Janet doesn't deny the occurrence of panic attacks in some cases of psychasthenia (cf., for example, his interesting description of nocturnal panic attacks; p. 247). But these can only be accounted for by the assumption of a temporary and more severe collapse of the psychological tension, leading to disturbances at the third and fourth levels. Fear, on the other hand, is a more complex and differentiated emotion, involving psychic activity of the higher levels, such as imagination, perception and goal-directed behavior. Fear as such, however, is the expression of activity at the fourth level of psychic functioning.

From a psychological point of view, Janet was far ahead of his time, by pointing to the importance of disturbances in the domain of attention and perception and their relation to the sense of the self. Psychology and psychiatry had to wait till the 1980s, before "attentional bias" became a topic of some interest in empirical research of the anxiety disorders.

CLINICAL STUDIES

After 1900, relatively few psychiatric monographs were devoted exclusively to anxiety and anxiety disorders. One exception was the profound clinical study by Störring (1934). Several authors occupied themselves with conceptual questions, based on clinical observations, for example Goldstein (1929) and Kronfeld (1935). Other names, which should be mentioned in this context, are those of Hoche (1911), Kornfeld (1902) and Oppenheim (1909).

Next, reference should be made to several studies arising from particular theoretical points of view. These include not only the psychoanalytical studies by Stekel (1932), Bitter (1948) and Riemann (1961), but also the anthropological studies of von Gebsattel (1954a, 1954b, 1954c) and Tellenbach (1976).

Finally, one should be reminded of those studies, which were carried out in the periods around both World Wars and which were exclusively devoted to traumatic forms of anxiety, such as the publications on "Schreckneurosen" and "Schreckpsychosen" (from the German *Schreck*: terror) (cf. Bonhoeffer, 1919; Kleist, 1918; Panse, 1952).

Instead of summarizing these studies, I will focus the discussion on two themes: the rejection of the James–Lange theory of emotion and the debate about the distinction between fear and anxiety.

With regard to the first theme, there seemed to be a significant resistance amongst clinicians to the James–Lange theory of emotions. Bodily changes, according to this theory, instead of resulting from subjective feelings, are actually the cause of feeling and emotion. Sensory perceptions transform into emotion by the awareness of bodily changes (cf. James, 1884, pp. 189, 204, 1890, p. 450). It is usually assumed that James postulated a temporal sequence between bodily changes and emotional perceptions. Although this is not entirely correct, interpreters have focused mainly on this side of the Jamesian account. Perhaps this was the result of the association of James' view with the theory of the Dane Lange, who indeed emphasized the temporal priority of bodily changes.

Clinicians criticized the James–Lange theory just on this point, by referring to the immediacy of the experience of anxiety. According to Störring, the experience of anxiety is not mediated by prior bodily perception. Kornfeld (1902) (not to be confused with Kronfeld) and Hoche (1911) lodged the same objection, on descriptive grounds. Störring, however, was not entirely consistent on this point since he also spoke of anxiety as a reaction to, or a processing of, sensations associated with specific organs, thus suggesting a temporal priority of organic changes (Störring, 1934, pp. 24, 32). Kraepelin and Lange's authoritative handbook rejected the James–Lange theory on theoretical grounds, both because of its psychophysical dualism and its disregard for central regulatory processes. An emotion such as fear of suffocation could be both somatic and psychological in origin. According to Kraepelin and Lange, the origin of this fear (whether lack of oxygen, hypercapnia, acidosis or frightening events) is irrelevant to the quality of the emotion itself. In all cases, the central issue is a threat to the patient's existence as a biological entity rather than any perception of bodily changes (Kraepelin and Lange, 1927, p. 470). It should be noted, however, that James was too much of a Darwinist to be accused of psychophysical dualism.

In summary, it can be said that clinical psychiatrists resisted the James–Lange theory mainly on clinical grounds. Clinical observation simply contradicted the presumed primacy of bodily changes.

In discussing the second theme, that of the distinction between anxiety and fear, consideration should be given to Kurt Goldstein's observations of patients with organic brain damage. The majority of Goldstein's patients were victims of World War I. He observed (1929) that, when faced with overly complex tasks, these patients displayed a catastrophic reaction consisting of a wide range of physiological and psychomotor symptoms. Goldstein believed that, even though it was not subjectively experienced as such, this condition could best be interpreted as an expression of anxiety.

Whilst Goldstein's patients were unaware of the fact of their anxiety, the appearance of their physical symptoms coincided with the failure to accomplish their tasks. Strictly speaking, their anxiety was neither a reaction to failure nor a reaction to an awareness of failure. Anxiety—and this was the essence of Goldstein's interpretation—was quite literally the actual manifestation of failure. Goldstein concludes that generally spoken anxiety is the expression of a frustrated urge for self-realization.

This reference to the urge for self-realization was particularly popular amongst those contemporary authors who drew their inspiration from vitalism. Although similar references can also be found in Freud's later work (Freud, 1933), it was actually the colossal presence of Charles Darwin behind the scenes which inspired this line of thought. However, Goldstein was not thinking of the survival of the species, or that of the individual, in purely Darwinian terms. The urge towards self-realization was more than a purely biological reality. It also found expression, for example, in the productive creativity shown by children and adults in mastering the world. Anxiety was referred to as a disruption of the stability of personality ("Erschütterung (des) Bestandes der Persönlichkeit"; cf. Goldstein, 1929, pp. 415–416). Ultimately, however,

Goldstein failed to fully clarify the conceptual status of this urge towards self-realization.

In conceptually more explicit accounts by other authors we find a scheme in which personality is divided into an impersonal (biological) substructure and a personal superstructure. The substructure is described in vitalistic terms whilst the superstructure is analyzed in terms derived from existential phenomenology. Examples of this can be found in work by Arthur Kronfeld, Felix Krueger, Philipp Lersch, and, to a lesser extent, H. C. Rümke. According to Kronfeld (1935), anxiety is based upon a disintegration of the personal superstructure. In its most extreme form, this disintegration is expressed as psychotic anxiety. However, the type of anxiety which Kronfeld preferred to have in mind was existential rather than psychotic:

> Anxiety is the mental expression of the existential annihilation of the integrity ("Einheitsform") of the person. Its archetype is the fear of death, the anxiety related to vital destruction. (Kronfeld, 1935, p. 378; translation by the author)

Such statements only become comprehensible when it is realized that Kronfeld rejected the link between anxiety and threat, or, in other words, the relation between object-less anxiety and object-related fear. Anxiety, in the true sense of the word, is not the counterpart of safety, but of the synthetic activity of the I, the person in its striving for one-ness and meaningfulness. In the same way, anxiety is not an intensified form of fear, nor the result of the perception of a threatening situation. It is a fragmentation of the self, leading to the outbreak of chaotic and formless biological forces.

The work of these anthropologically inspired clinicians is still of considerable interest, as a contrast to mainstream psychiatric thinking, at that time and nowadays, which tends to favor a biological interpretation of objectless anxiety.

ON THE WAY TO DSM-III

The study of anxiety was not a high priority in the period from 1930 to 1960. In addition to the previously mentioned influence of psychoanalysis, which described anxiety as a non-specific phenomenon, the assumption that anxiety occupied a low position in the hierarchy of psychiatric symptoms also had a part in this (Tyrer, 1984). Not only did anxiety occur in practically all psychopathological syndromes, it also marked the lower boundary of psychopathology, where this bordered on normality.

Jablensky (1985) adds to this that classification traditionally has been an area of interest for institutional psychiatry. The relative neglect of the classification of anxiety disorders can be seen as a reflection of the fact that, as a rule, patients with neurotic anxiety were never hospitalized.

This status quo gradually changed during the 1950s. At that time, the psychophysiological investigation of emotions continued along the lines of the

James–Lange theory. Ax (1953), for instance, attempted to draw a distinction between the emotions of anxiety and anger, on the basis of their peripheral physiological symptoms. In the same period, the anxiolytic effect of benzodiazepines was discovered, resulting in a flood of research into the effects of these chemicals on the central nervous system (Sternbach, 1980). Wolpe (1958) introduced systematic desensitization as a form of behavior therapy, thereby giving new impetus to the treatment of people with anxiety and phobic disorders. Roth (1959) described a form of depersonalization associated with severe anxiety and phobic phenomena. This was the so-called "phobic anxiety–depersonalization syndrome". Although it usually developed in the wake of a psychotrauma, this picture could sometimes occur spontaneously. The EEGs of one-sixth of all patients revealed the presence of temporal epileptic symptoms.

Finally, at the end of the 1950s Klein discovered that panic attacks in agoraphobic patients could be blocked using imipramine (Klein, 1964, 1980). This marked the beginning of an immense stream of experimental, pharmacological, clinical, longitudinal, epidemiological, genetic and familial research into the existence and course of panic disorder.

With this expansion of psychopharmacological research, increasingly stringent criteria for the definition of psychiatric syndromes were drawn up. Thus, psychopharmacological and biological psychiatric research constituted a powerful impetus for the development of the Feighner Criteria (Feighner et al., 1972). These, together with the Research Diagnostic Criteria (Spitzer et al. 1975, 1978) formed the basis of the DSM-III-R (American Psychiatric Association Committee on Nomenclature and Statistics, 1980, 1987). The emphasis on descriptive precision led to the demarcation of various forms of anxiety and to an abandonment of the concept of neurosis, which was considered to be too vague. Neurasthenic neurosis was discarded. Anxiety neurosis, phobic neurosis and obsessive-compulsive neurosis were combined under the heading of anxiety disorders. Post-traumatic stress disorder, a newcomer, was added to the anxiety disorders. Anxiety neurosis was subsequently split up into panic disorder and generalized anxiety disorder, whilst phobic neurosis was divided up into agoraphobia, simple phobias and social phobia (cf. Spitzer and Williams, 1985).

In spite of the non-theoretical nature of DSM-III, this change nevertheless heralded in a fundamentally different approach to the psychopathology of anxiety. DSM-III bode farewell, not only to the psychodynamic conflict model, but also to a broader tradition in which anxiety was associated with more or less subtle disruptions of personality structure. It was replaced by a finely grained description and classification of more superficial symptomatology. This resulted in a shift from the predominantly dimensional or dispositional approach which characterized the neurosis model, to a typological or categorical approach to psychopathology. Panic disorder represents the most outstanding example of this development.

SUMMARY AND CONCLUSION

Looking back at our historical review, one may discern three lines in the interpretation of pathological anxiety which are still of topical interest today.

First and foremost, there is the medical tradition, which from Antiquity until
now dominates the theoretical literature on anxiety and which, at least in the
last 150 years, tends to favor a biological approach.

Secondly, the concept of anxiety as an inner threat can be recognized, a concept
which is defended by psychoanalysts and contemporary cognitive psychologists.

Finally, the existential concept of anxiety is worth mentioning, a concept
which dates from the seventeenth (Pascal) and nineteenth (Kierkegaard) centuries, and which via existential phenomenology inspires the work of anthropological psychiatrists and existential psychotherapists in our age.

These three traditions are not at all on their way to converge. Contemporary
psychiatry gives the appearance that medical tradition is still enlarging its
domain, at the expense of the psychoanalytic and existential traditions.

It should be noted, however, that psychiatry as a medical discipline has
incorporated elements of the psychoanalytic tradition, besides all sorts of
behavioral and cognitive explanations. Behind the surface, consequently, some
of the old controversies are still under discussion, for instance those concerning
the role of bodily perception in the genesis of panic, those concerning the primacy of biological or psychological explanations, and, not to mention more,
those concerning the nature of classification.

The classification debate itself may serve as an example of the shifting
boundaries of psychiatry. One of the issues in this debate is where to draw the
boundary between normality and pathology. We have noticed to what extent this
boundary was influenced by social conditions, such as war circumstances
(effort syndrome), and the appreciation of the pressures of daily life (neurasthenia).

Clinicians and researchers are currently fascinated with the biological
approach to anxiety. As such, this comes as no surprise, since this approach
seems to bring the promise of control and of tangible results. It is the relation
between psychiatry as a science and psychiatry as a clinical enterprise which is
especially at stake here. As scientific disciplines, neurobiology and pharmacology tackle problems abstractively and objectively. This implies that there is, by
definition, a gap between the research findings in these disciplines and clinical
reality. Scientific constructs do not relate to this reality in its entirety, but merely to aspects of psychopathological syndromes. Identification of these constructs with reality, i.e. reification, almost inevitably leads to distortions in
description and diagnosis. The conceptual history of anxiety illustrates the
repeated recurrence of forgotten ideas. These were eliminated in the process of
abstraction, only to return via the back door. One may recall, for instance,
Westphal's and Freud's view on fear of anxiety as the nucleus of agoraphobia;
MacKenzie's and Wood's emphasis on the causative role of cognitive attribu-

tions; Janet's description of disturbances in attention and perception as central phenomena in psychasthenia.

The gap between scientific explanation and clinical reality, rather than being a barrier to our understanding, offers a space for creative insight and heuristic probing. This gap, instead of short-circuiting it, should be kept open.

REFERENCES

American Psychiatric Association Committee on Nomenclature and Statistics (1980). *Diagnostic and Statistical Manual of Mental Disorders*, 3rd edn. American Psychiatric Association, Washington.

American Psychiatric Association Committee on Nomenclature and Statistics (1987). *Diagnostic and Statistical Manual of Mental Disorders*, 3rd edn, revised. American Psychiatric Association, Washington.

Ax, A. (1953). The physiological differentiation between fear and anger in humans. *Psychosom. Med.*, **15**, 433–442.

Beard, G. M. (1884). *Sexual Neurasthenia (Nervous Exhaustion). Its Hygiene, Causes, Symptoms, and Treatment* (ed. A. D. Rockwell). E. B. Treat, New York.

Beard, G. M. (1890). *A Practical Treatise on Nervous Exhaustion (Neurasthenia). Its Symptoms, Nature, Sequences, Treatment* (ed. A. D. Rockwell). H. K. Lewis, London.

Beck, A. T. (1976). *Cognitive Therapy and the Emotional Disorders*. New American Library, New York.

Beck, A. T., Emery, G. with Greenberg, R. L. (1985). *Anxiety Disorders and Phobias. A Cognitive Perspective*. Basic Books, New York.

Benedikt, M. (1870). Über "Platzschwindel". *Allgemeine Wiener Med. Zeitung*, **15**, 488–489.

Bitter, W. (1948). *Die Angstneurose. Entstehung und Heilung. Mit 2 Analysen nach Freud und Jung*. Hans Huber, Bern.

Bonhoeffer, K. (1919). Zur Frage der Schreckpsychosen. *Monatschr. Psychiatrie und Neurol.*, **22**, 143–156.

Burton, R. (1621; edition 1896). *The Anatomy of Melancholy*, Vols I–III (ed. A. R. Shilleto). George Bell, London.

Culpin, M. (1920). The psychological aspect of the effort syndrome. *Lancet*, **ii**, 184–186.

Da Costa, J. M. (1871). On irritable heart: a clinical study of a form of functional cardiac disorder and its consequences. *Am. J. Med. Sci.*, **71**, 17–52.

Feighner, J. P., Robins, E., Guze, S. B. *et al.* (1972). Diagnostic criteria for use in psychiatric research. *Arch. Gen. Psychiatry*, **26**, 57–63.

Freud, S. (1894). Draft E. In *Standard Edition*, Vol. I, pp. 189–195.

Freud, S. (1895a). Über die Berechtigung, von der Neurasthenie einen bestimmten Symptomen-komplex als "Angstneurose" abzutrennen. In *Gesammelte Werke*, Band I, pp. 315–342.

Freud, S. (1895b). Obsessions et phobies. In *Gesammelte Werke*, Band I, pp. 343–355.

Freud, S. (1895c). Zur Kritik der Angstneurose. In *Gesammelte Werke*, Band I, pp. 355–376.

Freud, S. (1926). Hemmung, Symptom und Angst. In *Gesammelte Werke*, Band XIV, pp. 111–205.

Freud, S. (1933). Neue Folge der Vorlesungen zur Einfürung in die Psychoanalyse. In *Gesammelte Werke*, Band XV, pp. 1–197.

Galenus (1976). On the affected parts. In *Galen on the Affected Parts*, translation from the Greek text with explanatory notes (ed. R. E. Siegel). Karger, Basel.

Goldstein, K. (1929). Zum Problem der Angst. *Allgemeine Arztl. Z. Psychother. Psychische Hyg.*, **2**, 409–437.

18   ADVANCES IN THE NEUROBIOLOGY OF ANXIETY DISORDERS

Hecker, E. (1893). Ueber larvirte und abortive Angstzustände bei Neurasthenie. *Zentralb. Nervenheilk.*, **16**, 565–572.
Hoche, A. E. (1911). Pathologie und Therapie der nervösen Angstzustände. *Dtsch. Z. Nervenheilk.*, **41**, 194–204.
Jablensky, A. (1985). Approaches to the definition and classification of anxiety and related disorders in European psychiatry. In *Anxiety and the Anxiety Disorders* (eds A. H. Tuma and J. Maser), pp. 735–758. Erlbaum, Hillsdale, NJ.
James, W. (1884). What is an emotion? *Mind*, **9**, 188–205.
James, W. (1890). *Principles of Psychology*, 2 vols. Dove, New York.
Janet, P. (1903). *Les obsessions et la Psychasthénie*. Alcan, Paris.
Jones, M. (1948). Physiological and psychological responses to stress in neurotic patients. *J. Ment. Sci.*, **94**, 392–427.
Jones, M. and Lewis, A. (1941). Effort syndrome. *Lancet*, **i**, 813–818.
Klein, D. F. (1964). Delineation of two drug-responsive anxiety syndromes. *Psychopharmacologia*, **5**, 397–408.
Klein, D. F. (1980). Anxiety reconceptualized. *Compr. Psychiatry*, **21**, 411–427.
Kleist, K. (1918). Schreckpsychosen. *Allgemeine Z. Psychiatrie*, **75**, 432–510.
Kornfeld, S. (1902). Zur Pathologie der Angst. *Jahrb. Psychiatrie Neurol.*, **22**, 411–442.
Kraepelin, E. (1899). *Psychiatrie. Ein Lehrbuch für Studirende und Aertzte* (sechste, vollständig umgearbeitete Auflage). Johann Ambrosius Barth, Leipzig.
Kraepelin, E. and Lange, J. (1927). *Psychiatrie. Band I* (neunte Auflage). Johann Ambrosius Barth, Leipzig.
Kronfeld, A. (1935). Über Angst. *Ned. Tijdschr. Psychol.*, **3**, 366–387.
Lewis, A. (1967). Problems presented by the ambiguous word "anxiety" as used in psychopathology. *Isr. Ann. Psychiatry Relat. Disc.*, **5**, 105–121.
MacKenzie, J. (1916). The soldier's heart. *Br. Med. J.*, **i**, 117–119.
MacKenzie, J. (1920). The soldier's heart and war neurosis: a study in symptomatology. *Br. Med. J.*, **i**, 491, 530–534.
Oppenheim, H. (1909). Zur Psychopathologie der Angstzustände. *Berl. Klin. Wochenschr.*, **46**, 1293–1295.
Panse, F. (1952). *Angst und Schreck in klinisch-psychologischer und sozialmedizinischer Sicht. Dargestellt an Hand von Erlebnis-berichten aus dem Luftkrieg*. Georg Thieme Verlag, Stuttgart.
Riemann, F. (1961). *Grundformen der Angst und die Antinomien des Lebens*, Ernst Reinhardt Verlag, München/Basel.
Roth, M. (1959). The phobic anxiety–depersonalization syndrome. *Proc. R. Soc. Med.*, **52**, 587–595.
Schmidt-Degenhard, M. (1986). Angst: problemgeschichtliche und klinische Aspekte. *Fortschr. Neurol. Psychiatrie*, **54**, 321–339.
Spitzer, R. L. and Williams, J. B. W. (1985). Proposed revisions in the DSM-III classification of anxiety disorders based on research and clinical experience. In *Anxiety and the Anxiety Disorders* (eds A. H. Tuma and J. Maser), pp. 759–773. Erlbaum, Hillsdale, NJ.
Spitzer, R. L., Endicott, J., Robins, E. *et al.* (1975). Preliminary report of the reliability of Research Diagnostic Criteria applied to psychiatric case records. In *Predictability in Psychopharmacology: Preclinical and Clinical Correlations* (eds A. Sudilovsky, S. Gershon and B. Beer), pp. 1–44. Raven Press, New York.
Spitzer, R. L., Endicott, J. and Robins, E. (1978). Research Diagnostic Criteria: rationale and reliability. *Arch. Gen. Psychiatry*, **35**, 773–782.
Stekel, W. (1932). *Nervöse Angstzustände und ihre Behandlung*, Urban & Schwarzenberg, Vienna.
Sternbach, L. H. (1980). The benzodiazepine story. In *Benzodiazepines. Today and tomorrow* (eds R. G. Priest, U. Vianna Filho, R. Amrein and M. Skreta), pp. 5–18. MTP Press, Lancaster.

Störring, G. E. (1934). *Zur Psychopathologie und Klinik der Angstzustände*, Abhandlungen aus der Neurologie, Psychiatrie, Psychologie und ihren Grenzgebieten. Beihefte zur Monatschrift für Psychiatrie und Neurologie, Heft 72, Karger, Berlin.

Tellenbach, H. (1976). *Melancholie. Problemgeschichte, Endogenität, Typologie, Pathogenese, Klinik* (dritte erweiterte Auflage). Springer-Verlag, Berlin.

Tyrer, P. J. (1984). Classification in anxiety. *Br. J. Psychiatry*, **144**, 78–83.

von Gebsattel, V. E. Freiherr (1954a). Anthropologie der Angst. In *Prolegomena einer medizinischen Anthropologie. Ausgewählte Aufsätze*, pp. 378–389. Springer-Verlag, Berlin.

von Gebsattel, V. E. Freiherr (1954b). Zur Psychopathologie der Phobien. Die psychasthenische Phobie. In *Prolegomena einer medizinischen Anthropologie. Ausgewählte Aufsätze*, pp. 42–74. Springer-Verlag, Berlin.

von Gebsattel, V. E. Freiherr (1954c). Die Welt des Zwangskranken. In *Prolegomena einer medizinischen Anthropologie. Ausgewählte Aufsätze*, pp. 74–128. Springer-Verlag, Berlin.

Westphal, C. (1872). Die Agoraphobie, eine neuropathische Erscheinung. *Arch. Psychiatrie Nervenkr.*, **3**, 138–161.

Wolpe, J. (1958). *Psychotherapy by Reciprocal Inhibition*, Stanford University Press, Stanford.

Wood, P. (1941). Da Costa's syndrome (or effort syndrome). *Br. Med. J.*, 767–772, 805–811, 845–851.

2 Phenomenology of Anxiety Disorders: Clinical Heterogeneity and Comorbidity

STEPHEN M. STAHL
Clinical Neuroscience Research Center and University of California, San Diego, California, USA

INTRODUCTION

The phenomenology of anxiety disorders is evolving at a rapid pace. Originally, the concept of anxiety as a psychiatric disorder evolved in order to set a threshold to distinguish pathological anxiety from anxiety as a normal emotion. Descriptive features were also added to this concept in order to separate a generalized disorder of anxiety from depression (DSM-II) (Brown *et al.*, 1993; Barlow *et al.*, 1986). This was particularly useful during the era when the first anxiolytics and the first antidepressants were being introduced into clinical practice and criteria were required for determining which patients to treat with an anxiolytic and which to treat with an antidepressant (Downing and Rickels, 1974; Stahl, 1993, 1996).

Today, however, the trend is far different. One of the principal current influences upon the phenomenology of anxiety disorders is the fragmentation of the original concept of a single generalized type of anxiety disorder into several discrete subtypes of anxiety disorder (DSM-IV) (Rickels and Schweizer, 1990; Wittchen, 1994). Notably, for example, panic disorder has broken out of the category of generalized anxiety disorder, and social phobia in turn from panic disorder. Phobias and post-traumatic stress disorder are also discrete entities and not generalized forms of anxiety. Even generalized anxiety associated with symptoms of depression is being considered as a possible separate disorder of mixed anxiety depression.

The modern forces which have structured criteria to distinguish specific diagnostic subtypes of anxiety disorders from generalized anxiety disorder have led in general to better criteria for epidemiological, natural history and treatment studies of the specific anxiety disorder subtypes. However, this trend has not necessarily been as useful for what has become a residual category of generalized anxiety disorder (GAD—formerly anxiety neurosis). Indeed, the modern

Advances in the Neurobiology of Anxiety Disorders. Edited by H. G. M. Westenberg, J. A. Den Boer and D. L. Murphy
©1996 John Wiley & Sons Ltd

category of generalized anxiety disorder has evolved into a residual category which is now very different from the original version as conceived several decades ago.

What makes GAD controversial today is that the evolution of this residual category is very different depending upon one's perspective. Thus, psychiatric practitioners may see modern GAD as nothing more than an undiagnosed anxiety condition whereas psychiatric nosologists may see GAD as a distinct entity with important differences from the specific diagnostic subtypes of anxiety disorders as well as from other major psychiatric disorders with which GAD frequently coexists. Psychopharmacologists may wonder whether today's patients with "pure" GAD—i.e., that minority of GAD patients who have no other major psychiatric disorder and only have subthreshold symptoms of any of the other discrete anxiety disorders—resemble those who participated in drug trials 15–30 years ago when diagnostic criteria were less rigid and emphasis was on distinguishing anxiety from depression and not generalized anxiety from specific anxiety subtypes. General practitioners and other non-psychiatric practitioners may see more subsyndromal generalized anxiety and rarely use the diagnosis of GAD.

Thus, the new category has created intense debates, since it is not clear that the "Balkanization" of the state of anxiety has left a "rump state" residual disorder useful to all those who approach this entity from various unique perspectives. The phenomenology of anxiety disorders is thus currently a series of competing trends, and these will be reviewed in this chapter.

ANXIETY: A NORMAL EMOTION, A DISTURBING SYMPTOM OR A PSYCHIATRIC DISORDER?

Despite long-standing debates on what constitutes the difference between anxiety as a normal, healthy or even necessary emotion and anxiety as a disabling psychiatric disorder, nosologists continue to wrestle with how to make this distinction. Defining a disorder of anxiety reawakens classical debate between psychoanalytic and medical points of view, since the former sees anxiety as an outgrowth of neurotic conflict, and the latter as a disorder of neuronal functioning (see Figure 1).

Existentialism states that being alive in the world equates to a state of anxiety. Psychoanalytic notions of "angst" propose that anxiety makes freedom possible, and without the individual's struggle with anxiety, growth is not possible (Freud, 1961). Medical points of view, especially by non-psychiatric physicians, look instead for objective pathology and "real" illness rather than existential suffering or neurotic conflicts. Thus, the symptoms of anxiety in the absence of physical indicators of disease may be assumed to be trivial or irrelevant to a medical practitioner trying to investigate complaints which are caused by diagnosable and treatable pathologies.

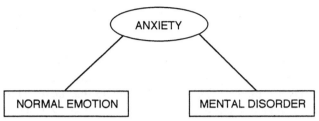

Figure 1 Competing trends in defining anxiety as part of a mental disorder versus a normal emotion

Practitioners have long recognized, however, that some states of anxiety are truly disabling and not trivial, yet not caused by diagnosable physical diseases. An assumed neurobiological mechanism underlies such states (Tallman *et al.*, 1980) but the vagueness with which the biological basis can be demonstrated may lead to skepticism about whether any specific individual has a "disease" or has "emotional weakness." Psychopharmacologists have also long recognized that symptoms of anxiety can be relieved by anxiolytic drugs. However, since the advent of symptomatic treatments for anxiety, it has never been clear where to draw the line for determining a threshhold of use for anxiolytic agents. Too liberal use of anxiolytics in the 1960s in order to reduce symptoms of anxiety associated with anxiety neurosis led by the 1980s to claims of an "overmedicated society" to the detriment of existential being, self-actualization and personal growth (Tallman *et al.*, 1980). Too restrictive diagnostic criteria and use of treatments in reaction to this have led in some cases to trivializing anxiety disorders and confusing the lack of personal growth which can occur from choosing not to try to manage stress with the disability of a mental illness which cannot be overcome with effort.

Thus, the diagnosis of an anxiety disorder is the product of two competing trends: one tending to raise the threshold and the other tending to lower it. Those forces which act to set a high threshold for an anxiety disorder seek to define discrete clinical entities which are legitimate mental disorders with social and occupational disability, with the implication of a unique biological basis, and a unique genetic basis compared to other mental disorders such as depression. Those forces which try to define a lower threshold for an anxiety disorder attempt to separate normal emotions or mere discomfort from a mental disorder of anxiety. Finding the line between an anxiety disorder and normal anxiety and fear is especially problematic given popular misconceptions and stigma which perceive that mental illness is not a disease of neurobiological dysfunctioning but rather that it is due to emotional weakness; due to bad parenting; that it is the victim's fault and the victim could will it away if he really wanted to be well; that it is incurable and that it is the consequence of sinful behavior.

ANXIETY VERSUS DEPRESSION: COMORBID STATES OR MIXED STATES?

While psychoanalysts and biological psychiatrists debate whether a given anxiety state is normal or pathological, psychopharmacologists have sought diagnostic criteria to determine which subjects with presumed pathological anxiety to treat with an anxiolytic and which to treat with an antidepressant. Thus the competing trends here have been whether to separate anxiety and depression into distinct disorders with separate treatments, or to merge anxiety and depression into mixed categories and comorbid states.

The original trend was to separate anxiety from depression (Figure 2) in order to facilitate investigation of new therapeutic agents targeted selectively to either depression or anxiety (DSM-II) (Downing and Rickels, 1974; Stahl, 1993). This ushered in the era of "lumping" subjects as suffering either from a disorder of anxiety or from depression. Thus, the category of anxiety neurosis evolved about the same time as the discovery of the benzodiazepines, the first anxiolytics which were anxioselective and not just sedating and tranquilizing. The diagnostic criteria separating anxiety neurosis from depression at that time were helpful in proving the anxioselectivity of this new class of therapeutic

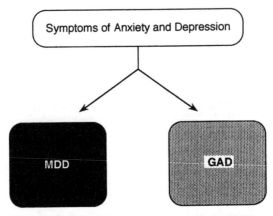

Figure 2 Classical separation of symptoms of anxiety and depression into either anxiety neurosis/generalized anxiety disorder (GAD) or major depressive disorder (MDD)

agents (DSM-II). Concomitantly, the diagnostic criteria separating anxiety neurosis from depression were key in helping to prove that the tricyclic antidepressants and monoamine oxidase (MAO) inhibitors have antidepressant properties distinct from major tranquilizers used to treat psychosis and distinct from anxiolytics used to treat generalized states of anxiety. The early diagnostic criteria for depression and anxiety neurosis were thus extremely helpful in showing the early antidepressants to be the first effective drug treatments for mood disorder and the first anxiolytics to be anxioselective as opposed to non-specific tranquilization by all drugs of all emotional symptoms associated with mood disorder, anxiety and psychosis (Stahl, 1996).

As time has progressed, the ability to lump patients into only a category of generalized anxiety or a category of depression began to unravel. Foremost was the recognition that symptoms of anxiety and depression frequently coexist (Figure 3) (Stahl, 1993; Rickels and Schweizer, 1990; Boulenger and Lavallee, 1993; Wittchen and Essau, 1993). This has generated a competing trend of

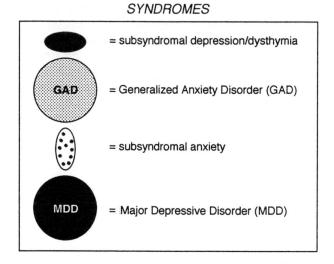

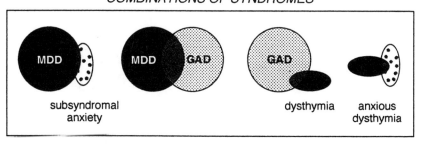

Figure 3 Modern classification of symptoms of anxiety and depression either as a single mixed syndrome or a comorbid combination of two syndromes

"splitting" symptoms of anxiety and depression within individuals into discrete and separate multiple syndromes (Figure 3). Thus, some patients suffer both from major depressive disorder and generalized anxiety disorder/anxiety neurosis (i.e., an anxiety disorder and a depressive disorder which are comorbid). Adding to the complexity, however, is the fact that in most individuals the mixed symptoms of anxiety and depression fail to exceed diagnostic thresholds for both disorders (Wittchen, 1994; Boulenger and Lavallee, 1993; Wittchen and Essau, 1993). Symptoms which fail to exceed diagnostic thresholds are categorized as "subsyndromal" and come perilously close to what some would define as normal emotions (see discussion above and Figure 1). Furthermore, mixed symptoms of anxiety and depression are often not stable over time, with *subthreshold* symptoms sometimes increasing to meet full diagnostic criteria or diminishing to resolve entirely, and with *threshold* diagnostic entities sometimes diminishing to a subsyndromal state rather than resolving entirely (Boulenger and Lavallee, 1993; Wittchen and Essau, 1993).

The current debate in combining not only depression and anxiety disorders, but also subsyndromal states with threshold diagnostic entities, centers on whether patients with mixed syndromes differ from patients with "pure" syndromes in terms of their natural history, disease progression and treatment response. Although in the past patients were lumped as predominantly a "pure" anxiety disorder, or as predominantly a "pure" depressive disorder, today the recognition of mixed states has rendered the diagnostic process much more complex but perhaps more descriptively exact. It is not yet clear whether the current "splitting" trend of making multiple diagnoses and then combining these as mixed syndromes creates additional categories which are different in

Anxious Dysthymia can be a precursor to many other syndromes

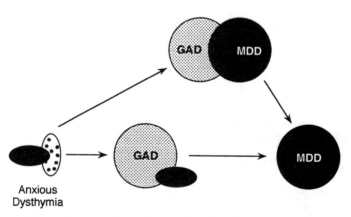

Figure 4 Subsyndromal anxiety mixed with subsyndromal depression, sometimes called "anxious dysthymia", may be a precursor to a variety of psychiatric disorders, including generalized anxiety disorder (GAD) mixed with symptoms of depression, generalized anxiety disorder plus major depressive disorder (MDD), or major depressive disorder itself

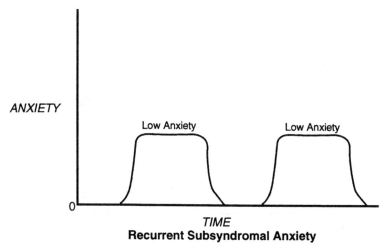

ANXIETY

TIME
Recurrent Subsyndromal Anxiety

Figure 5 Recurrent subsyndromal anxiety, never reaching the threshold of a diagnosable psychiatric disorder, and fluctuating between subsyndromal symptoms of anxiety and normal functioning

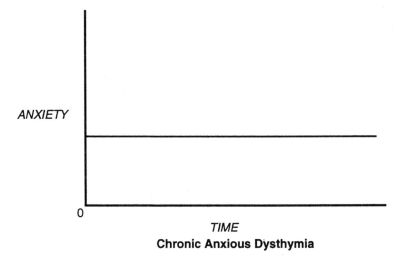

ANXIETY

TIME
Chronic Anxious Dysthymia

Figure 6 Chronic unremitting subsyndromal anxiety with neither decompensation into a diagnosable psychiatric disorder, nor return to normal functioning

prevalence, stability, natural history and treatment compared to the "pure" disorders, but numerous studies are in progress to address these issues.

One promising hypothesis is that subsyndromal symptoms are not trivial even though they are very close to normal emotional states. That is, chronic unremitting subsyndromal mixtures of anxiety and depression (anxious dysthymia or subsyndromal mixed anxiety depression) may be a harbinger for breakdown into a full criteria mental disorder of anxiety and/or depression, par-

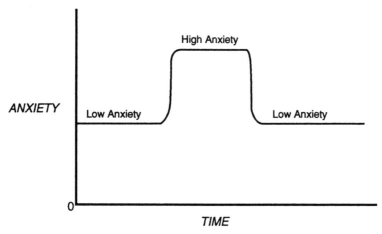

Figure 7 Double anxiety syndrome characterized by fluctuation between subsyndromal anxiety and generalized anxiety disorder, but never returning to normal functioning

ticularly in response to stressful life events (Figure 4) (Stahl, 1993; Boulenger and Lavallee, 1993; Wittchen and Essau, 1993; Blazer *et al.*, 1987). Thus, there is an important emphasis on the chronicity of symptoms in such cases, and the stability of symptoms over time.

In the case of subsyndromal anxiety which is intermittent with full return to asymptomatic functioning, such patients may be exhibiting more or less normal emotions (Figure 5). However, in the case of subsyndromal anxiety which is very persistent over time, this may indicate a vulnerable subject at risk for developing a full threshold anxiety disorder, with less than complete recovery over time back to a state of subsyndromal symptoms, but not to a level of being completely normal (Figure 6). Such vulnerable states may begin even in childhood as what was previously known as overanxious disorder but is now merged into the concept of modern GAD. This latter case of vulnerable states of low-grade anxiety decompensating into a full GAD syndrome may be conceptualized as "double anxiety" analogous to "double depression" in which chronic low-grade depression (dysthymia) decompensates intermittently into major depressive disorder, followed by incomplete recovery to dysthymia (Figure 7). Although longitudinal modifiers have been introduced into diagnostic use in the DSM-IV for the affective disorders, they have not yet been proposed for the anxiety disorders. Further research may very well demonstrate the utility of longitudinal disease descriptors for chronic anxiety disorders analogous to their use for the affective disorders.

PHENOMENOLOGY OF GENERALIZED ANXIETY: CAN GAD SURVIVE AS A CONCEPT?

Clearly, the concept of a generalized disorder of anxiety has been useful in the past.

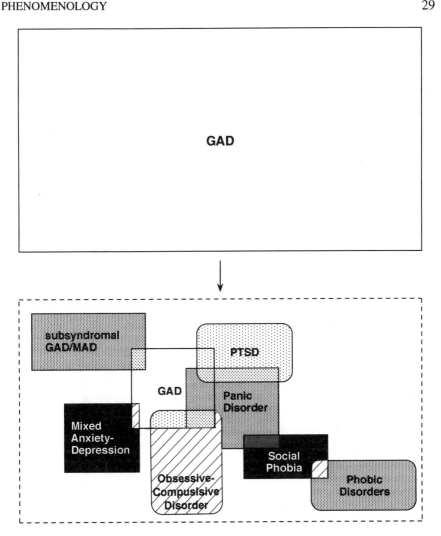

Figure 8 Fragmentation of the original concept of generalized anxiety disorder (GAD)/anxiety neurosis into anxiety disorder subtypes

As discussed above, it undoubtedly assisted in defining major depressive disorder, and in establishing the original utility of anxiolytic versus antidepressant drugs. However, the concept of a generalized disorder of anxiety has seriously begun to unravel as the original concept is now broken down into at least seven discrete subtypes of anxiety disorder plus whatever remains of GAD (Figure 8). Thus, is a patient with GAD an undiagnosed anxiety disorder awaiting proper diagnostic categorization as a "real" anxiety disorder, or is it "anxiety disorder if you don't have a specific anxiety disorder?"

Perhaps leading the pack in the exit from GAD was panic disorder with or without agoraphobia when it was recognized that a discrete entity existed with frequent panic attacks and which was not anxiety neurosis (DSM-III). The carved out entity of panic disorder was recognized to have a unique syndromal cluster with agoraphobia, phobic avoidance, anticipatory anxiety and interepisode generalized anxiety and was therefore extracted from GAD, where it undoubtedly resided and was misdiagnosed as GAD/anxiety neurosis previously.

Another example of the fragmentation of the original concept of GAD is social phobia, which not only fragments GAD, but also the original concept of panic disorder. Social phobia was extracted from both GAD and panic disorder when it was increasingly recognized that panic attacks can be expected or unexpected, and that expected panic attacks in the context of social phobia differed from unexpected panic attacks associated with panic disorder (DSM-IV). Thus, panic disorder now requires that some of the attacks be unexpected. Frequently, expected panic attacks are associated with social phobia.

Panic disorder and social phobia are examples of how the various entities of anxiety disorder subtypes are leaving the original category of GAD as better clinical descriptions become available (Figure 8). This raises the question whether there will be a useful category of GAD left once the dust has settled. The evolution of diagnostic criteria to distinguish anxiety disorder subtypes from GAD is not merely a useless renaming exercise, because experience with the newly defined anxiety disorder subtypes establishes that each has a different natural history, epidemiology, and especially, pharmacologic and psychotherapeutic treatment. Such differences in fact became evident only after the identification of diagnostic criteria for subtyping anxiety disorders which allowed them to be extracted from GAD.

In the past, it is likely that loose diagnostic criteria were applied to many subjects with anxiety disorder subtypes who were misdiagnosed as a generalized form of anxiety disorder and treated with a generalized anxiolytic, especially a benzodiazepine. Now, new diagnostic categories have clarified how various so-called "antidepressants" such as MAO inhibitors, tricyclic antidepressants and especially serotonin selective reuptake inhibitors are effective "anxiolytic" treatments for selected subtypes of anxiety disorder (Stahl, 1993, 1996; Rickels and Schweizer, 1990, 1993). It is unlikely that this could have happened in the absence of distinguishing diagnostic criteria for anxiety disorder subtypes.

The fragmentation of classical GAD/anxiety neurosis, although perhaps good for panic disorder and social phobia, has nevertheless caused confusion about how to characterize and treat patients who have the residual category of modern GAD (Brown et al., 1993; Rickels and Schweizer, 1990). Thus, shifting the concept of anxiety neurosis and then GAD from the 1960s to the 1990s has raised questions as to whether those subjects treated with anxiolytic medications and studied in trials of new antianxiety agents in the 1990s any longer resemble those studied when the original benzodiazepines were introduced into practice in the 1960s. It should perhaps be no surprise that by the 1990s there have evolved great difficulties in showing drug–placebo differences in the use of anxiolytic agents when studied in the entity called generalized anxiety disorder in the 1990s, whereas drug–placebo differences were much more readily demonstrable using the same agents in clinical drug trials in the 1960s. Negative clinical trials tend not to be published and are often only publicly available in the summary basis of approval from the US Food and Drug Administration after marketing of a compound for anxiety. Studies in progress as well as drugs dropped from further development are generally not published. Thus, one can get a very distorted view of anxiolytic drug efficacy from reading merely the published literature.

To the extent that the modern diagnostic category of GAD is intended to identify a unique anxiety state differentiated from other anxiety states and depression, and which denotes those subjects most likely to respond to anxiolytic medication, the modern diagnostic category of GAD has therefore been a failure. GAD as currently defined usually does not occur as a single entity, since comorbidity, especially with other specified anxiety disorders, medical disorders and psychiatric disorders, is the rule and not the exception (Brown and Barlow, 1992; Sanderson and Barlow, 1990). It has been exceedingly difficult to use "GAD populations purified of comorbid psychiatric and medical states but which meet threshhold criteria GAD rather than mere symptoms of anxiety" as a target population to demonstrate efficacy of anxiolytic medications. For example, in the past two decades, only one therapeutic agent has been approved for the treatment of generalized anxiety in the USA, and none in the past 10 years. This is not the result of the lack of trying or a dearth of novel anxiolytic medications based upon preclinical and early clinical trials. It is largely the result that studies of GAD frequently fail to show any difference between drug and placebo. The ongoing pattern is for large multicenter trials of many hundred patients per trial to show drug–placebo differences about half the time, but large placebo responses to obscure drug effects about half the time as well. This is also the case with established anxiolytics used as comparator agents, which far more consistently showed drug–placebo differences when studies were performed employing diagnostic categories in use in the 1960s.

Given the migrating diagnostic criteria for a generalized disorder of anxiety of the past several decades, and the dilution of apparent efficacy of anxiolytic agents which used to work consistently better than placebo, it is no wonder that it is difficult to ascertain whether there is such a disorder or what the utility of the concept of modern GAD is. Does GAD exist or are generalized anxiety and its syndromal components just outgrowths of any number of specific anxiety disorders and depression? Is there any difference between subjects with pure GAD and the GAD component of subjects with comorbid states? What is the prognostic significance of subsyndromal states of GAD? What is the utility of making such distinctions from a diagnostic or treatment perspective? These and many other questions fuel the debate and define the competing trends for GAD, but currently there is little consensus on such issues among experts approaching GAD from different perspectives.

PHENOMENOLOGY OF ANXIETY DISORDERS IN PSYCHIATRIC PRACTICE

Ambiguity and lack of immediate pragmatic answers to these questions have led non-psychiatric practitioners to largely reject the notion of GAD, to trivialize the importance of anxiety when seen outside of the context of depression, and to neglect it when seen in the context of true physical disease. However, some surprises are present when one analyzes recent studies of GAD in psychiatric settings where it is usually not a single "pure" entity but rather exists in a patient with comorbid additional psychiatric disorders. Specifically, GAD in modern psychiatric practices is usually associated with comorbid psychiatric disorders, and is relatively chronic and not only poorly diagnosed (i.e., GAD may not even be diagnosed since diagnostic emphasis is given to the comorbid disorder which is generally considered primary) but relatively poorly managed (i.e., treatment is aimed at the primary disorder) (Rickels and Schweizer, 1990, 1993; Boulenger and Lavallee, 1993; Wittchen and Essau, 1993; Blazer *et al.*, 1987; Brown and Barlow, 1992; Sanderson and Barlow, 1990; Massion *et al.*, 1993; Keller, 1994; Hirschfeld, 1994; Noyes *et al.*, 1980; Krieg *et al.*, 1987; Woodruff *et al.*, 1972).

Looking at GAD longitudinally suggests that indeed it is not trivial (Massion *et al.*, 1993; Keller, 1994; Hirschfeld, 1994; Noyes *et al.*, 1980; Krieg *et al.*, 1987; Woodruff *et al.*, 1972). That is, patients with GAD in psychiatric practice appear to have about the same degree of occupational and social dysfunctioning associated as experienced by patients with depression, the latter of which is comparable to the physical and social disability associated with advanced coronary artery disease (Wells *et al.*, 1989). GAD is also associated with frequent suicide attempts (Massion *et al.*, 1993; Keller, 1994). In terms of treatment effectiveness, many GAD patients "respond" to anxiolytic treatments by improving to just below the threshold for the diagnostic criteria for GAD only to relapse to a full syndrome in several months. Thus, the treatment success of

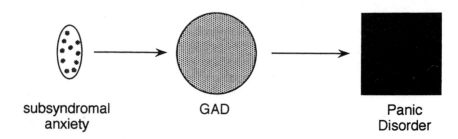

| subsyndromal anxiety | GAD | Panic Disorder |

Subsyndromal Anxiety can be a precursor to GAD or Panic disorder

Figure 9 Subsyndromal anxiety may serve as a precursor to generalized anxiety disorder (GAD), and GAD may serve as a precursor to panic disorder

der or major depressive disorder? The debate rages on, but no resolution of this issue is at hand to guide the practitioner. In an era of health care rationing, such subjects may well be neglected until clear diagnostic and treatment guidelines evolve.

PHENOMENOLOGY OF ANXIETY DISORDERS IN THE MARKETPLACE

Prevalence studies of anxiety disorders differ widely depending upon whether the population surveyed is one from the general population, a psychiatric practice, or a non-psychiatric practice. Furthermore, epidemiological studies which are driven by the desire to identify subjects who meet the criteria for freshly minted nosological entities can come to far different conclusions than physician surveys or pharmaceutical market analyses which measure what is actually happening to patients with anxiety disorders, especially when it comes to the use of anxiolytic treatments. Also, the results of such studies can differ widely in different countries throughout the world.

For example, prevalence rates for GAD in the general population range from 2% to 6% and are similar in studies from the USA, England, Switzerland and Italy (Robins and Regier, 1991). If one estimates the size of a market which could benefit from a generalized anxiolytic on the basis of conservative prevalence estimates of GAD, for the population 15 and older, 4 to 5 million Americans are afflicted with GAD within a given 12-month period. On the other hand, most patients who consult physicians for chronic anxiety have a diagnosis of "anxiety not otherwise specified." According to the US National Center for Health Statistics (Gardocki, 1988), 54% of visits to psychiatrists for anxiety resulted in a diagnosis of "anxiety not otherwise specified" and only 31% resulted in a diagnosis of GAD with the remaining 15% being classified as panic disorder. This suggests that the number of patients with GAD may be as little as 36% of all patients with non-panic-related primary anxiety and that using the prevalence of GAD alone may significantly underestimate the problem of non-panic anxiety. If this is true, about 12 million Americans are afflicted with non-panic-related anxiety during any given year.

GAD is a term used in the USA but is seldom used in Europe. Nevertheless, by applying the same conservative estimates of GAD to the populations of the five largest European pharmaceutical markets (UK, France, Italy, Germany and Spain), the total number of persons afflicted with GAD in these countries is estimated to be 6 million. However, in 1992, Pharmacometrics, a German research and consulting firm (unpublished marketing report) estimated the prevalence of all primary anxiety states (GAD, panic and other) in these markets to be only 7.6 million. If GAD represents 31% of all anxiety states, one would expect a much larger number for all anxiety states. Although this discrepancy cannot be readily explained, it appears that non-panic-related anxiety afflicts at least 6 million people in these European markets, but the number may be as high as 16 million.

No prevalence studies of primary anxiety disorders have been published from Japan, but the great stigma of mental illness in that culture makes cross-cultural comparisons extremely difficult. There is no reason *a priori* to believe that prevalence rates would differ across industrialized nations, including Japan, and at least one study of Asians in Hong Kong suggests a lifetime prevalence rate of GAD of 11.1% (Chen *et al.*, 1993).

Assuming that the prevalence of GAD is approximately 2.7% in the general population, one estimate of anxiety in the major pharmaceutical markets (USA, Japan, and five European countries) would be 12 million persons afflicted. Assuming that patients with GAD represent only 36% of all patients with non-panic-associated anxiety conditions, another estimate of anxiety in the major pharmaceutical markets would be 35 million persons afflicted. The actual number afflicted is most likely to fall somewhere between these estimates, but shows the potential importance of anxiety as a common and frequently occurring disorder of the general population.

In the eight largest pharmaceutical markets in 1992 (USA, Canada, Japan, UK, France, Italy, Spain, Germany), there were approximately 50 million visits to physicians by patients with anxiety disorders, reflecting an annual growth rate of 2% during the years 1988–1992 (MIDAS IMS, Inc., 1992, unpublished marketing report). The most robust growth in the number of visits occurred in Japan (15%) and Germany (9%), and actually fell in the USA between 1992 and 1993. Japan and Germany have traditionally had far fewer anxiety visits compared to other major markets. That is, for every 100 persons in the country, there was only one visit to a physician annually by a patient with a primary diagnosis of anxiety in Germany, three in Japan, five in the USA and 16 in Canada, where there is the highest rate. This variance in the pattern of health services utilization between countries is influenced by several factors, which include the structure of the health care system, social stigma placed on psychiatric disorder, and perhaps most importantly, diagnostic differences between countries. This latter phenomenon is most clearly demonstrated in Japan and Germany where most patients who are treated with antianxiety agents typically do not receive an anxiety diagnosis.

In all major markets, patients with primary anxiety are more likely to be treated by a primary care practitioner than a psychiatrist (17–38% of visits seen by a psychiatrist; the rest by non-psychiatric physicians; MIDAS IMS, Inc., 1992, unpublished marketing report). In the USA, there is a progressive decline in the number of patients receiving anxiolytics for the diagnosis of a primary anxiety disorder, but no reduction in the number of overall prescriptions for anxiolytics. Anxiolytics are increasingly being prescribed for depression and other indications, and usually in combination with a second agent, generally an antidepressant. Raising consciousness about depression in the past decade in the context of the introduction of several effective and less bothersome antidepressants has shifted the focus away from anxiety as a symptom towards depression as a symptom. Thus, the concept can exist—especially among non-psychiatric practitioners—that if you are disabled you must have depression and may need an antidepressant. However, if you are anxious, your problem may be trivial or exaggerated, and you should work it out on your own without the need for a dependence-forming anxiolytic crutch. This point of view is somewhat encouraged by the turmoil as to what a primary generalized disorder of anxiety actually is, how to recognize and diagnose it in medical and psychiatric practices and how to treat it. Given the frequency of anxiety and the clear indications that many patients with anxiety are truly disabled, it appears important if not urgent to clarify the phenomenology of anxiety disorders so that treatment guidelines can be generated for patients with a potentially readily recognizable and treatable primary generalized disorder of anxiety.

REFERENCES

Barlow, D. H., Blanchard, E. B., Vermilyea, J. A. *et al.* (1986). Generalized anxiety and generalized anxiety disorder: description and reconceptualization, *Am. J. Psychiatry*, **143**, 40–44.

Barrett, J. E., Barrett, J. A., Oxman, T. E. and Gerber, P. D. (1988). The prevalence of psychiatric disorders in a primary care practice. *Arch. Gen. Psychiatry*, **45**, 1100–1106.

Blazer, D., Hughes, D. and George, L. K. (1987). Stressful life events and the onset of a generalized anxiety syndrome. *Am. J. Psychiatry*, **144**, 1178–1183.

Boulenger, J.-P. and Lavallee, Y.-J. (1993). Mixed anxiety and depression: diagnostic issues. *J. Clin. Psychiatry* **54**(1) (Suppl.), 3–8.

Brown, T. A. and Barlow, D. H. (1992). Comorbidity among anxiety disorders: implications for treatment and DSM-IV. *J. Consult. Clin. Psychol.*, **60**, 835–844.

Brown, T. A., O'Leary, T. A. and Barlow, D. H. (1993). Generalized anxiety disorder. In *Clinical Handbook of Psychological Disorders*, 2nd edn (ed. D. H. Barlow), pp. 137–188. Guilford Press, New York.

Chen, C.-N., Wong, J., Lee, N. *et al.* (1993). The Shatin community mental health survey in Hong Kong. *Arch. Gen. Psychiatry*, **50**, 125–133.

Downing, R. W. and Rickels, K. (1974). Mixed anxiety–depression: fact or myth? *Arch. Gen. Psychiatry*, **30**, 312–317.

Freud, S. (1961). Introductory lectures on psychoanalysis. In *The Standard Edition of the Complete Psychological Works of Sigmund Freud*, Vol. 15 (ed. J. Strachey). Hogarth Press, London.

Gardocki, G. J. (1988). National Center for Health Statistics, Vital and Health Statistics, 1988 Office visits to psychiatrists, series 13, number 94, DHHS Pub. No. (PHS) 88–1755. Public Health Service, US Government Printing Office, Washington, DC.

Hirschfeld, R. M. A. (1994). Epidemiology and clinical presentation of generalized anxiety disorder in the United States. *Neuropsychopharmacology*, **10**, 132S.

Katon, W., Von Korff, M., Lin, E. *et al.* (1990). Distressed high utilizers of medical care: DSM-III-R diagnoses and treatment needs. *Gen. Hosp. Psychiatry*, **12**, 355–362.

Keller, M. B. (1994). Long term course of generalized anxiety. *Neuropsychopharmacology*, **10**, 134S.

Krieg, J. C., Bronisch, T., Wittchen, H.-U. and von Zerssen, D. (1987). Anxiety disorders: a long term prospective and retrospective follow up study of former inpatients suffering from an anxiety neurosis or phobia. *Acta Psychiatr. Scand.*, **76**, 36–47.

Lepine, J.-P. (1994). Anxiety disorders in primary care. *Neuropsychopharmacology*, **10**, 133S.

38ADVANCES IN THE NEUROBIOLOGY OF ANXIETY DISORDERS

Massion, A. O., Warshaw, M. G. and Keller, M. B. (1993). Quality of life and psychiatric morbidity in panic disorder and generalized anxiety disorder. *Am. J. Psychiatry*, **150**, 600–607.

Noyes, R., Clancy, J., Hoenck, P. R. and Slymen, D. J. (1980). The prognosis of anxiety disorders. *Arch. Gen. Psychiatry*, **37**, 173–178.

Ormel, J., Van Den Brink, W., Koeter, M. W. J. *et al.* (1990). Recognition, management and outcome of psychological disorders in primary care: a naturalistic follow-up study *Psychol. Med.*, **20**, 909–923.

Regier, D. A., Narrow, W. E., Rae, D. S. *et al.* (1993). The de facto US mental and addictive disorders service system. *Arch. Gen. Psychiatry*, **50**, 85–94.

Rickels, K. and Schweizer, E. (1990). The clinical course and long-term management of generalized anxiety disorder, *J. Clin. Psychopharmacol.*, **10**(3) (Suppl.), 101S–110S.

Rickels, K. and Schweizer, E. (1993). The treatment of generalized anxiety disorder in patients with depressive symptomatology. *J. Clin. Psychiatry,* **54**(1) (Suppl.), 20–23.

Robins, L. N. and Regier, D. A. (1991). *Psychiatric Disorders in America.* Free Press, New York.

Sanderson, W. C. and Barlow, D. H. (1990). A description of patients diagnosed with DSM-III-R generalized anxiety disorder. *J. Nerv. Ment. Dis.*, **178**, 588–591.

Stahl, S. M. (1993). Mixed anxiety and depression: clinical implications, *J. Clin. Psychiatry*, **54**(1) (Suppl.), 33–38.

Stahl, S. M. (1996). *Essential Psychopharmacology*, Cambridge University Press, New York.

Tallman, J. F., Paul, S. M., Skolnick, P. and Gallager, D. W. (1980). Receptors for the age of anxiety: pharmacology of the benzodiazepines. *Science*, **207**, 274–281.

Von Korff, M., Shapiro, S., Burke, J. D. *et al.* (1987). Anxiety and depression in a primary care clinic. *Arch. Gen. Psychiatry*, **44**, 152–156.

Wells, K. B., Stewart, A., Hays, R. D. *et al.* (1989). The functioning and mental well-being of depressed patients: results from the medical outcomes study, *JAMA*, **262**, 914–919.

Wittchen, H.-U. (1994). Differences between the US and European view of the diagnosis of anxiety. *Neuropsychopharmacology*, **10**, 131s.

Wittchen, H.-U. and Essau, C. A. (1993). Comorbidity and mixed anxiety–depressive disorders: is there epidemiological evidence? *J. Clin. Psychiatry*, **54**(1) (Suppl.), 9–15.

Woodruff, R. H., Guze, S. B. and Clayton, P. J. (1972). Anxiety neurosis among psychiatric outpatients. *Compr. Psychiatry*, **13**, 165–170.

3 The Genetics of Anxiety Disorders

ANDREW MACKINNON AND DEBRA FOLEY

Mental Health Research Institute of Victoria, Parkville, Victoria, Australia

INTRODUCTION

While interest in the heritability of anxiety disorders has existed for as long as for other psychiatric disorders, research efforts have been both limited and scattered. This stands in stark contrast to genetic research into both mood disorders and psychoses, reviews of which can assemble a large body of research culminating in current efforts to scan the entire genome with the aim of identifying individual genes responsible for these disorders (see, for example, Mitchell *et al.*, 1993). The task of this review is thus to assemble and integrate the literature relating to genetic research into anxiety disorders, then to identify future research strategies and the possible impact of genetic research in this area. Because the genetics of anxiety disorders has been the subject of a number of reviews (see, for example, Foley and Hay, 1992), this chapter will emphasize the most recent research.

PHENOTYPES: THE CLASSIFICATION OF ANXIETY DISORDERS

The anxiety disorders underwent significant diagnostic revision with the publication of DSM-III (American Psychiatric Association, 1980; Frances *et al.*, 1993; Zal, 1988). As most recent family and twin studies of anxiety disorders have employed DSM-III/DSM-III-R criteria, this chapter will be organized according to this classification scheme. For a comparison of ICD and DSM definitions, however, see Torgersen (1986), and the respective nomenclatures for the full diagnostic criteria.

The characteristic features of the DSM-III-R anxiety disorders are symptoms of anxiety and avoidance behavior. These disorders comprise: Panic Disorder with Agoraphobia; Panic Disorder without Agoraphobia; Agoraphobia without a history of Panic Disorder; Social Phobia; Simple Phobia; Obsessive-Compulsive Disorder (OCD); Post-traumatic Stress Disorder and Generalized Anxiety Disorder. The classification of Post-traumatic Stress Disorder (PTSD) is considered controversial as the predominant symptom is the re-experiencing

Advances in the Neurobiology of Anxiety Disorders. Edited by H. G. M. Westenberg, J. A. Den Boer and D. L. Murphy
©1996 John Wiley & Sons Ltd

of trauma, not anxiety or avoidance behavior (American Psychiatric Association, 1987). The latter are, however, extremely common in PTSD, and symptoms of increased arousal are invariably present.

Changes in classification systems reflect the evolution and refinement of definitions and diagnostic criteria for the anxiety disorders. This is an ongoing process and other psychiatric nomenclature such as the International Classification of Diseases (ICD-9; ICD-10) apply a different classification system (Torgersen, 1986). That no single ICD-9 category corresponds to DSM-III panic disorder (PD) (Maier et al., 1986) highlights the difficulty of determining the relevant phenotypic features and correct diagnostic assignment of anxiety phenomenology.

This is not a trivial issue, particularly for genetics. Variation in diagnostic assignment can have a significant impact on genetic analyses (Torgersen, 1985). Without knowing how far the phenotype extends, identification of "affected" relatives remains problematic and familial/cotwin risk cannot be accurately characterized. This boundary problem is relevant to consider when evaluating reports of patient "comorbidity", familial disorder overlap, and the complex range of familial risk and twin concordances that necessarily arise in reports of twin and family studies of anxiety disorders, some of which will be outlined below. At least some of the disorder overlap is likely to reflect inappropriate diagnostic boundaries, or criteria that only partly tap the underlying latent traits involved. As genetic analysis requires accurate identification of affected individuals, this issue must be addressed if knowledge of the etiology of the anxiety disorders is to be advanced.

HISTORICAL PERSPECTIVE

Although the various diagnostic criteria and labeling of the anxiety disorders have changed over time, similar symptom clusters can be traced through the medical literature (Wooley, 1976). These provide insight into the relative importance attached to specific symptoms or subsets of symptoms over time (e.g., Culpin, 1920; Skerritt, 1983).

One fundamental change introduced by DSM-III, which has received widespread support, is the importance accorded to the spontaneous panic attack (American Psychiatric Association, 1980; Klein, 1981). This is the basis for the subdivision of anxiety neurosis (American Psychiatric Association, 1968) into generalized anxiety disorder (GAD) and panic disorder (PD). The validity of this subdivision is based on claims of unique phenomenology and natural history (Anderson et al., 1984), pharmacodissection (Klein, 1981), differential familial risk (Harris et al., 1983; Crowe et al., 1983; Gruppo Italiano Disturbi d'Ansia, 1989; Noyes et al., 1987), and a distinct response to various provocation agents (Pitts and McClure, 1967; Margraf et al., 1986; Cowley and Arana, 1990).

The evidence supporting the validity of these two "new" disorders, however, pertains largely to PD. GAD is less well characterized, and doubt has been expressed regarding its validity (Garvey *et al.*, 1988; Aronson, 1987; but cf. Noyes *et al.*, 1992), and appropriate diagnostic placement (Noyes *et al.*, 1987).

PHENOTYPIC BOUNDARIES: CONSIDERATION OF SEVERITY AND BREADTH

A key issue in genetic studies of anxiety disorders relates to the diagnostic cut-offs employed by DSM-III/DSM-III-R. It is important to consider the impact of varying phenotypic boundaries in two dimensions: severity and breadth. Examples from the PD literature may be used to illustrate both issues.

Evaluation of severity criteria requires consideration of the boundary between "normal" and "abnormal" states of anxiety. It must also be considered whether that boundary reflects etiologically discrete processes, or a threshold of distress that, if exceeded, leads to help seeking or categorization as a "case". The diagnostic cut-offs for PD employed by DSM-III produced the (artificial) category of sub-panic disorders or limited symptom attacks, formally recognized by DSM-III-R. The necessarily arbitrary nature of these criteria have been criticized (Katerndahl, 1990) and shown to contradict familial (Noyes *et al.*, 1986), experimental (Cowley *et al.*, 1987), and epidemiological data (von Korff *et al.*, 1985), which all suggest a severity spectrum.

RESEARCH DESIGNS AND ANALYSES

Genetic analyses proceed from a well-defined phenotype. A number of commonly used approaches to genetic research can be identified. All analyses rely on the collection of information about the occurrence of the phenotype (illness) within pedigrees with known patterns of genetic covariation. Environmental covariation is also controlled in certain designs. Studies of anxiety disorders have involved families of probands or the study of twins. Recent advances in molecular genetics have increased the range of methods by which specific genetic sites associated with a disorder may be identified.

Research designs in human genetic investigations may be thought of as following a path from establishing familiality (a necessary condition for heritability) to the demonstration that observed patterns of familiality are due to genetic rather than environmental causes and, finally, to the location or modeling of the gene or genes involved.

The investigation of the patterns of illness among family members is the most common type of study. The aim of these studies is to demonstrate that the disorder concerned is familial, having a higher prevalence in relatives of ill individuals than in the general population. Families are recruited into studies through an affected proband. Information about the illness status of relatives is obtained directly by interview with each relative (the family study method), or, less satisfactorily, by interviewing the proband or other informant about relatives (the family history method). Prevalence rates for relatives of different degrees of genetic similarity may then be compared to prevalence rates for the same disorder in the population. Higher prevalence rates in the families of ill probands are indicative of familiality. Prevalence rates for psychiatric disorders vary according to recruitment methods and the methods used to diagnose disorders. Family studies can be methodologically strengthened by using prevalence in families recruited through a control proband as the basis for comparison rather than relying on population estimates.

Family studies demonstrate the possibility of genetic transmission but, because environmental exposure tends to covary with degree of genetic similarity, other causes of an excess of cases cannot be ruled out by this approach. Adoption studies are one method of breaking the nexus between genes and environment. This approach has not been used in any study of anxiety disorders. The study of twins remains a practical means of determining whether covariation of disorders in relatives is due to genetic or environmental causes.

The classical twin design relies on the comparison of monozygotic (MZ) twins, who are genetically identical, with dizygotic (DZ) twins, who share, on average, half their genes. In most studies of illness, twins are ascertained through an affected proband. The concordance rates for MZ and DZ twins are calculated and compared statistically. Significantly higher concordance in MZ than DZ twins is evidence for a genetic effect (see Gottesman and Carey, 1983). Other effects, such as the importance of environmental factors unique to each twin or shared between, may also be tested (see Neale and Cardon, 1992).

Twins may also be selected randomly (specifically, unconditioned on a proband with the disorder) from sources such as twin registries. This allows the direct estimation of heritabilities and other sources of variation but is generally only suitable for traits that are common or continuously distributed in the population. This approach also allows multivariate analyses to be undertaken in which strength of genetic and environmental factors common to two or more traits or disorders can be estimated.

GENETIC MODELING

The research designs discussed above provide evidence for the role of genes in a disorder. A further step is to determine the mechanism of the genes involved. As psychiatric disorders do not display simple Mendelian patterns of segregation, quantitative models of transmission have relied on the abstraction of a continuous latent variable referred to as liability. Individuals whose liability exceeds a threshold value exhibit the disorder while those whose liability is below the threshold do not. Models can be divided into those in which a large number of genetic and environmental factors are assumed to make small, additive contributions to liability (multifactorial polygenic models (MFP)) and those in which a single gene is posited as responsible (single major locus (SML)).

The fitting of specific models to family pedigrees is referred to as segregation analysis. Linkage analysis attempts to associate a putative gene responsible for a disorder with a gene whose site on the human genome is known. While these techniques have been widely employed in the study of mood disorders and psychoses (see Mitchell *et al.*, 1993) only a few investigators have used them in the study of anxiety disorders.

PANIC DISORDER

FAMILY STUDIES OF PANIC DISORDER

Early family history studies (e.g. Oppenheimer and Rothschild, 1918; McInnes, 1937) are of largely historical interest, as the disorders they describe are not synonymous with PD (Aronson, 1987). They do, however, indicate that the diagnostic precursors of DSM-III PD were also familial.

Family studies of PD/agoraphobia have yielded a range of familial risk estimates. Some of the methodological features likely to contribute toward these discrepant reports have been previously summarized (see Table 1 in Foley and Hay, 1992). Despite the variation across studies, it is apparent that there is an increased risk of homotypic disorder in adult relatives of PD probands. Reports of risk range between 8% to 31% in family interview studies and from 4% to 36% in family history studies. Most reports range between 10% and 25%, which is significantly in excess of the median lifetime prevalence rate, which for PD is 1.4% (males 0.9%; females 1.8%) and for agoraphobia is 4.1% (males 1.5%; females 6.4%) (Robins *et al.*, 1984). Several family studies report an increased risk for PD/agoraphobia only (or mainly) in females (Noyes *et al.*, 1978; Crowe *et al.*, 1980; Cloninger *et al.*, 1981; Crowe *et al.*, 1983; Moran and Andrews, 1985; Gruppo Italiano Disturbi d'Ansia, 1989).

LINKAGE STUDIES

PD is the only anxiety disorder in which linkage analysis has been attempted. These analyses have been undertaken by Crowe's group in the USA. Crowe *et al.* (1987) investigated 26 PD pedigrees, testing 29 red cell antigens and protein polymorphisms as genetic markers. They excluded linkage to 18 loci, but found evidence suggestive of linkage to α-haptoglobin (located in chromosomal region 16q22) with a lod score of 2.27. (A lod score is the base-10 logarithm of the odds of linkage. Lod scores greater than 3 are taken to support linkage.) In 1990, however, the same group (Crowe *et al.*, 1990) analyzed 10 new pedigrees alone and in combination with the previous 26. On this occasion, they demonstrated exclusion of close linkage to α-haptoglobin, a finding which suggests that the earlier result reflected a type I error. Wang *et al.* (1992) failed to establish linkage between the disorder and any of five adrenergic receptor loci. Schmidt *et al.* (1993) excluded linkage to another candidate site, the γ-aminobutyric acid β1 locus. Kendler *et al.* (1993) comment that PD due to a highly penetrant single major locus detectable by linkage analysis, may exist but if it does, individuals with this etiology constitute a modest proportion of the general population who meet lifetime criteria for PD.

TWIN STUDIES OF PANIC DISORDER

Earlier twin studies of neurosis provide support for a heritable component. However, they applied broad, often poorly documented criteria for proband selection and determination of concordance. These studies have been reviewed elsewhere (Miner, 1973; Slater and Shields, 1969; Torgersen, 1983b). There are few recent twin studies of clinically ascertained PD probands (Torgersen, 1983a; Skre et al., 1993).

Torgersen (1983a) conducted the first twin study of PD. It comprised 13 MZ (five with PD and eight with PD and agoraphobia) and 16 DZ (six with PD and 10 with PD and agoraphobia) Norwegian same-sex twins admitted to psychiatric institutions. Concordance for panic disorder with or without agoraphobia was 2/13 (15.4%) for MZ and 0/16 (0.0%) for DZ pairs. For cotwin concordance based on the presence of any anxiety disorders the respective MZ and DZ concordances were 6/13 (46.2%) and 4/16 (25%). More recently Skre et al. (1993) reported the prevalence of anxiety disorders, including PD, in 20 MZ and 29 DZ cotwins of anxiety disorder probands (who overlap with the sample described in Torgersen, 1983b, defined in 1983a), and compared them with a group of cotwins of 12 MZ and 20 DZ twin probands with other non-psychotic mental disorders. Concordances for PD in MZ and DZ cotwins of PD probands were 5/12 (41.6%) and 3/18 (16.6%), respectively. The rate of PD in cotwins of "pure GAD" probands (i.e., GAD without PD, but with a mood disorder) was 0/5 and 0/7 for MZ and DZ pairs, and in the comparison group (which included seven pairs with anxiety probands, four with social phobia, three with simple phobia and one with agoraphobia) the MZ and DZ concordances were 1/15 (6.6%) and 2/24 (8.3%).

Data on the lifetime prevalence and concordance in MZ and DZ twins for DSM-III anxiety disorders, major depression and dysthymia diagnosed by the Diagnostic Interview Schedule (DIS) were reported by Andrews et al. (1990a). Their 446 pairs were volunteers, ascertained from the community and the Australian Twin Registry (ATR) unconditional on either twins' status for any disorder. Focusing only on pairs with PD with or without agoraphobia, the concordance rate in MZ and DZ cotwins was 1/11 (9.1%) and 1/23 (4.3%), respectively. The MZ and DZ concordance for any anxiety disorder was 7/11 (63.6%) and 10/23 (43.5%), respectively. In this sample multiple diagnoses were common, with no apparent pattern to their co-occurrence. These MZ concordance figures are lower than those reported in the Norwegian series which surveyed mostly inpatients, and lower than the rates reported in a larger population survey by Kendler et al. (1993). Also, the DZ rates are lower than those found in first-degree relatives, as are those of the Norwegians. Kendler's concordance figures are closer to the rates in the family studies, although at the low end of the range.

A population-based survey of female twins from the Virginian Twin Registry (VTR) found a more modest familial aggregation for PD than reported for families of clinically ascertained probands (Kendler *et al.*, 1993). The relatively small number of twins who met the various criteria of PD employed did not allow for resolution of competing models of transmission. Kendler analyzed the data using a variety of diagnostic approaches (based on DSM-III-R and using the SCID computer algorithm and clinician rating of all information collected subdivided into narrow (definite and probable) and broad (definite, probable and possible cases) categories of diagnoses) and reported estimates of the heritability of liability ranging from 30% to 40% for most of the diagnostic approaches. For the computer "narrow" diagnosis the concordance rate in MZ and DZ twins was not significantly different, yielding significant estimates of only shared and unique environment components in subsequent model fitting. The relative risk for PD in cotwins of affected twins versus the entire twin population was 1.5–2.0 in DZ and 3.0 in MZ twins, averaged across the various definitions of PD employed.

Kendler *et al.* (1993) reported that PD with phobic avoidance appeared to represent a more severe form of panic without phobic avoidance, based on the fit of multiple threshold models incorporating the presence of phobic avoidance. This accords with some (Noyes *et al.*, 1986), but not all, views of agoraphobia (cf. Fyer, 1987). Agoraphobia without panic, which Eaton and Keyl (1990) found to be more common in the general population than in clinical settings, was not surveyed. As other clinical and population surveys (Lelliott *et al.*, 1989; Eaton and Keyl, 1990, respectively) document persons with agoraphobia who deny any history of PD, incorporation of such data in threshold models such as those reported by Kendler would be of interest.

Likewise, consideration of subclinical or limited symptom panic attacks in these threshold models would also be illuminating. Katerndahl (1990) noted the arbitrary nature of DSM-III regarding the distinction between infrequent and limited symptom panic attacks and those meeting full DSM criteria. As phobic avoidance did not differ between limited symptom and full-blown attacks the severity threshold may be more complex than the available data can determine. The evaluation of a multiple threshold model incorporating subclinical PD (where criteria for number of symptoms and/or frequency of attacks required by the DSM is not met), PD, and PD with various levels of phobic avoidance, would be valuable as it would assist critical evaluation of appropriate boundaries of PD, and the relationship among non-recurrent episodes of panic in the general population which are much more common than PD, and which may or may not reflect a continuum in the normal population regarding anxiety (see Norton *et al.*, 1992). Evaluation of the position of agoraphobia without panic attacks on such a continuum would help clarify the relationship between phobic behavior and episodes of panic anxiety.

Given the concordance observed between twins it must be recognized that environmental factors are also important for this disorder and may indeed interact with gene action. Kendler *et al.* (1992a) investigated the relationship between parental loss prior to age 17 and adult psychopathology in female VTR twins. Risk varied with the kind of loss, the parent involved and the form of adult psychopathology. PD was associated with parental death and maternal, but not paternal, separation. Risk for phobia was associated with parental death only.

OVERLAP WITH OTHER DISORDERS

Family data have highlighted the complex relationship among PD, agoraphobia, GAD and major depression (Crowe *et al.*, 1983; Harris *et al.*, 1983; Leckman *et al.*, 1983a; Noyes *et al.*, 1986; Noyes *et al.*, 1987; Coryell *et al.*, 1988; Gruppo Italiano Disturbi d'Ansia, 1989; Coryell *et al.*, 1992). The work of both Leckman and Coryell and their colleagues has emphasized the importance of characterizing the phenotypic breadth evident in both probands and their relatives, explicitly outlining inclusion and exclusion criteria applied to proband populations, the temporal relationship among "comorbid" diagnoses, and the impact of diagnostic hierarchies on calculations of risk.

An elevated risk of major depression in relatives of PD probands has been found in most (Bowen and Kohout, 1979; Munjack and Moss, 1981; Leckman *et al.*, 1983a; Mellman and Uhde, 1987; Coryell *et al.*, 1988), but not all (Harris *et al.*, 1983; Crowe *et al.*, 1983; Noyes *et al.*, 1986), family studies of PD. Again, it is worth noting that calculation of risk in relatives varies across studies, due to the variable use and/or reporting of diagnostic hierarchies or application of "primary" diagnoses.

The presence of both PD and major depression in probands was associated with a significantly elevated risk to relatives for a range of disorders: major depression, PD, phobia and alcoholism. Leckman found this risk was elevated irrespective of the temporal relationship of PD and depression in the proband. Coryell *et al.* (1988) found the temporal relationship between anxiety disorders and depression did predict differential patterns of familial risk. A recent report consolidates this view (Coryell *et al.*, 1992).

An elevated risk of alcoholism among relatives of probands with PD with or without agoraphobia has been found in a number of studies (Munjack and Moss, 1981; Leckman *et al.*, 1983a; Noyes *et al.*, 1986; Mellman and Uhde, 1987; Coryell *et al.*, 1988); others have not (Pauls *et al.*, 1979; Gruppo Italiano Disturbi d'Ansia, 1989). Male relatives have the highest risk (Harris *et al.* 1983; Noyes *et al.*, 1978). Standard criteria for assessment of alcoholism were not always applied, although more recent studies have been more consistent. Further, it is difficult to determine the temporal relationship between alcoholism and other disorders, especially given the difficulty of identifying age of onset in the former.

Various hypotheses have been proposed to account for the overlap of PD and alcoholism. Alcohol consumption as an attempt at self-medication for chronic anticipatory anxiety has been suggested (Quitkin *et al.*, 1972). Alcohol abuse may, however, predate the onset of PD/agoraphobia (Kushner *et al.*, 1990), and may, in some cases, be a cause and not a consequence of neurosis (Mullan *et al.*, 1986).

OTHER PHOBIAS

There have been few studies of the heritability of simple phobic disorders. Fyer *et al.* (1990) investigated the relatives of simple phobics. They demonstrated that simple phobia occurs in 31% of the relatives of simple phobic probands compared with 11% of the relatives of controls. There was no difference in the rates of depression or other anxiety disorders. Specifically, there was no evidence for increased rates of other phobic disorders, suggesting a genetic specificity for simple phobics.

Twin studies conducted using self-report questionnaires of fears have found moderate heritability (Rose and Ditto, 1983). Multivariate analyses of such data by Phillips *et al.* (1987) showed that a genetic rather than social model could account for patterns of parent–child transmission. Specificity of the object of fear was also analyzed by Phillips *et al.*(1987). They concluded that both a general tendency towards a fearful reaction and fear of specific objects were separately transmitted. Marks (1986) has reported strong familial transmission of blood phobia, but the symptomatology of this condition differs from other phobias.

OBSESSIVE-COMPULSIVE DISORDER

Early family studies of disorders comparable to the DSM-III-R classification of OCD generally found rates in first-degree relatives in excess of the then accepted prevalence rate in the population (see Mackinnon and Mitchell, 1994). Generally, these studies can all be criticized for not employing controls. In addition, knowledge of the diagnosis in the proband, the lack of a universally adopted definition of the disorder, and the lack of structured interviews make the results of these studies difficult to interpret.

Furthermore, it had been generally accepted that OCD is a relatively uncommon disorder, with prevalence in the general population estimated as 0.05%. More recently, the Epidemiological Catchment Area (ECA) studies have estimated the prevalence of OCD diagnosed to DSM-III criteria as 2.6% in the North American population (Robins and Regier, 1991). Thus prevalence in relatives in some of these studies may not be significantly elevated over this population prevalence estimate.

Five studies have employed DSM-III or Research Diagnostic Criteria (RDC) for diagnosis. Of these, studies by Insel *et al.* (1983) and Rasmussen and Tsuang (1986) share the same methodological limitations as earlier investigations. While the prevalence of 7% found by Rasmussen and Tsuang (1986) is consistent with earlier studies, Insel *et al.*'s failure to find any cases of OCD in parents of their patients may reflect their small sample size or use of the family history method. While no control group was used, the finding of case rates of 25% in fathers and 9% in mothers of probands in Lenane *et al.*'s (1990) study is strongly suggestive of familiality. This finding must be tempered by the fact that probands in this study were children and adolescents recruited from a specialized child clinic. It may not be possible to generalize these findings to populations with onset of OCD in later adolescence or adulthood.

The study of Black *et al.* (1992) lacks many of the limitations of early investigations: the family study method was used, with DSM-III diagnoses made using the DIS (see Robins and Regier, 1991). Unlike previous studies, Black *et al.* (1992) present age-corrected risk of disorders. The risk of 2.6% in 120 first-degree relatives of their 32 probands was not significantly higher than for the relatives of their controls (2.4%). Both rates are very close to that found in the ECA studies. The risk of symptoms not reaching criteria (subsyndromal OCD) amongst relatives of probands was higher than for controls (18% vs 12.9%), but this difference was not significant. However, the risk of anxiety disorders was significantly higher in probands' compared to controls' relatives (30.8% vs 17.8%). This pattern was not found for mood or alcohol disorders. The two groups did not differ significantly on their scores on the scales of the Leyton Obsessional Inventory.

Young *et al.* (1971) calculated the heritability of eight obsession-related items from the Middlesex Hospital Questionnaire as 0.43 on a sample of 32 twins. Clifford *et al.* (1984) calculated similar heritabilities from the Trait and Symptom scales of the Brief Leyton Obsessional Inventory as 0.47 and 0.44. As the result of multivariate genetic analysis of these two scales and EPQ Neuroticism, Clifford *et al.* (1984) concluded that the genetic transmission of obsessive tendencies involved a general neurotic tendency as well as specific obsessional genetic factors.

Reports of concordance for OCD in twins have largely been confined to series of case studies of concordant MZ pairs. Marks *et al.* (1969) calculated the chance of finding a concordant MZ twin pair as 1 in 6–800 million, based on prevalence rate of 0.05% and 1 in 120 to 200 live births being MZ twins. Thus the existence of even a small number of reliably diagnosed twins has been taken as evidence for non-independence in the etiology of the disorder. Using the much higher lifetime prevalence estimate of 2.6% found in the ECA studies (Robins and Regier, 1991) leads to an estimate of chance concordance of more than 1 in 300 000. Using this figure, all reports of concordant twins could be explained by chance and thus this estimate must cause reappraisal of the impact of reports of small numbers of concordant twins: given interest in MZ twins concordant for particular disorders, the possibility that the cases in the literature have arisen by chance is more difficult to refute. It should also be noted that the reasoning behind this calculation does not exclude environmental transmission as the determinant of concordance.

Twin studies of clinically defined OCD have principally comprised individual case reports or very small numbers (see Black, 1974; Carey and Gottesman, 1981). Considerable doubt exists about the nature of the diagnoses made in a number of these studies, with speculation that the literature may be biased towards the reporting of concordant MZ cases. Nevertheless, concordance is greater for MZ than DZ twins. Carey and Gottesman reported the largest single twin study of OCD, involving 15 MZ and 15 DZ pairs derived from the Maudsley Twin Register. Although MZ concordance was not significantly greater than DZ, MZ/DZ concordance ranges from 33%/7% for treated conditions involving obsessional symptoms to 87%/47% for both treated and untreated obsessional symptoms or features were found.

Even though total numbers are small and doubts must remain about ascertainment bias and diagnostic validity, the likelihood of familial aggregation and the higher concordance in MZ than DZ twins suggests that genetic factors are involved in this disorder.

Andrews et al.'s (1990a) study of 446 unselected twin pairs failed to find any MZ or DZ pairs concordant for OCD. Broadening concordance to include other anxiety disorders produced elevated concordance for MZ twins over DZ twins (2/18=11.2% MZ, 1/20=5.0% DZ, 0/10 DZ opposite sex) but this difference was not significant.

A cautious summary of research into the genetics of this disorder must emphasize the lack of reliable knowledge and contradictory research findings. The findings of twin studies must be considerably qualified. The scientific impact of small numbers of concordant MZ pairs is heavily dependent on assumptions of the prevalence of OCD. While concern has been expressed about actual zygosity of the twins in some reports, the effects of recruitment bias, diagnostic reliability and independence are probably greater threats to the higher levels of concordance in MZ over DZ twins that can be achieved by aggregating reports. The inability to test models in which one twin provides a learning environment for the other is a source of frustration.

Based on recent well-conducted studies, some confidence can be had in suggesting that a general tendency to anxiety disorders or symptoms is transmitted genetically. This finding could explain why older family and twin studies using looser definitions of illness found evidence of familiality. Also in accord with this conclusion are the findings of Clifford et al. (1984) using a self-report inventory. It is, however, difficult to hypothesize a genetic diathesis model that would not predict an excess of cases of OCD itself in addition to other disorders. The only defence to this point is the lack of power arising from the same sample sizes used: there is an obvious need for a large family study to address this issue.

POST-TRAUMATIC STRESS DISORDER

PTSD is unique within the classification of anxiety disorders in its incorporation of exposure to a distressing event as the key criterion in its DSM-III-R specification. This poses great difficulty in the design of genetic studies of the disorder. Consequently the few studies that have been undertaken of PTSD have used veterans of military service as subjects.

Davidson and his colleagues carried out two family studies of PTSD using World War II, Korean War and Vietnam War veterans. While elevated levels of psychopathology amongst relatives of probands were found in the initial study (Davidson *et al.*, 1985), a larger, better-controlled study (Davidson *et al.*, 1989) failed to replicate these findings.

By virtue of its size and method of ascertainment, the American Vietnam Era Twin Registry (Eisen *et al.*, 1987) has allowed unique analyses relevant to PTSD to be undertaken. First, using MZ twins concordant and discordant for combat exposure, it was demonstrated that subsequent symptoms of PTSD were significantly related to this exposure (Goldberg *et al.*, 1990). Combat exposure was also related to zygosity. This necessitated the construction of models incorporating genetic and environmental effects. After adjusting for differences in combat exposure, genetic factors accounted for between 13% and 34% of the variance in individual symptoms of PTSD. No common environment effects were found.

The study of Comings *et al.* (1991) illustrates an alternative approach to investigating the genetics of PTSD. They showed an increased frequency of the A1 allele of the Taq I polymorphism of the dopamine D_2 receptor gene in patients with PTSD compared to controls. As this gene has been proposed as a major locus for alcoholism (Noble, 1993), Comings *et al.*'s (1991) findings must be tempered by their selection of PTSD patients with comorbid alcoholism.

The above studies share a number of important limitations. All involve only males and reflect a restricted range of events as their trigger. There is a long period between the events and the symptoms as assessed in the studies. This implies that severe or chronic manifestations of the disorder only are being studied. In the studies of Davidson *et al.* (1985, 1989) and Comings *et al.* (1991), all subjects had additional psychiatric diagnoses, including alcoholism and major depression. The specificity of the relationship between PTSD and study findings therefore appears uncertain.

The prospects for undertaking genetic research into PTSD using traditional family or twin methods seem poor. Advancement in this area is more likely to occur indirectly. This may involve establishing a relationship between PTSD and personality traits such as neuroticism whose genetic basis is well established. Alternatively, the identification of biochemical markers related to PTSD may lead to studies of heritability of these markers.

GENERALIZED ANXIETY DISORDER

FAMILY STUDIES

Although the earlier family studies (Harris *et al.*, 1983; Crowe *et al.*, 1983) are often cited as supporting the distinctness of PD from GAD, the application of diagnostic hierarchies following DSM-III or "primary" diagnoses may have partly obscured what seems to be a more complex relationship when relatives of probands with a range of "comorbid" diagnoses were investigated (Leckman *et al.*, 1983a; Coryell *et al.*, 1988).

Leckman *et al.* (1983a) reported a significantly increased risk of GAD among relatives of probands with depression and PD (10.5%) compared with relatives of probands with depression but no anxiety disorder (6.2%). Relatives of probands with depression and GAD had an increased risk of depression (19.8%) compared with the relatives of probands with depression only (10.7%), or the relatives of controls (5.6%). Coryell *et al.* (1988) reported that relatives of probands with both PD and depression had a higher risk for GAD (13.3%) than the relatives of probands with depression and panic attacks (10.4%) or depression without panic attacks (6.3%).

In contrast, evidence supporting the distinction of GAD and PD is provided by the only family interview study of GAD conducted to date. Noyes *et al.* (1987) reported a 19.5% risk of GAD in relatives of community volunteers with GAD, but no increased risk for other disorders. The risk of GAD to relatives of medical outpatients with PD and agoraphobia was 5.4% and 3.9% respectively, and among relatives of controls was 3.5%. A family study utilizing clinically ascertained GAD patients and their relatives would be valuable for confirmation of Noyes *et al.'s* (1987) findings. Noyes *et al.* (1992) collected family history data for GAD and PD probands. GAD subjects had more relatives with GAD than did subjects with PD (10.0% vs 3.8% "possible" plus "definite" diagnoses, respectively). PD probands had more relatives with PD (11.8% vs 1.8% with "possible" and "definite" diagnoses). Rates of depression and alcoholism were similar across both GAD and PD probands' relatives (5.4% vs 3.8% and 11.3% vs 10.8%, respectively).

From a familial perspective the boundary between PD and GAD is still unclear and will require further evaluation of the longitudinal nature of both disorders (see, for example, Garvey *et al.*, 1988). There has been only one family interview study (Noyes *et al.*, 1987), and one recent twin study (Kendler *et al.*, 1992b) of GAD, although its overlap with other DSM-III-R disorders has been documented in a number of other family studies of depression or other anxiety disorders (e.g. Coryell *et al.*, 1992). Noyes *et al.* (1987) reported a 19.5% risk of GAD among the first-degree relatives of GAD probands who were community volunteers. There was no increase in risk for other disorders. As yet there have been no reports of the risk of GAD in relatives of clinically ascertained GAD probands. The relationship between GAD and the other anxiety disorders is unresolved.

TWIN STUDIES

The four published twin studies (Torgersen, 1983a; Andrews *et al.*, 1990a; Kendler *et al.*, 1992b; Skre *et al.*, 1993) have considered GAD and its overlap with other disorders to varying degrees.

Kendler *et al.*'s (1992b) population-based female twin study of GAD defined comorbidity, for the purposes of their report, as restricted to syndromes that co-occurred in time. The twins were subdivided into those who met criteria for GAD only when criteria for major depression or PD was not met simultaneously, versus those who had only GAD or no disorder. Overlaying this consideration of hierarchical effects in temporal overlap was a division based on length of GAD criterion symptoms (one and six months). Applying no hierarchy, and including all who met criteria for one month's duration of symptoms, the tetrachoric correlations for GAD were: MZ 0.35 (SE=0.07) and DZ 0.12 (SE=0.08).

Of nine definitions of GAD employed (including three threshold models with and without hierarchies for PD and depression) the genes plus individual environment model provided the best overall fit. For six-month GAD, diagnosed without hierarchy or with major depression above GAD in the hierarchy, the shared plus individual environment models provided the best fit. The difference in preferred models may be due to the smaller numbers of twins who met criteria for GAD with six months duration, given the threshold model incorporating one- and six-month criteria for GAD fit the data well. Evidence of genetic effects in shorter-, rather than longer-duration GAD would otherwise be hard to reconcile. Kendler *et al.* (1992b) also note the unexpectedly higher risk for one-month GAD diagnosed without hierarchy in DZ compared to MZ twins.

Torgersen's (1983a) clinical sample fails to support a significant genetic predisposition to GAD. Torgersen (1983a) reported concordances for GAD among pairs as follows: MZ 0% (0/12) and DZ 5% (1/20). Any evidence for a genetic effect in Andrews *et al.*'s (1990a) data is equivocal (27% for MZ, 9% for same-sex DZ twins but 24% for opposite-sex DZ twins).

OVERLAP AND NON-SPECIFICITY OF TRANSMISSION

A recurrent finding for both family and twin studies is the lack of specificity of transmission. Prevalence for individual disorders in relatives of probands may or may not be raised, but increased prevalence has frequently been observed for a broader spectrum of anxiety disorders. Similarly, in twin studies, although concordance for specific anxiety disorders is often low, broadening the definition of the disorder considered often increases concordance beyond what would be predicted on the basis of the necessarily increased prevalence of a broader category of disorders alone.

A GENERAL NEUROTIC SYNDROME

The concept of a general neurotic syndrome is a formal model that posits a single diathesis to all disorders with specific, possibly environmental factors determining which disorder is manifest. The twin study of Andrews *et al.* (1990a) provides support for this view. Lifetime diagnoses for DSM-III-R anxiety disorders, dysthymia and major depressive episode were made for each twin using a standardized interview. Phenotypically, substantial correlations in liability ranging from 0.41 to 0.77 were observed between all disorders (Andrews *et al.*, 1990b). It was also demonstrated that a single common factor model provided a good fit to the correlations. The number of cases of each disorder detected preclude the testing of a multivariate model involving a genetic common factor. Cotwins of probands had an elevated risk of various disorders, with concordance for any disorder being significantly greater for MZ than DZ twins. The breakdown of individual diagnoses is striking in showing the lack of specific concordance or pattern of concordance among twins who had any anxiety disorder. When specific concordance was observed it was often because one twin had multiple diagnoses, with the cotwin having just one of these disorders. This suggests a common heritable tendency to neurotic disorders rather than to specific disorders.

Torgersen's analyses of his Norwegian twin study also support this view, with specific concordance being low, while broader concordance was greater with the pattern of MZ/DZ concordance supporting a heritable factor. The concept of a general syndrome might best be viewed as approximation only. Clusters of genetically related disorders may exist, rather than all anxiety disorders being equally genetically related.

OVERLAP WITH OTHER DISORDERS

As discussed above, elevated rates of depression and alcoholism have frequently been found in probands with anxiety disorders and their relatives. An association between Tourette's syndrome and OCD has also been posited (see Apter *et al.*, 1993). Multivariate models are capable of determining whether these relationships are due to the action of common genes. An analysis of self-report symptoms of anxiety and depression in Australian twins by Kendler *et al.* (1987) demonstrated this approach. They concluded that a common set of genes was responsible for symptoms of anxiety and depression, but that the two sets of symptoms resulted from different environmental effects.

More recently, Kendler and colleagues' longitudinal survey of VTR twins used similar techniques to show that essentially the same genes were involved in diagnoses of major depression and generalized anxiety disorder. In contrast, major depression and phobias appear to share only a small percentage of common gene action (see Kendler *et al.*, 1992b).

Ultimately methods that identify the specific genes involved may further illuminate the shared etiology of disorders. It should be noted that the demonstration of unshared gene action in phenologically similar disorders may be as important as finding common genetic diatheses. For instance, demonstrating that the genes responsible for Tourette's syndrome were not involved in OCD without Tourette's would establish the co-occurrence of symptoms as simply being part of the syndrome.

FUTURE ISSUES CONCERNING OVERLAP

While comorbidity has been investigated in family and twin studies, the issue of contingency or temporal ordering is rarely considered. Kendler's approach of defining comorbidity of other disorders with GAD as being temporally comorbid is unusual. Most studies accumulate lifetime prevalence of disorders that may be widely separated in time and do not collect data relating to patterns of onset. The two studies of PD that have considered this issue have produced conflicting conclusions (see Leckman *et al.*, 1983b, and Coryell *et al.*, 1988). Although recording the chronological sequence of multiple diagnoses increases the complexity of data collection, this step will be important in understanding both genetic and environmentally determined relationships between disorders.

FUTURE RESEARCH DIRECTIONS

The future contribution of genetics to many areas of medical research is seen as centering around recent developments in molecular genetics. We make the suggestion that, in contrast, progress in the genetics of anxiety disorders will be underpinned by developments in quantitative genetics. The application of multivariate techniques by Kendler and his colleagues, first to self-report symptom data and more recently to DSM-III-R diagnoses, exemplifies one important method. This approach is essentially dimensional, based on correlations in liability of dichotomous diagnoses. Eaves *et al.* (1993) have demonstrated an alternative approach based on latent class analysis. Applied illustratively to conduct disorder in adolescent male twins, this approach could be employed with clusters of disorders or symptoms. Depending on prevalence rates, sample size requirements may be lower than for the dimensional approach. This method allows the fitting of a variety of models, including those that allow for environmental and genetic heterogeneity and gene–environment interaction in the etiology of symptoms or disorders. The growing availability of these models and computer software to fit them is likely to play a central role in future research.

It seems that no single gene is responsible for any anxiety disorder in the majority of cases. This implies that linkage techniques are unlikely to be successfully applied to anxiety disorder data in the future. It is possible that association studies might be undertaken and lead to the detection of genes responsible for moderate-sized effects on vulnerability to anxiety disorders. Association studies of the D_2 dopamine receptor gene exemplify this type of research (see Noble, 1993) and could provide a model for anxiety disorders. The construction of categorical disorders relies on relatively arbitrary cut-points along severity dimensions. Models that retain the quantitative characteristics of a disorder and relate this dimension to specific loci would have obvious application in this area. Quantitative trait loci (QTL) have been successfully applied in plant and non-human genetics, relating dimensional traits to genes having a moderate effect on them (see McClearn *et al.*, 1991). So far the only example of the application of QTL in humans is by Fulker *et al.* (1991) to twin data on reading ability. QTL detection will be a means of combining molecular and quantitative approaches to complex behavior genetics.

New methods of analysis bring their own requirements for study designs. Nevertheless a few general points can be made about this aspect of research. Some disorders, such as OCD, still await large, carefully controlled family studies to satisfactorily demonstrate familiality. Available studies appear to over-represent females. Sometimes this is by design, as in the case of Kendler's VTR study. Sometimes it is due to reliance on clinical samples. While the study of clinically ascertained cases has a role in research, it is well recognized that only a small, and possibly biased, proportion of individuals with anxiety disorders seek treatment (Kendler, 1993). Population-based research is likely to be important in future research, but this will require large samples, particularly in the investigation of relatively rare conditions.

CONCLUSION

Genetics cannot offer psychiatry the "Holy Grail" of the single gene responsible for any anxiety disorder. Nonetheless this review can point to a resurgence of interest in the genetics of anxiety disorders. Better study designs, together with the application of recently developed models, offer the prospect of refining the classification of the disorders, understanding the relationship between them and with other disorders. Finally, emerging methods of detecting individual genes that play a role in the development of anxiety disorders may lead to substantial advances in the understanding of their etiology.

REFERENCES

American Psychiatric Association (1968). *Diagnostic and Statistical Manual of Mental Disorders*, 2nd edn. American Psychiatric Association, Washington, DC.
American Psychiatric Association (1980). *Diagnostic and Statistical Manual of Mental Disorders*, 3rd edn. American Psychiatric Association, Washington, DC.
American Psychiatric Association (1987). *Diagnostic and Statistical Manual of Mental Disorders*, 3rd edn, revised. American Psychiatric Association, Washington, DC.
Anderson, D. J., Noyes, R., Jr and Crowe, R. R. (1984). A comparison of panic disorder and generalized anxiety disorder. *Am. J. Psychiatry*, **141**, 572–575.
Andrews, G., Stewart, G., Allen, R. and Henderson, A. S. (1990a). The genetics of six neurotic disorders: a twin study. *J. Affect. Disord.*, **19**, 23–29.
Andrews, G., Stewart, G., Morris-Yates, A. *et al.* (1990b). Evidence for a general neurotic syndrome. *Br. J. Psychiatry*, **157**, 6–12.
Apter, A., Pauls, D. L., Bleich, A. *et al.* (1993). An epidemiological study of Gilles de la Tourette's syndrome in Israel. *Arch. Gen. Psychiatry*, **50**, 734–738.
Aronson, T. A. (1987). Is panic disorder a distinct diagnostic entity? A critical review of the borders of a syndrome. *J. Nerv. Ment. Dis.*, **175**, 595–598.
Black, A. (1974). The natural history of the obsessional states. In *Obsessional States* (ed. H. R. Beech), pp. 20–54. Methuen, London.

Black, D. W., Noyes, R., Jr, Goldstein, R. B. and Blum, N. (1992). A family study of obsessive-compulsive disorder. *Arch. Gen. Psychiatry*, **49**, 362–368.

Bowen, R. C. and Kohout, J. (1979). The relationship between agoraphobia and primary affective disorders. *Can. Psychiatr. Assoc. J.*, **24**, 317–322.

Carey, G. and Gottesman, I. I. (1981). Twin and family studies of anxiety, phobic and obsessive disorders. In *Anxiety: New Research and Changing Concepts* (eds D. F. Klein and J. Rabkin), pp. 117–136. Raven Press, New York.

Clifford, C. A., Murray, R. M. and Fulker, D. W. (1984). Genetic and environmental influences on obsessional traits and symptoms, *Psychol. Med.*, **14**, 791–800.

Cloninger, C. R., Martin, R. L., Clayton, P. and Guze, S. B. (1981). A blind follow up and family study of anxiety neurosis: preliminary analysis of the St Louis 500. In *Anxiety: New Research and Changing Concepts* (eds D. F. Klein and J. G. Rabkin), pp. 137–150. Raven Press, New York.

Comings, D. E., Comings, B. G., Muhleman, D. *et al.* (1991). The dopamine D2 receptor locus as a modifying gene in neuropsychiatric disorders. *JAMA*, **266**, 1793–1800.

Coryell, W., Endicott, J., Andreasen, N. C. *et al.* (1988). Depression and panic attacks: the significance of overlap as reflected in follow-up and family study data. *Am. J. Psychiatry*, **145**, 293–300.

Coryell, W., Endicott, J. and Winokur, G. (1992). Anxiety syndromes as epiphenomena of primary depression: outcome and familial psychopathology. *Am. J. Psychiatry*, **149**, 100–107.

Cowley, D. S. and Arana, G. W. (1990). The diagnostic utility of lactate sensitivity in panic disorder. *Arch. Gen. Psychiatry*, **47**, 277–284.

Cowley, D. S., Dager, S. R., Foster, S. I. and Dunner, D. L. (1987). Clinical characteristics and response to sodium lactate of patients with infrequent panic. *Am. J. Psychiatry*, **144**, 795–798.

Crowe, R. R., Pauls, D. L., Slymen, D. and Noyes, R., Jr (1980). A family study of anxiety neurosis: morbidity risk in families of patients with and without mitral valve disorder. *Arch. Gen. Psychiatry*, **37**, 77–79.

Crowe, R. R., Noyes, R., Jr, Pauls, D. L. and Slymen, D. (1983). A family study of panic disorder. *Arch. Gen. Psychiatry*, **40**, 1065–1069.

Crowe, R. R., Noyes, R., Jr, Wilson, A. F. *et al.* (1987). A linkage study of panic disorder. *Arch. Gen. Psychiatry*, **44**, 933–937.

Crowe, R. R., Noyes, R., Jr, Samuelson, S. *et al.* (1990). Close linkage between panic disorder and alpha-haptoglobin excluded in 10 families, *Arch. Gen. Psychiatry*, **47**, 377–380.

Culpin, M. (1920). The psychological aspects of the effort syndrome. *Lancet*, **ii**, 184–186.

Davidson, J., Swartz, M., Storck, M. *et al.* (1985). A diagnostic and family study of post-traumatic stress disorder. *Am. J. Psychiatry*, **142**, 90–93.

Davidson, J., Smith, R. and Kudler, H. (1989). Familial psychiatric illness in chronic post-traumatic stress disorder. *Compr. Psychiatry*, **30**, 339–345.

Eaton, W. W. and Keyl, P. M. (1990). Risk factors for the onset of Diagnostic Interview Schedule/DSM-III agoraphobia in a prospective, population-based study. *Arch. Gen. Psychiatry*, **47**, 819–824.

Eaves, L. J., Silberg, J. L., Hewitt, J. K. *et al.* (1993). Analyzing twin resemblance in multi-symptom data: genetic applications of a latent class model for symptoms of conduct disorder in juvenile boys. *Behav. Genet.*, **23**, 5–19.

Eisen, S. A., True, W. R., Goldberg, J. *et al.* (1987). The Vietnam Era Twin (VET) Registry: method of construction. *Acta Genet. Med. Gemellol. (Roma)*, **36**, 61–66.

Foley, D. and Hay, D. A. (1992). Genetics and the nature of the anxiety disorders. In *Contemporary Issues and Prospects for Research in Anxiety* (eds G. D. Burrows, M. Roth and R. Noyes Jr), pp. 21–56. Elsevier, Amsterdam.

Frances, A., Pincus, H., Manning, D. and Widiger, T. (1993). Classification of anxiety states in DSM-III and perspectives for its classification in DSM-IV. In *Anxiety: Psychobiology and Clinical Perspectives* (eds N. Sartorius, V. Andreoli, G. Cassano *et al.*). Hemisphere, New York.

Fulker, D. W., Cardon, L. R., Defries, J. C. *et al.* (1991). Multiple regression analysis of sibpair data on reading to detect quantitative trait loci. *Reading Writing*, **3**, 299–313.

Fyer, A. J. (1987). Agoraphobia, *Mod. Probl. Pharmacopsychiatry*, **22**, 91–126.

Fyer, A. J., Mannuzza, S., Gallops, M. S. *et al.* (1990). Familial transmission of simple phobias and fears: a preliminary report. *Arch. Gen. Psychiatry*, **47**, 252–256.

Garvey, M. J., Cook, B. and Noyes, R., Jr (1988). The occurrence of a prodrome of generalized anxiety in panic disorder. *Compr. Psychiatry*, **29**, 445–449.

Goldberg, J., True, W. R., Eisen, S. A. and Henderson, W. (1990). A twin study of the effects of the Vietnam war on posttraumatic stress disorder. *JAMA*, **263**, 1227–1232.

Gottesman, I. I. and Carey, G. (1983). Extracting meaning and direction from twins data. *Psychiatr. Dev.*, **1**, 35–50.

Gruppo Italiano Disturbi d'Ansia (1989). Familial analysis of panic disorder and agoraphobia. *J. Affect. Disord.*, **17**, 1–8.

Harris, E. L., Noyes, R., Jr, Crowe, R. R. and Chaudhry, D. R. (1983). Family study of agoraphobia. *Arch. Gen. Psychiatry*, **40**, 1061–1064.

Insel, T. R., Hoover, C. and Murphy, D. L. (1985). Parents of patients with obsessive-compulsive disorder. *Psychol. Med.*, **13**, 807–811.

Katerndahl, D. A. (1990). Infrequent and limited symptom panic attacks. *J. Nerv. Ment. Dis.*, **178**, 313–317.

Kendler, K. S. (1993). Twin studies of psychiatric illness: current status and future directions. *Arch. Gen. Psychiatry*, **50**, 905–915.

Kendler, K. S., Heath, A. C., Martin, N. G. and Eaves, L. J. (1987). Symptoms of anxiety and symptoms of depression: same genes, different environments? *Arch. Gen. Psychiatry*, **44**, 451–457.

Kendler, K. S., Neale, M. C., Kessler, R. C. *et al.* (1992a). Childhood parental loss and adult psychopathology in women: a twin study perspective. *Arch. Gen. Psychiatry*, **49**, 109–116.

Kendler, K. S., Neale, M. C., Kessler, R. C. *et al.* (1992b). Generalized anxiety disorder in women: a population-based twin study. *Arch. Gen. Psychiatry*, **49**, 267–272.

Kendler, K. S., Neale, M. C., Kessler, R. C. *et al.* (1993). Panic disorder in women: a population-based twin study. *Psychol. Med.*, **23**, 397–406.

Klein, D. F. (1981). Anxiety reconceptualized. In *Anxiety: New Research and Changing Concepts* (eds D. F. Klein and J. G. Rabkin), pp. 235–264. Raven Press, New York.

Kushner, M. G., Sher, K. J. and Beitman, B. D. (1990). The relation between alcohol problems and the anxiety disorders, *Am. J. Psychiatry*, **147**, 685–695.

Leckman, J. F., Weissman, M. M., Merikangas, K. R. *et al.* (1983a). Panic disorder and major depression: increased risk of depression, alcoholism, panic, and phobic disorders in families of depressed probands with panic disorder, *Arch. Gen. Psychiatry*, **40**, 1055–1060.

Leckman, J. F., Merikangas, K. R., Pauls, D. L. *et al.* (1983b). Anxiety disorders and depression: contradictions between family study data and DSM-III conventions. *Am. J. Psychiatry*, **140**, 880–882.

Lelliott, P., Marks, I., McNamee, G. and Tobena, A. (1989). Onset of panic disorder with agoraphobia: toward an integrated model. *Arch. Gen. Psychiatry*, **46**, 1000–1004.

Lenane, M. C., Swedo, S. E., Leonard, H. *et al.* (1990). Psychiatric disorders in first degree relatives of children and adolescents with obsessive compulsive disorder. *J. Am. Acad. Adolesc. Psychiatry*, **29**, 407–412.

Mackinnon, A. and Mitchell, P. B. (1994). The genetics of anxiety and depression. In *The Handbook of Depression and Anxiety* (eds J. A. den Boer and A. Sitsen), pp. 71–118. Marcel Dekker, New York.

Maier, W., Buller, R., Sonntag, A. and Heuser, I. (1986). Subtypes of panic attacks and ICD-

9 classification. *Eur. Arch. Psychiatry Neurol. Sci.*, **235**, 361–366.

Margraf, J., Ehlers, A. and Roth, W. T. (1986). Sodium lactate infusions and panic attacks: a review and critique. *Psychosom. Med.*, **48**, 23–51.

Marks, I. M. (1986). Genetics of fear and anxiety disorder. *Br. J. Psychiatry*, **149**, 406–418.

Marks, I. M., Crowe, M., Drewe, E. *et al.* (1969). Obsessive-compulsive neurosis in identical twins. *Br. J. Psychiatry*, **115**, 991–998.

McClearn, G. E., Plomin, R., Gora-Maslak, G. and Crabbe, J. C. (1991). The gene chase in behavioral science. *Psychol. Sci.*, **2**, 222–229.

McInnes, R. G. (1937). Observations of heredity in neurosis. *Proc. R. Soc. Med.*, **30**, 895–904.

Mellman, T. A. and Uhde, T. W. (1987). Obsessive-compulsive symptoms in panic disorder, *Am. J. Psychiatry*, **144**, 1573–1536.

Miner, G. D. (1973). The evidence for genetic components in the neuroses: a review. *Arch. Gen. Psychiatry*, **29**, 111–118.

Mitchell, P., Mackinnon, A. and Waters, B. (1993). The genetics of bipolar disorder. *Aust. NZ J. Psychiatry*, **27**, 560–580.

Moran, C. and Andrews, G. (1985). The familial occurrence of agoraphobia. *Br. J. Psychiatry*, **146**, 262–267.

Mullan, M. J., Gurling, H. M. D., Oppenheim, B. E. and Murray, R. M. (1986). The relationship between alcoholism and neurosis: evidence from a twin study. *Br. J. Psychiatry*, **148**, 435.

Munjack, D. J. and Moss, H. B. (1981). Affective disorder and alcoholism in families of agoraphobics. *Arch. Gen. Psychiatry*, **38**, 869–871.

Neale, M. C. and Cardon, L. C., (1992). *Methodology for Genetic Studies of Twins and Families.* Kluwer, Dordrecht.

Noble, E. P. (1993) The D$_2$ dopamine receptor gene: a review of association studies in alcoholism. *Behav. Genet.*, **23**, 119–129.

Norton, G. R., Cox, B. J. and Malan, J. (1992). Nonclinical panickers: a critical review. *Clin. Psychol. Rev.*, **12**, 121–139.

Noyes, R., Jr, Clancy, J., Crowe, R. R. *et al.* (1978). The familial prevalence of anxiety neurosis, *Arch. Gen. Psychiatry*, **35**, 1057–1059.

Noyes, R., Jr, Crowe, R. R., Harris, E. L. *et al.* (1986). Relationship between panic disorder and agoraphobia: a family study. *Arch. Gen. Psychiatry*, **43**, 227–232.

Noyes, R., Jr, Clarkson, C., Crowe, R. R. *et al.* (1987). A family study of generalized anxiety disorder. *Am. J. Psychiatry*, **144**, 1019–1024.

Noyes, R., Jr, Woodman, C., Garvey, M. J. *et al.* (1992). Generalized anxiety disorder vs. panic disorder: distinguishing characteristics and patterns of comorbidity. *J. Nerv. Ment. Dis.*, **180**, 369–379.

Oppenheimer, B. S. and Rothschild, M. A. (1918). The psychoneurotic factor in the irritable heart of soldiers, *JAMA*, **70**, 1919–1922.

Pauls, D. L., Noyes, R., Jr and Crowe, R. R. (1979). The familial prevalence in second-degree relatives of patients with anxiety neurosis (panic disorder). *J. Affect. Disord.*, **1**, 279–285.

Phillips, K., Fulker, D. W. and Rose, R. J. (1987). Path analysis of seven fear factors in adult twin and sibling pairs and their parents. *Genet. Epidemiol.*, **4**, 345–355.

Pitts, F. N., Jr and McClure, J. N., Jr (1967). Lactate metabolism in anxiety neurosis. *N. Engl. J. Med.*, **277**, 1329–1336.

Quitkin, F. M., Rifkin, A., Kaplan, J and Klein, D. F. (1972). Phobic anxiety syndrome complicated by drug dependence and addiction: a treatable form of drug abuse, *Arch. Gen. Psychiatry*, **27**, 159–162.

Rasmussen, S. A. and Tsuang, M. T. (1986). Clinical characteristics and family history in DSM-III obsessive-compulsive disorder, *Am. J. Psychiatry*, **143**, 317–322.

Robins, L. N. and Regier, D. A. (1991). *Psychiatric Disorders in America: The*

Epidemiologic Catchment Area Study. Free Press, New York.

Robins, L. N., Helzer, J. E., Weissman, M. *et al.*, (1984). Lifetime prevalence of specific psychiatric disorders in three sites. *Arch. Gen. Psychiatry*, **41**, 949–958.

Rose, R. J. and Ditto, W. B. (1983). A developmental-genetic analysis of common fears from early adolescence to early adulthood, *Child Dev.*, **54**, 361–368.

Schmidt, S. M., Zoëga, T. and Crowe, R. R. (1993). Excluding linkage between panic disorder and the gamma-aminobutyric acid beta 1 receptor locus in five Icelandic pedigrees. *Acta Psychiatr. Scand.*, **88**, 225–228.

Skerritt, P. W. (1983). Anxiety and the heart: a historical review. *Psychol. Med.*, **13**, 17–25.

Skre, I., Onstad, S. I., Torgersen, S. *et al.* (1993). A twin study of DSM-III-R anxiety disorders. *Acta Psychiatr. Scand.*, **88**, 85–92.

Slater, E. and Shields, J. (1969). Genetical aspects of anxiety. In *Studies of Anxiety* (ed. M. H. Lader), pp. 62–71. British Journal of Psychiatry Special Publication, No. 3, Headley Ashford, UK.

Torgersen, S. (1983a). Genetic factors in anxiety disorders. *Arch. Gen. Psychiatry*, **40**, 1085–1089.

Torgersen, S. (1983b). Genetics of neurosis: the effects of sampling variation upon the twin concordance ratio. *Br. J. Psychiatry*, **142**, 126–132.

Torgersen, S. (1985). Hereditary differentiation of anxiety and affective neuroses. *Br. J. Psychiatry*, **146**, 530–534.

Torgersen, S. (1986). Anxiety neuroses and DSM-III. *Acta Psychiatr. Scand.*, **73** (Suppl. 328), 54–56.

von Korff, M. R., Eaton, W. W. and Keyl, P. M. (1985). The epidemiology of panic attacks and panic disorder. *Am. J. Epidemiol.*, **122**, 970–981.

Wang, Z. W., Crowe, R. R. and Noyes, R., Jr (1992). Adrenergic receptor genes as candidate genes for panic disorder: a linkage study. *Am. J. Psychiatry*, **149**, 470–474.

Wooley, C. F. (1976). Where are the diseases of yesteryear: Da Costa's syndrome, soldiers heart, the effort syndrome, neurocirculatory asthenia and the mitral valve prolapse syndrome (Editorial). *Circulation*, **53**, 749–751.

Young, J. P. R., Fenton, G. W. and Lader, M. H. (1971). The inheritance of neurotic traits: a twin study of the Middlesex Hospital Questionnaire. *Br. J. Psychiatry*, **119**, 393–398 (1971).

Zal, M. (1988). From anxiety to panic disorder: a historical perspective, *Contemp. Psychiatry*, **18**, 367–371.

4 New Developments in Animal Tests of Anxiety

SANDRA E. FILE, NICK ANDREWS AND SANDY HOGG

Psychopharmacology Research Unit, Guy's Hospital, London, UK

INTRODUCTION

Animal tests of anxiety are used both to screen new compounds for potential anxiolytic action and to study the neural substrates of anxiety. Contact with the clinical literature is vital with regard to the efficacy of new products and to the issues of diagnostic classification. Unfortunately, there is an inevitably long delay between testing a new compound in animal tests and finally having clear evidence as to its clinical efficacy. Clinical data are now available for some of the 5-HT$_{1A}$ receptor agonists, but it is too soon to judge the clinical efficacy of the other potential anxiolytic compounds reviewed in this chapter. The recent changes in the diagnostic classification of anxiety disorders are beginning to be reflected in our thinking about animal tests. The DSM-III-R classification recognizes several separate anxiety disorders: generalized anxiety disorder; panic disorder (with or without agoraphobia); simple phobias; obsessive-compulsive disorder; social phobia; post-traumatic stress disorder. These distinctions are reflected in the organization of the sections in this book. The clinical acceptance of the heterogeneity of anxiety disorders suggests that there are distinct neurobiological substrates for each and it is therefore necessary to examine whether different animal tests might reflect these differences.

There is already evidence that distinctions exist among animal tests of anxiety. For example, factor analysis studies have shown that there is no single factor which is measured by the social interaction, elevated plus-maze and punished drinking tests of anxiety (File, 1991). We also have recent evidence that exposure to different tests of anxiety results in different patterns of neurotransmitter release (File *et al.*, 1992, 1993a). With these sorts of approaches we hope that we will eventually be able to use behavioral and/or genetic manipulations to induce in animals neurobiological states that closely parallel those occurring in the anxiety disorders.

Matching particular tests of anxiety to particular anxiety disorders is an extremely difficult task. However, psychiatrists base their diagnosis of anxiety

Advances in the Neurobiology of Anxiety Disorders. Edited by H. G. M. Westenberg, J. A. Den Boer and D. L. Murphy
©1996 John Wiley & Sons Ltd

disorders at least partly on non-verbal behavioral and physiological responses (restlessness, avoidant behaviors, body posture, tremor, sweating); behavioral pharmacologists make similar inferences from animal behavior. The success of these inferences will depend on the careful selection and interpretation of the animal tests, based on a detailed ethological knowledge of the species selected for use. There has been a recent explosion in the number of new tests proposed as tests of anxiety and the importance of validating each new test cannot be stressed too highly. However, it is lamentable that even among the well-established and widely used tests only two (the social interaction test (File and Hyde, 1978; File, 1980) and the elevated plus-maze (Pellow *et al.*, 1985)) have been extensively validated using behavioral, physiological and pharmacological measures.

Even when this is achieved, can the animal's response ever be abnormal in the sense that pathological anxiety states appear to be? At the present moment the answer has to be "no," but it is possible that future behavioral genetic research will approach the question of *trait* anxiety in animals. Strains of rat have been selectively bred to show a high or low response of defecation to the stress of being placed in a large, brightly lit arena (Broadhurst, 1975), or to show high or low activity levels in response to electric shock (Bignami, 1965). These strains are not considered to reflect high or low "anxiety" levels, but the same method of selective breeding could be applied to the behavioral responses in selected animal tests of anxiety. For the present we are restricted to studying an animal's response to conditions that are selected to generate an internal state akin to the human *state* anxiety. This chapter will review the tests that might best reflect generalized anxiety disorder and simple phobias. Other chapters in this book review animal tests of panic disorder and obsessive-compulsive disorder.

GENERALIZED ANXIETY DISORDER

From the mid-1940s until the mid-1970s animal tests of anxiety consisted of delivering electric shock as a punishment, most often for an operant lever-press response. These tests were developed as screening tests for the pharmaceutical industry and their usefulness has recently been reviewed (Howard and Pollard, 1991). They were successful at detecting and discriminating amongst drugs acting at the γ-aminobutyric acid (GABA)–benzodiazepine receptor complex, but failed to detect clear anxiolytic activity of newer compounds. These tests have received extensive study with regard to the experimental parameters necessary to produce reliable responding, but the question of whether they best reflect generalized anxiety or one of the other anxiety disorders has never been explicitly addressed. Indeed, since they are based on the punishment of a specific response in a specific situation it is more likely that these tests generate a state of conditioned fear, rather than anxiety. The same point can be made with respect to the potentiated startle test and Davis (1991) explicitly discusses similarities and differences between conditioned fear and anxiety.

Crawley (1981) developed a test in which the number of transitions made by mice between a light and a dark compartment is used as a measure of anxiety.

The mice are faced in this test with a conflict between the desire to explore a novel area and their aversion to bright light. An increase in transitions, without an increase in general locomotor activity, is taken to indicate anxiolytic activity. Interestingly, only certain strains of mouse (those with a high baseline rate of transition) show this effect, thus raising the possibility of exploring differences in trait anxiety (Crawley and Davis, 1982). There have been several recent modifications to this test, involving the relative sizes of the light and dark compartments and the behavioral measures used; the potential importance of these parametric changes has not yet been assessed. Costall defined an anxiolytic action as an increase in rearing and locomotor activity in the light compartment and/or a decrease in these behaviors in the dark compartment (Costall *et al.*, 1987). They also use an increase in the percentage of time in the light area and/or an increase in the latency to go from the light to the dark area (Barnes *et al.*, 1992a). This definition was based on the effects seen with the benzodiazepines, but this does not necessarily mean that the effect represents an anxiolytic action. Several of the new anxiolytic candidates have been assessed in this test and the results will be reviewed in a later section.

The social interaction test of anxiety exploits the uncertainty and anxiety generated by placing rats in an unfamiliar or brightly lit environment. The dependent variable is the time that pairs of male rats spend in active social interaction (mostly social investigation) and both the familiarity and the light level of the test arena are manipulated. Undrugged rats show the highest level of social interaction when the test arena is familiar and is lit by low light. Less time is spent in social interaction if the arena is unfamiliar to the rats or is brightly lit; anxiolytic drugs prevent this decline. The overall level of motor activity is also measured so that the specificity of changes in social behavior can be assessed. The test probably best reflects generalized anxiety disorder, since the behavior is controlled by manipulating the features of the test arena to generate uncertainty. Social interaction is simply the dependent variable. The test is not one of social phobia, since novel partners generate more interaction than do familiar ones. This is one of the few animal tests of anxiety that has been validated behaviorally and physiologically, as well as pharmacologically (File and Hyde, 1978; File, 1980, 1988). In order to validate the test behaviorally, measures indicative of anxiety and stress such as defecation, self-grooming and displacement activities were associated with the reductions in social interaction; and other causes of response change (e.g. exploration of the environment, odor changes) were excluded. In order to validate the test physiologically, changes in adrenocorticotropic hormone (ACTH), corticosterone and hypothalamic norepinephrine were measured. Attempts to develop a similar test of social interaction in mice have not proved successful, mainly because of the predominance of aggressive attacks in mice, but also because mice failed to respond to manipulations of the familiarity of the test arena. It also seems that the test may not be valid for female rats, which respond less than male rats to changes in familiarity of the test arena (Johnston and File, 1991). This test was developed and validated with males and it is not too surprising that the function of social investigation is different in males and females.

The elevated plus-maze uses conflict between exploration and aversion to elevated open places. In this test, the anxiety is generated by placing the animal on an elevated open arm; here it is the height and openness of the arms, rather than the light level, that is crucial for generating behavioral and physiological changes. The apparatus is in the shape of a plus sign with two open arms and two arms enclosed by high walls. The rat has free access to all arms and anxiolytics increase the percentage of time that the animals spend on the open arms and the percentage of all entries made into the open arms. This test has been validated behaviorally and physiologically in the rat (Pellow et al., 1985) and has also proved applicable to mice (Lister, 1987), suggesting that aversion to elevated, open places is a feature of both species. The relative importance of height versus the open aspects of the arms remains controversial (Treit et al., 1993). A detailed ethological analysis of the various behaviors in this test has recently been conducted (Rodgers and Cole, 1993). The elevated plus-maze has proved sensitive to a wide range of anxiolytic and anxiogenic treatments and thus seems to have good predictive value for drugs that are effective in generalized anxiety disorder. The effects of putative novel anxiolytics in this test will be reviewed later in this chapter. However, as will be discussed below, when animals are tested more than once in this test, the nature of the anxiety state is changed. It has been suggested that by trial 2 this test may be generating a state more akin to phobic anxiety (Rodgers et al., 1992; File and Zangrossi, 1993; File et al., 1993b). This possibility will be discussed in detail below.

SIMPLE PHOBIAS

It is fairly easy to produce conditioned fear in rodents. Typically, a previously neutral stimulus is paired with an electric shock. Subsequent presentations of the stimulus disrupt ongoing behavior and produce avoidance or defence (Davis, 1991). A more ethological version of conditioned fear has been developed by Treit (1985), in which an electrified probe is placed in the rat's home cage and the species-specific response to this is to bury the probe. Unfortunately these tests cannot provide animal models of simple phobias, because phobias differ from conditioned fears in that the phobias do not extinguish, do not respond to symbolic intervention and respond poorly to anxiolytic drug treatment (Klein, 1981). Simple phobias are defined as persistent and recognizably irrational fears of a circumscribed object or situation; the phobic response includes significant distress and a compelling desire to avoid the object/situation (Weiss and Uhde, 1990). Patients with generalized anxiety disorder do not necessarily develop phobic avoidances (Klein, 1981) or experience spontaneous panic attacks, although a situational specific panic can sometimes occur (Zitrin et al., 1981).

The set of phobic stimuli is limited and non-arbitrary, the phobic object can easily be identified and phobias are often acquired as a result of an identifiable frightening experience. In humans, phobias of animals have the earliest age of onset and a heritability of phobia liability of about 30% (Kendler *et al.*, 1992). Experience specific to the individual plays an important role in the determination of the phobic object. In animals, some phobias are very easily and rapidly acquired, e.g. phobic responses to sudden loud noises in dogs (Hothersall and Tuber, 1979); others are innate, e.g. fear of snakes in monkeys (Mineka, 1985). One particular animal model that may prove especially relevant to innately based phobias is described below.

Blanchard's group (Blanchard *et al.*, 1990) has studied the behavior of wild and laboratory rats in burrows in the presence of a natural predator (a cat) and after its removal. They distinguish between defensive behaviors that are fear-related, i.e. exhibited during the presence of the cat, and those that are anxiety-related, i.e. are manifest after exposure to the cat and reflect risk assessment. In an extension of this idea, Zangrossi and File (1992a) have shown that as well as detecting behavioral avoidance responses in laboratory rats *during* exposure to cat odor it is also possible to detect resulting anxiogenic effects in the social interaction and elevated plus-maze tests, even when these are carried out 1 h later in a room never associated with cat odor. It is therefore possible that this model can be used both to study innately based phobic responses and to study the subsequent generalization of anxiety to other situations. Interestingly, whilst chlordiazepoxide was effective at reducing the generalized anxiety responses, even at high doses it was ineffective against the direct phobic avoidance (Zangrossi and File, 1992b). Exposure to cat odor also led to an elevation in plasma corticosterone concentrations (File *et al.*, 1993c) and although this corticosterone response habituated after five successive exposures, the behavioral avoidance did not (File *et al.*, 1993c). Further studies revealed a bimodal distribution of responders and non-responders to cat odor, with the responders showing behavioral, neurochemical and corticosterone responses. Such a striking difference in responses could form the basis of future selective breeding and genetic studies. Interestingly, when the rats with a marked avoidance response to the first cat odor exposure were given a long (60 min) exposure to the odor they then showed a generalization of avoidance to the test situation (Zangrossi and File, 1994).

Our laboratory rats have never been exposed to a cat and therefore their response to cat odor is innate. Other phobic responses can be acquired and a series of recent experiments with the elevated plus-maze suggests that this may be a situation in which the rat readily acquires a phobic response. Thus, whereas exposure to the plus-maze for the first time might generate a state similar to that in generalized anxiety, it has become clear that trial 2 evokes a different neurochemical state (File *et al.*, 1992). Rather than showing habituation of their corticosterone response to the plus-maze, rats given a second trial maintain a high response (File *et al.*, 1993d). Furthermore, in contrast to their efficacy on trial 1, benzodiazepines have little effect on trial 2, although the scores of the control animals show little change (Lister, 1987; File, 1990). A factor analysis showed that the scores on trial 1 reflected a different factor than did those from trial 2. The change in response is not dependent on the drug state on trial 1, or on the intertrial interval, and generalizes across mazes of different materials; it is dependent on experience of the open arms (File *et al.*, 1990). It is therefore possible that during the first 5 min exposure to the elevated plus-maze the rat rapidly acquires a fear of heights and/or open space and that on the next trial its behavior reflects phobic, rather than generalized, anxiety. Even if this particular suggestion proves wrong it is important to note that experience of the plus-maze undoubtedly changes the nature of the state that it evokes.

DRUG EFFECTS IN THE BLACK–WHITE CROSSING TEST

It can be seen from Table 1 that the black–white crossing test is extremely reliable in detecting positive effects of the 5-HT_3 receptor antagonists across a wide dose range. Although positive effects of cholecystokinin (CCK) antagonists have been reported, they all come from a single study and it will be important to see if this same pattern is maintained across laboratories and different CCK antagonists. This test has also detected positive effects of 5-HT_{1A} agonists, including those at doses which appear to be anxiogenic in the elevated plus-maze.

DRUG EFFECTS IN THE SOCIAL INTERACTION TEST

Table 2 shows that social interaction test is sensitive to the effects of 5-HT_{1A} receptor agonists, but the effects are not as strong or as reliable as those of the benzodiazepines. One of the problems is that although rats treated with buspirone showed less decrease in social interaction in response to high light or unfamiliarity (indicating an anxiolytic effect), their scores were all depressed compared with the control group; the same pattern was found for low doses of neuroleptics (File, 1984). The test provides much more variable results with the 5-HT_3 receptor antagonists and often it is only one or two doses of a wide range that give positive results.

DRUG EFFECTS IN THE ELEVATED PLUS-MAZE

Table 3 shows that there is extensive agreement that the 5-HT_{1A} receptor agonists have *anxiogenic* effects in this test. The only reports of anxiolytic activity come from the study by Dunn *et al.* (1989). This is particularly puzzling since the doses Dunn *et al.* report as being anxiolytic are the same as those reported by other groups as being anxiogenic. The elevated plus-maze has detected anxiolytic activity of the 5-HT_3 receptor antagonists, the reported inactivity coming mainly from studies by File's group.

5-HT$_{1A}$ RECEPTOR AGONISTS

The animal tests described above have been able to detect positive effects of the 5-HT$_{1A}$ receptor agonists, but the effects are neither strong nor robust. At higher doses anxiogenic effects are found and the detection of these has been more reliable and have been seen best in the plus-maze. Conflict tests have in general been insensitive to the effects of 5-HT$_{1A}$ receptor agonists, except in pigeons. The reason for this species difference is unknown, but may relate to differences in postsynaptic receptors, or in the metabolism of the compounds.

However, there is one test that reliably detects an effect of this class of drug. The learned helplessness test has traditionally been considered as an animal test of depression, since it is sensitive to the actions of antidepressant drugs. Following exposure to an uncontrollable shock of high intensity there is a marked disturbance of avoidance behavior, which is ameliorated by antidepressant drugs. Anxiolytics are also effective, if given prior to the inescapable shock, whereas antidepressants are effective if given after the shock. The 5-HT$_{1A}$ receptor agonists are effective in the same way as antidepressant drugs (Thiebot and Martin, 1991). It is therefore possible that this experimental situation provides a test that is sensitive to the anxiolytic action of antidepressants, or to drugs that are effective in anxious depression.

Thus, from their profile in animal tests, this class of drug would be considered as antidepressant with anxiolytic properties. The clinical results are in agreement with this. Although buspirone was marketed as an anxiolytic, it is clear that its profile is similar to that of an antidepressant. Its anxiolytic actions are weaker than those of the benzodiazepines, its onset of efficacy shows a delay of two to three weeks and it has antidepressant actions (Deakin, 1993).

5-HT$_3$ RECEPTOR ANTAGONISTS

These compounds are reliably detected in the black–white crossing test, over wide dose ranges. They are less well detected by the social interaction and elevated plus-maze tests, although anxiolytic effects of limited doses have been reported. The important question is whether this class of drug has any significant anxiolytic effects in patients. So far there have been no significant effects reported. The only published study found ondansetron to be no different from placebo (Lader, 1991). Since many years have passed since these compounds were reported to have anxiolytic effects in animal tests it would seem more and more unlikely that they will prove to be powerful anxiolytic agents in the clinic. This then raises the important question of what action the black–white crossing test is so reliably detecting.

CHOLECYSTOKININ ANTAGONISTS

Because CCK precipitates panic attacks in patients with panic disorder, the main

Table 1. Summary of studies investigating the effects of putative anxiolytics on behavior in the mouse black–white crossing test. All doses are expressed per kilogram body weight. Doses with a significant anxiolytic effect (+) are shown in **bold**, no effect at any dose is shown by 0, doses with a significant anxiogenic effect (−) are shown in ***bold italics***

Class of drug	Drug	Dose	Route	Effect	Reference
5-HT$_{1A}$ agonist	Buspirone	0.06, 0.125 mg	i.p.	+	Costall *et al.* (1988a)
		0.25–2 mg	i.p.	+	Kilfoil *et al.* (1989)
		0.1–10.0 mg	s.c.	+	Onaivi and Martin (1989)
		1.0–5.0 mg			
	Umespirone	10 ng; **0.1 µg–10 mg**	i.p.	+	Barnes *et al.* (1991)
		0.125 mg; **0.25–1 mg**	i.p.	+	Costall *et al.* (1992)
	E 4424	**0.1 µg–0.5 mg**	i.p.	+	Costall *et al.* (1992)
	Ipsapirone	0.5; **1, 5 mg**	i.p.	+	Costall *et al.* (1992)
5-HT$_3$ antagonist	(*S*)-RS-42358	0.01 ng; **0.1 ng–10 mg**	p.o.	+	Costall *et al.* (1993)
	DAU 6215	0.01–1 mg	i.p.	+	Borsini *et al.* (1993)
	WAY 100289	1–10 µg, **0.1, 1 and 10 mg**	p.o.	+	Bill *et al.* (1992)
		10, **100 µg**, 1, 10 mg	s.c.	+	Bill *et al.* (1992)
	ICS 205-930	1,10 ng; **100 ng–0.3 mg**	i.p.	+	Kilfoil *et al.* (1989)
		0.001–1.0 mg	i.p.	+	Onaivi and Martin (1989)
		10 ng–1 µg	i.p.	+	Costall *et al.* (1989)
		1, 10, 100 µg and 1 mg	s.c.	+	Bill *et al.* (1992)
	Ondansetron	0.01; **0.05–10 µg**	i.p.	+	Jones *et al.* (1988)
		0.1, 1, 10, 100 µg and 1 mg	s.c.	+	Bill *et al.* (1992)
	Zacopride	**0.0001–10 mg**	i.p.	+	Costall *et al.* (1988b)
		0.1 and 1 µg; **10 µg and 1 mg**	s.c.	+	Bill *et al.* (1992)
	(*R*)-Zacopride	1 ng; **10 ng–10 mg**	i.p.	+	Young and Johnson (1991)
		1 ng; **10 ng–10 mg**	p.o.	+	Young and Johnson (1991)
		1 ng; **10 ng–10 mg**	i.p.	+	Barnes *et al.* (1992a)
	(*S*)-Zacopride	1 ng–1 µg; **10 µg–1 mg**	i.p.	+	Young and Johnson (1991)
		1 ng–10 µg; **100 µg–1 mg**	p.o.	+	Young and Johnson (1991)
		1 ng–10 mg	i.p.	0	Barnes *et al.* (1992a)

	Dose	Route	Effect	Reference
Granisetron	10 ng; **1 µg–1 mg**	i.p.	+	Barnes et al. (1992b)
CCK antagonist				
MDL 72222	0.001–1.0 mg	i.p.	+	Onaivi and Martin (1989)
PD 134308	0.01 µg; **0.1 µg–30 mg**	s.c.	+	Hughes et al. (1990)
	0.01 µg; **0.1µg–10 mg**	p.o.	+	Hughes et al. (1990)
PD 13158	0.01 µg; **0.1 µg–30 mg**	s.c.	+	Hughes et al. (1990)
Others				
Idazoxan	0.5–4 mg; *8–16 mg*	i.p.	–	Venault et al. (1993)
Sulpiride	5–40 mg	i.p.	–	Simon et al. (1992)
Anpirtoline	**1 ng–1 mg**	i.p.	+	Metzenauer et al. (1992)
Dup 753	1–10; **0.1–1000 µg**	p.o.	+	Barnes et al. (1990)
Captopril	0.1; **1–50 mg**	i.p.	+	Costall et al. (1990)
Ceranapril	0.1 and 1 µg; **0.01–10 mg**	i.p.	+	Costall et al. (1990)
Ritanserin	0.05–10 mg	i.p.	0	Costall et al. (1988a)
Metergoline	0.05–10 mg	i.p.	0	Costall et al. (1988a)
Methysergide	0.05–10 mg	i.p.	0	Costall et al. (1988a)

Table 2. Summary of studies investigating the effects of putative anxiolytics on behavior in the rat social interaction test. All doses are expressed per kilogram body weight. Doses with a significant anxiolytic effect (+) are shown in **bold**, no effect at any dose is shown by 0, doses with a significant anxiogenic effect (−) are shown in ***bold italics***

Class of drug	Drug	Dose	Route	Effect	Reference
5-HT$_{1A}$ agonist	Buspirone	0.25–2.5 mg	i.p.	0	File (1984)
		5.0–20.0 mg	p.o.	+	Guy and Gardner (1985)
	8-OH-DPAT	**0.125–0.25 mg**	i.p.	+	Dunn et al. (1989)
	E4424	0.1; **1–500 µg**	i.p.	+	Costall et al. (1992)
	Ipsapirone	0.5; **1, 5 mg**	i.p.	+	Costall et al. (1992)
5-HT$_3$ antagonist	Ondansetron	***0.001–1.0 mg***	p.o.	+	Jones et al. (1988)
		0.01, 0.1, 1.0 mg	p.o.	0	Johnston and File (1988c)
		0.1, 1.0, 10 mg	p.o.	+	Piper et al. (1988)
		0.1, 1.0 mg	p.o.	0	File and Johnston (1989)
		0.1, 1 µg; **0.01, 0.1 mg**	s.c.	+	Blackburn et al. (1993)
	BRL 46470A	0.01 µg; **0.1 µg–0.1 mg**	s.c and p.o.	+	Blackburn et al. (1993)
	Granisetron	**0.1 and 1.0 mg**	p.o.	+	Piper et al. (1988)
		0.01 and 0.1; **1.0 mg**	p.o.	+	Johnston and File (1988c)
		0.1, 1.0 mg	p.o.	0	File and Johnston (1989)
	ICS205–930	0.01–1.0 µg	p.o.	+	Tyers et al. (1987)
		0.01, **0.1**, 1.0 mg	p.o.	+	Johnston and File (1988c)
	MDL72222	**1.0–100 µg**	p.o.	+	Tyers et al. (1987)
	Zacopride	0.01, 0.1, 1.0 mg	i.p.	0	File and Johnston (1989)
	(S)-RS 42358	0.01 ng; **0.1 ng–1 mg**	i.p.	+	Costall et al. (1993)
CCK antagonist	PD 134308	0.01 µg; **1µg–1 mg**	s.c.	+	Hughes et al. (1990)
Other	Captopril	**1 and 50 mg**	i.p.	+	Costall et al. (1990)
	Ceranapril	**0.01** and 10 mg	i.p.	+	Costall et al. (1990)
	MK-801	**0.05**; 10 mg	i.p.	+	Dunn et al. (1989)
	R-(+)-HA966	**5 and 10 mg**	i.p.	+	Dunn et al. (1992)
	F 2692	**3, 10 and 30 mg**	i.p.	+	File and Andrews (1994)

Table 3. Summary of studies investigating the effects of putative anxiolytics on behavior in the elevated plus-maze. All doses are expressed per kilogram body weight. Doses with a significant anxiolytic effect (+) are shown in **bold**, no effect at any dose is shown by 0, doses with a significant anxiogenic effect (−) are shown in ***bold italics***

Class of drug	Drug	Dose	Route	Effect	Reference
5-HT$_{1A}$ agonist	Buspirone	*0.5 mg*	s.c.	−	Pellow and File (1986)
		0.5, 1 and 2; *4 and 8 mg*	s.c.	−	Pellow et al. (1987)
		0.5; **1 mg**	i.p.	+	Dunn et al. (1989)
		1 mg	s.c.	−	Moser (1989)
		0.15–0.5; *1 and 2 mg*	s.c.	−	Moser et al. (1990)
		1 mg	s.c.	−	Klint (1991)
		0.1–0.4; *0.8 mg*	s.c.	−	File and Andrews (1991)
		2.5, 5, 10 and 20 mg	s.c.	0	Wada and Fukuda (1991)
		0.1; *0.2 mg*	s.c.	−	Andrews and File (1993)
	Gepirone	**1 mg**	i.p.	+	Dunn et al. (1989)
		1; *3, 5.6 and 10 mg*	i.p.	−	Motta et al. (1992)
	Ipsapirone	10 mg	s.c.	−	Moser (1989)
		1.25; *2.5 mg*	s.c.	−	Pellow et al. (1987)
	8-OH DPAT	*0.0125–0.5 mg*	i.p.	−	Critchley and Handley (1987)
		0.0625 and 0.125 mg	s.c.	0	Pellow et al. (1987)
		0.1; **0.2 mg**	i.p.	+	Dunn et al. (1989)
		0.0125–0.1; *0.2 mg*	s.c.	−	Moser et al. (1990)
		0.1 and 1 mg	s.c.	−	Klint (1991)
5-HT$_3$ antagonist	Ondansetron	0.025; **0.05 and 0.1 mg**	i.p.	+	Dunn et al. (1991)
	Zacopride	0.01, 0.1 and 1 mg	p.o.	0	Johnston and File (1988c)
		0.01, 0.1 and 1 mg	p.o.	0	Johnston and File (1988c)
		0.03; **0.1 and 0.3 mg**	i.p.	+	Dunn et al. (1991)
	(R)-Zacopride	0.001, 0.1 and 1 mg	i.p.	0	File and Andrews (1993)
	(S)-Zacopride	0.001, 0.1 and 1 mg	i.p.	0	File and Andrews (1993)
	BRL 46470A	0.1 and 1; **10 and 100 µg**	p.o.	+	Blackburn et al. (1993)
	(S)-RS 42358	**0.01 and 100 ng**	i.p.	+	Costall et al. (1993)

Table 3 (*continued*)

Class of drug	Drug	Dose	Route	Effect	Reference
	ICS 205930	0.01, 0.1 and 1 mg	p.o.	0	Johnston and File (1988c)
	MDL 2222	0.125; **0.25 and 0.5 mg**	i.p.	+	Dunn *et al.* (1991)
		5; **10 mg**	i.p.	+	Dunn *et al.* (1991)
CCK antagonist	PD 134308	**0.01 and 1 mg**	s.c.	+	Hughes *et al.* (1990)
Others	MK 801	0.05; **0.1 mg**	i.p.	+	Dunn *et al.* (1989)
	R-(+)-HA966	**5 and 10 mg**	i.p.	+	Dunn *et al.* (1992)
	F 2692	0.3 and 1; **3–100 mg**	i.p.	+	Assié *et al.* (1993)

interest in developing CCK antagonists has turned to the possible treatment of panic disorder. The relevance of testing these compounds in tests of generalized anxiety might therefore be questioned. Recent psychiatric research has focused on whether generalized anxiety disorder should be distinguished from panic disorder. One of the main reasons to support this distinction was the claim that, whereas benzodiazepines were effective in the former disorder, they were ineffective against panic attacks, and these were best treated with antidepressants (Klein, 1981). These views have been challenged because of the clinical overlap between generalized anxiety, panic disorder and depression and because high doses of benzodiazepines, in particular alprazolam, *have* now been shown to be effective against panic attacks (Ballenger *et al.*, 1988). An alternative view is therefore that panic disorder is just an extreme form of anxiety.

If panic disorder is to be regarded simply as a severe form of generalized anxiety, then the animal tests that have proved sensitive to anxiogenic agents should also be sensitive to propanic agents. Apart from the effects of yohimbine, which may cause generalized anxiety rather than panic, we found little effect of panic-inducing agents in the social interaction or elevated plus-maze tests (Johnston and File, 1988a). Since these tests do not elicit any behaviors similar to those seen in panic disorder, the logic of using them as a screen for potential antipanic compounds is not clear. The black–white crossing, social interaction and plus-maze tests have all detected anxiolytic effects of CCK antagonists, but there has been insufficient work to establish how strong and reliable such results are. However, since the clinically used antipanic compounds also have anxiolytic effects in generalized anxiety, it may be these latter aspects that are being detected.

Alprazolam, a triazolobenzodiazepine, is an effective antipanic agent and the elevated plus-maze is more sensitive to triazolobenzodiazepines than is the social interaction test (Johnston and File, 1988b). The efficacy of antidepressants in preventing panic attacks has not been questioned, and these compounds have positive effects in the learned helplessness test; but animal tests of anxiety have not generally detected their anxiolytic activity. However, weak anxiolytic effects of the monoamine oxidase inhibitor, phenelzine, have been detected in the plus-maze (Johnston and File, 1988b). Clonidine has been used to treat panic attacks, but has no anxiolytic action in the social interaction test or in the plus-maze. The general insensitivity of these animal tests to pro- and antipanic compounds does suggest that the mechanism of actions of these drugs differs from those of the benzodiazepines and other drugs acting at the GABA–benzodiazepine receptor complex. It would therefore seem to be more appropriate to test the effects of CCK antagonists in animal tests more likely to reflect panic disorder, such as stimulation of the dorsal periaqueductal gray (Graeff, 1991). However, all animal tests of panic disorder will suffer from the limitation that they are unlikely to include the catastrophic interpretation of bodily sensations that is often seen as crucial in panic disorder (Clark, 1988).

CONCLUSIONS

With the growing body of pharmacological data available for putative animal tests of generalized anxiety disorder these tests will gain further pharmacological validation as soon as the clinical evidence for some of the new compounds becomes more widespread. Validation of putative tests of simple phobias will be harder, at least with regard to pharmacological studies, since drug treatment of simple phobias is not well established. One of the aspects that has been neglected in all of the available animal tests is the important one of sex differences.

There is a higher incidence of anxiety disorders in women than in men and it is therefore pertinent to ask whether there are sex differences in animal tests of anxiety. The sex differences in the level of ambulation and rearing (higher levels shown by female rats) were taken to indicate that female rats were less anxious than male rats (Gray, 1971). However, this interpretation was severely criticized because other physiological differences, such as body weight, could have explained the differences and ambulation in the open field is influenced by several factors other than anxiety (e.g. exploration and locomotor activity level). In an attempt to determine whether there were any general sex differences in animal tests of anxiety, Johnston and File (1991) tested male and female rats of equal weight in three different tests (social interaction; elevated plus-maze; punished drinking), but no systematic sex differences emerged. Female rats had scores in the plus-maze indicating lower anxiety, and in another study they were found to have a lower anxiogenic response in the plus-maze after exposure to inescapable shock (Steenbergen *et al.*, 1990); both these results could have been partly influenced by overall differences in level of activity. A major concern also emerged as to whether the social interaction test was valid for female rats. Certainly more research using female rats would seem to be warranted, including the exploration of possible sex differences in tests of simple phobias.

With age, humans become more sensitive to the sedative effects of the benzodiazepines and similar findings have been reported in the rat (Komiskey *et al.*, 1987; File, 1990). However, interestingly, old rats were *less* sensitive to the anxiolytic effects of benzodiazepines in a punished lever-pressing test (Komiskey *et al.*, 1987) and in the elevated plus-maze test of anxiety (File, 1990). It is difficult to see how a pharmacokinetic explanation could account for the simultaneously observed increased sensitivity to the sedative effects and decreased sensitivity to the anxiolytic effects. As well as observing an age-related change in benzodiazepine sensitivity, File (1990) found that old rats had scores in the plus-maze indicative of increased anxiety. If an age-related increase in need for anxiolytic medication, but a reduced therapeutic window of response to benzodiazepines, also exists clinically, then the elderly would seem a group most likely to benefit from the newer non-sedative anxiolytics. Again, it would be useful to explore possible age-related changes in the other tests of anxiety.

REFERENCES

Andrews, N. and File, S. E. (1993). Handling history of rats modifies behavioural effects of drugs in the elevated plus-maze test of anxiety. *Eur. J. Pharmacol.*, **235**, 109–112.

Assié, M. B., Chopin, P., Stenger, A. *et al.* (1993). Neuropharmacology of a new potential anxiolytic compound F 2692, 1-(3'-trifluoro-methylphenyl)1, 4-dihydro 3-amino 4-oxo 6-methyl pyridazine. 1. Acute and in-vitro effects. *Psychopharmacology*, **110**, 13–18.

Ballenger, J. C., Burrows, G. D., DuPont, R. L. *et al.* (1988). Alprazolam in panic disorder and agoraphobia: results from a multicenter trial. I: Efficacy in short-term treatment. *Arch. Gen. Psychiatry*, **45**, 413–422.

Barnes, N. M., Costall, B., Kelly, M. E. *et al.* (1990). Anxiolytic-like action of DuP753, a non-peptide angiotensin II receptor antagonist. *Neuroreport*, **1**, 15–16.

Barnes, N. M., Costall, B., Domeney, A. M. *et al.* (1991). The effects of umespirone as a potential anxiolytic and antipsychotic agent. *Pharmacol. Biochem. Behav.*, **40**, 89–96.

Barnes, N. M., Costall, B., Ge, J. *et al.* (1992a). The interaction of R(+)-and (S)-zacopride with PCPA to modify rodent aversive behaviour. *Eur. J. Pharmacol.*, **218**, 15–26.

Barnes, N. M., Cheng, C. H. K., Costall, B. *et al.* (1992b). Profiles of interaction of R(+)-/S(–)-zacopride and anxiolytic agents in mouse model. *Eur. J. Pharmacol.*, **218**, 91–100.

Bignami, G. (1965). Selection for high rates and low rates of avoidance conditioning in the rat. *Anim. Behav.*, **13**, 221–227.

Bill, D. J., Fletcher, A., Glenn, B. D. and Knight, M. (1992). Behavioural studies on WAY 100289, a novel 5-HT$_3$ receptor antagonist, in two animal models of anxiety. *Eur. J. Pharmacol.*, **218**, 324–334.

Blackburn, T. P., Baxter, G. S., Kennett, G. A. *et al.* (1993). BRL 46470A: a highly potent, selective and long-acting 5-HT$_3$ receptor antagonist with anxiolytic-like properties. *Psychopharmacology*, **110**, 257–264.

Blanchard, R. J., Blanchard, D. C., Rodgers, R. J. and Weiss S. M. (1990). The characterization and modelling of antipredator defensive behavior. *Neurosci. Biobehav. Rev.*, **14**, 463–472.

Borsini, F., Brambilla, A., Cesana, R. and Donetti, A. (1993). The effect of DAU 6215, a novel 5-HT$_3$ antagonist, in animal models of anxiety. *Pharmacological Res.*, **27**, 151–164.

Broadhurst, P. L. (1975). The Maudsley reactive and non-reactive strains of rats: a survey. *Behav. Genet.*, **5**, 299–319.

Clark, D. M. (1988). A cognitive model of panic attacks. In *Panic, Psychological Perspectives* (eds S. Rachman and J. D. Maser), pp. 79–81. Erlbaum, Hillsdale, NJ.

Costall, B., Hendrie, C. A., Kelly, M. E. and Naylor, R. J. (1987). Actions of sulpiride and tiapride in a simple model of anxiety in mice. *Neuropharmacology*, **26**, 195–200.

Costall, B., Kelly, M. E., Naylor, R. J. and Onaivi, E. S. (1988a). Actions of buspirone in a putative model of anxiety in the mouse. *J. Pharm. Pharmacol.*, **40**, 494–500.

Costall, B., Domeney, A. M., Gerrard, P. A. *et al.* (1988b). Zacopride: anxiolytic profile in rodent and primate models of anxiety. *J. Pharm. Phamacol.*, **40**, 302–305.

Costall, B., Kelly, M. E., Naylor, R. J. *et al.* (1989). Neuroanatomical sites of action of 5-HT$_3$ receptor agonist and antagonists for alteration of aversive behaviour in the mouse. *Br. J. Pharmacol.*, **96**, 325–332.

Costall, B., Domeney, A. M., Gerrard, P. A. *et al.* (1990). Effects of captopril and SQ 29, 852 on anxiety-related behaviours in rodent and marmoset. *Pharmacol. Biochem. Behav.*, **36**, 13–20.

Costall, B., Domeney, A. M., Farre, A. J. *et al.* (1992). Profile of action of a novel 5-hydroxytryptamine 1A receptor ligand E-4424 to inhibit aversive behaviour in the mouse, rat and marmoset. *J. Pharmacol. Exp. Ther.*, **262**, 90–98.

Costall, B., Domeney, A. M., Kelly, M. E. *et al.* (1993). The effect of the 5-HT$_3$ receptor antagonist, RS-42358-197, in animal models of anxiety. *Eur. J. Pharmacol.*, **234**, 91–99.

Crawley, J. N. (1981). Neuropharmacological specificity of a simple animal model for the behavioral actions of benzodiazepines. *Pharmacol. Biochem. Behav.*, **15**, 695–699.

Crawley, J. N. and Davis, L. G. (1982). Baseline exploratory activity predicts anxiolytic responsiveness to diazepam in five mouse strains. *Brain Res. Bull.*, **8**, 609–612.

Critchley, M. A. E. and Handley, S. L. (1987). 5-HT$_{1A}$ ligand effects in the X-maze anxiety test. *Br. J. Pharmacol.*, **92**, 660P.

Davis, M. (1991). Animal models of anxiety based on classical conditioning: the conditioned emotional response and the fear-potentiated startle effect. In *Psychopharmacology of Anxiolytics and Antidepressants* (ed. S. E. File), pp. 187–212. Pergamon Press, New York.

Deakin, J. F. W. (1993). A review of clinical efficacy of 5-HT$_{1A}$ agonists in anxiety and depression. *J. Psychopharmacol.*, **7**, 283–290.

Dunn, R. W., Corbett, R. and Fielding, S. (1989). Effects of 5-HT$_{1A}$ receptor agonists and NMDA receptor antagonists in the social interaction test and the elevated plus-maze. *Eur. J. Pharmacol.*, **169**, 1–10.

Dunn, R. W., Carlezon, W. A. and Corbett, R. (1991). Preclinical anxiolytic versus antipsychotic profiles of the 5-HT$_3$ antagonists ondansetron, zacopride, 3α-tropanyl-1H-indole-3-carboxylic acid ester, and 1αH, 3α, 5αH-tropan-3-yl-3, 5-dichlorobenzoate. *Drug Dev. Res.*, **23**, 289–300.

Dunn, R. W., Flanagan, D. M., Martin, L. L. *et al.* (1992). Stereoselective R(+) enantiomer of HA-966 displays anxiolytic effects in rodents. *Eur. J. Pharmacol.*, **214**, 207–214.

File, S. E. (1980). The use of social interaction as a method of detecting anxiolytic activity of chlordiazepoxide-like drugs. *J. Neurosci. Meth.*, **2**, 219–238.

File, S. E. (1984). Neurochemistry of anxiety. In *Drugs in Psychiatry. Volume 2. Antianxiety agents* (eds G. D. Burrows, T. Norman and B. Davies), pp. 13–30. Elsevier Biochemical Press, Amsterdam.

File, S. E. (1988). How good is social interaction as a test of anxiety? In *Selected Models of Anxiety, Depression and Psychosis* (eds P. Simon, P. Soubrie and D. Wildlocher), pp. 151–166. Karger, Basel.

File, S. E. (1990). Age and anxiety: increased anxiety, decreased anxiolytic, but enhanced sedative, response to chlordiazepoxide in old rats. *Hum. Psychopharmacol.*, **5**, 169–173.

File, S. E. (1991). The biological basis of anxiety. In *Current Practices and Future Developments in the Pharmacotherapy of mental disorders* (eds H. Y. Meltzer and D. Nerozzi), pp. 159–166. Elsevier, Amsterdam.

File, S. E. and Andrews, N. (1991). Low but not high doses of buspirone reduce the anxiogenic effects of diazepam withdrawal. *Psychopharmacology*, **105**, 578–582.

File, S. E. and Andrews, N. (1993). Enhanced anxiolytic effect of zacopride enantiomers in diazepam-withdrawn rats. *Eur. J. Pharmacol.*, **237**, 127–130.

File, S. E. and Andrews, N. (1994). F 2692: flumazenil-reversible anxiolytic effects but inactive on [^{3}H]-Ro 15-4513 binding. *Pharmacol. Biochem. Behav*, **48**, 223–228.

File, S. E. and Hyde, J. R. G. (1978). Can social interaction be used to measure anxiety? *Br. J. Pharmacol.*, **62**, 19–24.

File, S. E. and Johnston, A. L. (1989). Lack of effects of 5-HT$_3$, receptor antagonists in the social interaction and elevated plus-maze tests of anxiety in the rat. *Psychopharmacology*, **99**, 248–251.

File, S. E. and Zangrossi, H. (1993). "One-trial tolerance" to the anxiolytic actions of benzodiazepines in the elevated plus-maze, or the development of a phobic state? *Psychopharmacology*, **110**, 240–244.

File, S. E., Mabbutt, P. S. and Hitchcott, P. K. (1990). Characterisation of the phenomenon of "one-trial tolerance" to the anxiolytic effect of chlordiazepoxide in the elevated plus-maze. *Psychopharmacology*, **102**, 98–101.

File, S. E., Andrews, N., Wu, P.-Y. *et al.* (1992). Modification of chlordiazepoxide's behavioural and neurochemical effects by handling and plus-maze experience. *Eur. J. Pharmacol.*, **218**, 9–14.

File, S. E., Zangrossi, H. and Andrews, N. (1993a). Social interaction and elevated plus-maze tests: changes in release and uptake of 5-HT and GABA. *Neuropharmacology*, **32**, 217–221.

File, S. E., Zangrossi, H., Viana, M. and Graeff, F. G. (1993b). Trial 2 in the elevated plus-maze: a different form of fear? *Psychopharmacology*, **111**, 491–494.

File, S. E., Zangrossi, H. Sanders, F. L. and Mabbutt, P. S. (1993c) Dissociation between behavioral and corticosterone responses on repeated exposures to cat odor. *Physiol. Behav*, **54**, 1109–1111.

File, S. E., Zangrossi, H., Sanders, F. L. and Mabbutt, P. S. (1993d). Raised corticosterone in the rat after exposure to the elevated plus-maze. *Psychopharmacology*, **113**, 543–546.

Graeff, F. G. (1991). Neurotransmitters in the dorsal periaqueductal grey and animal models of panic anxiety. In *New Directions in Anxiety* (eds M. Briley and S. E. File), pp. 288–319. Macmillan, London.

Gray, J. A. (1971). Sex differences in emotional behaviour in mammals including man: endocrine bases. *Acta Psychol.*, **35**, 29–46.

Guy, A. P. and Gardner, C. R. (1985). Pharmacological characterization of a modified social interaction model of anxiety in the rat. *Neuropsychobiology*, **13**, 194–200.

Hothersall, D. and Tuber, D. S. (1979). Fears in companion dogs: characteristics and treatment. In *Psychopathology in Animals. Research and Clinical Implications* (ed. J. D. Keehn), pp. 239–255. Academic Press, New York.

Howard, J. L. and Pollard, G. T. (1991). Effects of drugs on punished behavior: pre-clinical test for anxiolytics. In *Psychopharmacology of Anxiolytics and Anti-depressants* (ed. S. E. File), pp. 131–153. Pergamon Press, New York.

Hughes, J., Boden, P., Costall, B. *et al.* (1990). Development of a class of selective cholecystokinin type B receptor antagonists having potent anxiolytic activity. *Proc. Natl Acad. Sci. USA*, **87**, 6728–6732.

Johnston, A. L. and File, S. E. (1988a). Can animal tests of anxiety detect panic-promoting agents? *Hum. Psychopharmacol.*, **3**, 149–152.

Johnston, A. L. and File, S. E. (1988b). Profiles of the antipanic compounds, tri-azolobenzodiazepines and phenelzine, in two animal tests of anxiety. *Psychiatry Res.*, **25**, 81–90.

Johnston, A. L. and File, S. E. (1988c). Effects of 5-HT$_3$ antagonists in two animal tests of anxiety. *Neurosci Lett.*, **32**, S44.

Johnston, A. L. and File, S. E. (1991). Sex differences in animal tests of anxiety. *Physiol. Behav.*, **49**, 245–250.

Jones, B. J., Costall, B., Domeney, A. M. *et al.* (1988). The potential anxiolytic activity of GR 38032F, a 5-HT$_3$ receptor antagonist. *Br. J. Pharmacol.*, **93**, 985–993.

Kendler, K. S., Neale, M. C., Kessler, R. C. *et al.* (1992). The genetic epidemiology of phobias in women. *Arch. Gen. Psychiatry*, **49**, 273–281.

Kilfoil, T., Michel, A., Montgomery, D. and Whiting, R. L. (1989). Effects of anxiolytic and anxiogenic drugs on exploratory activity in a simple model of anxiety in mice. *Neuropharmacology*, **28**, 901–905.

Klein, D. F. (1981). Anxiety reconceptualized. In *Anxiety: New Research and Changing Concepts* (eds D. F. Klein and J. Rabkin), pp. 235–263. Raven Press, New York.

Klint, T. (1991). Effects of 8-OH DPAT and buspirone in a passive avoidance test and in the elevated plus-maze test in rats. *Behav. Pharmacol.*, **2**, 481–489.

Komiskey, H. L., Buck, M. A., Mundinger, K. L. *et al.* (1987) Effect of aging on anticonflict and CNS depressant activity of diazepam in rats. *Psychopharmacology*, **93**, 443–448.

Lader, M. H. (1991). Ondansetron in the treatment of anxiety. In *Biological Psychiatry*, Vol. 2, (eds G. Racagni, N. Brunello and T. Fukud), pp. 885–887. Excerpta Medica, Amsterdam.

Lister, R. G. (1987). The use of a plus-maze to measure anxiety in the mouse. *Psychopharmacology*, **92**, 180–185.

Metzenauer, P., Barnes, N. M., Costall, B. *et al.* (1992). Anxiolytic-like actions of anpirtoline in a mouse light–dark aversion paradigm. *Neuroreport*, **3**, 527–529.

Mineka, S. (1985). Animal models of anxiety-based disorders. In *Anxiety and Anxiety Disorders* (eds A. H. Tuma and J. D. Maser), pp. 199–244. Erlbaum, Hillsdale, NJ.

Moser, P. C. (1989). An evaluation of the elevated plus-maze test using the novel anxiolytic buspirone. *Psychopharmacology*, **99**, 48–53.

Moser, P. C., Tricklebank, M. D., Middlemiss, D. N. *et al.* (1990). Characterization of MDL 73005EF as a 5-HT$_{1A}$ selective ligand and its effects in animal models of anxiety: comparison with buspirone, 8-OH-DPAT and diazepam. *Br. J. Pharmacol.*, **99**, 343–349.

Motta, V., Maisonnette, S., Morato, S. *et al.* (1992). Effects of blockade of 5-HT$_2$ receptors and activation of 5-HT$_{1A}$ receptors on exploratory activity of rats in the elevated plus-maze. *Psychopharmacology*, **107**, 135–139.

Onaivi, E. S. and Martin, B. R. (1989). Neuropharmacological and physiological validation of a computer-controlled two-compartment black and white box for the assessment of anxiety. *Prog. Neuropsychopharmacol. Biol. Psychiatry*, **13**, 963–976.

Pellow, S. and File, S. E. (1986). Anxiolytic and anxiogenic drug effects on exploratory activity in an elevated plus-maze: a novel test of anxiety in the rat. *Pharmacol. Biochem. Behav.*, **24**, 525–529.

Pellow, S., Chopin, P., File, S. E. and Briley, M. (1985). Validation of open:closed arm entries in an elevated plus-maze as a measure of anxiety in the rat. *J. Neurosci. Meth.*, **14**, 149–167.

Pellow, S., Johnston, A. L. and File, S. E. (1987). Selective agonists and antagonists for 5-hydroxytryptamine receptor subtypes, and interactions with yohimbine and FG 7142 using the elevated plus-maze test in the rat. *J. Pharm. Pharmacol.*, **3**, 917–928.

Piper, D., Upton, N., Thomas, D. and Nicholson, J. (1988). The effects of 5-HT$_3$ receptor antagonists BRL 43694 and GR 38032F in animal behavioural models of anxiety. *Br. J. Pharmacol.*, **94**, 314P.

Rodgers, R. J. and Cole, J. C. (1993). Anxiety enhancement in the murine elevated plus-maze by immediate prior exposure to social stressors. *Physiol. Behav*, **53**, 383–388.

Rodgers, R. J., Lee, C. and Shepherd, J. K. (1992). Effects of diazepam on behavioural and antinociceptive responses to the elevated plus-maze in male mice depend upon treatment regimen and prior maze experience. *Psychopharmacology*, **106**, 102–110.

Simon, P., Panissaud, C. and Costentin, J. (1992). Sulpiride anxiogenic-like effect inhibition by a D$_1$ dopamine receptor antagonist. *Neuroreport*, **3**, 941–942.

Steenbergen, H. L., Heinsbroek, R. P. W., Van Hest, A. and Van De Poll, N. E. (1990). Sex-dependent effects of inescapable shock administration on shuttlebox-escape performance and elevated plus-maze behavior. *Physiol. Behav.*, **48**, 571–576.

Thiebot, M. -H. and Martin, P. (1991). Effects of benzodiazepines, 5-HT1A agonists and 5-HT3 antagonists in animal models sensitive to antidepressant drugs. In *5-HT1A Agonists, 5-HT3 Antagonists and Benzodiazepines: Their Comparative Behavioural Pharmacology* (eds R. J. Rodgers and S. J. Cooper), pp. 159–194. Wiley, Chichester.

Treit, D. (1985). Animal models for the study of anti-anxiety agents: a review. *Neurosci. Biobehav. Rev.*, **9**, 203–222.

Treit, D., Menard, J. and Royan, C. (1993). Anxiogenic stimuli in the elevated plus-maze. *Pharmacol. Biochem. Behav.*, **44**, 463–469.

Tyers, M. B., Costall, B., Domeney, A. M. *et al.* (1987). The anxiolytic activities of 5-HT$_3$, antagonists in laboratory animals. *Neurosci. Lett.*, **29**, S68.

Venault, P., Jacquot, F., Save, E. and Chapouthier, G. (1993). Anxiogenic-like effects of yohimbine and idazoxan in two behavioural situations in mice. *Life Sci.*, **52**, 639–645.

Wada, T. and Fukuda, N. (1991). Effects of DN-2327 a new anxiolytic, diazepam and buspirone on exploratory activity of the rat in an elevated plus-maze. *Psychopharmacology*, **104**, 444–450.

Weiss, S. R. B. and Uhde, T. W. (1990). Animal models of anxiety. In *Neurobiology of Panic Disorder* (ed. J. C. Ballenger), pp. 3–27. Wiley–Liss, New York.

Young, R. and Johnson, D. N. (1991). Anxiolytic-like activity of R(+)- and S(–)-zacopride in mice. *Eur. J. Pharmacol.*, **201**, 151–155.

Zangrossi, H. and File, S. E. (1992a). Behavioral consequences in animal tests of anxiety and exploration of exposure to cat odor. *Brain Res. Bull.*, **29**, 381–388.

Zangrossi, H. and File, S. E. (1992b). Chlordiazepoxide reduces the generalised anxiety, but not the direct responses, of rats exposed to cat odor. *Pharmacol. Biochem. Behav.*, **43**, 1195–1200.

Zangrossi, H. and File, S. E. (1994). Habituation and generalization of phobic responses to cat odor. *Brain Res. Bull,* **33**, 189–194.

Zitrin, C. M., Woerner, M. G. and Klein, D. F. (1981). Differentiation of panic anxiety from anticipatory anxiety and avoidance behavior. In *Anxiety: New Research and Changing Concepts* (eds D. F. Klein and J. Rabkin), pp. 27–46. Raven Press, New York.

Part II

PANIC DISORDER

5 Potential Animal Models for the Study of Antipanic and Antiphobic Treatments

BEREND OLIVIER,[1,2] **ELLEN MOLEWIJK,**[1] **LUCIANNE GROENINK,**[2] **ROSEMARIE JOORDENS,**[2] **THEO ZETHOF**[1] **AND JAN MOS**[1]

[1]*CNS Research, Solvay Duphar BV, DA Weesp, and* [2]*Department of Psychopharmacology, Faculty of Pharmacy, Utrecht University, Utrecht, The Netherlands*

INTRODUCTION

Anxiety seems an almost inevitable component of mental illness. It is present most purely in the so-called anxiety disorders, but it can also be a component of depression, schizophrenia, and personality disorders. The DSM-III-R distinguishes four major types of anxiety disorders: panic disorder with or without agoraphobia (PD); other phobias; generalized anxiety disorders (GAD); and obsessive-compulsive disorder (OCD). Pathological anxiety is difficult to model in animal experimental paradigms, although an abundant number of animal models of anxiety are in use. However, most, if not all, have no clear face and/or predictive validity with respect to the various DSM-III-R categories, and presumably primarily reflect normal anxiety/fear processes instead of pathological processes. Although no standard animal (behavioral) models for the study of antipanic and antiphobic treatments are available, a number of anxiolytic tests have been described with potential use in discriminating between the various anxiety categories. In this contribution, after a short introduction, a selected number of animal paradigms will be dealt with to exemplify how and to what extent animal models of anxiety may be of help to find antipanic and antiphobic drugs.

ANIMAL MODELS OF ANXIETY

Basically, two types of animal behavior models are used to detect putative anxiety-reducing drugs. Such models can be based on conditioned behavior and involve responses controlled by operant conditioning procedures. The other type of model involves unconditioned behavior, relying on natural behavioral reactions and not requiring specific training. Often the latter models rely on species-specific responses (e.g. social interaction, ultrasonic vocalization) and

Advances in the Neurobiology of Anxiety Disorders. Edited by H. G. M. Westenberg, J. A. Den Boer and D. L. Murphy
©1996 John Wiley & Sons Ltd

Table 1. Animal behavior models frequently used in the study of anxiolytic drug effects

Conditioned models	Unconditioned models
Conflict procedures	Light–dark exploration
Fear-potentiated startle	Elevated plus-maze
Periaqueductal gray stimulation	Ultrasonic vocalization in pups
Conditioned taste aversion	Social interaction
Conditioned defensive burying	Defeat-induced analgesia
Conditioned place preference	Stress-induced hyperthermia
Conditioned adult ultrasonic vocalization	Predator exposure
Conditioned suppression of drinking	Open field (neophobia)
Active/passive avoidance response	Stretched attention posture
Schedule-induced polydipsia	Noise test
Go–no go paradigm	

are sometimes referred to as "ethologically based" models. Table 1 summarizes those models currently in use to study the anxiolytic effects of drugs.

Some of the more frequently used procedures, like the conflict procedures, fear-potentiated startle, elevated plus-maze, social interaction test and light–dark exploration, will be shortly summarized. Instead of a very broad overview of all models used, we chose to focus on some newly developed animal models with attractive features for some anxiety categories. One of them, conditioned ultrasonic vocalization by adult rats, seems a model with predictive validity for panic disorder. A second model, stress-induced hyperthermia, measures different aspects of anxiety (anticipatory) from the other models and could be interesting as a putative model for phobias. A third model, exposure to a predator, could be a promising model to study panic-like reactions of animals.

PD is characterized by episodes of intense anxiety accompanied by severe autonomic symptoms (e.g. sweating, heart-beating, trembling). These episodes are referred to as panic attacks. In PD patients the panic attacks can either emerge spontaneously ("out of the blue") or in relation to a specific environmental context ("situational panic attacks"). Cognitive factors play an important role in the development and maintenance of situational panic attacks: the environmental stimuli associated with earlier experienced panic attacks may become potent triggers for new panic attacks (Swinson and Kuch, 1990).

Pharmacological treatments currently used against PD are the triazolobenzodiazepine alprazolam (Ballenger et al., 1988; Chouinard et al., 1982; Sheehan, 1982), the serotonin (5-HT) uptake inhibitors fluvoxamine (Cassano et al., 1988; Den Boer et al., 1987; Westenberg and Den Boer 1989, 1990) and clomipramine (e.g. Den Boer et al., 1987; McTavish and Benfield, 1990) and the mixed 5-HT/norepinephrine (NE) uptake inhibitor imipramine (Mavissakalian and Michelson, 1986; Zitrin et al., 1980). Classical benzodiazepines, like diazepam (Dunner et al., 1986; Noyes et al., 1984) or chlordiazepoxide (McNair and Kahn, 1981) have only moderate therapeutic effects and at much higher doses than those required to treat GAD. The NE uptake inhibitors maprotiline (Westenberg and Den Boer, 1989, 1990) and desipramine (Kalus et al., 1991) have been found ineffective in reducing panic attacks.

Drug treatment for phobias is less clear. Treatment of agoraphobia largely parallels that of PD (Levin and Liebowitz, 1987), whereas social phobia is treated primarily with β-blockers or monoamine oxidase (MAO) inhibitors (Levin and Liebowitz, 1987).

CONFLICT MODELS

In conflict models ongoing behavior is suppressed by aversive stimulation. Suppressed behavior is either lever-pressing for food in hungry rats (Geller and Seifter, 1960), water-licking in thirsty rats (Vogel et al., 1971), key-pecking by hungry pigeons (Barrett et al., 1986) or exploration by mice of a new environment, as in the four-plate test (Aron et al., 1971). Signaled or unsignaled electric shock may be used as aversive stimulation. The release of suppressed behavior without affecting the levels of punished responding following pharmacological intervention is considered as the "anxiolytic" effect. In rodents, pigeons and primates benzodiazepines are consistently found to be effective in these models (Barrett, 1991), but non-benzodiazepine anxiolytics like the 5-HT_{1A} receptor agonists, the specific serotonin reuptake inhibitors (SSRIs) and other putative anxiolytics are difficult to detect using such conflict procedures. Therefore, such models are not adequate for finding new antipanic or antiphobic treatments.

FEAR-POTENTIATED STARTLE RESPONSE

The startle response of a rat to a loud tone can be augmented by prior Pavlovian fear-conditioning (Davis et al., 1993). During the fear-conditioning phase a light stimulus, serving as the conditioned stimulus, signals the presence of a shock (unconditioned stimulus). During the startle response presentation of the light augments the startle amplitude. Benzodiazepines (BZDs) have an anxiolytic effect in this paradigm as they inhibit the augmented startle amplitude without affecting the basal startle (Davis et al., 1993). Several other putative anxiolytics, like the 5-HT_{1A} agonists, seem to work in the fear-potentiated startle response (FPS), whereas no data are yet known for SSRIs. Neither acute nor chronic (three weeks) imipramine altered baseline startle or FPS (Cassella and Davis, 1985). Because imipramine is an effective antipanic agent, the FPS does not appear a promising model for PD.

ELEVATED PLUS-MAZE

The elevated plus-maze, first described by Handley and Mithani (1984), is an exploratory behavior model in which rats are placed in an elevated maze, consisting of two (opposite) open and two closed alleys. The animals will explore the different alleys (total number of entries). The open arms are more aversive to the rats than the closed ones, as revealed by a preference of the animals to explore the closed alleys. Anxiolytic drugs will help to overcome the fear-induced inhibition of open-alley exploration. The ratio of open versus total arm entries gives a sensitive measure of the anxiolytic effect of a drug.

In this model BZDs show up as reliable anxiolytics. However, other putative anxiolytics, like the 5-HT$_{1A}$ agonists, the SSRIs and the 5-HT$_3$ antagonists, are sometimes active, sometimes not, or sometimes even anxiogenic (Barrett, 1991). Therefore, this model does not seem to have specific qualities as an antipanic or antiphobic paradigm.

SOCIAL INTERACTION TEST

In this test, first described by File and Hyde (1979) and File (1980), either rats or mice unfamiliar to each other are placed in pairs in an open arena, which may be either familiar or unfamiliar to the animals, and may be brightly or dimly lit. The most aversive situation is obviously a brightly lit, unfamiliar environment in which low levels of social interaction between two conspecifics occur. The time spent by the animals in social interaction is measured as well as locomotor activity. Again, benzodiazepines can easily be detected as anxiolytics in this model, as they increase the time spent in social interaction. For other putative anxiolytics ambivalent data have been reported and the model does not properly model for antipanic, antiphobic or anti-OCD properties of drugs (Barrett, 1991).

CONDITIONED ULTRASONIC DISTRESS VOCALIZATIONS IN ADULT MALE RATS AS A BEHAVIORAL MODEL OF PANIC DISORDER

We have evaluated conditioned ultrasonic vocalizations (CUSV) produced by rats as a behavioral paradigm to screen for antipanic drugs (Molewijk *et al.*, 1993, 1995). CUSV can be recorded in a range of threatening situations. For instance, rat pups emit ultrasounds (approx. 35 kHz) when separated from their mother and littermates (Gardner, 1985; Hofer and Shair, 1987; Insel *et al.*, 1986; Mos and Olivier, 1989). Adult rats may produce ultrasonic distress vocalizations (USV) (approx. 22 kHz), for example, in the presence of a predator (Blanchard *et al.*, 1991), a dominant male (Tornatzky and Miczek, 1992; Van der Poel and Miczek, 1991; Vivian and Miczek, 1993), after a painful (Tonoue *et al.*, 1986; Van der Poel *et al.*, 1989) or a loud acoustic (Kaltwasser, 1991; Miczek and Vivian, 1993) stimulus. Interestingly, rats can also produce USV in association with a prior aversive event, without the actual physical presence of threat. This feature may have face validity towards situational panic attacks, where environmental stimuli may acquire aversive properties and become triggers for panic attacks. In this study, USV are elicited by reintroducing adult male rats into the environment in which they previously received inescapable footshocks. During the USV test no electrical current is applied. The sensitivity of these CUSV to various psychopharmacological treatments was assessed. The specificity of reduction in CUSV emission was determined by measuring spontaneous locomotor activity in an open field.

Table 2 shows the results of the various drugs on the number of vocalizations in the CUSV test in rats.

Table 2. Effects of various psychoactive drugs on the number of ultrasonic vocalizations (USV) in the adult rat. Activity indicates measurement of locomotion in an open field. $\downarrow$ *(x)* indicates a suppression at the indicated dose and higher doses. Specificity indicates if USV is decreased before activity (+), simultaneously or the reverse (–); n.t. = not tested; n.d. = not determinable

Drug	Dose range	USV	Activity	Specificity
BZD receptor ligands				
Diazepam	(0.3, 1, 3, 10, 30)	$\downarrow$(30)	$\downarrow$(10, 30)	–
Chlordiazepoxide	(1, 3, 10)	–	n.t.	n.d.
Alprazolam	(0.3, 1 , 3)	$\downarrow$(3)	$\downarrow$3	–
Bretazenil	(1, 3, 10)	–	n.t	n.d.
Alpidem	(2.5, 5, 10)	–	–	n.d.
Zolpidem	(0.5, 1, 2)	–	$\downarrow$(2)	–
Flumazenil	(1, 3, 10)	–	n.t.	n.d.
5-HT$_{1A}$ receptor ligands				
8-OH-DPAT	(0.01, 0.03, 0.1, 0.3)	$\downarrow$(0.03)	$\uparrow$(0.1)	+?
Flesinoxan	(0.1, 0.3, 1)	$\downarrow$(0.3)	–	+
Buspirone	(0.3, 1, 3)	$\downarrow$(1)	$\downarrow$(1)	–
Ipsapirone	(0.3, 1, 3)	$\downarrow$(3)	n.t.	n.d.
BMY 7378	(0.3, 1, 3)	$\downarrow$(3)	n.t.	n.d.
5-HT and NE uptake inhibitors				
Fluvoxamine	(0.3, 1, 3)	$\downarrow$(3)	–(3)	+
Clomipramine	(5, 10, 20)	$\downarrow$(10)	$\downarrow$(10)	–
Imipramine	(5, 10, 20)	$\downarrow$(10)	n.t.	n.d.
Maprotiline	(5, 10, 20)	–	n.t.	n.d.
Desipramine	(1, 3, 10)	–	$\downarrow$(10)	–?
Miscellaneous				
Clonidine	(0.03, 0.1, 0.3)	$\downarrow$(0.1)	$\downarrow$(0.03)	–
Yohimbine	(0.3, 1, 3)	$\downarrow$(1)	n.t.	n.d.
Ondansetron	(0.001, 0.01, 0.1)	–	–	n.d
Haloperidol	(0.3, 1, 3)	$\downarrow$(3)	$\downarrow$(<1)	–

The classical BZD receptor agonists diazepam (0.3, 1, 3, 10, 30 mg/kg i.p.) and chlordiazepoxide (1, 3, 10 mg/kg i.p.) did not reduce the CUSV produced by adult rats or only at a very high dose (diazepam at 30 mg/kg). A reduction of motor activity was observed after diazepam 10 and 30 mg/kg i.p. In contrast, the triazolobenzodiazepine alprazolam dose-dependently and efficaciously suppressed USV, with a lowest effective dose (LED) of 3 mg/kg i.p. This dose also reduced locomotor activity. The partial BZD agonists bretazenil (1, 3, 10 mg/kg i.p.), alpidem (2.5, 5, 10 mg/kg i.p.) and zolpidem (0.5, 1, 2 mg/kg i.p.) had no effect on CUSV. Alpidem had no effect on locomotion, whereas zolpidem (2 mg/kg i.p.) reduced locomotor activity. The BZD antagonist flumazenil (1, 3, 10 mg/kg i.p.) did not affect CUSV. The full 5-HT_{1A} receptor agonists 8-hydroxy-2-(di-n-propylamino)tetralin (8-OH-DPAT) and flesinoxan potently and efficaciously reduced CUSV. 8-OH-DPAT suppressed CUSV at 0.03 mg/kg s.c., whereas complete abolition occurred at 0.1 and 0.3 mg/kg s.c., concurrent with stimulation of motor activity. Flesinoxan suppressed the number of CUSV at 0.3 and 1 mg/kg i.p., but had no effect on locomotion. The partial 5-HT_{1A} receptor agonists buspirone, ipsapirone and BMY 7378 produced clear dose-dependent inhibition of CUSV (LED 1, 3 and 3 mg/kg i.p. respectively). Buspirone also reduced locomotor activity at these dose levels (LED 1 mg/kg i.p.). The 5-HT uptake inhibitors fluvoxamine and clomipramine reduced CUSV at LEDs of 3 and 10 mg/kg i.p. respectively. Fluvoxamine did not affect locomotor activity at the dose suppressing CUSV. Clomipramine reduced locomotion at 10 and 20 mg/kg i.p. The mixed 5-HT/NE uptake inhibitor imipramine dose-dependently reduced CUSV (LED 10 mg/kg i.p.). On the other hand, the NE uptake inhibitors maprotiline and desipramine had no (significant) effect on CUSV in adult rats. Desipramine, however, reduced locomotor activity at 10 mg/kg i.p.

The α_2-adrenergic agonist clonidine as well as the α_2-adrenergic antagonist yohimbine potently reduced CUSV (LED 0.1 and 1 mg/kg i.p. respectively). Clonidine reduced motor activity at all doses tested. The 5-HT_3 receptor antagonist ondansetron (0.001, 0.01, 0.1 mg/kg i.p.) had no effect on CUSV. The dopamine D_2 receptor antagonist haloperidol suppressed the number of ultrasonic vocalizations only at a very high dose (LED 3 mg/kg i.p.). Haloperidol reduces locomotor activity at 1 mg/kg i.p.

The drugs currently used to treat PD, like the triazolobenzodiazepine alprazolam, the 5-HT uptake inhibitors fluvoxamine and clomipramine and the mixed 5-HT/NE uptake inhibitor imipramine, reduced the number of ultrasonic vocalizations in this model. The anxiolytic effect of imipramine probably results from uptake inhibition of 5-HT rather than NE, since only 5-HT (not NE) uptake inhibitors are active both in this CUSV model and in PD. The classical BZDs diazepam and chlordiazepoxide, which are only moderately active in PD at doses well above anxiolytic doses used in GAD, did not reduce CUSV at anxiolytic doses found in most animal models of anxiety. A reduction of CUSV occurred only after a very high dose (30 mg/kg i.p.) of diazepam. Other

BZD ligands like bretazenil, alpidem, zolpidem and flumazenil had no effect on CUSV. The partial BZD receptor agonist bretazenil (which has not been tested in PD) was characterized as an anxiolytic drug only in some animal models (Sanger et al., 1985). Considering the low potency of the classical BZD receptor agonists in this model and in PD, the low intrinsic activity of bretazenil possibly makes it less suitable for treating panic-like states. The same probably holds for the partial $\omega_{1/3}$ agonist alpidem (Langer et al., 1990); Zivkovic et al., 1990). The first study with alpidem in PD did not reveal clear therapeutic effectiveness (Schneier et al., 1993). Zolpidem is described as a hypnotic agent (Sanger et al., 1987) whose effects in PD are unknown. The BZD receptor antagonist flumazenil was either inactive (Woods et al., 1991) or anxiogenic in PD patients (Nutt et al., 1990).

The partial 5-HT_{1A} receptor agonists and anxiolytic agents buspirone (Goa and Ward, 1986) and ipsapirone (Martin and Mason, 1987), as well as the full 5-HT_{1A} receptor agonists 8-OH-DPAT (Hjörth et al., 1982) and flesinoxan (Wouters et al., 1988), potently and efficaciously reduced ultrasound emission in the adult rat. Also the weak partial 5-HT_{1A} receptor agonist BMY 7378 (Yocca et al., 1987) suppressed CUSV. This suggests that 5-HT_{1A} receptor agonists could be effective treatments against PD. Preliminary clinical results with buspirone, however, did not reveal a reduction of the number of panic attacks (Robinson et al., 1989; Sheehan et al., 1990, 1993). On the other hand, Lesch et al. (1992) demonstrated a reduced hypothermic and neuroendocrine response to a challenge dose of ipsapirone in panic patients, suggesting a subsensitivity of 5-HT_{1A} receptors in the pathophysiology of PD. Whether or not 5-HT_{1A} receptor agonists are false positives in this model depends on further clinical data.

The NE uptake inhibitors maprotiline and desipramine, which are most probably not effective in preventing panic attacks, did not affect CUSV in this model.

The α_2-adrenergic agonist clonidine, as well as the α_2-adrenergic antagonist yohimbine, reduced CUSV. Clonidine is reported to have short-lasting antipanic properties (Ko et al., 1983; Uhde et al., 1989), whereas yohimbine acts as a panic provocative agent in PD patients (Charney et al., 1984). Both here and in the study of De Vry et al. (1992) yohimbine potently and efficaciously reduced USV in adult rats. Furthermore, in drug discrimination procedures in rats yohimbine generates, and generalizes to, a 5-HT_{1A} receptor agonist cue (Winter and Rabin, 1992; Ybema et al., 1993). Possibly the CUSV reduction after yohimbine can be attributed to these 5-HT_{1A} receptor agonistic properties.

The 5-HT_3 receptor antagonist ondansetron, whose anxiolytic properties have been reported in some models of anxiety (Costall et al., 1989), had no effect on USV in this model or in other CUSV models (De Vry et al., 1992; Sanchez, 1993). The effect of ondansetron in PD has not been investigated.

The dopamine D_2 receptor antagonist haloperidol did not reduce USV except at a very high dose (3 mg/kg i.p.), whereas locomotor behavior was already reduced at 1 mg/kg i.p. There are no data on the effects of haloperidol in PD patients.

For the main classes of effective drugs in PD, viz. the triazolobenzodiazepine and 5-HT uptake inhibitors, and also the main classes of ineffective drugs, viz. classical BZD and NE uptake inhibitors, a very high correlation between the clinical effect in PD and the effect on CUSV was found. This suggests that this CUSV model has high predictive validity towards the psychopharmacology of PD and thus could be used as a behavioral paradigm to screen for antipanic treatments. It should, however, be noted that therapeutic effects in humans are usually observed after chronic administration and not after single doses (as in the USV model). Also panic provocatives like CCK_4, lactate and carbon dioxide have to be evaluated on CUSV.

STRESS-INDUCED HYPERTHERMIA

In a recently described animal paradigm (Borsini et al., 1989) it was found that in group-housed mice removed one by one from their housing cage, mice removed last always had higher rectal temperatures than those removed first. This phenomenon is called stress-induced hyperthermia (SIH) and has been interpreted as being caused by anticipatory fear or stress of an aversive event (handling, disturbance in the cage). We were able to replicate these findings (Zethof et al., 1991, 1994). The body temperature of group-housed rats also increases when they are handled and recorded sequentially (Eikelboom and Stuart, 1979; Poole and Stephenson, 1977). Such findings have been considered as a conditioned response in anticipation to handling and/or insertion of the rectal probe (Eikelboom, 1986). Temperature rises can be conditioned to stimuli occurring in anticipation of events such as forced exercise (Gollnick and Ianuzzo, 1968), microwave radiation (Bermant et al., 1979) or drug injections and rotarod measurements (York and Regan, 1982). Interactions between body temperature and emotional states occur in man also (Reeves et al., 1985; Yoshiue et al., 1989) and it is customary to include changes in autonomic functioning (like temperature) in the diagnosis of GAD and PD (e.g. in DSM-III-R). Moreover, the stress-induced rise in rectal temperature could be prevented by administration of BZDs, but not by antidepressants or neuroleptics (Borsini et al., 1989; Zethof et al., 1991), supporting the view that SIH may be considered as an animal model representing some form of (anticipatory) anxiety. We used the SIH paradigm to study various putative anxiolytic drugs from different drug classes, like BZD receptor agonists, $5-HT_{1A}$ receptor agonists, antidepressants including SSRIs and $5-HT_3$ receptor antagonists.

Basically, the SIH test is a simple and robust paradigm. Male mice are housed in groups of 10 animals per cage. Mice are randomly marked by a dye (1–10) one day prior to the actual test. The rectal temperature of each of the group-housed mice was measured sequentially at 1 min intervals. The rectal temperatures of the successive 10 mice (mean of eight cages) are depicted in Figure 1.

It can be seen that picking up and temperature measurement of a mouse from

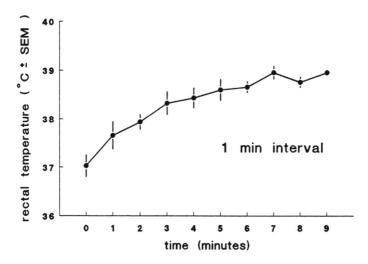

Figure 1 The rectal temperature of male NMRI mice housed in a cage with 10 mice (eight cages). The temperature of mice 1 to 10 was measured sequentially using a 1 min interval. After temperature measurement animals were not returned to the cage, the number of remaining mice decreasing from 10 to one. Each point is the mean temperature ($\pm$ SEM) of eight mice

the cage (they are not returned in the cage) leads to an enhancement of the temperature of the next mouse, until approximately 8–10 min after picking up the first mouse the maximal temperature has been reached. This is a very reliable and robust phenomenon, with maximal temperature increases of 1.3–1.8°C. This maximal rise in temperature has a certain delay. Increasing the interval between measurement of mouse 1 and mouse 2 from 1 to 2, 5 or 10 min clearly shows that in all cases the maximum is reached at about 8–10 min (Zethof *et al.*, 1994).

We were able to show that the increase in temperature in SIH was paralleled by increases in adrenocorticotropic hormone (ACTH), corticosterone and glucose levels (Figure 3) in blood plasma (Groenink *et al.*, 1994), supporting the idea that SIH reflects a stress-related phenomenon.

To further study the SIH model as an animal anxiety paradigm we injected group-housed mice with a drug 60 min before testing. The test consisted of sequential temperature measurement of 10 mice using the 1 min time interval. Figure 2 shows the effects of five compounds, orally administered 60 min before testing.

Diazepam has an effect on the basal temperature (mouse 1), although only significant at 12 mg/kg p.o. Diazepam potently and dose-dependently reduces the SIH (mouse 10). Because the effect on SIH is much stronger than on baseline temperature, it can be concluded that diazepam exerts a potent anxiolytic effect with an ED_{50} of approximately 5 mg/kg p.o. Similar results were found for alprazolam, with an ED_{50} in SIH of approximately 0.7 mg/kg p.o. Alcohol

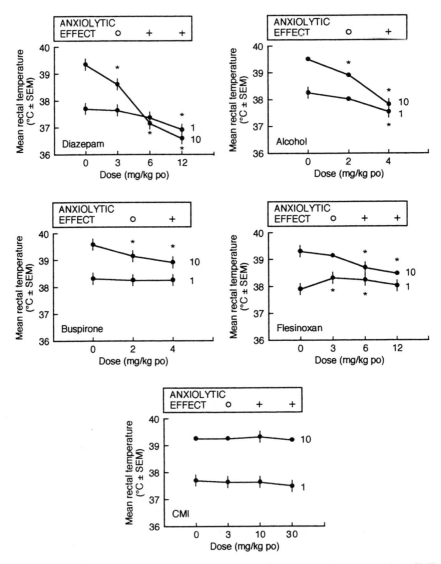

Figure 2 The effect of diazepam, alcohol, buspirone, flesinoxan and clomipramine (CMI) (orally administered 60 min before testing) on the rectal temperature of male group-housed mice in the SIH paradigm. The temperature of mouse 1 and mouse 10 (*N*=8 each) is shown. Asterisks indicate a significant difference from the corresponding vehicle. In the rectangle at the top of each figure is indicated whether a drug exerts anxiolytic activity (more effect on increased than on basal temperature). The dose of alcohol is in grams per kilogram

(Figure 2) also exerts an anxiolytic effect in this paradigm. Classical anxiolytics (BZDs, alcohol) can therefore easily be detected in this anxiety paradigm. Another putative class of anxiolytic agents, the 5-HT$_{1A}$ receptor agonists, are

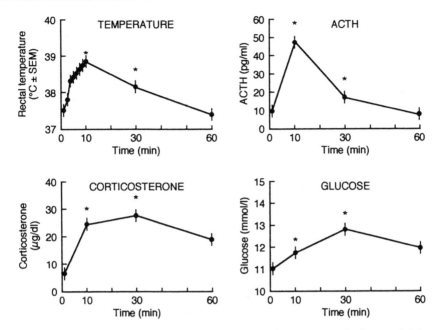

Figure 3 In group-housed mice (N=10 per cage) the rectal temperature of mice nos 2–9 has been measured sequentially using a 1 min interval. Mice nos 1 and 10 were decapitated and their blood was collected for hormone assays. The rectal temperature of mouse no. 8 was remeasured 30 or 60 min after the start of the experiment, whereas mouse no. 9 was decapitated 30 or 60 min after starting the experiment. Effects of the SIH procedure on rectal temperature, plasma ACTH levels (pg/ml), plasma corticosterone levels (μg/dl) and plasma glucose levels (mmol/l) are shown. Each point is the mean (±SEM) of 16 mice, except at 30 and 60 min (N=8). Asterisks denote a significant increase (p<0.05) from 0 min

also anxiolytic in this paradigm, but have a slightly different profile of action. Buspirone (Figure 2) has no effect on the basal temperature in group-housed or isolated mice (unpublished) up to 20 mg/kg. At doses of 10, but certainly at 20 mg/kg p.o., buspirone exerts anxiolytic activity, although the effect is less strong than that of the BZDs. For another 5-HT$_{1A}$ receptor agonist, ipsapirone, we could not find any anxiolytic activity up to 20 mg/kg p.o. (data not shown), but another, full and potent 5-HT$_{1A}$ receptor agonist, flesinoxan, has anxiolytic effects, but again less potent than the BDZ receptor agonists (Figure 2).

5-HT$_3$ receptor antagonists (ondansetron) had no effects on SIH (and basal temperature) over a wide range of doses, suggesting that 5-HT$_3$ receptor antagonists do not exert anxiolytic properties in this paradigm (data not shown). Another class of putative anxiolytic agents, the SSRIs, including fluvoxamine and clomipramine (CMI) are basically without effect in SIH. Figure 2 shows the effects of CMI over a wide dose range (3–30 mg/kg p.o.). No effects whatsoever were seen.

In summary, SIH appears a very promising paradigm to study stress-related processes and putative antistress or anxiolytic properties of drugs. Because the model simultaneously measures the effects of a drug on baseline temperature (mouse 1) and SIH (mouse 10), anxiolytic effects can be dissected very elegantly.

PHYSIOLOGICAL AND BEHAVIORAL RESPONSES IN RATS AFTER EXPOSURE TO A PREDATOR

Rats exposed to aversive or stressful stimuli show behavioral and physiological responses, such as freezing (Buwalda et al., 1992; Steenbergen et al., 1989; Van Dijken et al., 1992a, 1992b), ultrasonic vocalizations (Cuomo et al., 1992; Molewijk et al., 1993; Mos and Olivier, 1989), as well as changes in heart rate (Bohus, 1974; Buwalda et al., 1992; Diamant et al., 1991; Hagan and Bohus, 1984; Steenbergen et al., 1989; Wan et al., 1992) and core temperature (Diamant et al., 1991; Kluger et al., 1987; Long et al., 1990; Nakamori et al., 1993; Singer et al., 1986; Wan et al., 1990). Commonly used aversive stimuli are arbitrary stimuli, such as an electric shock or a loud noise. It has been suggested that presentation of an ecologically relevant aversive stimulus, a natural predator or its odor, might be a useful tool in studying anxiety (Blanchard and Blanchard, 1989), because of its innate character. Exposure to the calls of predators of mice was reported to activate defensive behavior and inhibit consummatory behavior (Hendrie and Neill, 1991). The vicinity of a cat induced movement arrest and high rates of risk assessment in rats, whereas non-defensive behaviors, such as eating and drinking, were inhibited (Blanchard et al., 1992b, 1993). Rats living in a visible burrow system emitted ultrasonic sounds while hiding in the burrows after presentation of a cat (Blanchard et al., 1989, 1990a, 1990b, 1992b). Moreover, rats exposed to the odor of a cat showed high rates of risk assessment, including flat back approach and stretched attend behaviors orienting towards the aversive stimulus (Blanchard et al., 1990a, 1990b), and spent more time sheltering (File and Zangrossi, 1993; Zangrossi and File, 1992b). Therefore, the presentation of a predator to rodents seems to be a strong unconditioned aversive stimulus, which could be used to gain insight into the underlying mechanisms of anxiety. We investigated the effects of exposure to an ecologically relevant stimulus, such as a cat, on heart rate (HR) and core temperature (CT) in male rats. To this purpose, HR and CT were measured in freely moving rats using a telemetry system consisting of implantable transmitters and a receiver (Clement et al., 1989). In addition, the effects of the 5-HT$_{1A}$ receptor agonist flesinoxan, which is supposed to exert anxiolytic activity (Mos and Olivier, 1989), on behavioral and physiological cat-induced responses were analyzed. The measurement of HR and CT in freely moving rats using telemetry devices allows an integrated approach to the study of anxiety in laboratory animals. In this experiment a small macrolon cage with the experimental rat was placed in a large wooden observation cage (80×60×50 cm). After 15 min basal monitoring, a cat or a rabbit was introduced

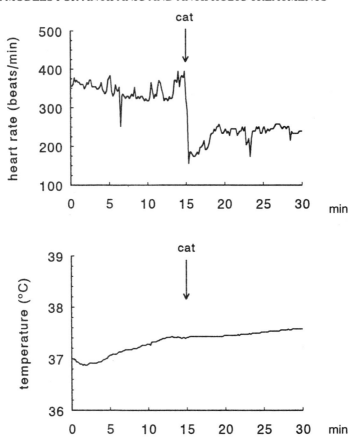

Figure 4 A typical example of the effect of exposure to a cat on heart rate (beats/min) and core temperature (°C) in a rat. The cat was introduced into the cage after 15 min basal monitoring and remained in the cage until the end of the session

into the observation cage for a period of 15 min. Both the cat and the rabbit were familiarized with rats and did not engage in interactions with the rat, which was shielded by the grid of the macrolon cage.

Figure 4 shows a prototypical example of the effect of exposure of a rat to a cat on HR and CT. Cat exposure led to a considerable bradycardia, lasting for the whole exposure period. No such dramatic effect was seen on CT (Figure 4).

When rats were exposed three successive times to a cat at intervals of three to four days, no adaptation in the cat exposure-induced bradycardia occurred (Figure 5). No clear effects were observed on CT.

Confrontation of the rats with a rabbit, a non-predator, also led to some bradycardia, but significantly less than when confronted with a cat (Figure 6). A similar pattern was seen with CT, where some hyperthermia occurred.

When flesinoxan (0.1 or 0.5 mg/kg i.p.) was given, no attenuation of the cat-induced bradycardia was observed. However, simultaneous measurement of

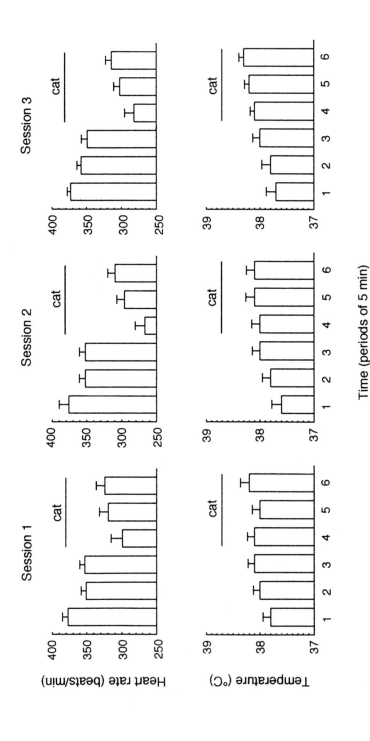

Figure 5 Mean course of heart rate (HR) and core temperature (CT) in rats (*N*=8) during three successive exposures to a cat. In each session a cat was presented for a period of 15 min, after 15 min basal monitoring. The three sessions were performed at intervals of three and four days. HR data was expressed as mean HR (beats/min) ± SEM. CT data were expressed as mean CT (°C) ± SEM

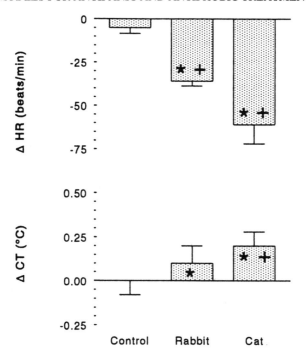

Figure 6 Effects of exposure to no animal (control), a rabbit and a cat on heart rate (HR) and core temperature (CT) in rats ($N=8$). HR data were expressed as mean change in HR (beats/min)±SEM as compared to basal HR, and CT data were expressed as mean change in CT (°C)±SEM as compared to basal CT. *$p<0.05$ as compared to the change in HR or CT in the control session (without exposure to a cat or a rabbit); [+]$p<0.05$ as compared to basal HR or CT

ultrasound production by the rat showed that flesinoxan was able to reduce the cat-induced USV in the rats (Figure 7).

No such USV was detected in control sessions, neither after introduction of a rabbit. It can be concluded that rats suddenly confronted with a cat show a pronounced bradycardia, which is not subject to habituation or sensitization over three successive confrontations. The observed bradycardia was not specifically related to a predator, since the presence of a rabbit also induced bradycardia. However, the cat-induced bradycardia was stronger and was accompanied by ultrasound production, a signal of fear or anxiety. Therefore this model could be used to study physiological aspects of fear-induced behavior and as such could be a model for panic-like behavior.

A diversity of aversive stimuli can produce fear bradycardia in animals and man. For example, the presence of a natural predator, a snake, induced bradycardia in wild rodents of six different species (Myron and Hofer, 1970). An immediate bradycardiac response was seen in rats after sudden elimination of background noise (Steenbergen et al., 1989). Repeated exposure of rats living in a visible burrow system to a predator (cat) showed that no habituation or

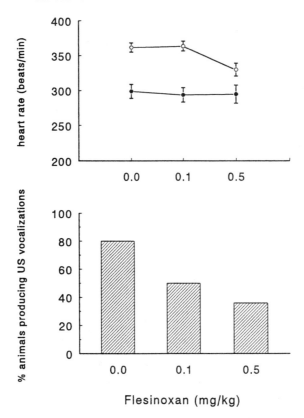

Figure 7 Effect of acute treatment with saline, 0.1 mg/kg and 0.5mg/kg flesinoxan (i.p.) on heart rate and the percentage of rats producing cat-induced US vocalizations (N=14)

sensitization occurred to repeated exposure to the predator (Blanchard *et al.*, 1990, 1991). From an ethological point of view one could expect this, because perception and reaction to life-threatening stimuli seem of vital importance (Bolles, 1970).

The findings of fear-induced bradycardia in combination with ultrasound production and concomitant behavioral responses seem to open a putative model to test antipanic and antiphobic drugs. Thus far no such studies have been reported, but the model seems to have at least good face validity.

CONCLUSIONS

Most, if not all, animal models of anxiety/fear are very sensitive and valuable in detecting drugs acting via the γ-aminobutyric acid–benzodiazepine receptor complex but are less, or even not at all, sensitive to anxiolytic drugs with different mechanisms of action, like 5-HT$_{1A}$ receptor agonists.

Table 3. Anxiolytic potential of drug classes

	BZD agonists	5-HT$_{1A}$ agonists	SSRIs	Imipramine	5-HT$_3$ antagonists	Prediction for human anxiety disorder
Conflict	+++	+/0	+/0	0	0	GAD
Elevated plus-maze	+++	+/0/ −	+/0	0	0/+	GAD
Social interaction	++	+	+/0	0	+/0	GAD
Light/dark	+++	++	+/0	0	++/0	GAD
Fear-potentiated Startle	++	+	?	0	+	GAD
Pup UV	++	+++	++	0	0	GAD/OCD/ phobias
CUSV	+/0	+++	++	++	0	PD/OCD ?
SIH	+++	++	0	0	0	GAD

+++, very strong anxiolytic; ++, strong anxiolytic; +, moderate anxiolytic; 0, no effect; −, anxiogenic.
Pup UV, ultrasonic pup vocalization; SIH, stress-induced hyperthermia; CUSV, conditioned ultrasonic vocalization.

Another shortcoming of animal anxiety models is that they have never been developed as models of the various anxiety disorders as recognized in DSM-III-R. No specific animal models predict antipanic, antiphobic or anti-OCD properties of newly developed drugs, although certainly attempts have been made.

By studying the effects of clinically relevant drugs in the various animal models, one could get some insight into whether different anxiety models differentiate the various drugs. This may lead to a delineation of animal models of anxiety predicting for the various anxiety disorders.

Table 3 tries to summarize the various animal anxiety models and the anxiolytic potential of the different drug classes in them. As can be seen, almost all models are very sensitive towards classical BZDs, except CUSV.

PD seems to differ from GAD in that classic BZDs are not active or only weakly so, although alprazolam, a triazolobenzodiazepine, is specifically aimed at PD. Furthermore, imipramine and SSRIs are antipanic in contrast to other antidepressants. The CUSV model seems to fit nicely with this profile and has attractive features to detect putative panicolytic properties of drugs. It is as yet unclear whether 5-HT$_{1A}$ receptor agonists will show clear antipanic properties, but if not, this class of drugs would show up as false positive in this test.

The ultrasonic pup vocalization model is interesting because it picks up, besides BZD and 5-HT$_{1A}$ agonists, SSRIs but not imipramine. This suggests that this model may be predictive for GAD, and maybe phobias and OCD, but not for PD.

The SIH test, on the other hand, is insensitive to SSRIs and tricyclic antidepressants, thereby presumably reflecting anti-GAD properties.

In conclusion, prediction of putative antipanic, anti-OCD, antiphobia or anti-GAD properties of drugs, based on outcome in animal models, is not yet possible.

Some promising models for PD seem to emerge (CUSV), but have to be used cautiously.

It is proposed to test new psychoactive drugs in a range of animal anxiety paradigms to obtain an "anxiolytic profile," a kind of fingerprint which may point to putative activity in a certain anxiety disorder.

ACKNOWLEDGMENTS

We thank Marijke Mulder and Ruud van Oorschot for technical support.

REFERENCES

Aron, C., Simon, P. and Boissier, J. R. (1971). Evaluation of a rapid technique for detecting minor tranquilizers. *Neuropharmacologia*, **10**, 459–469.

Ballenger, J. C., Burrows, G. D. and DuPont, R. (1988). Alprazolam in panic disorder and agoraphobia: results from a multicentre trial, I: Efficacy in short-term treatment. *Arch. Gen. Psychiatry*, **45**, 413–422.

Barrett, J. E. (1991). Animal behavioral models in the analysis and understanding of anxiolytic drugs at serotonin receptors. In *Animal Models in Psychopharmacology* (eds B. Olivier, J. Mos and J. L. Slangen), pp. 37–52. Birkhäuser Verlag, Basel.

Barrett, J. E., Witkins, J. M., Mansbach, R. S. *et al.* (1986). Behavioral studies with anxiolytic drugs. III. Antipunishment actions of buspirone in the pigeon do not involve benzodiazepine receptor mechanism. *J. Pharmacol. Exp. Ther.*, **238**, 1009–1013.

Bermant, R. I., Levinson, D. M. and Justesen, D. R. (1979). Classical conditioning of microwave-induced hyperthermia in rats. *Radio Sci.*, **14**, 201–207.

Blanchard, R. J. and Blanchard, D. C. (1989). Antipredator defensive behaviors in a visible burrow system. *J. Comp. Psychol.*, **103**, 70–82.

Blanchard, R. J., Blanchard, D. C. and Hori, K. (1989). An ethoexperimental approach to the study of defense. In *Ethoexperimental Approaches to the Study of Behavior* (eds R. J. Blanchard, P. F. Brain, D. C. Blanchard and S. Parmigiani), pp. 114–136. Kluwer, Dordrecht.

Blanchard, R. J., Blanchard, D. C., Rodgers, J. and Weiss, S. M. (1990a). The characterization and modelling of antipredator defensive behavior. *Neurosci. Biobehav. Rev.*, **14**, 463–472.

Blanchard, R. J., Blanchard, D. C., Weiss, S. M. and Meyer, S. (1990b). The effects of ethanol and diazepam on reactions to predatory odors. *Pharmacol. Biochem. Behav.*, **35**, 775–780.

Blanchard, R. J., Blanchard, D. C., Agullana, R. and Weiss, S. M. (1991). Twenty-two kHz alarm cries to presentation of a predator, by laboratory rats living in visible burrow systems. *Physiol. Behav.*, **50**, 567–572.

Blanchard, D. C., Shepherd, J. K., Rodgers, R. J. and Blanchard, R. J. (1992a). Evidence for differential effects of 8-OH-DPAT on male female rats in the Anxiety/Defense Test Battery. *Psychopharmacology*, **106**, 531–539.

Blanchard, R. J., Agullana, R., McGee, L. *et al.* (1992b). Sex differences in the incidence and sonografic characteristics of antipredator ultrasonic cries in the laboratory rat (Rattus norvegicus). *J. Comp. Psychol.*, **106**, 270–277.

Blanchard, R. J., Shepherd, J. K., Rodgers, R. J. *et al.* (1993). Attenuation of antipredator defensive behavior in rats following chronic treatment with imipramine. *Psychopharmacology*, **110**, 245–253.

Bohus, B. (1974). Telemetered heart rate responses of the rat during free and learned behavior. *Biotelemetry*, **1**, 193–201.

Bolles, R. C. (1970). Species specific defense reactions (SSDR) and avoidance learning. *Psychol. Rev.*, **77**, 32–48.

Borsini, F., Lecci, A., Volterra, G. and Meli, A. (1989). A model to measure anticipatory anxiety in mice? *Psychopharmacology*, **98**, 207–211.

Buwalda, B., Nyakas, C., Koolhaas, J. M. *et al.* (1992). Vasopressin prolongs behavioral and cardiac responses to mild stress in young but not in aged rats. *Physiol. Behav.*, **52**, 1127–1131.

Cassano, G. B., Petracca, A., Perugi, G. *et al.* (1988). Clomipramine for panic disorder: I. The first 10 weeks of a long-term comparison with imipramine. *J. Affect. Disord.*, **14**, 123–127.

Cassella, J. V. and Davis, M. (1985). Fear-enhanced acoustic startle is not attenuated by acute and chronic imipramine treatment in rats. *Psychopharmacology*, **87**, 278–282.

Charney, D. S., Heninger, G. R. and Breier, A. (1984). Noradrenergic functioning in panic anxiety: effects of yohimbine in healthy subjects and patients with agoraphobia and panic disorder. *Arch. Gen. Psychiatry*, **41**, 751–763.

Chouinard, G., Annable, L., Fontaine, R. and Solyon, L. (1982). Alprazolam in the treatment of generalized anxiety and panic disorders: a double-blind, placebo-controlled study. *Psychopharmacology*, **77**, 229–233.

Clement, J. G., Mills, P. and Brockway, B. (1989). Use of telemetry to record body temperature and activity in mice. *J. Pharmacol. Meth.*, **21**, 129–140.

Costall, B., Jones, B. J., Kelly, M. E. *et al.* (1989). Exploration of mice in a black and white test box: validation as a model of anxiety. *Pharmacol. Biochem. Behav.*, **32**, 777–785.

Cuomo, V., Cagiano, R., De Salvia, M. *et al.* (1992). Ultrasonic vocalization as an indicator of emotional state during active avoidance learning in rats. *Life Sci.*, **50**, 1049–1055.

Davis, M., Falls, W. A., Campeau, S. and Kim, S. (1993). Fear-potentiated startle: a neural and pharmacological analysis. *Behav. Brain Res.*, **58**, 175–198.

Den Boer, J. A., Westenberg, H. G. M., Kamerbeek, W. D. J. *et al.* (1987). Effect of serotonin uptake inhibitors in anxiety disorders: a double-blind comparison of clomipramine and fluvoxamine. *Int. Clin. Psychopharmacol.*, **2**, 21–32.

De Vry, J., Benz, U., Schreiber, R. and Traber, J. (1992). Shock-induced ultrasonic vocalization in young adult rats: an animal model for testing the anxiolytic activity of putative anti-anxiety drugs. In *Behavioural Pharmacology of 5-HT$_{1A}$ receptor ligands: Studies on the mechanism of action* (ed. R. Schreiber), pp. 65–83. Krips, Meppel.

Diamant, M., Croiset, G., de Zwart, N. and de Wied, D. (1991). Shock-prod burying test in rats: autonomic and behavioral responses. *Physiol. Behav.*, **50**, 23–31.

Dunner, D. L., Ishiki, D., Avery, D. H. *et al.* (1986). Effect of alprazolam and diazepam on anxiety and panic attacks in panic disorder: a controlled study. *J. Clin. Psychiatry*, **47**, 458–460.

Eikelboom, R. (1986). Learned anticipatory rise in body temperature due to handling. *Physiol. Behav.*, **37**, 649–653.

Eikelboom, R. and Stuart, J. (1979). Conditioned temperature effects using morphine as the unconditioned stimulus. *Psychopharmacology*, **61**, 31–38.

File, S. E. (1980). The use of social interaction as a method for detecting anxiolytic activity of chlordiazepoxide-like drugs. *J. Neurosci. Meth.*, **2**, 219–238.

File, S. E. and Hyde, J. R. G. (1979). A test of anxiety that distinguishes between the actions of benzodiazepines and those of other minor tranquilizers and of stimulants. *Pharmacol. Biochem. Behav.*, **11**, 65–69.

File, S. E. and Zangrossi, H., Jr (1993). "One-trail tolerance" to the anxiolytic actions of benzodiazepines in the elevated plus-maze, or the development of a phobic state? *Psychopharmacology*, **110**, 240–244.

Gardner, C. R. (1985). Distress vocalization in rat pups: a simple screening method for anxiolytic drugs. *J. Pharmacol. Meth.*, **14**, 181–187.

Geller, I. and Seifter, J. (1960). The effects of meprobamate, barbiturates, d-amphetamine and promazine on experimentally induced conflict in the rat. *Psychopharmacologia*, **1**, 482–492.

Goa, K. L. and Ward, A. (1986). Buspirone: a preliminary review of its pharmacological properties and therapeutic efficacy as an anxiolytic. *Drugs*, **32**, 114–129.

Gollnick, P. D. and Ianuzzo, C. D. (1968). Colonic temperature response of rats during exercise. *J., Appl. Physiol.*, **24**, 747–750.

Groenink, L., van der Gugten, J., Zethof, T. *et al.* (1994). Stress-induced hyperthermia in mice: hormonal correlates. *Physiol. Behav.*, **56**, 747–749.

Hagan, J. J. and Bohus, B. (1984). Vasopressin prolongs bradycardiac response during orientation. *Behav. Neural Biol.*, **41**, 77–83.

Handley, S. L. and Mithani, S. (1984). Effects of alpha-adrenoceptor agonists and antagonists in a maze-exploration model of "fear"-motivated behaviour. *Naunyn-Schmiedeberg's Arch. Pharmacol.*, **327**, 1–5.

Hendrie, C. A. and Neill, J. C. (1991). Exposure to the calls of predators of mice activates defensive mechanisms and inhibits consummatory behavior in an inbred mouse strain. *Neurosci. Biobehav. Rev.*, **15**, 479–482.

Hjörth, S., Carlsson, A., Lindberg, P. *et al.* (1982). 8-Hydroxy-2-(di-n-propylamino)tetralin, 8-OH-DPAT, a potent and selective simplified ergot congener with central 5-HT-receptor stimulating activity. *J. Neural Transm.*, **55**, 169–188.

Hofer, M. A. and Shair, H. N. (1987). Isolation distress in two-week old rats: influence of home cage, social companions, and prior experience with littermates. *Dev. Psychobiol.*, **20**, 465–476.

Insel, T. R., Hill, J. L. and Mayor, R. B. (1986). Rat pup isolation calls: possible mediation by the benzodiazepine receptor complex. *Pharmacol. Biochem. Behav.*, **24**, 1263–1267.

Kaltwasser, M. T. (1991). Acoustic startle induced ultrasonic vocalizations in the rats: a novel animal model of anxiety? *Behav. Brain. Res.*, **43**, 133–137.

Kalus, O., Asnis, G. M., Rubinson, E. *et al.* (1991). Desipramine treatment in panic disorder. *J. Affect. Disord.*, **21**, 239–244.

Kluger, M. J., O'Reilly, B., Shope, T. R. and Vander, A. J. (1987). Further evidence that stress hyperthermia is a fever. *Physiol. Behav.*, **39**, 763–766.

Ko, G. N., Elsworth, J. D., Roth, R. H. *et al.* (1983). Panic-induced elevations of plasma MHPG levels in phobic-anxious patients: effects of clonidine and imipramine. *Arch. Gen. Psychiatry*, **40**, 425–450.

Langer, S. Z., Arbilla, S., Tan, S. *et al.* (1990). Selectivity for omega-receptor subtypes as a strategy for the development of anxiolytic drugs. *Pharmacopsychiatry*, **23**, 103–107.

Lesch, K. P., Wiesman, M., Hoh, A. *et al.* (1992). 5-HT$_{1A}$ receptor-effector system responsivity in panic disorder. *Psychopharmacology*, **106**, 111–117.

Levin, A. P. and Liebowitz, M. R. (1987). Drug treatment of phobias: efficacy and optimum use. *Drugs*, **34**, 504–514.

Long, N. C., Vander, A. J. and Kluger, M. J. (1990). Stress-induced rise of body temperature in rats is the same in warm and cool environments. *Physiol. Behav.*, **47**, 773–775.

Martin, K. F. and Mason, R. (1987). Ipsapirone is a partial agonist at 5-hydroxytryptamine$_{1A}$ receptors in the rat hippocampus: electrophysiological evidence. *Eur. J. Pharmacol.*, **141**, 479–484.

Mavissakalian, M. and Michelson, L. (1986). Agoraphobia: relative and combined effectiveness of therapist-assisted in vivo exposure and imipramine. *J. Clin. Psychiatry*, **47**, 117–122.

McNair, D. M. and Kahn, R. J. (1981). Imipramine compared with a benzodiazepine for agoraphobia. In *Anxiety: New Research and Changing Concepts* (eds D. F. Klein and J. Rabkin), pp. 69–80. Raven Press, New York.

McTavish, T. and Benfield, P. (1990). Clomipramine: an overview of its pharmacological properties and a review of its therapeutic use in obsessive compulsive disorder and panic disorder. *Drugs*, **39**, 136–153.

Miczek, K. A. and Vivian, J. A. (1993). Automated quantification of withdrawal from 5-day diazepam in rats: ultrasonic distress vocalizations and hyperreflexia to acoustic startle stimuli. *Psychopharmacology*, **110**, 379–382.

Molewijk, H. E., Van der Poel, A. M., Vedder, A. W. and Olivier, B. (1993). Suppression of ultrasonic vocalizations in adult rats by flesinoxan, ipsapirone, alprazolam, clonidine and fluvoxamine. *Behav. Proc.*, **29**, 120.

Molewijk, H. E., Van der Poel, A. M., Mos, J. *et al.* (1995). Conditioned ultrasonic distress vocalizations in adult male rats as a behavioural paradigm for screening anti-panic drugs. *Psychopharmacology*, **117**, 32–40.

Mos, J. and Olivier, B. (1989). Ultrasonic vocalizations by rat pups as an animal model for anxiolytic activity: effects of serotonergic drugs. In *Behavioural Pharmacology of 5-HT* (eds P. Bevan, A. R. Cools and T. Archer), pp. 361–366. Erlbaum, Hillsdale, NJ.

Myron, A. and Hofer, M. D. (1970). Cardiac and respiratory function during sudden prolonged immobility in wild rodents. *Psychosom. Med.*, **32**, 633–647.

Nakamori, T., Morimoto, A., Morimoto, K. *et al.* (1993). Effects of α-and β-adrenergic antagonists on rise in body temperature induced by psychological stress in rats. *Am. J. Physiol.*, **264**, R156–R161.

Noyes, R., Jr, Anderson, D. J. and Clancy, J. (1984). Diazepam and propranolol in panic disorder and agoraphobia. *Arch. Gen. Psychiatry*, **41**, 287–292.

Nutt, D. J., Glue, P., Lawson, C. and Wilson, S. (1990). Flumazenil provocation of panic attacks: evidence for altered benzodiazepine receptor sensitivity in panic disorder. *Arch. Gen. Psychiatry*, **47**, 917–925.

Poole, S. and Stephenson, J. D. (1977). Core temperature: some shortcomings of rectal temperature measurements. *Physiol. Behav.*, **18**, 203–205.

Reeves, D. L., Levinson, D. M., Justesen, D. R. and Lubin, B. (1985). Endogenous hyperthermia in normal human subjects: experimental study of emotional states (II). *Int. J. Psychosom.*, **32**, 18–23.

Robinson, D. S., Shrotriya, R. C., Alms, D. R. *et al.* (1989). Treatment of panic disorder: nonbenzodiazepine anxiolytics including buspirone. *Psychopharmacol. Bull.*, **25**, 21–26.

Sanchez, C. (1993). Effect of serotonergic drugs on footshock-induced ultrasonic vocalization in adult male rats. *Behav. Pharmacol.*, **4**, 269–277.

Sanger, D. J., Joly, D. and Zivkovic, B. (1985). Behavioral effects of nonbenzodiazepine anxiolytic drugs: a comparison of CGS 9896 and zopiclone with chlordiazepoxide. *J. Pharmacol. Exp. Ther.*, **232**, 831–837.

Sanger, D. J., Perrault, G., Morel, E. *et al.* (1987). The behavioural profile of zolpidem, a novel hypnotic drug of imidazopyridine structure. *Physiol. Behav.*, **41**, 235–240.

Schneier, F. R., Carrasco, J. L., Hollander, E. *et al.* (1993). Alpidem in the treatment of panic disorder. *J. Clin. Psychopharmacol.*, **13**, 150–153.

Sheehan, D. V. (1982). Current views in the treatment of panic and phobic disorders. *Drug Ther. Hosp.*, **7**, 74–93.

Sheehan, D. V., Raj, A. B., Sheehan, K. H. and Soto, S. (1990). Is buspirone effective for panic disorder? *J. Clin. Psychopharmacol.*, **10**, 3–11.

Sheehan, D. V., Raj, A. B., Harnett Sheehan, K. *et al.* (1993). The relative efficacy of high-dose buspirone and alprazolam in the treatment of panic disorder: a double-blind placebo-controlled study. *Acta Psychiatr. Scand.*, **88**, 1–11.

Singer, R., Harker, C. T., Vander, A. J. and Kluger, M. J. (1986). Hyperthermia induced by open-field stress is blocked by salicylate. *Physiol. Behav.*, **36**, 1179–1182.

Steenbergen, J. M., Koolhaas, J. M., Strubbe, J. H. and Bohus, B. (1989). Behavioral and cardiac responses to a sudden change in environmental stimuli: effect on forced shift in food intake. *Physiol. Behav.*, **45**, 729–733.

Swinson, R. P. and Kuch, K. (1990). Clinical features of panic and related disorders. In *Clinical Aspects of Panic Disorder* (ed. J. C. Ballinger), pp. 13–30. Wiley–Liss, New York.

Tonoue, T., Ashida, Y., Makino, H. and Hata, H. (1986). Inhibition of shock-elicited ultrasonic vocalization by opioid peptides in the rat: a psychotropic effect. *Psychoneuroendocrinology*, **11**, 177–184.

Tornatzky, W. and Miczek, K. A. (1992). Behaviour and telemetered autonomic responses to alcohol and social stress. *Soc. Neurosci. Abstr.*, **18**, 715.

Uhde, T. W., Stein, M. B., Vittone, B. J. *et al.* (1989). Behavioural and physiological effects of short-term and long-term administration of clonidine in panic disorder. *Arch. Gen. Psychiatry*, **46**, 170–177.

Van der Poel, A. M. and Miczek, K. A. (1991). Long ultrasonic calls in male rats following mating, defeat, aversive stimulation: frequency modulation and bout structure. *Behaviour*, **119**, 127–142.

Van der Poel, A. M., Noach, E. J. K. and Miczek, K. A. (1989). Temporal pattern of ultrasonic distress calls in the adult rat: effects of morphine and benzodiazepines. *Psychopharmacology*, **97**, 147–148.

Van Dijken, H. H., Van der Heyden, J. A. M., Mos, J. and Tilders, F. J. H. (1992a). Inescapable footshocks induce progressive and long-lasting behavioral changes in male rats. *Physiol. Behav.*, **51**, 787–794.

Van Dijken, H. H., Mos, J., Van der Heyden, J. A. M. and Tilders, F. J. H. (1992b). Characterization of stress-induced long-term behavioral changes in rats: evidence in favor of anxiety. *Physiol. Behav.*, **52**, 945–951.

Vivian, J. A. and Miczek, K. A. (1993). Diazepam and gepirone selectively attenuate either 20–32 or 32–64 kHz ultrasonic vocalizations during aggressive encounters. *Psychopharmacology*, **112**, 66–73.

Vogel, J. R., Beer, B. and Coldy, D. E. (1971). A simple and reliable conflict procedure for testing anti-anxiety agents. *Psychopharmacologia*, **21**, 1–7.

Wan, R., Diamant, M., De Jong, W. and De Wied, D. (1990). Changes in heart rate and body temperature during passive avoidance behavior in rats. *Physiol. Behav.*, **47**, 493–499.

Westenberg, H. G. M. and Den Boer, J. A. (1989). Selective monoamine uptake inhibitors and a serotonin antagonist in the treatment of panic disorder. *Psychopharmacol. Bull.*, **25**, 119–123.

Westenberg, H. G. M. and Den Boer, J. A. (1990). Guidelines to ensure antipanic drugs are effective. *Clin. Neuropharmacol.*, **13**, 655–656.

Winter, J. C. and Rabin, R. (1992). Yohimbine as a serotonergic agent: evidence from receptor binding and drug discrimination. *J. Pharmacol. Exp. Ther.*, **263**, 682–689.

Woods, S. W., Charney, D. S., Silver, J. M. *et al.* (1991). Behavioural, biochemical and cardiovascular responses to the benzodiazepine receptor antagonist flumazenil in panic disorder. *Psychiatry Res.*, **36**, 155–172.

Wouters, W., Hartog, J. and Bevan, P. (1988). Flesinoxan. *Drug Dev. Rev.*, **6**, 71–83.

Ybema, C. E., Slangen, J. L., Olivier, B. and Mos, J. (1993). Dose-dependent discriminative stimulus properties of 8-OH-DPAT. *Behav. Pharmacol.*, **4**, 610–624.

Yocca, F. D., Hyslop, D. K., Smith, D. W. and Maayani, S. (1987). BMY 7378, a buspirone analogue with high affinity, selectivity and low intrinsic activity at the $5-HT_{1A}$ receptor in rat and guinea pig hippocampal membranes. *Eur. J. Pharmacol.*, **137**, 293–294.

York, J. L. and Regan, S. G. (1982). Conditioned and unconditioned influences on body temperature and ethanol hypothermia in laboratory rats. *Pharmacol. Biochem. Behav.*, **17**, 199–142.

Yoshiue, S., Yoshizawa, H., Ito, H. *et al.* (1989). Analysis of body temperature at different sites in patients having slight fever caused by psychogenic stress. In *Thermoregulation: Research and Clinical Applications* (eds P. Lomax and S. Schönbaum), pp. 169–172. Karger, Basel.

Zangrossi, H., Jr and File, S. E. (1992). Chlordiazepoxide reduces the generalized anxiety, but not the direct responses, of rats exposed to cat odor. *Pharmacol. Biochem. Behav.*, **43**, 1195–1200.

Zethof, T. J. J., van der Heyden, J. A. M. and Olivier, B. (1991). A new animal model for anticipatory anxiety? In *Animal Models in Psychopharmacology* (eds B. Olivier, J. Mos and J. L. Slangen), pp. 65–68. Birkhäuser Verlag, Basel.

Zethof, T. J. J., van der Heyden, J. A. M., Tolboom, J. T. B. M. and Olivier, B. (1994). Stress-induced hyperthermia in mice: a methodological study. *Physiol. Behav.*, **55**, 109–115.

Zitrin, C. M., Klein, D. F. and Woerner, M. G. (1980). Treatment of agoraphobia with group exposure in vivo and imipramine. *Arch. Gen. Psychiatry*, **37**, 63–72.

Zivkovic, B., Morel, E., Joly, D. *et al.* (1990). Pharmacological and behavioural profile of alpidem as an anxiolytic. *Pharmacopsychiatry*, (Suppl.) **23**, 108–113.

6 A Critical Review of the Role of Norepinephrine in Panic Disorder: Focus on its Interaction with Serotonin

ANDREW W. GODDARD[1], SCOTT W. WOODS[1] AND DENNIS S. CHARNEY[2]

[1]*Yale University Department of Psychiatry, New Haven, and* [2]*Veterans Administration Medical Center, West Haven, Connecticut, USA*

INTRODUCTION

The recognition of panic disorder (PD) as a discrete psychiatric syndrome in the 1960s, prompted by the discovery of the efficacy of imipramine in patients with panic episodes, launched the modern era of research in PD. The presence of autonomic symptoms during panic attacks such as palpitations, sweating, tremulousness, flushing, and dizziness, together with the clinical efficacy of imipramine, have led investigators to pursue abnormalities in the norepine-phrine (NE) system to explain the pathophysiology and natural history of PD. Although our current state of knowledge suggests that there are probably a vari-ety of dysfunctions in multiple neurotransmitter systems in PD (Nutt and Lawson, 1992), the NE system, and more recently the serotonin (5-HT) system, have occupied a prominent place in recent research efforts. This review will evaluate the evidence supporting an NE hypothesis of PD. The role of the 5-HT system in PD will also be examined. Finally, preclinical and clinical data impli-cating 5-HT modulation of NE function will be presented and its relevance to the pathophysiology and treatment of PD outlined.

THE NOREPINEPHRINE SYSTEM IN PANIC DISORDER

PRECLINICAL STUDIES

Anatomy

The NE neuronal system projects from the locus coeruleus (LC), the major NE nucleus in the brain, to multiple brain target areas implicated in anxiety and fear

Advances in the Neurobiology of Anxiety Disorders. Edited by H. G. M. Westenberg, J. A. Den Boer and D. L. Murphy
©1996 John Wiley & Sons Ltd

behaviors such as the amygdala, hippocampus, and cortex and spinal cord (Fillenz, 1990). The LC receives afferent inputs from the sensory systems which monitor the internal and external environments (Cedarbaum and Aghajanian, 1978; Aston-Jones and Ennis, 1988; Aston-Jones et al., 1986, 1991a, 1991b; Rasmussen and Aghajanian, 1989a, 1989b; Craig, 1992). Thus, the NE system is well situated anatomically to integrate and coordinate fear responses to threatening stimuli. The hypothesis that the LC–NE system functions as a fear/alarm system in animals was first advanced by Redmond and Huang (1979).

Fear behavior and norepinephrine function

A series of experiments has examined the relationship between fear behaviors and LC activity. Electrical stimulation of the LC produced fear behaviors in stump-tailed monkeys (Redmond and Huang, 1979; Redmond et al., 1976), while exposure of freely moving cats to dangerous or threatening situations (restraint, exposure to a dog) resulted in increased LC firing (Abercrombie and Jacobs, 1987a, 1987b; Rasmussen et al., 1986; Levine et al., 1990). In contrast, elevated LC firing rates were not observed in cats following exposure to activating but non-stressful stimuli such as administration of food or exposure to inaccessible rats (Abercrombie and Jacobs, 1987a). This response to fear-provoking stimuli appears to be specific to the LC since there was no evoked increase in electrical activity in cells of the dorsal raphe nuclei or substantia nigra under similar conditions (Strecker and Jacobs, 1985; Wilkinson and Jacobs, 1988). The increased firing rate of the LC following administration of the α_2-adrenergic antagonist, yohimbine, has also been associated with fear states in animals (Redmond and Huang, 1979). Conversely, agents that decrease NE function via suppression of LC activity such as clonidine have tended to decrease fear in non-human primates, and inhibit the behavioral effects of electrical stimulation of the LC (Gold and Redmond, 1977). Bilateral lesions of the LC in the stump-tailed monkey were associated with decreases in fear behaviors found in a social group (Redmond et al., 1976), and in response to threatening human behavior (Huang et al., 1976).

Other investigators, also using direct recording techniques of LC neurons in awake animals, have reported increased phasic LC activity to a variety of environmental sensory stimuli associated with novelty and fear (Foote and Bloom, 1979; Foote et al., 1980; Aston-Jones and Bloom, 1981). In these studies LC activity level was positively correlated with vigilance. Conversely, vegetative activities such as sleeping, grooming and sweet water consumption, by comparison, were associated with low levels of LC activity. Thus, the LC–NE system may also function as an orienting system, which focuses brain activity on external stimuli relevant to survival.

Parallel functioning of the central and peripheral norepinephrine systems

The central and peripheral NE systems function in a parallel fashion, a fact which has important implications for human anxiety disorders. Elam *et al.* (1986) observed parallel activation of the LC and splanchnic sympathetic neurons following cutaneous noxious and non-noxious thermal stimuli. Furthermore, an elegant series of studies has documented the existence of peripheral autonomic regulation of LC neurons in a variety of contexts (Svensson, 1987), implicating the LC as a monitor of interoceptive stimuli. Specifically, acute reductions in blood volume and blood pressure, hypoxia, hypercapnia, and acute visceral distension (bladder, distal colon, rectum, stomach) have been observed to produce parallel activations in peripheral sympathetic and LC activity. Given its sensitivity to both the external and internal environments, the LC may function as an integrative system, which orients the behavior of the organism towards salient external or internal stimuli which could be life-threatening.

These data have considerable relevance to the pathophysiology and treatment of PD. Interoceptive cues are known to trigger clinical panic in many patients, and PD patients are frequently somatically preoccupied early in the course of their illness. Conversely, these patients are often sensitive to mild external stressors and are prone to develop phobias as a result. A hypothesis of overactivity in the LC–NE system in PD helps to explain these clinical phenomena. In addition, effective pharmacologic and behavioral treatments for PD tend to reduce the sensitivity of patients to internal and external environmental cues.

Behavioral stress and norepinephrine function

Preclinical studies have documented significant increases in central NE function following a variety of stressors. Immobilization stress in rats increased NE turnover in the forebrain, which effect was blocked by benzodiazepines (Corrodi *et al.*, 1971). Controllable shock stress to rats either caused no change or a decrease in NE turnover, while uncontrollable shock stress increased brain NE turnover (Tsuda and Tanaka, 1985). In this series of studies rats were also able to reverse the elevation in NE turnover during a shock stress by mastering a task which reduced the shock intensity. Recent studies of behavioral sensitization suggest the involvement of NE mechanisms. For example, prior chronic stress in rats produced enhanced NE synthesis and release in the hippocampus following exposure to a novel stress (Nisenbaum *et al.*, 1991). Repeated shock stress was observed to decrease the shock stimulus required to produce a given increase in NE function (Irwin *et al.*, 1986). A recently conducted *in vivo* dialysis study in rats reported stress-induced sensitization of NE release in medial frontal cortex (Finlay and Abercrombie, 1991). These mechanisms may be relevant to the pathogenesis of PD. In particular the relationship of stressful life events to the onset of panic, the tendency for patients to have a chronic course (perhaps related to chronic uncontrollable stress due to repeated panic attacks), and the acquisition of phobias may be explained by these basic processes.

Fear conditioning and the norepinephrine system

The NE system has also been implicated in fear conditioning of animals. For example, it has been reported that an intact NE system may be required for the acquisition of conditioned fear responses in rats (Tsaltas *et al.*, 1987; Cole and Robbins, 1987). Neutral stimuli which have been previously paired with a shock have been observed to produce similar increases in NE metabolism and behavioral impairments to those seen during exposure to shock alone (Cassens *et al.*, 1981; Tanaka *et al.*, 1986). Increased LC firing rate in response to a previously neutral acoustic stimulus was observed following fear conditioning in freely moving cats (Rasmussen *et al.*, 1986). These data raise the possibility that the NE system is instrumental in the development of phobic acquisition in PD patients. Furthermore, a fear-potentiated startle paradigm has been used to evaluate fear conditioning and anticipatory fear in rats (Davis, 1990). Administration of the α_2-adrenoreceptor antagonist, yohimbine, has been found to augment startle responses in this paradigm (Davis *et al.*, 1979), suggesting that NE hyperactivity (which is hypothesized to be present in PD) may precipitate abnormal anticipatory fear in humans.

Antipanic medications and norepinephrine function

The clinical efficacy of imipramine (Zitrin *et al.*, 1983), an NE reuptake blocker, and the monoamine oxidase inhibitor (MAOI), phenelzine (Tyrer *et al.*, 1973), indirectly suggests underlying abnormalities of NE function in PD. In animal studies both tricyclics and MAOIs have a variety of inhibitory effects on NE function including reduction in LC firing rates, NE turnover, tyrosine hydroxylase activity and postsynaptic β-receptor number and functioning (Charney *et al.*, 1981; Sugrue, 1983; Sulser, 1984; Nyback *et al.*, 1975; Svensson and Usdin, 1978; Keith *et al.*, 1986). However, these compounds may also affect 5-HT function (Blier *et al.*, 1987), and other neural systems, and therefore their therapeutic mechanism of action in PD may be complex.

CLINICAL STUDIES OF NOREPINEPHRINE IN PANIC DISORDER

Introduction

In this section clinical biological studies of NE function in PD will be reviewed. Studies of platelet NE function in PD will be briefly mentioned. Then neurobiologic challenge studies addressing this topic will be described. Finally, a genetic study examining adrenoreceptor abnormalities in PD will be discussed. A critique of the role of NE in PD will conclude the clinical NE section.

Platelet studies

Clinical studies comparing PD patients to healthy control subjects have reported abnormalities in the α_2-adrenoreceptor in PD patients. For example, Cameron *et al.* (1984, 1990) observed a reduction in the density (B_{max}) of platelet α_2-receptors in PD patients. However, these changes have not been replicated by other groups (Nutt and Fraser, 1987; Norman *et al.*, 1987; Charney *et al.*, 1989a). These findings suggest that some peripheral indices of NE function are not consistently abnormal in PD.

Neurobiologic challenge studies

Pharmacologic challenge studies (summarized in Table 1) have also attempted to evaluate adrenoreceptor functioning in PD. A series of studies has evaluated central α_2-receptor functioning in PD with the selective antagonist, yohimbine. A subgroup of PD patients (63%) experienced increased anxiety and panic symptoms in response to oral (Charney and Heninger, 1985; Charney *et al.*, 1987a) or intravenous (Charney *et al.*, 1992) administration of yohimbine, together with elevated plasma 3-methoxy-4-hydroxyphenethyleneglycol (MHPG) and cortisol, elevated blood pressure and heart rate. These behavioral and neuroendocrine findings have been well replicated (see Table 1). Questions have been raised about whether or not systemic administration of yohimbine influences presynaptic α_2-receptor functioning in the way that these clinical studies assume. However, a recent study in rats, which simultaneously measured brain and plasma NE and MHPG in response to yohimbine 1 mg/kg i.v., found enhanced brain release of NE and elevated brain and plasma levels of titrated MHPG following yohimbine, consistent with inhibition of the somatodendritic α_2-autoreceptor (Szemeredi *et al.*, 1991).

Another clinical probe of NE function in PD has been the α_2-adrenoreceptor agonist, clonidine. Clonidine administration caused greater hypotension, greater decreases in plasma MHPG, and less sedation in panic patients than in controls (Charney and Heninger, 1986a). These findings have also been consistently replicated (see Table 1; also Nutt, 1989; Coplan *et al.*, 1993). Panic patients who had manifested yohimbine-induced panic were found to be more likely to have the response to clonidine described above compared to controls (Charney *et al.*, 1992). These data suggest that presynaptic α_2-adrenoreceptor sensitivity is increased in PD. In addition the growth hormone (GH) response to clonidine has been found to be blunted in PD patients in relation to controls (Uhde *et al.*, 1986; Charney and Heninger, 1986a; Nutt, 1989), suggesting subsensitivity of central postsynaptic α_2-adrenoreceptors in PD. The GH finding is not specific to PD and has also been reported in depression and generalized anxiety disorder (Abelson *et al.*, 1991). In conclusion, panic patients have consistently abnormal responses to α_2-adrenoreceptor agonists and antagonists. However, no simple explanation can account for the sensitivity of PD patients to both clonidine and yohimbine. Possibilities include a primary dysregulation in the α_2-adrenoreceptor itself, dysregulation of intracellular second and third messenger systems

Table 1. Neurobiologic challenge studies of norepinephrine function in panic disorder

Agent	Reference	Design	Measures	Results
Yohimbine	Charney and Heninger (1984)	P=39, C=20 Yohimbine 20 mg p.o.	Mood, panic symptoms BP, HR, MHPG[a]	↑ Anxiety, ↑ physical Sx P>C ↑ Sitting systolic BP, MHPG P>C
	Charney et al. (1987a)	P=68, C=20 Yohimbine 20 mg p.o.	Mood, panic attacks and symptoms BP, HR, MHPG and cortisol	Panic attacks in 54% P vs 5% C ↑ MHPG and cortisol in panicking P vs C ↑ Systolic BP and HR in panicking P vs C
	Gurguis and Uhde (1990)	P=11, C=7 Yohimbine 20 mg p.o.	Mood, MHPG, GH	↑ Anxiety, ↑ MHPG P>C Anxiety and MHPG Δ is correlated in P
	Woods et al. (1991)	P=14, C=11 Yohimbine 0.4 mg/kg i.v.	Mood, panic attacks MHPG, cortisol	Panic attacks in 63% P vs 9% C Bilateral ↓ in frontal CBF P vs C ↑ MHPG and cortisol P>C
	Charney et al. (1992)	P=38, C=15 Yohimbine 0.4 mg/kg i.v.	Mood, panic attacks BP, HR, MHPG, cortisol	Panic attacks in 63% P vs 7% C Replicated ↑ MHPG in panicking P>C
	Albus et al. (1992)	P=15, C=12 Yohimbine 20 mg p.o.	Mood, BP, HR, skin temp., NE, cortisol	↑ Anxiety, ↑ panic feelings P>C ↑ HR & ↓ skin temp, ↑ NE P>C
Clonidine	Charney and Heninger (1986a)	P=26, C=21 Clonidine 0.15 mg i.v.	Mood, sedation, BP, HR MHPG, GH	↓ BP, ↓ MHPG P>C Blunted GH response P vs C, sedation P<C
	Nutt (1989)	P=8, C=8 Clonidine 1.5 µg/kg i.v.	BP, HR	↓ BP and HR post clonidine P>C
	Uhde et al. (1986)	P=11, P(D)=11, C=11 Clonidine 2 µg/kg i.v.	GH	Blunted GH response in P and P(D) vs C
	Charney et al. (1992)	P=38, C=15 Clonidine 2µg/kg i.v.	GH, MHPG, HR, BP	Blunted GH response, greater ↓ MHPG from baseline in panicking P vs C

Isoproterenol	Rainey et al. (1984)	P=11, C=10 Isoproterenol infusion 1 μg/min i.v.	Panic symptoms		Panic attacks in 74% P vs 6% C
	Nesse et al. (1984)	P=14, C=6 Isoproterenol 0.06–4.0 μg i.v. bolus	Panic symptoms GH and cortisol, HR, BP		Anxiety responses P=C GH & cortisol ↑ in P vs C Blunted HR response in P vs C
	Pohl et al. (1988)	P=86, C=45 Isoproterenol infusion 1 μg/min i.v.	Panic symptoms		Panic attacks in 66% P vs 9% C

BP, blood pressure; C, healthy controls; GH, growth hormone; HR, heart rate; i.v., intravenous; p.o., orally; CBF, cerebral blood flow; MHPG, 3-methoxy-4-hydroxyphenylglycol; NE, norepinephrine; P, panic patients; P(D), depressed patients.
[a]All neuroendocrine measures are plasma measures.

linked to this receptor, or dysregulation of other non-NE neurotransmitter systems with significant input to the LC, in panic patients (Redmond, 1987).

β-Adrenoreceptor functioning has also been an object of study in PD. Infusion of isoproterenol, a peripherally acting compound that is selective for the β-adrenoreceptor, has been reported to trigger anxiety responses in panic patients compared to controls (Rainey et al., 1984; Pohl et al., 1985, 1988). Successful treatment of panic patients with tricyclic antidepressants blunted isoproterenol-induced anxiety and systolic blood pressure responses (Pohl et al., 1990). These studies are consistent with the hypothesis of increased β_1-adrenoreceptor sensitivity in PD, which is normalized by effective pharmacotherapy. However, Nesse et al. (1984) observed no differences between drug-free panic patients and controls in behavioral responses to intravenous isoproterenol. The mechanism of isoproterenol-induced panic remains to be clarified by future research.

Genetic studies

Given the wealth of clinical evidence linking PD to dysfunctions in the NE system, adrenergic receptor genes have been used as candidate genes in a recent linkage study of PD (Wang et al., 1992). Fourteen multiplex pedigrees with DSM-III PD or agoraphobia with panic attacks were studied, and loci for the α_1 and α_2, and β_1 and β_2-adrenoreceptors were included in the genetic analysis. No evidence of linkage was found to any of the loci studied (all lod scores <−2.0). These data do not support a mutation in the above adrenoreceptors as the cause of PD in the families studied. However, the possibility remains that there may be abnormalities in second and third messenger systems within NE neurons, or abnormalities in other receptor subtypes such as the β_3-receptor (Emorine et al., 1989) in PD. In addition some abnormalities in receptor functioning may not be identified by genetic studies.

CRITIQUE OF THE NOREPINEPHRINE HYPOTHESIS OF PANIC DISORDER

While the NE theory of PD continues to have utility as a working hypothesis, some data do not support the theory. For example, sodium lactate did not seem to affect the NE system since it did not alter plasma MHPG (Carr et al., 1986) and clonidine only partially reversed lactate-induced panic (Coplan et al., 1992). Also, contrary to the prediction of the NE hypothesis, phobic exposure of panic patients did not significantly alter plasma MHPG (Woods et al., 1987). However, it should be emphasized that plasma MHPG is not thought to be an accurate and sensitive measure of central NE function. In addition about a third of PD patients are insensitive to yohimbine testing. Yohimbine-induced panic, however, is relatively specific to PD (Charney et al., 1984; Glazer et al., 1987; Heninger et al., 1988; Rasmussen et al., 1987; Charney et al., 1989b), although a recent study has demonstrated that patients with post-traumatic stress disorder may also experience yohimbine-induced panic attacks (Southwick *et al.*, 1993). The latter finding is not unexpected given the preclinical data reviewed earlier, linking stress to changes in NE function.

Chronic treatment with the antipanic agent imipramine, which significantly decreases NE function, did not block yohimbine-induced panic in 11 patients (Charney and Heninger, 1985). However, preclinical data (Svensson and Usdin, 1978) has documented decreased LC firing after chronic administration of imipramine in rats, which is reversed by single-dose administration of yohimbine 2 mg/kg i.v. Part of the mechanism of action of imipramine may involve sustained inhibition of the presynaptic α_2-autoreceptor from elevated synaptic concentrations of endogenous NE, an effect which is temporarily interrupted by yohimbine. This may explain the breakthrough panic finding of Charney and Heninger (1985). Finally, the clinical response of PD to a variety of pharmacotherapeutic agents, including benzodiazepines (Ballenger *et al.*, 1988), tricyclics (TCAs) (Zitrin *et al.*, 1983), MAOIs (Tyrer *et al.*, 1973), serotonin reuptake inhibitors (SRIs) (Beaumont, 1977; Den Boer *et al.*, 1987; Den Boer and Westenberg, 1990a, 1990b; Evans *et al.*, 1986), and cognitive-behavioral treatments (Barlow, 1988), suggests the involvement of other neurotransmitter systems beyond NE in PD.

THE SEROTONIN SYSTEM IN PANIC DISORDER

Preclinical studies using various methods including electrical stimulation, anatomic lesioning and pharmacologic manipulation have suggested an important role for the 5-HT system in the expression of fear in animals (Kahn *et al.*, 1988a, 1988b).

Clinical neurobiologic studies of 5-HT function in PD, however, have produced mixed results. Platelet imipramine binding (a marker of the serotonin reuptake site) has generally been normal in PD (Uhde *et al.*, 1987; Innis *et al.*, 1987), while platelet 5-HT uptake in PD has been reported to be elevated (Norman *et al.*, 1986), normal (Balon *et al.*, 1987), or reduced (Pecknold *et al.*, 1988). Thus, no clear pattern of abnormality in 5-HT function in PD has emerged from analysis of peripheral blood elements. Alternatively, measurement of plasma 5-HT levels (Schneider *et al.*, 1987) indicated that PD patients had lower levels of circulating 5-HT in comparison to controls. The authors speculated that decreased 5-HT function may be part of the pathophysiology of PD, and that SRI medications, therefore, may be preferred treatments for the disorder.

To date, pharmacologic challenge studies of 5-HT in PD (summarized in Tables 2 and 3) have also been unable to establish a definite role for 5-HT in the pathophysiology of panic. Challenges with the 5-HT precursors L-tryptophan (Charney and Heninger, 1986b) and 5-hydroxytryptophan (5-HTP) (Den Boer and Westenberg, 1990b) did not discriminate between PD and controls on neuro-endocrine measures. Conversely, tryptophan depletion was not anxiogenic in unmedicated PD patients (Goddard et al., 1994). However, challenge with the 5-HT releasing agent, fenfluramine, has been reported to be anxiogenic and to increase plasma prolactin and cortisol in PD compared to controls (Targum and Marshall, 1989). Studies with the 5-HT agonist m-chlorophenylpiperazine (mCPP), a probe of postsynaptic 5-HT$_{1C}$ and 5-HT$_2$ receptor function, have produced equivocal findings. Increases in anxiety and plasma cortisol in PD patients compared to controls have been reported with oral (Kahn et al., 1988a, 1988b) but not intravenous administration of mCPP (Charney et al., 1987b; Germine et al.,1994).

Recent advances in 5-HT receptor pharmacology have identified at least three distinct families of 5-HT receptor and multiple subtypes within those families (Schmidt and Peroutka, 1989). The challenge studies reviewed above have manipulated "global" 5-HT functioning in PD or have used probes that lack selectivity (e.g. mCPP) without taking into account the full complexity of the 5-HT system and subsystems. In an attempt to address this problem a more recent study used the selective 5-HT$_{1A}$ partial agonist ipsapirone (IPS) as a challenge agent (Lesch et al., 1992; see Table 2). Corticotropin (ACTH), cortisol, and hypothermic responses to IPS were blunted in PD patients, but anxiety responses did not differ from controls. These data, if replicated, would implicate 5-HT$_{1A}$ receptor subsensitivity in the pathophysiology of PD. In conclusion the 5-HT system or one of its subsystems may have a role in the pathophysiology of PD, the precise nature of which needs to be delineated by further investigation.

In contrast to the uncertainty about the role of 5-HT in the pathogenesis of PD, there is a well-established role for 5-HT in the treatment of panic. Many compounds which affect 5-HT function are associated with clinical improvement of panic symptomatology. These include the serotonin precursor 5-HTP (Kahn and Westenberg, 1985), the SRIs fluvoxamine (Den Boer et al., 1987; Den Boer and Westenberg, 1990a), fluoxetine (Gorman et al., 1987), zimelidine (Evans et al., 1986), clomipramine (Beaumont, 1977; Den Boer et al., 1987), and other drugs which may increase net 5-HT neurotransmission such as TCAs and MAOIs (De Montigny et al., 1990; Blier et al., 1987). There are two studies that suggest that SRIs may even be superior in efficacy to medications which influence NE function (Den Boer and Westenberg, 1988; Modigh et al., 1992).

INTERACTIONS BETWEEN SEROTONIN AND NOREPINEPHRINE IN PANIC DISORDER

INTRODUCTION

The considerable body of evidence implicating NE dysfunction in the pathophysiology of PD, together with the convincing reports of clinical efficacy of SRI medications in the treatment of this disorder, raise the interesting question

Table 2. Neurobiologic challenge studies of serotonin function in panic disorder

Agent	Reference	Design	Measures	Results
mCPP	Charney et al. (1987b)	P=23, C=19 mCPP 0.1 mg/kg i.v.	Mood, panic symptoms GH, PRL, cortisol[a]	Panic episodes in 52% P vs 31% C ↑ GH, PRL, cortisol P=C
	Kahn et al. (1988b)	P=10, C=11, P(D)=10 mCPP 0.25 mg/kg p.o.	Mood, panic attacks	Panic attacks in 60% P vs 0% C, P(D)
	Kahn et al. (1988a)	P=13, C=15, P(D)=17 mCPP 0.25 mg/kg p.o.	Cortisol	↑ Cortisol release in P vs C and P(D)
	Germine et al. (1994)	P=27, C=22, mCPP 0.05 mg/kg i.v.	Mood, panic symptoms GH, PRL, cortisol GH,	↑ Anxiety P=C ↑ GH, PRL, cortisol responses P=C
Tryptophan	Charney and Heninger (1986b)	P=23, C=21 Tryptophan 7 g i.v. Pre & post alprazolam treatment 9/23 P	PRL	↑ PRL P=C PRL responses not altered by alprazolam treatment
Fenfluramine	Targum and Marshall (1989)	P=9, C=9, P(D)=9 Fenfluramine 60 mg p.o.	Mood, PRL, cortisol	↑ Anxiety in P>C and P(D) ↑ PRL, ↑ cortisol P>C and P(D)
IPS	Lesch et al. (1992)	P=14, C=14 IPS 0.3 mg/kg p.o.	Mood, temperature, plasma cortisol, ACTH	No consistent mood Δ P=C ↓ Temperature P>C ACTH, cortisol responses blunted P vs C

ACTH, adrenocorticotropic hormone, GH, growth hormone, IPS, ipsapirone; PRL, prolactin, i.v., intravenous; mCPP, *m*-chlorophenylpiperazine; p.o. orally; P, panic patients, P(D),
depressed patients. c, control; Δ = change.
[a]All neuroendocrine measures are plasma measures.

of whether or not the SRIs may affect NE function in PD via specific central 5-HT/NE interactions. Also of interest is the possibility that dysfunctional 5-HT/NE interactions may have a role in the pathophysiology of PD. Preclinical studies strongly suggest the existence of 5-HT/NE interactions at multiple neuroanatomic sites relevant to anxiety. This section will review the evidence supporting an anatomic basis for such interactions in the LC, hippocampus, amygdala, and neocortex. In addition neurophysiologic and neuropharmacologic data indicating functionally significant 5-HT/NE interactions at each of these sites will be examined. Studies evaluating 5-HT effects on NE function will be emphasized. In the second part of this section clinical studies pertinent to the theme of 5-HT/NE interactions in PD will be reviewed.

PRECLINICAL STUDIES

Locus coeruleus

Anatomy

A considerable body of evidence indicates the existence of 5-HT afferent innervation of the LC. The LC contains a substantial amount of 5-HT (Palkovits *et al.*, 1974; Pujol *et al.*, 1978) and its synthetic enzyme tryptophan hydroxylase (Renson, 1973; Brownstein *et al.*, 1975). A significant amount of 5-HT binding in LC has been demonstrated (Weismann-Nanopoulos *et al.*, 1985), as has 5-HT uptake into LC tissue (Leger and Descarries, 1978; McCrae-Degueurce *et al.*, 1981). 5-HT fibres and terminals have been found to project to the LC in rodents (Pickel *et al.*, 1978; Leger and Descarries, 1978; Steinbusch, 1984; Pieribone *et al.*, 1989) and primate (Pieribone *et al.*, 1988). A number of investigators have observed that the majority of 5-HT afferents to the LC are from dorsal raphe (DR) neurons (Palkovits *et al.*, 1974; Leger *et al.*, 1980; Morgane and Jacobs, 1979; Imai *et al.*, 1986). However, more recently another group has suggested that DR neurons do not have a large input to the LC (Aston-Jones *et al.*, 1986, 1990; Pieribone and Aston-Jones, 1988; Pieribone *et al.*, 1988, 1989) and that the 5-HT innervation is mainly from local 5-HT neurons in the pericoerulear central gray (Pieribone and Aston-Jones, 1990). Despite evidence of a rich 5-HT innervation of LC, electron micrographic studies suggest that only 10% of 5-HT terminals at the LC have the morphologic characteristics of synapses, and these appear to be mainly axodendritic (McRae-Degueurce *et al.*, 1985). In summary, there is much evidence documenting an anatomical substrate for 5-HT/NE interactions at the level of the pontine LC. The location of 5-HT neurons providing most of the afferent innervation remains controversial. In addition, the small number of morphologically developed 5-HT terminals suggests a neuromodulatory role of 5-HT on NE function.

Physiology

There also appear to be significant functional interactions between DR and LC neurons (Leger *et al.*, 1979; Baraban and Aghajanian, 1980; McRae-Degueurce *et al.*, 1985). For example, electrical stimulation of the DR inhibited the LC firing usually seen following presentation of a noxious stimulus (Segal, 1979). In the same study 5-HT, when applied iontophoretically to the LC, was found to inhibit basal LC firing. Alternatively, the neurons of the DR may exert a phasic inhibitory effect on the LC. In a recent *in vivo* study (Aston-Jones *et al.*, 1991a) 5-HT did not alter spontaneous LC discharge substantially, but did attenuate glutamate-evoked activation of LC neurons. The authors concluded that 5-HT may modulate activity in a major afferent to the LC, an excitatory amino acid pathway from the nucleus paragigantocellularis. In brief, there is some evidence that 5-HT has inhibitory effects on LC function, which could be physiologically significant. These data require replication. These effects may occur in response to excessive activity in important excitatory afferent projections to the LC.

Biochemistry

Data from biochemical studies provide further evidence of 5-HT inhibition of LC/NE function. Electrolytic lesions of either DR or raphe centralis neurons produced elevations in tyrosine hydroxylase activity in LC, but led to a slight decrease in the NE metabolite, 3,4-dihydroxyphenylethyleneglycol (DOPEG), in hippocampal and cortical target areas (McRae-Degueurce *et al.*, 1982). However, it was observed that lesions to both DR and raphe centralis nuclei caused a considerable rise in DOPEG in these terminal areas. Destruction of 5-HT terminals by the neurotoxin 5,6-dihydroxytryptamine also led to elevations in LC tyrosine hydroxylase activity (McRae-Degueurce and Pujol, 1979). Overall the biochemical data support the concept of inhibitory 5-HT control of LC function.

Neuropharmacology

Neuropharmacologic studies have observed a variety of inhibitory effects of serotonergic compounds on LC function. Acute administration of indirect 5-HT agonists, such as *d*-fenfluramine, sertraline, and fluoxetine, attenuated LC neuronal opiate withdrawal in anesthetized rats (Akaoka and Aston-Jones, 1993). Moreover, chronic treatment of rats with the selective and potent SRI, fluvoxamine, was associated with a significant downregulation of tyrosine hydroxylase within the LC (Nestler *et al.*, 1990). Bobker and Williams (1989), using a slice preparation, reported that acute administration of 5-HT and 5-HT agonists inhibited electrically stimulated, glutamate and GABA synaptic potentials in the LC. These *in vitro* data are consistent with the findings of Aston-Jones *et al.* (1991a) mentioned previously to the extent that 5-HT was found to be a potent inhibitor of glutamatergic stimulation of LC neurons. Bobker and Williams (1989) concluded that the location of this effect was presynaptic since neither 5-HT nor the other agonists had any effects on the membrane properties of the cells studied, and two 5-HT agonists did not alter response to exogenously applied glutamate or GABA, an important difference from the Aston-Jones *et al.* (1991a) report. Aston-Jones *et al.* (1991a) were unable to draw firm conclusions about the location of the 5-HT effect they observed as their method of local administration of 5-HT could have led to pre- or postsynaptic effects. 5-HT reuptake blockers have also been reported to have inhibitory or antagonist effects on two peptides, corticotropin-releasing factor (CRF) (Valentino *et al.*, 1990; Melia and Duman, 1991) and substance P (Riley *et al.*, 1993), that are excitatory to LC neurons. In summary, the pharmacologic data, with remarkable consistency, suggest that serotonergic agents, and SRIs in particular, exert inhibitory effects on LC function via a variety of mechanisms.

The precise 5-HT receptor subtype(s) and their role in mediating 5-HT effects on the LC are currently unclear. Several groups have postulated an inhibitory role of 5-HT$_{1A}$ receptors on LC activity (Bobker and Williams, 1989; Charlety *et al.*, 1991), while the observations of other workers contradict this claim (Clement *et al.*, 1992). With respect to 5-HT$_2$ receptors three groups have reported inhibitory effects of 5-HT$_2$ agonists on spontaneous LC firing rate (Aghajanian, 1980; Rasmussen and Aghajanian, 1986; Gorea and Adrien, 1988; Done and Sharp (1992). In addition, Rasmussen and Aghajanian (1986) reported a paradoxical increase in unit LC response to sciatic nerve stimulation following hallucinogen administration. Further work is required to clarify the function and location of 5-HT receptor subtypes that influence NE function.

Summary

An impressive body of preclinical evidence documents the presence of 5-HT modulation of NE function in the mammalian brain at the level of the LC. The modulatory effects of 5-HT on NE described thus far are inhibitory. Pharmacologic agents that augment 5-HT functioning such as the SRIs appear to downmodulate NE functioning in a variety of ways. Some of these structure/function relationships are depicted schematically in Figure 1.

Amygdala

Anatomy and physiology

The amygdala, another brain structure that has been implicated in fear responses in animals, may be regulated by converging monoamine systems. Anatomically, 5-HT (Andén *et al.*, 1966; Li *et al.*, 1990) and NE terminals (Davis, 1992) converge upon the amygdala from the DR and LC nuclei respectively. Recently, an inhibitory 5-HT pathway to the lateral amygdala has been described (Kheck *et al.*, 1991). The 5-HT and NE systems in general have an inhibitory effect on amygdala neurons (Davis, 1992). However, recent work by Sugita *et al.* (1992) has identified a fast, excitatory synaptic potential mediated by 5-HT in brain slices of lateral amygdala, apparently via 5-HT$_3$ receptors.

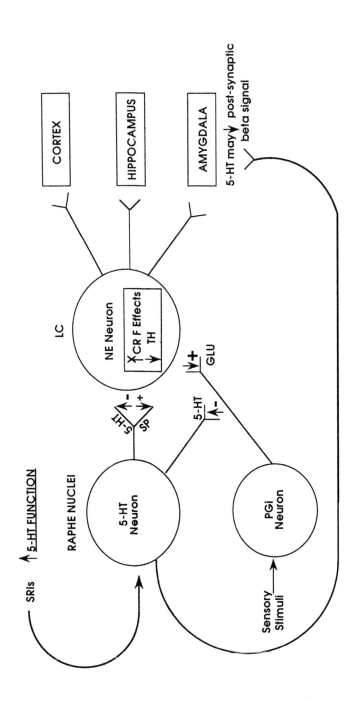

Figure 1 Potential effects of SRIs on noradrenergic function. CRF, corticotropin releasing factor; GLU, glutamate; LC, locus ceruleus; PGi, nucleus paragigantocellularis; SP, substance P; TH, tyrosine hydroxylase

While there is little data describing 5-HT/NE interactions in this region it is clear that there is a neuronal substrate, which could permit such interactions to occur.

Neuropharmacology

Little work has been done examining effects of serotonergic drugs on NE functioning at the level of the amygdala. One study on this topic (Ordway *et al.*, 1991) observed that repeated administration of a variety of antidepressants, including TCAs, MAOIs, and atypical agents (mianserin and trazodone), produced significant reductions in β_1-adrenoreceptor binding in the basolateral and lateral nuclei of the amygdala in addition to a number of other brain regions. In contrast, the SRIs citalopram and sertraline did not have this effect. Whether SRIs affect NE function in the amygdala via other adrenoreceptors or via NE intracellular mechanisms remains to be seen. Further studies specifically designed to evaluate 5-HT/NE interactions in the amygdala are needed to enhance our understanding about the nature, direction, and behavioral consequences of these putative interactions.

Hippocampus

Anatomy and physiology

The hippocampus receives NE input solely from the LC (Foote *et al.*, 1983; Fillenz, 1990), while 5-HT afferents to hippocampus come from both the DR and median raphe (MR) nuclei (Pratt, 1992). Physiologically, LC–NE activation is inhibitory to hippocampal neurons (Segal and Bloom, 1976; Segal, 1981). 5-HT also exerts an inhibitory (hyperpolarizing) effect on hippocampal pyramidal cells. α_2-Heteroreceptors have been identified on 5-HT terminals in the hippocampus (Frankhuyzen and Mulder, 1980, 1982), which may regulate local release of 5-HT (Rao and Hjorth, 1992; Mongeau *et al.*, 1993). Thus, there appears to be a substrate for potential 5-HT/NE interactions within the mammalian hippocampus.

Neuropharmacology

One behavioral pharmacologic study observed that the anxiogenic agent, tetrahydro-β-carboline, increased both 5-HT and NE release in hippocampus, following acute local administration (Huttunen *et al.*, 1985). The heightened release of 5-HT and NE may have profoundly inhibited hippocampal neuronal function, resulting in behavioral effects. The subpopulation of neurons within the hippocampus involved in fear responses and the precise local mechanisms by which these neurons are regulated by 5-HT and NE merit further investigation.

Cortex

Anatomy and physiology

Cortical neuronal function may be significantly influenced by 5-HT/NE interactions. Anatomic studies in rat and monkey suggest that the NE and 5-HT systems may overlap in layer III of the neocortex (Fillenz, 1990; Lidow *et al.*, 1989), providing a rich substrate for interactions between these two systems. The function of the NE innervation of the cortex is inhibition of spontaneous neuronal activity (Foote *et al.*, 1975; Armstrong-James and Fox, 1983), together with enhancement of neuronal responsiveness to excitatory or inhibitory inputs (Waterhouse *et al.*, 1982). 5-HT also appears to be inhibitory in prefrontal cortex, as demonstrated by studies using direct iontophoretic application of 5-HT (Aghajanian *et al.*, 1987). However, recently it has been observed in human cortical pyramidal cells that individual ionic currents are influenced by several different neurotransmitters, and that a given neurotransmitter, e.g. 5-HT, may have more than one postsynaptic effect (McCormick and Williamson, 1989). Thus, the control of cortical neuronal activity by systems such as 5-HT and NE is likely to be much more complex than the simple scheme outlined above.

Neuropharmacology

Pharmacologic studies suggest that 5-HT may exert inhibitory effects on cortical NE functioning. A number of studies had implicated 5-HT (Stockmeier *et al.*, 1985; Gillespie *et al.*, 1988) or 5-HT neurons (Nimgaonkar *et al.*, 1985) in the downregulation of β-receptor functioning in rat forebrain. Accordingly, an intact 5-HT system was said to be necessary for antidepressants to produce downregulation of β receptors. However, more recent work has contested this notion because of the lack of selectivity of ligands used to identify the β-receptor in earlier studies (Gillespie *et al.*, 1989; Hensler *et al.*, 1991). Also chronic administration of the SRIs citalopram and sertraline had no effect on β_1-receptor levels in rat cortex (Ordway *et al.*, 1991). However, regulation may occur beyond the synapse. For instance, 5-HT may regulate NE function by antagonizing β-mediated events at the second messenger level (Eiring *et al.*, 1992). In conclusion, while there is little firm data indicating that serotonergic medications downmodulate cortical adrenoreceptors, the possibility remains that medications such as the SRIs could downmodulate second and third messenger systems linked to the β-receptor (see Figure 1).

CLINICAL STUDIES OF SEROTONIN AND NOREPINEPHRINE IN PANIC DISORDER

Introduction

There are relatively few clinical studies of PD patients which have evaluated functional interrelationships or interactions between the 5-HT and NE systems. The existing studies will be described in some detail and their implications discussed. A model outlining potential therapeutic effects of SRIs via the NE system will be discussed.

Platelet studies

NE and 5-HT function in PD were separately assessed in a treatment study of 66 PD patients and 50 age- and sex-matched controls using a variety of platelet indices and a lymphocyte index (Butler *et al.*, 1992). The patients were evaluated before treatment and then during treatment with clomipramine or lofepramine (an NE reuptake blocker) for up to six months. The investigators found a number of abnormalities in these peripheral markers of 5-HT and NE function which persisted despite clinical improvement. In particular, 5-HT-evoked platelet aggregation was reduced, platelet 5-HT uptake (V_{max}) was reduced, and 5-HT$_2$ receptor density was increased compared to controls during most of the study. With respect to the NE system, NE-evoked aggregation was somewhat increased, and platelet α_2-receptor density and lymphocyte β-receptor density-were both increased, for the duration of the study. There was no differential effect of treatment condition on these parameters.

In summary, 5-HT functioning as measured by these peripheral markers was reduced while NE function was slightly elevated. The authors argued that their findings indicated trait abnormalities in 5-HT and NE function in PD, which could be pertinent to the pathogenesis and course of the disorder. The data are consistent with the concept of NE hyperactivity in the pathophysiology PD, a concept which already has considerable empirical support. They are also consistent with the data of Schneider *et al.* (1987) implicating decreased 5-HT function in the pathophysiology of this disorder.

Cerebrospinal fluid studies

A study conducted by Eriksson *et al.* (1991) examined cerebrospinal fluid (CSF) monoamine metabolites in 17 PD patients not on standing medications, and 17 age- and sex-matched healthy volunteers. This study did not directly assess interactions between the 5-HT and NE systems in PD, but aimed to measure CSF monoamine metabolites of 5-HT, NE and dopamine (DA). Levels of 5-hydroxyindoleacetic acid (5-HIAA), homovanillic acid (HVA) and MHPG did not differ between the two groups, suggesting that, in the resting state, none of these systems was functioning abnormally in PD (assuming that metabolite levels are a reliable index of neuronal function). Concentrations of MHPG were positively correlated with 5-HIAA and HVA concentrations in the patients but not the controls. The authors concluded that this may indicate that the NE system interacts more actively with other transmitter systems in anxiety patients than non-anxious controls. To the extent that these correlations of CSF metabolites represent interactions between transmitter systems, it appears that the level of NE function in PD in the non-panicking state may be accompanied by similar levels of functioning in the 5-HT and DA systems.

The study also reported on the effects of treatment on these CSF measures in five patients. Successful treatment with clomipramine (n=4) or imipramine (n=1) (at least two months of therapy) was associated with significant reductions in CSF concentrations of 5-HIAA, and smaller but significant reductions in MHPG, but no significant change in HVA levels. The effect of clomipramine and imipramine on 5-HIAA levels is probably related to their 5-HT reuptake blockade effects, which result in less 5-HT being exposed to MAO enzymes located in the synaptic terminal (Bowden *et al.*, 1985). Another CSF study in obsessive-compulsive disorder patients chronically treated with the SRI, fluvox-amine, reported a substantial decrease in CSF 5-HIAA, a smaller but significant decrease in MHPG, and no change in HVA (Wayne K. Goodman, personal communication). The effect of SRIs on CSF MHPG levels may be due to inhibition of NE function via some of the mechanisms mentioned in the preclinical part of this section (see Figure 1).

Neurobiologic challenge studies

The pharmacologic challenge studies that have assessed 5-HT/NE interactions or interrelationships in PD are summarized in Table 3. Manipulation of 5-HT function by 5-HTP challenge (Den Boer and Westenberg, 1990b) or tryptophan depletion (Goddard *et al.*, 1994) did not alter anxiety symptoms or plasma MHPG in unmedicated, non-panicking PD patients. These findings tend to argue against the concept of a trait deficit (Schneider *et al.*, 1987; Butler *et al.*, 1992) or hyperactivity in 5-HT functioning in PD, since if either were the case one would have expected to see changes in panic symptomatology during these challenges. Also with respect to the model of 5-HT modulation of NE function presented earlier (Figure 1) these data are not consistent with the notion of tonic presynaptic inhibitory control of NE function by 5-HT, as there are challenge effects on plasma MHPG. One possible explanation for the lack of effect on MHPG is that plasma MHPG is an insensitive index of central NE function.

An interesting alternative explanation of the above data is that inhibitory 5-HT modulation of NE may only be recruited during surges of NE hyperactivity as may occur during a naturalistic or chemical panic attack. In this case, one would not expect to observe behavioral changes or MHPG changes in PD patients in the non-panicking state. Empirical support for this idea comes from a recent study by our group in healthy subjects (Goddard *et al.*, 1995). Eleven subjects had significant increases in subjective nervousness following a tryptophan depletion/yohimbine 0.4 mg/kg i.v. challenge. This effect was much greater than the behavioral effect observed during each challenge alone and during a placebo challenge. However, the depletion/yohimbine challenge did not uniquely affect physiologic or biochemical (MHPG and cortisol) measures. We speculate that tryptophan depletion impaired the normal compensatory effect of 5-HT on an episode of NE hyperactivity, leading to breakthrough anxiety symptoms. Why MHPG and physiologic measures were not similarly augmented is unclear, but it is possible that cortical or limbic 5-HT/NE interactions may account for the dissociation of these effects from behavior (Figure 1). Work by Asnis *et al.* (1992) (see Table 3) is also consistent with the concept of a joint disturbance in 5-HT and NE function in PD and depression, i.e. a dysfunctional 5-HT/NE interaction.

Table 3. Neurobiologic challenge studies evaluating 5-HT/NE interrelationships in panic disorder

Agent	Reference	Design	Measures	Results
5-HTP	Den Boer and Westenberg (1990b)	P=20, C=20 5-HTP 60 mg i.v.	Mood, panic symptoms, plasma MHPG, cortisol, β-endorphin, melatonin[a]	No Δ in anxiety P=C, ↑ Cortisol, β-endorphin, and melatonin, P=C, MHPG- no Δ P=C
mCPP/DMI	Asnis et al. (1992)	P=22, C=10, P(D)=17 mCPP 0.25 mg/kg p.o. DMI 75 mg i.m.	Cortisol responses to mCPP and DMI	Cortisol responses to mCPP and DMI were negatively correlated, particularly in the patient groups
Yohimbine	Goddard et al. (1993a)	P=16 Pre and post fluvoxamine tests. Yohimbine 0.4 mg/kg i.v.	Mood, panic symptoms, BP, HR, MHPG and cortisol	Fluvoxamine blunted yohimbine-induced anxiety ↑ BP, MHPG and cortisol, no Δ
Clonidine	Coplan et al. (1995)	P=13, C=13, Pre and post fluoxetine tests (pts). Clonidine 0.15 mg p.o.	GH, MHPG	Blunted GH response observed in P vs C. Persists in spite of effective treatment MHPG ↓ in P>C. Trend for MHPG responses to normalize in best treatment responders
TRP depletion	Goddard et al. (1994)	P=8 TRP depletion with AA mixture	Mood, panic symptoms, BP, HR, MHPG, TRP	No effect of depletion on anxiety or panic No effect on BP, HR, MHPG

BP, blood pressure; C, healthy controls; DMI, desipramine; GH, growth hormone; 5-HTP, 5-hydroxytryptophan; HR, heart rate; i.v., intravenouss; mCPP, m-chlorophenylpiperazine; MHPG, 3-methoxy-4-hydroxyphenylglycol; P, panic patients; P(D), depressed patients; p.o., orally; TRP, Tryptophan; Δ = change.
[a]All neuroendocrine measures are plasma measures.

Mechanism of action of serotonin reuptake inhibitors in panic disorder

Chronic administration of an SRI is thought to increase net 5-HT neurotransmission via desensitization of the somatodendritic autoreceptor (Blier *et al.*, 1987). By augmenting 5-HT function SRIs may be increasing the inhibitory effects of 5-HT on LC–NE function described in the preclinical review and summarized in Figure 1. This interaction with NE function may be a part of the therapeutic mechanism of action of SRIs in PD. Two studies have evaluated the effect of successful clinical treatment of PD patients with SRIs in relation to clinical tests of NE function (see Table 3). Coplan *et al.* (1995) studied the effect of chronic fluoxetine treatment on response to an oral clonidine challenge of 0.15 mg. The authors replicated the blunted GH response in the PD group found by other investigators (see Table 1), and observed that this abnormality persisted despite successful treatment with fluoxetine, an observation that has already been reported in relation to behavioral treatment of PD (Middleton, 1990). Patients demonstrated a significant decrease from baseline levels of MHPG in response to clonidine compared to controls, as reported elsewhere (Charney *et al.*, 1986a), an effect which persisted even after fluoxetine therapy. However, further analysis of the data has revealed that the patients with high clinical global improvement ratings after fluoxetine treatment tend to have normalization of the MHPG response to clonidine (Jeremy Coplan, personal communication), suggesting modulation of NE function by fluoxetine in a subgroup of treatment responders. Firm conclusions from this data are limited by the absence of a placebo control for either fluoxetine and clonidine. Data from our own laboratory suggests that the SRI, fluvoxamine, may influence NE functioning in PD patients (Goddard *et al.*, 1993). The main finding of this study was blunting of the anxiogenic response to yohimbine in the fluvoxamine-treated but not the placebo group following eight weeks of treatment. There was no effect of treatment condition on baseline MHPG or cortisol, or on biochemical or physiologic responses to yohimbine. Although conclusions from the study are limited by the small number of patients involved, the results suggest that fluvoxamine does influence NE functioning in PD patients (to the extent that the behavioral response to yohimbine is an index of NE function), and that the mechanism of clinical improvement could be related to this effect. The data from these two studies are consistent with the preclinical data indicating the SRIs' ability to suppress NE function (see Figure 1), and are consistent with the CSF data presented earlier documenting suppression of CSF MHPG by SRIs.

CONCLUSION

There is an impressive body of preclinical and clinical data implicating the NE system in the pathophysiology of PD. The role of the 5-HT system in the pathophysiology of this disorder is less clear, although medications that block reuptake of 5-HT are efficacious in the treatment of PD. There is growing preclinical and clinical evidence of significant interactions between the 5-HT and NE monoamine systems. These interactions are relevant to our understanding of the pathophysiology of PD and mechanism of treatment response in PD. Specifically, 5-HT modulates NE function in an inhibitory manner and treatments such as the SRIs, which increase 5-HT function, may inhibit NE system function, which is believed to be hyperactive in PD. Also, with respect to pathophysiology, the 5-HT system may function as a compensatory system that is recruited to inhibit surges of NE system activity that are postulated to occur during chemical and naturalistic panic. Abnormalities in this compensatory response may contribute to the pathogenesis of PD. An appreciation of 5-HT/NE interactions adds heuristic power to the earlier monoamine theories of PD. Future work focusing on interactions between these important brain systems should add to our understanding of brain function in panic and other human anxiety disorders, and should assist in the formulation and monitoring of novel anxiolytic therapies.

ACKNOWLEDGMENTS

This work was supported in part by Public Health Service Grants MH-36229, MH-30929, MH-40140, MH-50641, and by the State of Connecticut. Thanks to the expert staff of the Clinical Neuroscience Research Unit at the Connecticut Mental Health Center, New Haven (Elizabeth Kyle for manuscript preparation, Katherine Walton for table preparation and Elizabeth Ruff for graphics preparation) and the Staff of the National PTSD Center at the West Haven Veterans Administration Medical Center. The scientific expertise of George K. Aghajanian MD greatly contributed to the development of this review.

REFERENCES

Abelson, J. L., Glitz, D., Cameron, O. G. *et al.* (1991). Blunted growth hormone response to clonidine in patients with generalized anxiety disorder. *Arch. Gen. Psychiatry.*, **48**, 157–162.

Abercrombie, E. D. and Jacobs, B. L. (1987a). Single-unit response of noradrenergic neurons in the locus coeruleus of freely moving cats. I: Acutely presented stressful and nonstressful stimuli. *J. Neurosci.*, **7**, 2837–2843.

Abercrombie, E. D. and Jacobs, B. L. (1987b). Single-unit response of noradrenergic neurons in the locus coeruleus of freely moving cats. II: Adaptation to chronically presented stressful stimuli. *J. Neurosci.*, **7**, 2844–2848.

Aghajanian, G. K. (1980). Mescaline and LSD facilitate the activation of locus coeruleus neurons by peripheral stimuli. *Brain Res.*, **186**, 492–498.

Aghajanian, G. K., Sprouse, J. S. and Rasmussen, K. (1987). Physiology of the midbrain serotonin system. In *Psychopharmacology: The Third Generation of Progress* (ed. H. Y. Meltzer), pp. 141–149.

Akaoka, H. and Aston-Jones, G. (1993). Indirect serotonergic agonists attenuate neuronal opiate withdrawal. *Neuroscience*, **54**(3), 561–565.

Albus, M., Zahn, T. P. and Breier, A. (1992). Anxiogenic properties of yohimbine. I. Behavioral, physiological and biochemical measures. *Eur. Arch. Psychiatry Clin. Neurosci.*, **241**, 337–344.

Andén, N. E., Dahlström, A., Fuxe, K. *et al.* (1966). Ascending monoamine neurons to the telencephalon and diencephalon. *Acta Physiol. Scand.*, **67**, 313–326.

Armstrong-James, M. and Fox, K. (1983). Effects of ionophoresed noradrenaline on the spontaneous activity of neurones in rat primary somatosensory cortex. *J. Physiol. (Lond.)*, **335**, 427–447.

Asnis, G. M., Wetzler, S., Sanderson, W. C. *et al.* (1992). Functional interrelationship of serotonin and norepinephrine: cortisol response to MCPP and DMI in patients with panic disorder, patients with depression, and normal control subjects. *Psychiatry Res.*, **43**, 65–76.

Aston-Jones, G. and Bloom, F. E. (1981). Norepinephrine-containing locus coeruleus neurons in behaving rats exhibit pronounced responses to non-noxious environmental stimuli. *J. Neurosci.*, **1**, 887–900.

Aston-Jones, G. and Ennis, M. (1988). Sensory-evoked activation of locus coeruleus may be mediated by a glutamate pathway from the rostral ventrolateral medulla. In *Frontiers in Excitatory Amino Acid Research* (eds A. Cavalheiro, J. Lehmann and L. Turski), pp. 471–478. Liss, New York.

Aston-Jones, G., Ennis, M., Pieribone, V. A. *et al.* (1986). The brain nucleus locus coeruleus: restricted afferent control of a broad efferent network. *Science.*, **234**, 734–737.

Aston-Jones, G., Shipley, M. T., Ennis, M. *et al.* (1990). Restricted afferent control of locus coeruleus neurons revealed by anatomic, physiologic and pharmacologic studies. In *The Pharmacology of Noradrenaline in the Central Nervous System* (eds C. A. Marsden and D. J. Heal), pp. 187–247. Oxford University Press, Oxford.

Aston-Jones, G., Akaoka, H., Charléty, P. and Chouvet, G. (1991a). Serotonin selectively attenuates glutamate-evoked activation of noradrenergic locus coeruleus neurons. *J. Neurosci.*, **11**, 760–769.

Aston-Jones, G., Shipley, M. T., Chouvet, G. *et al.* (1991b). Afferent regulation of locus coeruleus neurons: anatomy, physiology and pharmacology. *Prog. Brain Res.*, **88**, 47–75.

Ballenger, J. C., Burrows, G. D., DuPont, R. L. J. *et al.* (1988). Alprazolam in panic disorder and agoraphobia: results from a multicenter trial. I. Efficacy in short-term treatment. *Arch. Gen. Psychiatry.*, **45**, 413–422.

Balon, R., Pohl., R., Yeragani, V. *et al.* (1987). Platelet serotonin levels in panic disorder. *Acta Psychiatr. Scand.*, **75**, 315.

Baraban, F. M. and Aghajanian, G. K. (1980). Suppression of firing activity of 5HT neurons in the dorsal raphe by alpha-adrenoreceptor antagonists. *Neuropharmacology,* **19**, 355–363.

Barlow, D. H. (1988). *Anxiety and its Disorders: The Nature and Treatment of Anxiety and Panic.* Guilford Press, New York.

Beaumont, G. (1977). A large open multicenter trial of clomipramine (Anafranil) in the management of phobic disorders. *J. Int. Med. Res.*, **5**, 116–123.

Blier, P., de Montigny, C. and Chaput, Y. (1987). Modifications of the serotonin system by antidepressant treatments: implications for the therapeutic response in major depression. *J. Clin. Psychopharmacol.*, 7(6, Suppl.), 24S–35S.

Bobker, D. H. and Williams, J. T. (1989). Serotonin agonists inhibit synaptic potentials in the rat locus ceruleus in vitro via 5-hydroxytryptamine 1A and 5-hydroxytryptamine 1B receptors. *J. Pharmacol. Exp. Ther.*, **250**, 37–43.

Bowden, C. L., Koslow, S. H., Hanin, I. *et al.* (1985). Effects of amitriptyline and imipramine on brain amine neurotransmitter metabolites in cerebrospinal fluid. *Clin. Pharmacol. Ther.*, **37**, 316–324.

Brownstein, M. J., Palkovits, M., Saavedra, J. M. and Kizer, J. S. (1975). Tryptophan hydroxylase in the rat brain. *Brain Res.*, **97**, 163–166.

Butler, J., O'Halloran, A. and Leonard, B. E. (1992). The Galway study of panic disorder II: Changes in some peripheral markers of noradrenergic and serotonergic function in DSM III-R panic disorder. *J. Affect. Disord.*, **26**, 89–100.

Cameron, O. G., Smith, C. B., Hollingsworth, P. F. *et al.* (1984). Platelet α2-adrenergic receptor binding and plasma catecholamines: before and during imipramine treatment in patients with panic anxiety. *Arch. Gen. Psychiatry*, **41**, 1144–1148.

Cameron, O. G., Smith, C. B., Lee, M. A. *et al.* (1990). Adrenergic status in anxiety disorders: platelet α2-adrenergic receptor binding, blood pressure, pulse and plasma catecholamines in panic and generalized anxiety disorder patients and in normal subjects. *Biol. Psychiatry*, **28**, 3–20.

Carr, D. B., Sheehan, D. V., Surman, O. S. *et al.* (1986). Neuroendocrine correlates of lactate-induced anxiety and their response to chronic alprazolam therapy. *Am. J. Psychiatry*, **143**, 483–494.

Cassens, G., Kuruc, A., Roffman, M. *et al.* (1981). Alterations in brain norepinephrine metabolism and behavior induced by environmental stimuli previously paired with inescapable shock. *Behav. Brain Res.*, **2**, 387–407.

Cedarbaum, J. M. and Aghajanian, G. K. (1978). Afferent projections to the rat locus coeruleus as determined by a retrograde tracing technique. *J. Comp. Neurol.*, **178**, 1–16.

Charlety, P., Aston-Jones, G., Akaoka, H. *et al.* (1991). 5-HT decreases glutamate-evoked activation of locus coeruleus neurons through 5-HT 1A receptors. *CR Acad. Sci.*, **312**, 421–426.

Charney, D. S. and Heninger, G. R. (1985). Noradrenergic function and the mechanism of action of antianxiety treatment. II. The effect of long-term imipramine treatment. *Arch. Gen. Psychiatry*, **42**, 473–481.

Charney, D. S. and Heninger, G. R. (1986a). Abnormal regulation of noradrenergic function in panic disorders: effects of clonidine in healthy subjects and patients with agoraphobia and panic disorders. *Arch. Gen. Psychiatry*, **43**, 1042–1054.

Charney, D. S. and Heninger, G. R. (1986b). Serotonin function in panic disorders: the effects of intravenous tryptophan in healthy subjects and panic disorder patients before and during alprazolam treatment. *Arch. Gen. Psychiatry*, **43**, 1059–1065.

Charney, D. S., Heninger, G. R. and Breier, A. (1984). Noradrenergic function in panic anxiety: effects of yohimbine in healthy subjects and patients with agoraphobia and panic disorder. *Arch. Gen. Psychiatry*, **41**, 751–763.

Charney, D. S., Menkes, D. B. and Heninger, G. R. (1981). Receptor sensitivity and the mechanism of action of antidepressant treatment. *Arch. Gen. Psychiatry*, **38**, 1160–1180.

Charney, D. S., Woods, S. W., Goodman, W. K. and Heninger, G. R. (1987a). Neurobiological mechanisms of panic anxiety: biochemical and behavioral correlates of yohimbine-induced panic attacks. *Am. J. Psychiatry*, **144**, 1030–1036.

Charney, D. S., Woods, S. W., Goodman, W. K. and Heninger, G. R. (1987b). Serotonin function in anxiety: II. Effects of the serotonin agonist MCPP in panic disorder patients and healthy subjects. *Psychopharmacology*, **92**, 14–24.

Charney D. S., Innis, R. B., Duman, R. S. *et al.* (1989a). Platelet alpha-2-receptor binding and adenylate cyclase activity in panic disorder. *Psychopharmacology*, **98**, 102–107.

Charney, D. S., Woods, S. W. and Heninger, G. R. (1989b). Noradrenergic function in generalized anxiety disorder: effects of yohimbine in healthy subjects and patients with generalized anxiety disorder. *Psychiatry Res.*, **27**, 173–182.

Charney, D. S., Woods, S. W., Krystal, J. H. *et al.* (1992). Noradrenergic neuronal dysregulation in panic disorder: the effects of intravenous yohimbine and clonidine in panic disorder patients. *Acta Psychiatr. Scand.*, **86**, 273–282.

Clement, H. W., Gemsa, D. and Wesemann, W. (1992). Serotonin–norepinephrine interactions: a voltammetric study on the effect of serotonin receptor stimulation followed in the N. raphe dorsalis and the locus coeruleus of the rat. *J. Neural Transm. (Gen. Sect.)*, **88**, 11–23.

Cole, B. J. and Robbins, T. W. (1987). Dissociable effects of lesions to dorsal and ventral noradrenergic bundle on the acquisition performance, and extinction of aversive conditioning. *Behav. Neurosci.*, **101**, 476–488.

Coplan, J. D., Liebowitz, M. R., Gorman, J. M. *et al.* (1992). Noradrenergic function in panic disorder: effects of intravenous clonidine pretreatment on lactate induced panic. *Biol. Psychiatry*, **31**, 135–146.

Coplan, J. D., Papp, L. A., Martinez, J. *et al.* (1995) Persistence of blunted growth hormone response to clonidine in fluoxetine-treated patients with panic disorder. *Am. J. Psychiatry*, **152**, 619–622.

Corrodi, H., Fuxe, K., Lidbrink, P. and Olson, L. (1971). Minor tranquillisers, stress and central catecholamine neurones. *Brain Res.*, **29**, 1–16.

Craig, A. D. (1992). Spinal and trigeminal lamina I input to the locus coeruleus anterogradely labeled with *Phaseolus vulgaris* leucoagglutinin (PHA-L) in the cat and the monkey. *Brain Res.*, **584**, 325–328.

Davis, M. (1990). Animal models of anxiety based upon classical conditioning: the conditioned emotional response and fear potentiated startle effect. *Pharmacol. Ther.*, **47**, 147–165.

Davis, M. (1992). The role of the amygdala in fear and anxiety. *Am. Rev. Neurosci.*, **15**, 353–375.

Davis, M., Redmond, D. E., Jr and Baraban, J. M. (1979). Noradrenergic agonists and antagonists: effects on conditioned fear as measured by the potentiated startle paradigm. *Psychopharmacology*, **65**, 111–118.

De Montigny, C., Chaput, Y. and Blier, P. (1990). Modification of serotonergic neuron properties by long-term treatment with serotonin reuptake blockers. *J. Clin. Psychiatry*, **51** (12, suppl. B).

Den Boer, J. A. and Westenberg, H. G. M. (1988). Effect of a serotonin and noradrenaline uptake inhibitor in panic disorder: a double-blind comparative study with fluvoxamine and maprotiline. *Int. Clin. Psychopharmacol.*, **3**, 59–74.

Den Boer, J. A. and Westenberg, H. G. M. (1990a). Serotonin function in panic disorder: a double blind placebo controlled study with fluvoxamine and ritanserin. *Psychopharmacology*, **102**, 85–94.

Den Boer, J. A. and Westenberg, H. G. M. (1990b). Behavioral, neuroendocrine, and biochemical effects of 5-hydroxytryptophan administration in panic disorder. *Psychiatry Res.*, **31**, 367–378.

Den Boer, J. A., Westenberg, H. G. M., Kamerbeek, W. D. J. *et al.* (1987). Effect of serotonin uptake inhibitors in anxiety disorders: a double-blind comparison of clomipramine and fluvoxamine. *Int. Clin. Psychopharmacol.*, **2**, 21–32.

Done, C. J. G. and Sharp, T. (1992). Evidence that 5-HT$_2$ receptor activation decreases noradrenaline release in rat hippocampus *in vivo*. *Br. J. Pharmacol.*, **107**, 240–245.

Eiring, A., Manier, D. H., Bieck, P. R. *et al.* (1992). The "serotonin/norepinephrine link" beyond the β adrenoceptor. *Mol. Brain Res.*, **16**, 211–214.

Elam, M., Svensson, T. H. and Thorén, P. (1986). Locus coeruleus neurons and sympathetic nerves: activation by cutaneous sensory afferents. *Brain Res.*, **366**, 254–261.

Emorine, I. J., Marullo, S., Briend-Sutren, M. M. *et al.* (1989). Molecular characterization of the human β$_3$-adrenergic receptor. *Science*, **245**, 1118–1121.

Eriksson, E., Westberg, P., Alling, C. *et al.* (1991). Cerebrospinal fluid levels of monoamine metabolites in panic disorder. *Psychiatry Res.*, **36**, 243–251.

Evans, L., Kenardy, J., Schneider, P. and Hoey, H. (1986). Effect of a selective serotonin uptake inhibitor in agoraphobia with panic attacks. *Acta Psychiatr. Scand.*, **73**, 49–53.

Fillenz, M. (1990). *Noradrenergic Neurons*, Cambridge University Press, Cambridge.

Finlay, J. M. and Abercrombie, E. D. (1991). Stress induced sensitization of norepinephrine release in the medial prefrontal cortex. *Soc. Neurosci. Abstr.*, **17**, 151.

Foote, S. and Bloom, F. E. (1979). Activity of norepinephrine-containing locus coeruleus neurons in the unanesthetized squirrel monkey. In *Catecholamines: Basic and Clinical Frontiers* (eds E. Usdin, I. Kopin and J. Barchas), pp. 625–627. Pergamon Press, New York.

Foote, S. L., Freedman, R. and Oliver, A. P. (1975). Effects of putative neurotransmitters on neuronal activity in monkey auditory cortex. *Brain Res.*, **86**, 229–242.

Foote, S. L., Aston-Jones, G. and Bloom, F. E. (1980). Impulse activity of locus coeruleus neurones in awake rats and monkeys is a function of sensory stimulation and arousal. *Proc. Natl. Acad. Sci. USA*, **77**, 3033–3037.

Foote, S. L., Bloom, F. E. and Aston-Jones, G. (1983). Nucleus locus ceruelus: new evidence of anatomical and physiological specificity. *Physiol. Rev.*, **63**, 844–914.

Frankhuyzen, A. L. and Mulder, A. H. (1980). Noradrenaline inhibits depolarization-induced ^{3}H-serotonin release from slices of rat hippocampus. *Eur. J. Pharmacol.*, **63**, 179–182.

Frankhuyzen, A. L. and Mulder, A. H. (1982). Pharmacological characterization of presynaptic α-adrenoceptors modulating [^{3}H]5-hydroxytryptamine release from slices of the hippocampus of the rat. *Eur. J. Pharmacol.*, **81**, 97–106.

Germine, M., Goddard, A. W., Sholomskas, D. E. *et al.* (1994). Response to *m*-chlorophenylpiperazine (MCPP) in panic disorder patients and healthy subjects: influence of reduction in intravenous dosage. *Psychiatry Res.*, **54**, 115–135.

Gillespie, D. D., Manier, D. H., Sanders-Bush, E. and Sulser, F. (1988). The serotonin/norepinephrine-link in brain. II. Role of serotonin in the regulation of beta adrenoceptors in the low agonist affinity conformation. *J. Pharmacol. Exp. Ther.*, **244**, 154–159.

Gillespie, D. D., Manier, D. H. and Sulser, F. (1989). Characterization of the inducible serotonin-sensitive dihydroalprenolol binding sites with low affinity for isoproterenol. *Neuropsychopharmacology*, **2**, 265–271.

Glazer, W. M., Charney, D. S. and Heninger, G. R. (1987). Noradrenergic function in schizophrenia. *Arch. Gen. Psychiatry*, **44**, 898–904.

Goddard, A. W., Germine, M., Woods, S. W. *et al.* (1995). Effects of tryptophan depletion on responses to yohimbine in healthy human subjects. *Biol. Psychiatry*, **38**, 74–85.

Goddard, A. W., Woods, S. W., Sholomskas, D. E. *et al.* (1993). Effects of the serotonin reuptake inhibitor fluvoxamine on noradrenergic function in panic disorder. *Psychiatry Res.*, **48**, 119–133.

Goddard, A. W., Goodman, W. K., Woods, S. W. *et al.* (1994). Effects of tryptophan depletion in panic disorder. *Biol. Psychiatry*, **36**, 775–777.

Gold, M. S. and Redmond, D. E., Jr (1977). Pharmacological activation and inhibition of noradrenergic activity alter specific behaviors in nonhuman primates. *Neurosci. Abstr.*, **3**, 250.

Gorea, E. and Adrien, J. (1988). Serotonergic regulation of noradrenergic coerulean neurons. *Eur. J. Pharmacol.*, **154**, 285–291.

Gorman, J. M., Liebowitz, M. R., Fyer, A. J. *et al.* (1987). An open trial of fluoxetine in the treatment of panic attacks. *J. Clin. Psychopharmacol.*, **7**, 329–332.

Gurguis, G. N. M. and Uhde, T. W. (1990). Plasma 3-methoxy-4-hydroxyphenylethylene glycol (MHPG) and growth hormone responses to yohimbine in panic disorder patients and normal controls. *Psychoneuroendocrinology*, **15**, 217–224.

Heninger, G. R., Charney, D. S. and Price, L. H. (1988). α_2-Adrenergic receptor sensitivity in depression: the plasma MHPG, behavioral, and cardiovascular responses to yohimbine. *Arch. Gen. Psychiatry*, **45**, 718–726.

Hensler, J. G., Ordway, G. A., Gambarana, C. *et al.* (1991). Serotonergic neurons do not influence the regulation of *beta* adrenoceptors induced by either desipramine or isoproterenol. *Pharmacol. Exp. Ther.*, **256**, 656–664.

Huang, Y. H., Redmond, D. E. J., Snyder, D. R. *et al.* (1976). Loss of fear following bilateral lesions of the locus coeruleus in the monkey. *Neurosci. Abstr.*, **3**, 250.

Huttunen, P., Spencer, B. A. and Myers, R. D. (1985). Monoamine transmitter release induced by tetrahydro-β-carboline perfused in hippocampus of the unrestrained rat. *Brain Res. Bull.*, **15**, 215–220.

Imai, H., Steindler, D. A. and Kitai, S. T. (1986). The organization of divergent axonal projections from the midbrain raphe nuclei in the rat. *J. Comp. Neurol.*, **243**, 363–380.

Innis, R. B., Charney, D. S. and Heninger, G. R. (1987). Differential 3H-imipramine platelet binding in patients with panic disorder and depression. *Psychiatry Res.*, **21**, 33–41.

Irwin, J., Ahluwalia, P. and Anisman, H. (1986). Sensitization of norepinephrine activity following acute and chronic footshock. *Brain Res.*, **379**, 98–103.

Kahn, R. S. and Westenberg, H. G. M. (1985). 1–5-hydroxytryptophan in the treatment of anxiety disorders. *J. Affect. Disord.*, **8**, 197–200.

Kahn, R. S., Asnis, G. M., Wetzler, S. *et al.* (1988a). Serotonin and anxiety revisited. *Biol. Psychiatry*, **23**, 189–208.

Kahn, R. S., Wetzler, S., van Praag, H. M. *et al.* (1988b). Behavioral indications for serotonin receptor hypersensitivity in panic disorder. *Psychiatry Res*, **25**, 101–104.

Keith, R. A., Howe, B. B. and Salama, A. L. (1986). Modulation of peripheral beta-1 and alpha-2 receptor sensitivities by the administration of the tricyclic antidepressant imipramine alone and in combination with alpha-2 antagonists in rats. *J. Pharmacol. Exp. Ther.*, **236**, 356–363.

Kheck, N. M., Barb, C. and LeDoux, J. E. (1991). A serotonin projection to the lateral amygdaloid nucleus from the dorsal raphe nucleus. *Soc. Neurosci. Abstr.*, **17**, 472.

Leger, L. and Descarries, L. (1978). Serotonin nerve terminals in the locus coeruleus of adult rat: a radioautographic study. *Brain Res.*, **145**, 1–13.

Leger, L., Wiklund, L., Descarries, L. and Persson, M. (1979). Description of an indolaminergic cell component in the cat locus coeruleus: a fluorescence histochemical and radioautographic study. *Brain Res.*, **168**, 43–56.

Leger, L., McRae-Degueurce, A. and Pujol, J. F. (1980). Origine de l'innervation sérotonergique du locus coeruleus chez le rat. *CR Acad. Sci. Paris*, **290**, 807–810.

Lesch, K. P., Wiesmann, M., Hoh, A. *et al.* (1992). 5-HT1A receptor-effector system responsivity in panic disorder. *Psychopharmacology*, **106**, 111–117.

Levine, E. S., Litto, W. J. and Jacobs, B. L. (1990). Activity of cat locus coeruleus noradrenergic neurons during the defense reaction. *Brain Res.*, **531**, 189–195.

Li, Y. Q., Jia, H. G., Rao, Z. R. and Shi, J. W. (1990). Serotonin-, substance P- or leucine-enkephalin-containing neurons in the midbrain periaqueductal gray and nucleus raphe dorsalis send projection fibers to the central amygdaloid nucleus in the rat. *Neurosci. Lett.*, **120**, 124–127.

Lidow, M. S., Goldman-Rakic, P. S., Gallager, D. W. and Rakic, P. (1989). Quantitative autoradiographic mapping of serotonin 5-HT1 and 5-HT2 receptors and uptake sites in the neocortex of the rhesus monkey. *J. Comp. Neurol.*, **280**, 27–42.

McCormick, D. A. and Williamson, A. (1989). Convergence and divergence of neurotransmitter action in human cerebral cortex. *Proc. Natl Acad. Sci. USA*, **86**, 8098–8102.

McRae-Degueurce, A. and Pujol, J. F. (1979). Correlation between the increase in tyrosine hydroxylase activity and the decreases in serotonin content in the rat locus coeruleus after 5,6-dihydroxytryptamine. *Eur. J. Pharmacol.*, **59**, 131–135.

McRae-Degueurce, A., Leger, L., Wiklund, L. and Pujol, J. P. (1981). Functional recuperation of the serotonergic innervation in the rat locus coeruleus. *J. Physiol. (Paris)*, **77**, 389–392.

McRae-Degueurce, A., Berod, A., Mermet, A. *et al.* (1982). Alterations in tyrosine hydroxylase activity elicited by raphe nuclei lesions in the rat locus coeruleus: evidence for the involvement of serotonin afferents. *Brain Res.*, **235**, 285–301.

McRae-Degueurce, A., Dennis, T., Leger L. and Scatton, B. (1985). Regulation of noradrenergic neuronal activity in the rat locus coeruleus by serotoninergic afferents. *Physiol. Psychol.*, **13**(3), 188–196.

Melia, K. R. and Duman, R. S. (1991). Involvement of corticotropin-releasing factor in chronic stress regulation of the brain noradrenergic system. *Proc. Natl Acad. Sci. USA*, **88**, 8382–8386.

Middleton, H. C. (1990). An enhanced hypotensive response to clonidine can still be found in panic patients despite psychological treatment. *J. Anx. Disord.*, **4**, 213–219.

Modigh, K., Westberg, P. and Eriksson, E. (1992). Superiority of clomipramine over imipramine in the treatment of panic disorder: a placebo-controlled trial. *J. Clin. Psychopharmacol.*, **12**, 251–261.

Mongeau, R., Blier, P. and de Montigny, C. (1993). In vivo electrophysiological evidence for tonic activation by endogenous noradrenaline of α-2 adrenoreceptors on 5-hydroxytryptamine terminals in the rat hippocampus. *Naunyn Schmiedebergs Arch. Pharmacol.*, **347**, 266–272.

Morgane, P. J. and Jacobs, M. S. (1979). Raphe projections to the locus coeruleus in the rat. *Brain Res. Bull.*, **4**, 519–534.

Nesse, R. M., Cameron, O. G., Cuirtis, G. C. *et al.* (1984). Adrenergic function in patients with panic anxiety. *Arch. Gen. Psychiatry*, **41**, 771–776.

Nestler, E. J., McMahon, A., Sabban, E. L. *et al.* (1990). Chronic antidepressant administration decreases the expression of tyrosine hydroxylase in the rat locus coeruleus. *Neurobiology*, **87**, 7522–7526.

Nimgaonkar, V. L., Goodwin, G. M., Davies, C. L. and Green, A. R. (1985). Down-regulation of β-adrenoceptors in rat cortex by repeated administration of desipramine, electroconvulsive shock and clenbuterol requires 5-HT neurones but not 5-HT. *Neuropsychopharmacology*, **24**(4), 279–283.

Nisenbaum, L. K., Zigmund, M. J., Sved, A. F. and Abercrombie, E. D. (1991). Prior exposure to chronic stress results in enhanced synthesis and release of hippocampal norepinephrine in response to a novel stressor. *J. Neurosci.*, **11**, 1478–1484.

Norman, T. R., Judd, F. K., Gregory, M. *et al.* (1986). Platelet serotonin uptake in panic disorder. *J. Affect. Disord.*, **11**, 69–72.

Norman, T. R., Kimber, N. M., Judd, F. K. *et al.* (1987). Platelet 3H-rauwolscine binding in patients with panic attacks. *Psychiatry Res.*, **22**, 43–48.

Nutt, D. J. (1989). Altered alpha-2-adrenoceptor sensitivity in panic disorder. *Arch. Gen. Psychiatry*, **46**, 165–169.

Nutt, D. J. and Fraser, S. (1987). Platelet binding studies in panic disorder. *J. Affect. Disord.*, **12**, 7–11.

Nutt, D. and Lawson, C. (1992). Panic attacks. a neurochemical overview of models and mechanism. *Br. J. Psychiatry*, **160**, 165–178.

Nyback, H. V., Walters, J. R., Aghajanian, G. K. and Roth, R. H. (1975). Tricyclic antidepressants: effects on the firing rate of brain noradrenergic neurons. *Eur. J. Pharmacol.*, **32**, 302–312.

Ordway, G. A., Gambarana, C., Tejani-Butt, S. N. *et al.* (1991). Preferential reduction of binding of 125I-iodopindolol to beta-1 adrenoceptors in the amygdala of the rat after antidepressant treatments. *J. Pharmacol. Exp. Ther.*, **257**, 681.

Palkovits, M., Brownstein, M. and Saavedra, J. M. (1974). Serotonin content of the brain stem nuclei of the rat. *Brain Res.*, **80**, 237.

Pecknold, J. C., Suranyi-Cadotte, B., Chang, H. and Nair, N. P. V. (1988). Serotonin uptake in panic disorder and agoraphobia. *Neuropsychopharmacology*, **1**, 173–176.

Pickel, V. M., Tong, H. J. and Reis, D. J. (1978). *Immunocytochemical Evidence for Serotonergic Innervation of Noradrenergic Neurons in Nucleus Locus Ceruleus*, pp. 369–382. Raven Press, New York.

Pieribone, V. A. and Aston-Jones, G. (1988). The iontophoretic application of fluoro-gold for the study of afferents to deep brain nuclei. *Brain Res.*, **475**, 259–271.

Pieribone, V. A., and Aston-Jones, G. (1990). Serotonergic innervation of the rat locus coeruleus. *Eur. J. Pharmacol.*, **3** (Supp.), 231.

Pieribone, V. A., Aston-Jones, G. and Bohn, M. C. (1988). Adrenergic and nonadrenergic neurons of the C1 and C3 areas project to locus coeruleus: a fluorescent double labeling study. *Neurosci. Lett.*, **85**, 297–303.

Pieribone, V. A., Van Bockstaele, E. J., Shipley, M. T. and Aston-Jones, G. (1989). Serotonergic innervation of rat locus coeruleus derives from non-raphe brain areas. *Soc.*

Neurosci. Abstr., **15**, 420.

Pohl, R., Rainey, J. M., Ortiz, A. *et al.* (1985). Isoproterenol-induced anxiety states. *Psychopharmacol. Bull.*, **21**, 424–427.

Pohl, R., Yeragani, V. K., Balon, R. *et al.* (1988). Isoproterenol-induced panic attacks. *Biol. Psychiatry*, **24**, 891–902.

Pohl, R., Yeragani, V. K. and Balon, R. (1990). Effects of isoproterenol in panic disorder patients after antidepressant treatment. *Biol. Psychiatry*, **28**, 203–214.

Pratt, J. A. (1992). The neuroanatomical basis of anxiety. *Pharmacol. Ther.*, **55**, 149–181.

Pujol, J. F., Keane, P., McRae, A. *et al.* (1978). Biochemical evidence for serotonergic control of the locus coeruleus. In *Interactions Between Putative Neurotransmitters in the Brain* (eds S. Garattini, J. F. Pujol and R. Samanin), pp. 401–410. Raven Press, New York.

Rainey, M., Jr, Ettedgui, E., Pohl, B. *et al.* (1984). The β-receptor: isoproterenol anxiety states. *Psychopathology*, **17**(3), 40–51.

Rao, R. and Hjorth, S. (1992). α_2-Adrenoceptor modulation of rat ventral hippocampal 5-hydroxytryptamine release in vivo. *Naunyn Schmiedebergs Arch. Pharmacol.*, **345**, 137–143.

Rasmussen, K. and Aghajanian, G. K. (1986). Effect of hallucinogens on spontaneous and sensory-evoked locus coeruleus unit activity in the rat: reversal by selective 5-HT2 antagonists. *Brain Res.*, **385**, 395–400.

Rasmussen, K. and Aghajanian, G. K. (1989a). Failure to block responses of locus coeruleus neurons to somatosensory stimuli by destruction of two major afferent nuclei. *Synapse*, **4**, 162–164.

Rasmussen, K. and Aghajanian, G. K. (1989b). Withdrawal-induced activation of locus coeruleus neurons in opiate-dependent rats: attenuation by lesions of the nucleus paragigantocellularis. *Brain Res.*, **505**, 346–350.

Rasmussen, K., Marilak, D. A. and Jacobs, B. L. (1986). Single unit activity of the locus coeruleus in the freely moving cat, I: During naturalistic behaviors and in response to simple and complex stimuli. *Brain Res.*, **371**, 324–334.

Rasmussen, S. A., Goodman, W. K., Woods, S. W. *et al.* (1987). Effects of yohimbine in obsessive-compulsive disorder. *Psychopharmacology*, **93**, 308–373.

Redmond, D. E. (1987). Studies of the nucleus locus coeruleus in monkeys and hypotheses for neuropsychopharmacology. In *Psychopharmacology: The Third Generation of Progress* (eds H. Y. Meltzer), pp. 967–975. Raven Press, New York.

Redmond, D. E., Jr and Huang, Y. H. (1979). New evidence for a locus coeruleus–norepinephrine connection with anxiety. *Life Sci.*, **25**, 2149–2162.

Redmond, D. E., Jr, Huang, Y. H., Snyder, D. R. and Maas, J. W. (1976). Behavioral effects of stimulations of the locus coeruleus in the stumptail monkey (Macaca arctoides). *Brain Res.*, **116**, 502–510.

Renson, J. (1973). Assays and properties of tryptophan 5-hydroxylase. In *Serotonin and Behavior* (eds. J. Barchas and E. Usdin), pp. 19–32 Academic Press, New York.

Riley, L. A., Jonakait, G. M. and Hart, R. P. (1993). Serotonin modulates the levels of mRNAs coding for thyrotropin-releasing hormone and preprotachykinin by different mechanisms in medullary raphe neurons. *Mol. Brain Res.*, **17**, 251–257.

Schmidt, A. W. and Peroutka, S. J. (1989). 5-hydroxytryptamine receptor "families". *FASEB J.*, **3**, 2242–2249.

Schneider, L. S., Munjack, D., Severson, J. A. and Palmer, R. (1987). Platelet 3H-imipramine binding in generalized anxiety disorder, panic disorder, and agoraphobia with panic attacks. *Biol. Psychiatry,* **21**, 33–41.

Segal, M. (1979). Serotonergic innervation of the locus coeruleus from the dorsal raphe and its action on responses to noxious stimuli. *J. Physiol. (Lond.)*, **286**, 401–415.

Segal, M. (1981). The action of norepinephrine in the rat hippocampus: intracellular studies in the slice preparation. *Brain Res.*, **206**, 107–128.

Segal, M. and Bloom, F. E. (1976). The action of norepinephrine in the rat hippocampus IV: The effect of locus coeruleus stimulation on evoked hippocampal activity. *Brain Res.*, **107**, 513–525.

Southwick, S. M., Krystal, J., Morgan, C. A. *et al.* (1993). Abnormal noradrenergic function in posttraumatic stress disorder. *Arch. Gen. Psychiatry*, **50**, 266–274.

Steinbusch, H. W. M. (1984). Serotonin-immunoreactive neurons and their targets in the CNS. In *Classical Transmitters and Transmitter Receptors in the CNS*, Pt II (eds A. Björklund, T. Hökfelt and M. J. Kuhar), pp. 68–118. Elsevier, Amsterdam.

Stockmeier, C. A., Martino, A. M. and Kellar, K. J. (1985). A strong influence of serotonin axons on beta adrenergic receptors in rat brain. *Science*, **230**, 323–325.

Strecker, R. E. and Jacobs, B. L. (1985). Substantia nigra dopaminergic unit activity in behaving cats: effect of arousal on spontaneous discharge and sensory evoked activity. *Brain Res.,* **361**, 339–350.

Sugita, S., Shen, K.-Z. and North, R. A. (1992). 5-hydroxytryptamine is a fast excitatory transmitter at 5-HT$_3$ receptors in rat amygdala. *Neuron*, **8**, 199–203.

Sugrue, M. F. (1983). Do antidepressants possess a common mechanism of action? *Biochem. Pharmacol.,* **32**, 1811–1817.

Sulser, F. (1984). Regulation and function of noradrenaline receptor systems in brain. *Neuropharmacology*, **23**, 255–261.

Svensson, T. H. (1987). Peripheral, autonomic regulation of locus coeruleus noradrenergic neurons in brain: putative implications for psychiatry and psychopharmacology. *Psychopharmacology*, **92**, 1–7.

Svensson, T. H. and Usdin, T. (1978). Feedback inhibition of brain noradrenaline neurons by tricyclic antidepressants: a-receptor mediation. *Science*, **202**, 1089–1091.

Szemeredi, K., Komoly, S., Kopin, I. J. *et al.* (1991). Simultaneous measurement of plasma and brain extracellular fluid concentrations of catechols after yohimbine administration in rats. *Brain Res.*, **542**, 8–14.

Tanaka, M., Ida, Y., Tsuda, A. and Nagasaki, N. (1986). Involvement of brain noradrenaline and opioid peptides in emotional changes induced by stress in rats. In *Emotions: Neural and Chemical Control* (ed. Y. Oomura), pp. 417–427. Scientific Societies Press, Tokyo.

Targum, S. D. and Marshall, L. E. (1989). Fenfluramine provocation of anxiety in patients with panic disorder. *Psychiatry Res.,* **28**, 295–306.

Tsaltas, E., Gray, J. A. and Fillenz, M. (1987). Alleviation of response suppression to conditioned aversive stimuli by lesions of the dorsal noradrenergic bundle. *Behav. Brain Res.*, **13**, 115–127.

Tsuda, A. and Tanaka, M. (1985). Differential changes in noradrenaline turnover in specific regions of rat brain produced by controllable and uncontrollable shocks. *Behav. Neurosci.*, **99**, 802–817.

Tyrer, P., Candy, J. and Kelly, D. (1973). A study of the clinical effects of phenelzine and placebo in the treatment of phobic anxiety. *Psychopharmacologia*, **32**, 237–254.

Uhde, T. W., Vittone, B. J., Siever, L. J. *et al.* (1986). Blunted growth hormone response to clonidine in panic disorder patients. *Biol. Psychiatry*, **21**, 1077–1081.

Uhde, T. W., Berrettini, W. H., Roy-Byrne, P. P. *et al.* (1987). Platelet 3H-imipramine binding in patients with panic disorder. *Biol. Psychiatry*, **22**, 52–58.

Valentino, R. J., Curtis, A. L., Parris, D. G. and Wehby, R. G. (1990). Antidepressant actions on brain noradrenergic neurons. *J. Pharmacol. Exp. Ther.*, **253**, 833–840.

Wang, Z. W., Crowe, R. R. and Noyes, R., Jr (1992). Adrenergic receptor genes as candidate genes for panic disorder: a linkage study. *Am. J. Psychiatry*, **149**, 470–474.

Waterhouse, B. D., Moises, H. C., Yeh, H. H. and Woodward, D. J. (1982). Norepinephrine enhancement of inhibitory synaptic mechanisms in cerebellum and cerebral cortex: mediation by beta adrenergic receptors. *J. Pharmacol. Exp. Ther.*, **221**, 495–506.

Weissmann-Nanopoulos, D., Mach, E., Magre, J. *et al.* (1985). Evidence for the localization of 5-HT1A binding sites on serotonin containing neurons in the raphe dorsalis and raphe centralis. *Neurochem. Int.*, **7**, 1061–1072.

Wilkinson, L. O. and Jacobs, B. L. (1988). Lack of response of serotonergic neurons in the dorsal raphe nucleus of freely moving cats to stressful stimuli. *Exp. Neurol.*, **101**, 445–457.

Woods, S. W., Charney, D. S., McPherson, C. A. *et al.* (1987). Situational panic attacks: behavioral, physiological, and biochemical characterization. *Arch. Gen. Psychiatry*, **44**, 365–375.

Woods, S. W., Hoffer, P. B., McDougle, C. J. *et al.* (1991). Effects of yohimbine on regional cerebral blood flow in panic disorder. *Soc. Neurosci. Abstr.*, 17, no. 293.8.

Zitrin, C. M., Klein, D. F., Woerner, M. G. and Ross, D. C. (1983). Treatment of phobias: comparison of imipramine and placebo. *Arch. Gen. Psychiatry*, **40**, 125–138.

7 Involvement of Serotonin Receptor Subtypes in Panic Disorder: A Critical Appraisal of the Evidence

JOHAN A. DEN BOER AND HERMAN G. M. WESTENBERG

Department of Psychiatry, University Hospital Utrecht, Utrecht, The Netherlands

INTRODUCTION

There is accumulating evidence from preclinical and clinical studies suggesting that disturbances in the regulation of serotonin (5-hydroxytryptamine, 5-HT) and norepinephrine (NE) are involved in a variety of psychiatric disorders. In this chapter the role of 5-HT and 5-HT receptor subtypes in the pathogenesis of panic disorder (PD) will be critically reviewed.

Our knowledge on the 5-HT-containing pathways is rapidly growing. To date the complexity of the 5-HT neuronal system in terms of morphological characteristics, receptor subtypes and biochemical linkages is extraordinary. In order to be able to comprehend the results of clinical studies described below we will first give a concise description of the serotonergic system and the current receptor nomenclature.

SEROTONERGIC PATHWAYS IN THE CENTRAL NERVOUS SYSTEM

The cell bodies of the 5-HT-containing neurons are located predominantly in the brain stem. From here, ascending and descending fibers innervate virtually all brain regions. 5-HT-containing cell bodies that give rise to ascending projections are predominantly housed in the dorsal and median raphe nuclei. It has been demonstrated in the rat that fibers emerging from the dorsal raphe and the median raphe are morphologically different: those arising from the dorsal raphe nucleus are fine, with small varicosities, while those derived from the median raphe nucleus are thicker. The morphological differences between the two systems may signify biochemical and functional differences. Thus, Manoumas and Molliver (1988) have shown that fibers from the dorsal raphe nucleus are more likely to be damaged by the neurotoxin, *p*-chloroamphetamine, than those from the median raphe nucleus.

Advances in the Neurobiology of Anxiety Disorders. Edited by H. G. M. Westenberg, J. A. Den Boer and D. L. Murphy
©1996 John Wiley & Sons Ltd

Whether this morphological and anatomical differentiation bears any relevance for the pathogenesis and treatment of anxiety is as yet unclear. Although both nuclei appear to innervate overlapping fields, there are also exceptions. Autoradiographic and microdialysis studies reveal that parts of the limbic system, especially the septohippocampal formation, are furnished for the most part by projections from the median raphe, while the dorsal raphe, in particular its rostral part, innervates with greater density the neostriatum and the thalamus (Bonvento et al., 1992). It is of interest that the locus coeruleus (LC), the principal NA-containing nucleus in the central nervous system (CNS), is reciprocally connected to the raphe nuclei. For example, 5-HT neurons in the dorsal raphe nucleus have anatomic connections with the LC (Descarrier and Léger, 1978; Morgane and Jacobs, 1979; Baraban and Aghajanian, 1980). In addition, there are also a number of functional interactions between the LC and the raphe nuclei. 5-HT appears to have an inhibitory effect on LC firing (Segal, 1979), while NA was found to have an excitatory effect on 5-HT activity in the dorsal raphe nucleus (Baraban and Aghajanian, 1980). Another anatomic site where 5-HT–NA interaction may occur is formed by the terminal areas that are innervated by both monoaminergic pathways. Of particular interest in this respect is the hippocampus, which receives dense innervation of both systems. Therefore, mutual interactions are also likely to occur in this region. 5-HT nerve terminals in the hippocampus are endowed with α_2-adrenoreceptors (Göthert et al., 1981) and there are indications of a modulation of the hippocampal 5-HT release by endogenous NA (Feuerstein et al., 1985). Lesion studies have suggested a pivotal role of 5-HT in the regulation of the density and function of central β-adrenoreceptors (Gillespie et al., 1988).

In view of these complex neuronal interaction—the connections described above give only a glimpse of all possible interactions—any theory relating a complex behavior, such as anxiety, to a single neurotransmitter or to a single receptor subtype is predestined to be an oversimplification.

SEROTONIN RECEPTOR SUBTYPES

At present four major-classes of 5-HT receptors have been identified in the brain; they are designated as 5-HT_1, 5-HT_2, 5-HT_3 and 5-HT_4 receptors. With the exception of the 5-HT_3 receptor, they all belong to the superfamily of G protein-linked receptors. These receptors transduce signals by activating G proteins, producing relatively slow responses through second messengers. The 5-HT_3 receptor is unique among the 5-HT receptors in that it is a ligand-gated ion channel, producing rapid depolarizing responses, when stimulated. The 5-HT_1 family can be subdivided into at least five different subtypes all of which appear to be seven transmembrane domain receptors. They are denoted as 5-HT_{1A}, 5-HT_{1B}, 5-HT_{1C}, 5-HT_{1D} and 5-HT_{1E}. In this chapter we will use the accepted new terminology of 5-HT receptor subtypes: 5-HT_2 receptors are now designated as 5-HT_{2A}, and 5-HT_{1C} receptors are named 5-HT_{2C} receptors (Humphrey et al., 1993).

The $5\text{-}HT_1$ receptors were originally identified by their high affinity for [^{3}H]5-HT. Although the relatively high affinity of the $5\text{-}HT_{2C}$ receptor for 5-HT resulted in its classification as a $5\text{-}HT_1$-like receptor, subsequent studies have called this classification into question. Unlike the other 5-HT receptors, the $5\text{-}HT_{2C}$ receptor is not negatively coupled to adenyl cyclase. Like the $5\text{-}HT_{2A}$ receptor, stimulation of the $5\text{-}HT_{2C}$ receptor (previously called $5\text{-}HT_{1C}$) promotes the hydrolysis of phosphoinositide. In addition to this analogy in signal transduction, both receptors appear to be closely related also from a molecular viewpoint; there appears to be a high degree of amino acid sequence homology. The $5\text{-}HT_{1A}$, $5\text{-}HT_{1B}$ and $5\text{-}HT_{1D}$ receptors are all negatively linked to adenyl cyclase activity. The $5\text{-}HT_{1E}$ is a novel 5-HT receptor subtype, also linked to adenyl cyclase, but whose exact localization and function in the brain are as yet unknown. Preliminary studies using *in situ* hybridization histochemistry revealed that this receptor subtype is present in the human brain in cortical areas, caudate, putamen and amygdala (Bruinvels, 1993). The $5\text{-}HT_{1B}$ receptor is found only in some rodents and has been suggested to represent the species equivalent of the $5\text{-}HT_{1D}$ receptor of higher species, where the $5\text{-}HT_{1B}$ receptors are absent (Hoyer and Middlemiss, 1989). This is supported by recent cloning work which has led to a further differentiation of this receptor subtype into a human $5\text{-}HT_{1D\alpha}$ and $5\text{-}HT_{1D\beta}$ site; a closely related rat $5\text{-}HT_{1D\alpha}$ clone is identical to the rat $5\text{-}HT_{1\alpha}$ receptor (Hartig, 1992). The $5\text{-}HT_4$ receptor represents a new receptor subtype for 5-HT (Dumuis *et al.*, 1988). As yet, the molecular structure of the $5\text{-}HT_4$ receptor has not been reported, but pharmacologically it seems to be closely linked to the $5\text{-}HT_1$ receptors, as it appears to be positively coupled to adenyl cyclase (Bockaert *et al.*, 1987).

Recently, several new 5-HT receptor subtypes have been cloned like the $5\text{-}HT_{5A}$, $5\text{-}HT_{5B}$, $5\text{-}HT_6$ and $5\text{-}HT_7$ receptor (Erlander *et al.*, 1993; Matthes *et al.*, 1993; Plassat *et al.*, 1992; Monsma *et al.*, 1993). In view of the fact that the pharmacological properties and physiological functions of these newer receptors are still completely unknown, they will not be discussed in the present chapter.

Considering the limited number of cell bodies present in the brain, this multifaceted nature of 5-HT receptors is astonishing. It might explain the diversity of behavioral and physiological processes in which 5-HT appears to play a role.

THE PHARMACOLOGICAL FEATURES OF 5-HT RECEPTORS

The $5\text{-}HT_1$ receptor family

The $5\text{-}HT_{1A}$ receptors are selectively labeled by 8-hydroxy-2-(di-n-propy-lamino)tetralin (8-OH-DPAT; see Hamon *et al.*, 1990). The distribution of the $5\text{-}HT_{1A}$ binding sites is well characterized. The $5\text{-}HT_{1A}$ receptor is highly expressed in the hippocampus, the lateral septum, frontal cortex and dorsal raphe nucleus in rat and human brain (Pazos and Palacios, 1985; Pazos *et al.*, 1986). $5\text{-}HT_{1A}$ receptors in the hippocampus and cortex are thought to be located postsynaptically (Palacios *et al.*, 1987; Hamon *et al.*, 1990). Stimulation of the 5-HT_{1A} receptor on these postsynaptic target cells inhibits hippocampal activity (Andrade *et al.*, 1986; Yocca, 1990) and reduces the glucose utilization as measured by autoradiographic techniques. Recently a new class of drugs, denoted as azapirones, have been developed for this receptor subtype. Compounds of this class, such as ipsapirone, gepirone and buspirone, have all been found to mimic the effects of 5-HT at the 5-HT_{1A} site and display an anxiolytic profile in animal models of anxiety (see Traber and Glaser, 1987). Analogous to 8-OH-DPAT, these drugs inhibit the neuronal activity in both the raphe neurons and the hippocampal formation (Yocca, 1990). They also attenuate the 5-HT release in hippocampal perfusates when administered systemically (Sharp *et al.*, 1989). In contrast to 8-OH-DPAT, they are considered as partial agonists on the postsynaptic 5-HT_{1A} receptors (Sprouse and Aghajanian, 1988). Despite this knowledge on the pharmacology of azapirones, the mechanism of action underlying their anxiolytic effects in man remains obscure. The pharmacological effects on 5-HT_{1A} receptors are immediate, but in several brain regions, especially in the dorsal raphe nucleus, also temporary, due to desensitization of the receptors (Blier and De Montigny, 1987; Fanelli and McMonagle-Strucko, 1992). In rats, anxiolytic activity is seen already after acute systemic or local administration in the dorsal raphe nucleus, suggesting that "turning off" 5-HT function is "anxiolytic" in rats (Higgins *et al.*, 1988). In contrast, the anxiolytic effects in man emerge over several weeks of treatment. This late onset of action in human, therefore, poses a serious theoretical problem. It has been argued, therefore, that the therapeutic effects of azapirones in man are mediated by the downregulation of the somatodendritic autoreceptors in the raphe nuclei. This is a parsimonious explanation, but it does not take into account the acute effects.

If this is so, why does acute administration not worsen the symptomatology? Moreover, downregulation following chronic treatment would only recuperate the normal firing rate. Another possibility is that these compounds are acting through the postsynaptic 5-HT_{1A} receptors.

The late onset of action would then be explained by assuming a downregulation of the postsynaptic 5-HT_{1A} receptors. A recent behavioral study in rats supports this notion. Fernández-Guasti and coworkers (1992) found that after intracerebroventricular lesioning of the 5-HT system by 5,7-dihydroxytryptamine the effects of buspirone and ipsapirone in the burying behavior test were not influenced, whereas the behavioral effects of 8-OH-DPAT were completely abolished. This suggests that the anxiolytic affects of ipsapirone and buspirone may be mediated via stimulation of postsynaptic receptors, and the behavioral effects of 8-OHD-PAT by autoreceptors. Electrophysiological studies have revealed, however, that the responsiveness of the postsynaptic 5-HT_{1A} receptors in the dorsal hippocampus is not altered after administration of 5-HT_{1A} agonists (Blier and De Montigny, 1990). Similar findings were found in autoradiography studies, although desensitization was found in other brain regions (Fanelli and

McMonagle-Strucko, 1992). It is also conceivable that the acute effects on the postsynaptic receptors may have been obliterated by acute effects at the presynaptic sites; from a functional point of view, presynaptic and postsynaptic 5-HT receptors have opposite effects. Another possibility for the delayed action in man would be adaptive changes in other serotonergic or non-serotonergic receptors. The possibility of one 5-HT receptor subtype to modulate the function of another subtype can likewise not be excluded (Glennon *et al.*, 1991). It is interesting to note, therefore, that azapirones have the ability to downregulate the $5-HT_{2A}$ receptors (Eison and Yocca, 1985), which have also been linked to anxiety, as will be discussed below. But we are faced with yet another problem.

Azapirones are partial agonists (Segal *et al.*, 1989). Therefore, it is difficult to ascertain whether they are acting as agonists or antagonists at the postsynaptic 5-HT receptors. Clinical studies with full agonists and antagonists are therefore required to further our understanding in this respect.

The $5-HT_2$ receptor family

Members of the $5-HT_2$ family of receptors share the ability to stimulate phosphoinositide hydrolysis. This class was originally differentiated from the $5-HT_1$ category on the basis of different affinities for $[^3H]5-HT$ and $[^3H]$spiperone. The two members of this family, $5-HT_{2C}$ and $5-HT_{2A}$, are both labeled by the antagonists $[^3H]$mesulergine and $[^3H]$mianserine. Neurons that express $5-HT_{2C}$ are found to be widely distributed in the brain (Julius, 1991). Aside from the choroid plexus, where it was originally discovered, high densities are seen in the hippocampus, particularly in pyramidal neurons in the ventral part of the hippocampus, the posterior thalamic subnuclei and in other subcortical regions rich in monoaminergic cells, such as the substantia nigra, LC and raphe nuclei. In general, the cortical labeling is sparse (Harrington *et al.*, 1992). These findings suggest that $5-HT_{2C}$ receptors are involved in both pre- and postsynaptic serotonergic mechanisms and may serve as autoreceptors in the somatodendritic region. In view of its expression in the periaqueductal gray, $5-HT_{2C}$ receptors are believed to be implicated also in the processing of afferent sensory information and regulation of nociception (Molineaux *et al.*, 1989; Julius, 1991). *m*-Chlorophenylpiperazine (mCPP), the major metabolite of trazodone, has been described as a potent $5-HT_{2C}$ agonist, but it is by no means a specific ligand. It has affinity for almost all 5-HT binding sites and it also binds potently to α_2-adrenoreceptors (Hoyer, 1988; Schoeffler and Hoyer, 1989; Kilpatrick *et al.*, 1987; Hamik and Peroutka, 1989). Particularly, its affinity for the $5-HT_3$ receptors, to which it binds as strongly as to $5-HT_{2C}$ sites, is noteworthy. However, constants for affinity *in vitro* do not necessarily reflect activity *in vivo*. Despite its limited specificity, mCPP is commonly used as probe for the 5-HT function in psychiatric research (Kahn and Wetzler, 1991).

The other member of this family, the $5-HT_{2A}$ receptor, shows the highest density in the frontal cortex, but it also occurs in the striatum, nucleus accumbens and tuberculum olfactorium (Leysen, 1985). Little or no labeling has been found in the thalamus, hippocampus or brain stem (Pazos *et al.*, 1987). 5-HT$_{2A}$ binding sites are also expressed in the periphery, including platelets and smooth muscles. They are selectively labeled by [^{3}H]ketanserin. Many antidepressants have high affinity for the postsynaptic 5-HT$_{2A}$ receptors and most of them share the ability to cause a gradual downregulation of 5-HT$_{2A}$ receptors in rat brain. This feature of antidepressants has long been considered pertinent to the antidepressant efficacy of this class of drugs, but recent findings have called the relevance of this finding into question (see Charney *et al.*, 1991). Ritanserin, a selective 5-HT$_{2A}$/5-HT$_{2C}$ receptor antagonist, has been found to possess an anxiolytic profile in some animal models of anxiety (Meert and Janssen, 1989) and to exert anxiolytic effects in patients (Ceulemans *et al.*, 1985).

The 5-HT$_3$ receptors

Kilpatrick *et al.* (1987) were the first to demonstrate the presence of this binding site in rat brain. They reported dense labeling in the entorhinal cortex of this species. Subsequent studies revealed the occurrence throughout the brain, including the hippocampus, amygdala and brain stem. Selective 5-HT$_3$ antagonists such as ICS 205–930, MDL 72222, ondansetron and zacopride have been synthesized and animal tests suggest they will have a variety of effects, including anxiolytic activity in man (Tyers, 1989; Costall *et al.*, 1988; Papp and Przegalinski, 1989; Apud, 1993). As yet, only preliminary reports of clinical trials have appeared, which are not unequivocal (Lader, 1991).

ANIMAL MODELS OF ANXIETY

A variety of paradigms have been used in the psychopharmacology of anxiety, involving unconditioned and conditioned procedures, models concentrating upon drug-induced discriminative states and brain stimulation paradigms (e.g. stimulation of the periaqueductal gray).

Several 5-HT-augmenting and -depleting agents have been used in different models of anxiety. The results obtained so far, although contradictory, suggest that increased 5-HT function results in a behavioral profile in rodents resembling anxiolytic activity and vice versa (for review see Westenberg and Den Boer, 1994).

CLINICAL STUDIES IN PANIC DISORDER

Clinical evidence on the role of 5-HT is mainly derived from treatment studies and challenge paradigms with (non-selective) serotonergic drugs. In addition surrogate measurements in accessible biological samples, including blood, cerebrospinal fluid and urine, are employed to assess the functionality of 5-HT systems in the human brain under pathological and normal conditions. In the following section, the role of 5-HT in PD will be critically discussed.

DIAGNOSTIC CONSIDERATIONS

Until the 1960s the term neurosis played a dominating role in the clinical description of anxiety and phobic disorders, but with the introduction of the DSM-III and the DSM-III-R (American Psychiatric Association, 1980, 1987), a refinement in the classification has taken place. According to the DSM-III-R, anxiety disorders can be divided into several main categories, including panic disorder (PD) with and without agoraphobia, generalized anxiety disorder (GAD), social phobia (SP), and obsessive-compulsive disorder (OCD). Anxiety symptoms also undoubtedly feature prominently in some subtypes of OCD, but there is little evidence to support its categorization as an anxiety disorder (Montgomery, 1992). Most data support its perception as a separate diagnostic entity. Of particular interest is the distinction between GAD and PD.

This distinction is originally based on the observation that antidepressants, such as imipramine, can block spontaneous panic attacks, whereas until recently benzodiazepines were considered to be relatively ineffective against panic attacks. GAD patients seem to respond best to anxiolytics, such as benzodiazepines (see Westenberg and Den Boer, 1993). The present chapter will focus on research involving 5-HT function and the involvement of 5-HT receptor subtypes in PD.

TREATMENT STUDIES SUPPORTING THE ROLE OF 5-HT

Selective 5-HT uptake inhibitors

The recognition that antidepressants exert beneficial effects in PD have prompted investigators to evaluate the efficacy of these drugs. The use of antidepressants in the treatment PD originates from the observation of Klein and Fink (1962), who reported that imipramine was effective in anxiety states. In subsequent studies they provided further evidence that imipramine could prevent panic attacks and that in most patients attenuation of panic attacks was ensued by a decrease in other psychopathological dimensions, such as phobic avoidance and anticipatory anxiety (Klein, 1964, 1967). Today several studies have confirmed the superiority of imipramine to placebo.

These studies have been reviewed in several articles (see Modigh, 1987); therefore we will not reiterate all those papers but rather address the issue of the pharmacological mechanism underlying this feature. There has been some debate whether effects on NE- or 5-HT-containing neurons comprise the site at which antidepressants exert the main proportion of their action. Mavissakalian and Perel (1989) have proposed that the efficacy of imipramine in PD may be due predominantly to the 5-HT-ergic action of the drug. In a study of PD patients who received imipramine, the plasma imipramine level, but not that of the desmethyl metabolite, correlated significantly with improvement. The parent compound, imipramine, potently inhibits the neuronal uptake of both 5-HT and NA, while the metabolite, desmethylimipramine, is a selective NA uptake blocker. Thus the antipanic effects of imipramine may be mediated through the 5-HT system.

Studies with (SSRIs) permit dissection and characterization of imipramine's mixed effects on these neurotransmitter systems and exploration of the role of 5-HT in the pathogenesis of PD. In keeping with the presumed role of 5-HT in the mechanism of action underlying imipramine's effect in PD, beneficial effects were obtained with clomipramine and zimeldine, two selective 5-HT uptake inhibitors in several open-label studies (Evans et al., 1980; Koczkas and Weissman, 1981; Gloger et al., 1981; Grunhaus et al., 1984) The results of several controlled studies with SSRIs confirm the antipanic efficacy of antidepressants and hint at the involvement of 5-HT (Table 1).

There is also evidence that newer drugs like fluoxetine could be effective in PD, but until now only open studies have been published (Gorman et al., 1987; Schneier et al., 1990). By and large these studies indicate that SSRIs are effective in reducing symptoms of panic and anxiety in patients with PD. Further support for the role of 5-HT in the mechanism of action of antidepressants came from a study with fluvoxamine, which selectively inhibits the uptake of 5-HT, and maprotiline, an antidepressant which has selective effects for the NA transporter (Den Boer and Westenberg, 1988). The number of panic attacks and the level of anxiety decreased significantly in patients on fluvoxamine. In the maprotiline group there was no significant change in the number of panic attacks and only a slight reduction in anxiety. Subjects in this study were carefully selected, excluding those with concomitant depressive symptoms, to find a "pure" PD sample. Therefore, the data indicate a specific antipanic effect for fluvoxamine, which may be related to its effect on 5-HT systems in the brain. Generally, SSRIs show a latency of two to four weeks before the therapeutic effect occurs. In addition, a transient increase in anxiety is seen in the majority of PD patients at the beginning of treatment.

This biphasic profile (Figure 1) suggests that SSRIs display an acute anxiogenic effect that is converted into an anxiolytic effect following chronic administration. These initial anxiogenic effects have also been interpreted as a cognitively mediated sequence of events, since patients suffering from PD are apprehensive concerning the effect of any drug, which may easily lead to a misinterpretation of effect as potentially dangerous (Clark, 1986). Interestingly, this is compatible with the theory of receptor involvement in the explanation of this phenomenon since, for example, a supersensitivity of any receptor subtype may lead to a lowered threshold for activation of brain defensive systems, and subsequently to anxiety (Ramos et al., 1993).

Similar anxiogenic effects have been reported for healthy volunteers. Studying the effect of clomipramine on anxiety induced in healthy volunteers by simulated public speaking, Zuardi (1990) found that this antidepressant facilitated the increase in anxiety score. In contrast, benzodiazepines and maprotiline decreased anxiety in this model. It may be tentatively suggested from these findings that the differential effects on 5-HT neurotransmission following acute and chronic administration of SSRIs are responsible for these

Table 1. Controlled studies with selective 5-HT uptake inhibitors in panic disorder

Reference	Diagnosis	Treatment	Therapeutic effect
Evans *et al.* (1986)	PD (25)	ZIM IMI PLAC	ZIM superior to PLA; PLA = IMI
Kahn *et al.* (1987)	PD (35) GAD (7)	5HTP CLO PLA	CLO and 5HTP superior to PLA
Den Boer *et al.* (1987)	APA (19) GAD (2) OCD (4) Ag (1)	CLO FLU	CLO = FLU; both effective
Den Boer and Westenberg (1988)	APA (37) PD (7)	FLU MAP	FLU superior to MAP
Cassano *et al.* (1988)	PD (59)	CLO IMI	CLO = IMI CLO more rapid onset
Johnston *et al.* (1988)	PD (108)	CLO PLA	CLO superior to PLA PLA
Den Boer and Westenberg (1990a)	PD (60)	FLU RIT PLA	FLU superior to RIT and PLA
Black *et al.* (1993)	PD (75)	FLU COGN THER and PLA	FLU superior to COGN THER
Hoehn Saric *et al.* (1993)	PD (50)	FLU	FLU superior to PLA
Asnis *et al.* (1994)	PD (188)	FLU PLA	FLU superior to PLA
Bakish *et al.* (1994)	PD (54)	FLU IMI PLA	Using LOCF analysis: NS difference between FLU/PLA Visit-wise: FLU/IMI better than PLA
Fawcett *et al.* (1994)	PD (124)	FLU PLA	Large PLA response; visit-wise analysis: FLU superior to PLA

5HTP, 5-hydroxytryptophan; ZIM, zimeldine; IMI, imipramine; FLU, fluvoxamine; CLO, clomipramine; MAP, maprotiline; RIT, ritanserin; PLA, placebo; APA, agoraphobia with panic attacks; GAD, generalized anxiety disorder; PD, panic disorder; Ag, agoraphobia.
COGN THER, cognitive therapy; Number of patients in parenthesis; LOCF, last observation carried forward; NS, not significant.

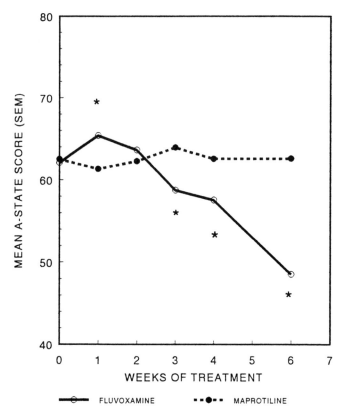

Figure 1 The effect of fluvoxamine and maprotiline in patients with panic disorder as assessed with the State Anxiety Inventory. *Significantly different from maprotiline ($p<0.01$) (Den Boer and Westenberg, 1988)

paradoxical effects. This concurs with experimental data, indicating that acute administration of SSRIs reduces the firing rate of 5-HT neurons, while due to desensitization of the somatodendritic 5-HT_{1A} autoreceptors an enhanced 5-HT function is seen after repeated administration (De Montigny and Aghajanian, 1978). These data also suggest that stimulation of an as yet unknown subset of 5-HT receptors may underlie the mechanism of action of SSRIs in PD.

Our original findings providing evidence for the antipanic efficacy of fluvox-amine have been confirmed in several (but not all) other studies (see Table 1).

Most recently, two double-blind placebo-controlled studies corroborated the anxiolytic and antipanic properties of fluvoxamine. The first study compared fluvoxamine, placebo and cognitive therapy under double-blind conditions (Black et al., 1993). It was found that fluvoxamine led to a significant reduction in the number of panic attacks, and was in fact reported to be of more benefit to patients compared to cognitive therapy. A second study of the same group was a placebo-controlled double-blind treatment study in which 93 PD patients were treated with fluvoxamine, and 95 with placebo. Similar to our original findings this group also found fluvoxamine to be significantly more effective in reducing the number of panic attacks (Asnis *et al.*, 1994). In this study the authors also reported that fluvoxamine did not just convert full-blown panic attacks into limited symptom attacks, but genuinely abolished acute attacks of anxiety.

Another study in which fluvoxamine (150–300 mg) was compared to placebo and imipramine (150–300 mg) failed to find differences between fluvoxamine and placebo. This may have been due to the fact that in this study (1) there were many drop-outs leading to only a 48.6% completion rate (completers per group were: fluvoxamine 18 (36%), imipramine 29 (60%), placebo 20 (40%), and (2) there was a widespread use of benzodiazepines in all treatment groups (Bakish *et al.*, 1994). Similar results were compared in a placebo-controlled study in 124 (included for analysis) PD patients with fluvoxamine by Fawcett *et al.* (1994; see Table 1). This group failed to find convincing confirmation for the efficacy of fluvoxamine in PD, possibly due to a high placebo response. However, week-by-week visit-wise analysis showed a consistent pattern of superiority of fluvoxamine over placebo for the frequency of panic attacks per week, as well as the severity of panic. There are several methodological differences between our own studies (Den Boer *et al.*, 1987; Den Boer and Westenberg, 1988, 1990a) and the recently conducted studies (Asnis *et al.*, 1994; Bakish *et al.*, 1994; Fawcett *et al.*, 1994). First, our studies were conducted in one centre; second, all psychometric evaluations were performed by one rater, thus avoiding interrater reliability problems; and third, we did not use newspaper advertising for the gathering of patients for this bears the risk of a recruitment bias which is almost impossible to control.

A selective therapeutic response of SSRIs, as opposed to other antidepressants such as desimipramine and amitriptyline, has also been demonstrated in OCD (Zohar and Insel, 1987; Goodman *et al.*, 1990). Several controlled studies with clomipramine, and the more selective SSRI, fluvoxamine, have all shown clear evidence of efficacy for these drugs in OCD (Clomipramine Collaborative Study Group, 1991; Goodman *et al.*, 1989, 1990; Jenike *et al.*, 1990; Perse *et al.*, 1987; Cottraux *et al.*, 1990; Fineberg *et al.*, 1992; Montgomery *et al.*, 1990). These findings point towards a role of 5-HT in OCD as well. Influence of NE cannot of course be ruled out with clomipramine, since this compound has an active NE-ergic metabolite, but the positive results from several controlled studies with fluvoxamine support the assumption that 5-HT is also of significance in the pathogenesis of OCD.

A ROLE FOR NOREPINEPHRINE IN PANIC DISORDER?

Based upon experiments with the α_2-adrenoreceptor antagonist yohimbine, a role for NE in PD has been suggested. Based upon the anxiogenic activity and the augmented (plasma) 3-methoxy-4-hydroxyphenethyleneglycol (MHPG) response to yohimbine in PD, it has been speculated that there exists an episodic overactivity of NE containing neural systems in the brain in PD (review: Charney *et al.*, 1994). If this were true it would be expected that maprotiline could exert robust anxiolytic effects in PD, as this compound downregulates β-adrenoreceptors, and subsequently reduces noradrenergic neurotransmission: clearly this is not the case (Den Boer and Westenberg, 1988).

In a recent placebo-controlled study in 65 patients with PD it was found that the NE uptake inhibitor desimipramine had anxiolytic effects (measured with the HAM-A) and possessed antipanic properties. In this study, 22 out of 26 (85%) were free of panic attacks at the end of treatment (week 12), whereas in the placebo group 13 out of 17 patients (76%) were panic-free (Lydiard *et al.*, 1993). The large placebo effects may have overshadowed the possible effects of desimipramine, but definitive conclusions about the efficacy of desimipramine are unwarranted.

The LC hypothesis rests firmly on the experiments with yohimbine and this also constitutes its weakness. Firstly, yohimbine, in addition to its noradrenergic effects, is also able to influence the level of 5-HT in the CNS (Papeschi and Theiss, 1975; Feuerstein *et al.*, 1975). Secondly, yohimbine may act as a 5-HT agonist at presynaptic receptors (Dwoskin *et al.*, 1988), while a recent receptor binding and drug discrimination study yielded evidence that yohimbine has affinity for 5-HT$_{1A}$ receptors (Winter and Rabin, 1992). Therefore, the anxiogenic effects of yohimbine could also, at least in part, be explained by virtue of its effects on serotonergic neurotransmission (Den Boer and Westenberg, 1993). Moreover, in a recent study it was found that treatment with the SSRI fluvoxamine in PD significantly reduced yohimbine-induced anxiety, whereas fluvoxamine was without effect on the increase in plasma MHPG invoked by yohimbine (Goddard *et al.*, 1993). In addition, lactate challenge in PD patients who panic after lactate administration does not lead to augmented plasma MHPG levels during full-blown panic attacks, whereas the LC hypothesis would predict that this would be the case (Den Boer *et al.*, 1989).

Nevertheless, a partial role for NE seems likely as older monoamine oxidase (MAO) inhibitors, which also influence NE-ergic systems, have been shown to be effective in the treatment of PD (Kelly *et al.*, 1970; Tyrer *et al.*, 1973).

In a recent study conducted in our centre we compared the effects of the selective MAO-A inhibitor brofaromine and the selective 5-HT uptake inhibitor fluvoxamine in a double-blind comparative study (Van Vliet *et al.*, 1994b). A similar anxiolytic was found as assessed with the Hamilton Anxiety Scale (Figure 2). A somewhat more rapid and slightly (although not statistically significant) larger antipanic effect was found for brofaromine compared to fluvoxamine (Figure 3). Therefore, one cannot rule out the possibility that this somewhat larger antipanic efficacy may have been accomplished by virtue of the effects of brofaromine on NE-ergic systems, in addition to its serotonergic effects.

Studies with SSRIs in GAD are lacking, but there are indications that patients suffering from social phobia may respond favorably to SSRIs as well. Recently, we have demonstrated the efficacy of fluvoxamine in a sample of social phobic patients (Van Vliet *et al.*, 1995).

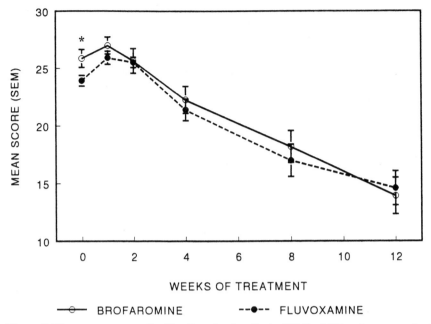

Figure 2 The mean score on the Hamilton Anxiety Scale (HAS) of PD patients treated with brofaromine or fluvoxamine. A significant baseline difference was present with respect to the HAS score (*$p<0.05$)

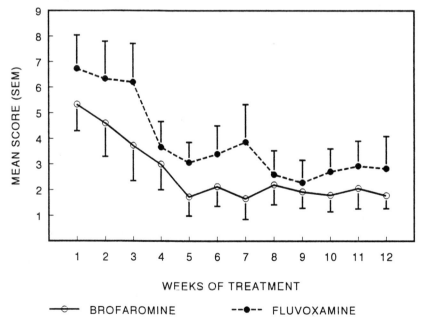

Figure 3 The number of panic attacks in patients suffering from panic disorder, treated with brofaromine or fluvoxamine. A significant time effect was present in the brofaromine group from week 5 on ($p<0.05$), and in the fluvoxamine group from week 4 ($p<0.05$)

In summary, SSRIs appear to be effective in various anxiety states, most notably in PD and OCD, whereas there is circumstantial evidence for their efficacy in social phobia (Den Boer *et al.*, 1992). The effects seem to be specific, viz. not secondary to their antidepressant effects, and are probably related to 5-HT functions in the brain. Preliminary evidence suggests that the selective MAO-A inhibitor brofaromine has anxiolytic and antipanic effects in PD.

DELAY OF ONSET OF ANTIDEPRESSANT TREATMENT IN PANIC DISORDER

The delay in onset of antidepressant or anxiolytic action of SSRIs and related compounds is still puzzling. Why does this delay occur when the inhibition of uptake is immediate? One consequence of the increased synaptic level of 5-HT would be activation of the somatodendritic and terminal autoreceptors, leading to a decreased neuronal firing and terminal release of 5-HT. Artigas *et al.* (1992), using *in vivo* brain microdialysis, reported that acute systemic administration of fluvoxamine or clomipramine resulted in a significant increase in the extracellular levels of 5-HT in the raphe nuclei but not in the frontal cortex, suggesting that the expected increase in 5-HT availability in the terminal area is compensated by a diminished impulse flow due to excessive activation of the somatodendritic or terminal autoreceptors. In keeping with this finding, electrophysiological findings have revealed that acute administration of SSRIs lead to a reduction in 5-HT neuronal firing, while long-term treatment will restore the normal impulse flow (De Montigny and Aghajanian, 1978; Chaput *et al.*, 1988; Blier *et al.*, 1988).

Autoradiographic studies have shown that chronic treatment with SSRIs may reduce the number of $5-HT_{1A}$ binding sites in the dorsal raphe nucleus (Welner *et al.*, 1989).

Moret and Briley (1990), studying the *in vitro* release of 5-HT, found that treatment with citalopram, a novel SSRI, for 21 days resulted also in a downregulation of the terminal 5-HT autoreceptors in rat brain slices. Desensitization of these autoreceptors would permit these neurons to restore their normal firing rate, resulting in a net gain in efficacy of synaptic signal transduction following long-term treatment. If this reasoning is correct one would predict SSRIs to exert their anxiolytic and antidepressant action by enhancing 5-HT neurotransmission. In keeping with this theory, Chaput *et al.* (1988) have reported that the response of hippocampal pyramidal cells to activation of the afferent 5-HT fibers in rats was unchanged after acute treatment with fluoxetine or citalopram, but markedly enhanced following chronic treatment with citalopram or zimeldine. Since direct microiontophoretic application of 5-HT did not reveal a heightened responsiveness after chronic treatment, it was concluded that SSRIs enhance 5-HT functioning by increasing the amount of 5-HT released per impulse and not by increasing the sensitivity of the postsynaptic 5-HT receptors. Interestingly, acute and long-term administration of gepirone, a $5-HT_{1A}$

agonist, mimicked the effects of SSRIs (Blier and De Montigny, 1990), suggesting that it possesses similar 5-HT-modifying characteristics. Obviously, processes beyond the 5-HT receptors must also be taken into account when a delayed onset of action is to be explained.

EFFECTS OF SELECTIVE 5-HT AGONISTS

Clinical evidence that 5-HT may be involved in GAD is mainly derived from studies with selective 5-HT_{1A} agonists. Studies with buspirone have revealed that this class of compounds possesses beneficial effects in GAD patients (Goldberg and Finnerty, 1987; Strand et al., 1990; Jacobson et al., 1985; Rickels et al., 1982; Feighner, 1987; Olajide and Lader, 1987; Böhm et al., 1990). Since the anxiolytic effects become apparent only after repeated administration, it is generally assumed that adaptive changes of 5-HT receptors are required to observe clinical relevant effects. Since somatodendritic receptors desensitize after chronic administration, resulting in a recuperation of the normal firing rate, anxiolytic effects might result from activation of the postsynaptic 5-HT_{1A} receptors, rather than from inhibition of 5-HT outflow resulting from stimulation of the somatodendritic autoreceptors. Studies with gepirone and ipsapirone, two relatively selective 5-HT_{1A} agonists, support the notion that 5-HT possibly plays a role in GAD (Borison et al., 1990; Harto et al., 1988). How full agonists compare to these partial agonists as antianxiety drugs remains to be seen. Clinical studies with flesinoxan, a compound that approximates 8-OH-DPAT in its affinity for the 5-HT_{1A} receptors, in GAD patients are currently in progress.

Studies with buspirone in PD are either inconclusive or negative (Schweizer and Rickels, 1988; Sheehan et al., 1988; Pohl et al., 1989; Robinson et al., 1989). In placebo-controlled trials a substantial improvement was seen, but the effect with buspirone was not different from placebo. It cannot be excluded that the huge placebo response seen in these trials may have obscured possible drug effects in PD, Preliminary evidence suggests that gepirone might be effective in PD, although so far only one open study has been published (Pecknold et al., 1993).

Recently, we have investigated the effects of the full 5-HT_{1A} agonist flesinoxan, which surpasses buspirone in affinity for this receptor subtype, in PD patients. Patients were treated with flesinoxan and placebo using a crossover design with a placebo run-in phase (Westenberg et al., 1992). In contrast to our expectations, treatment with 2.4 mg of flesinoxan, a dose that is usually well tolerated by healthy volunteers and GAD patients, resulted in a significant increase in anxiety (Figure 4).

In contrast to what is generally seen with SSRIs this deterioration did not lead to improvement following repeated administration. In a subsequent study in which lower dosages were used, flesinoxan was found to be indistinguishable from placebo. It is interesting to note that this drug did not increase the

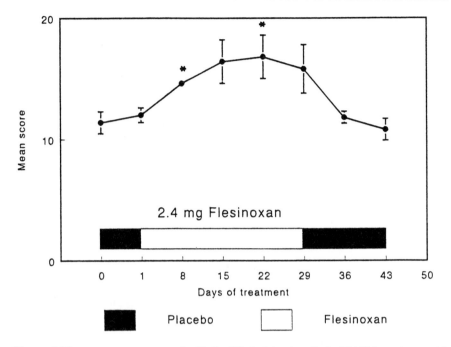

Figure 4 The mean score measured with the Clinical Anxiety Scale (CAS) in patients with panic disorder treated with 2.4 mg of flesinoxan and placebo. Flesinoxan appeared to be anxiogenic in this sample (*$p<0.05$)

frequency of panic attacks. It was anxiogenic, rather than panicogenic, in PD patients.

In summary, the efficacy of 5-HT$_{1A}$ agonists in GAD is currently the firmest clinical evidence for a role of 5-HT in this condition. The results of the partial 5-HT$_{1A}$ agonists like buspirone, ipsapirone and gepirone in PD are puzzling and require further investigation, because they may be lead to the mechanism of action underlying the paradoxical effects of SSRIs in this condition. The increase in anxiety seen in PD patients contrasts with the results in GAD and suggests a differential role of 5-HT$_{1A}$ receptors in these disorders.

The anxiogenic effects of the selective 5-HT$_{1A}$ agonist flesinoxan in PD raises the possibility that 5-HT$_{1A}$ antagonists might be effective anxiolytics, although at the present state of knowledge it is unclear in which anxiety disorder. No 5-HT$_{1A}$ antagonist is available for clinical use as yet, but there is a compound fulfilling the profile of a 5-HT$_{1A}$ antagonist. Recent studies have shown that the experimental compound WAY 100135 is a selective somato-dendritic and postsynaptic 5-HT$_{1A}$ antagonist (Fletcher et al., 1993; Routledge et al., 1993). Once this compound is available for clinical studies, it would be of interest to study its potential anxiolytic profile.

5-HT ANTAGONISTS IN THE TREATMENT OF PANIC DISORDER

Reasoning from the hypothesis that the effects of SSRIs and other antidepressants in PD may be due to their effect on postsynaptic 5-HT_{2A} receptors, one would expect selective 5-HT_{2A} antagonists to be efficacious with a more rapid onset of action in this condition, because of their direct blocking effect on the postsynaptic 5-HT_{2A} receptors. To validate this hypothesis, Den Boer and Westenberg (1990a) performed a placebo-controlled study with ritanserin and fluvoxamine in patients with PD. Clinical studies had indicated that GAD patients might benefit from treatment with ritanserin, suggesting that this receptor antagonist displays anxiolytic activity after chronic treatment (Ceulemans *et al.*, 1985). The reference drug, fluvoxamine, was significantly superior to placebo on several indexes of anxiety, on the frequency of panic attacks and on measures of phobic avoidance, but ritanserin had no effect on any of these measures. The outcome of this study suggests that $5\text{-HT}_{2A/2C}$ antagonists are not efficacious in PD. The presumed supersensitivity of these receptors in PD patients (Den Boer and Westenberg, 1988, 1990a) could hence not be validated by this study. This study suggested that $5\text{-HT}_{2A/2C}$ receptors are not critically altered in PD but allows no conclusions about other 5-HT receptor subtypes (Den Boer and Westenberg, 1991). Whether SSRIs exert their efficacy in PD through 5-HT_{2A} or 5-HT_{2C} receptors can, however, not be excluded. Studies with fluvoxamine and ritanserin or placebo as add-on medication are required to address this issue. A recent study combining fluvoxamine and ritanserin confirmed our findings, for adding ritanserin to fluvoxamine did not augment the effects of fluvoxamine plus placebo in a sample of PD patients (Pols *et al.*, 1993).

There is to date only one small study with ritanserin in OCD (Erzegovesi *et al.*, 1992). Patients in this study were treated with fluvoxamine and received ritanserin or placebo as add-on medication in a double-blind fashion. At the end of the trial a statistically significant difference was found between the treatment conditions, which was tentatively attributed by the authors to a worsening in the ritanserin group. This finding suggests that the effects of fluvoxamine in OCD can be antagonized by blocking the $5\text{-HT}_{2A/2C}$ receptors, suggesting a possible role for 5-HT_{2A} or 5-HT_{2C} receptors in mediating antiobsessive effects. Whether ritanserin alone also has an effect on the symptomatology in OCD patients is as yet unknown. Clearly, clinical studies with more selective 5-HT_{2A} and 5-HT_{2C} antagonists are required to confirm the differential effects of ritanserin in GAD (anxiolytic), PD (ineffective) and OCD (attenuating the efficacy of antiobsessive drugs).

Much less is known about the clinical effects of 5-HT_3 antagonists in anxiety states. Although animal data have yielded promising results, no conclusive clinical trials in PD have been published as yet. In one preliminary report on the efficacy of ondansetron in GAD patients, the efficacy of this putative anxiolytic was difficult to assess due to the high placebo response (Lader, 1991). A recent study reported anxiolytic effects of the 5-HT$_3$ antagonist tropisetron in GAD (Lecrubier et al., 1993).

CHALLENGE PARADIGMS

To elucidate the role of 5-HT, several investigators have used behavioral and neuroendocrine probes to evaluate 5-HT functions *in vivo*. This paradigm involves the administration of direct or indirect acting 5-HT agonists and the measurement of a function allegedly under 5-HT-ergic control. The pituitary–adrenal (e.g. the release of cortisol, prolactin and β-endorphin) response to 5-HT agonists is commonly used as a marker to assess the functional state of the 5-HT system in humans. This strategy promises to become increasingly useful as more selective drugs become available for clinical use. Other responses, besides the hormonal response, include body temperature and behavior. Measurement of the hormonal, physiological or behavioral effects following administration of 5-HT selective drugs permits an assessment of the responsivity of the 5-HT system in the brain involved in the effects under investigation. There is extensive pharmacological and neuroanatomical evidence that 5-HT-containing neurons regulate the hypothalamo–pituitary–adrenal (HPA) axis in rats (Fuller, 1990).

5-HT-containing nerve terminals make synaptic contacts with the corticotropin-releasing hormone (CRH)-containing cells in the hypothalamus and direct and indirect 5-HT agonists all increase adrenocorticotropic hormone (ACTH), β-endorphin and cortisol release. Another pituitary hormone that is regulated, in part, through 5-HT neurons is prolactin. There is circumstantial evidence that drugs that increase 5-HT function increase prolactin secretion as well.

m-CHLOROPHENYLPIPERAZINE CHALLENGE IN PANIC DISORDER

Using this so-called neuroendocrine strategy, Kahn et al. (1988a) studied the responsivity of 5-HT receptors in PD patients by measuring the cortisol release after administration of mCPP. When given orally (0.25 mg/kg), mCPP induced an augmented cortisol release in PD patients as compared with normal controls and depressed patients. mCPP was also found to increase anxiety in PD patients but not in healthy controls (Kahn et al., 1988b). Based on these findings the authors postulated that 5-HT receptors in PD patients might be supersensitive and that drugs that reduce 5-HT function should be useful therapeutic agents in PD. Anxiogenic effects of mCPP in PD patients were also seen by Klein et al. (1991). Considering the non-specificity of mCPP, it is not clear which receptor subtype would be functioning abnormally in PD. A recent study in normal controls revealed that pretreatment with ritanserin was able to diminish the mCPP-induced increase in anxiety and prolactin, and to abolish mCPP-induced corti-sol increase, suggesting that the neuroendocrine and behavioral responses to mCPP might be mediated by 5-HT$_{2C}$ receptors (Seibyl *et al.*, 1991).

FENFLURAMINE AND 5-HTP CHALLENGE IN PANIC DISORDER

A summary of serotonergic challenge studies in PD is depicted in Table 2. Targum and Marshall (1989), using an oral dose of 60 mg fenfluramine, an indi-rect 5-HT agonist, found significantly greater prolactin and cortisol responses in PD patients than in either depressed patients or healthy controls. PD patients also revealed a significantly greater anxiogenic response to fenfluramine administration than either depressed patients or healthy controls. Alterations in mood after administration of fenfluramine are unlikely to occur (Lichtenberg *et al.*, 1992). A more recent study reported an increased prolactin response to a single oral dose of 60 mg fenfluramine in PD patients compared to controls (Apostolopoulos *et al.*, 1993). These data offer circumstantial evidence for the hypothesis that an impaired 5-HT system must be considered as an important element in the pathophysiology of PD. These findings are consistent with the hypothesis of increased 5-HT receptor function in PD, although following a serotonergic challenge with fenfluramine it is not clear which receptor subtype is involved in mediating prolactin release. Animal experiments have implicated both 5-HT$_{2C}$, and 5-HT$_{2A}$ receptors in prolactin release. In human volunteers ritanserin appears to be able to abolish the fenfluramine anorectic effects, as well as the fenfluramine-induced increases in oral temperature and plasma pro-lactin, thus supporting the idea that 5-HT$_{2A}$ or 5-HT$_{2C}$ receptors mediate the effects of fenfluramine (Goodall *et al.*, 1993). Other investigators, however, have debated the idea that the 5-HT/HPA interaction is abnormal in PD patients. Charney *et al.* (1987), using 0.1 mg/kg mCPP intravenously, found similar cor-tisol and prolactin responses in PD patients and healthy controls. They also reported a similar anxiogenic effect of mCPP in PD patients and controls. Differences in design (dosage and routine of administration) may account for these discrepancies (Murphy *et al.*, 1989). Using prolactin as a hormonal probe of 5-HT activity, Charney and Heninger (1986) also reported similar increases in both patients and controls after loading with tryptophan. The validity of the latter test has been questioned by Van Praag *et al.* (1987), who contend that prolactin release after high doses of tryptophan can affect catecholamine as well as 5-HT neurons. It is contended to do so by competing with tyrosine for the same carrier mechanism in the blood–brain barrier, thereby reducing the tyrosine influx into the brain, which in turn could lead to decreased catecholamine levels.

Den Boer and Westenberg (1990b) evaluated the responsivity of the 5-HT system in PD patients and healthy controls by measuring the neuroendocrine and behavioral concomitants of 5-HTP administration. Cortisol and β-endor-phin plasma levels were used as hormonal probes of the 5-HT responsivity.

Table 2. Serotonergic challenges in panic disorder

Reference	Challenge	Route	Dose	Effects	Hormonal	Remarks
Den Boer and Westenberg (1990)	l-5-HTP Plac	i.v. 20 PD 20 C	60 mg	=	↑ Cortisol, β-endorphin	↑ Similar in PD and C, Severe GI side effects
Van Vliet et al. (1996a)	l-5-HTP Plac	i.v. 7 PD 7 C	10, 20, 40 mg	= = =	↑ Cort PD = C ↑ Cort PD = C ↑ Cort PD > C	All underwent four infusions (Plac, 10, 20, 40 mg 5-HTP). Mild GI side effects only in the 40 mg group
Charney and Heninger (1986)	Tryptophan Plac	i.v. 23 PD 21 C	7 g	=	↑ Prolactin	↑ Similar in PD vs C
Targum and Marshall (1989)	Fenfluramine Plac	Oral 9 PD 9 MDD 9 C	60 mg	PD ↑ MDD = C =	Prol/Cort ↑ PD>MDD =C	Suggests hyperresponsivity in PD
Apostolopoulos et al. (1993)	Fenfluramine Plac	Oral 11 PD ↑ 12 C	60 mg	ND	Prol PD ↑↑ C ↑	Indicative of 5-HT function
Kahn et al. (1988a)	mCPP	Oral 11 C 10 PD 10 MDD	0.25 mg/kg	PD ↑ C = MDD =	ND	↑ Depression, anxiety and hostility in PD. No criteria given for panic attacks

Study	Drug	Route/N	Dose	Behavioral	Hormone	Comments
Kahn et al. (1988b)	mCPP Plac	Oral 13 PD 17 MDD 15 C	0.25 mg/kg	ND	Cort ↑ PD	Augmented Cort response in PD vs other groups
Charney et al. (1987)	mCPP Plac	i.v. 23 PD 19 C	0.1 mg/kg	PD = C =	GH, Cort. Prol: PD=C	i.v. dose possibly too high
Klein et al. (1991)	mCPP Caffeine Plac	Oral 10 PD	0.5 mg/kg 480 mg	Anxiety caf> mCPP	mCPP: Cort ↑ Prol ↑ Caf: Cort = Prol ↑	mCPP: panic 70%, Caf: 70%
Lesch et al. (1991)	Ipsapirone Plac	Oral 14 PD 14 C	0.3 mg/kg	=	PD: Cort ↓ PD: ACTH ↓ C: both =	Slight increase in nervousness in C

Abbreviations: i.v., intravenous; C, healthy controls; MDD, major depressive disorder; Prol, prolactin; Cort, cortisol; Caf, caffeine; ND, not done; mCPP, m-chlorphenylpiparazine; UDP, unipolar depression; OCD, obsessive-compulsive disorder; ACTH, adrenocorticotropic hormone; GI, gastrointestinal.

Following an intravenous dose of 60 mg of 5-HTP in combination with 150 mg of carbidopa, a peripheral decarboxylase inhibitor, significant but similar increases of both hormones were found in patients and controls. Administration of 5-HTP appeared to decrease rather than to increase levels of anxiety in PD patients. Despite severe gastrointestinal side effects, most patients became less anxious by the end of the test. In contrast, controls did not consider 5-HTP administration as a relief; they developed a dysphoric mood with organic brain syndrome-like symptoms instead. The relatively high dose of 5-HTP and the side effects may have obscured differences in hormonal response; therefore we recently conducted a double-blind placebo-controlled 5-HTP dose–response study (Van Vliet et al., 1994a). In this study we administered 5-HTP in doses ranging from 10–40mg i.v. in PD patients and healthy controls. We found that 10 and 20 mg 5-HTP elicited dose-dependent but comparable rises in cortisol in patients with PD and controls. At dosages below 40 mg no side effects were reported, supporting the idea that the hormonal response was the result of 5-HTP-induced rather than stress-induced HPA activity. In the 40 mg dose, however, an augmented cortisol response was found in PD compared to controls, thus supporting the idea of an increased 5-HT receptor sensitivity in panic disorder (Van Vliet et al., 1996a).

DISCUSSION OF CHALLENGE STUDIES

A general problem of the neuroendocrine paradigm is the non-selectivity of the challenge agents used so far and the complexity of the mechanisms controlling the hormones allegedly under 5-HT control. There is considerable pharmacological evidence that activation of either 5-HT_{1A} or $5\text{-HT}_{2A}/5\text{-HT}_{2C}$ receptors leads to a stimulation of the HPA axis (Fuller, 1990). In man elevated plasma cortisol levels have also been observed after acute administration of selective 5-HT_{1A} ligands such as ipsapirone and gepirone (Lesch et al., 1990; Rausch et al., 1990). In contrast to mCPP, these selective 5-HT_{1A} ligands induce a blunted response in depressed patients (Lesch et al., 1990), suggesting that these effects may occur through separate pathways.

5-HTP affects HPA activity through stimulation of the 5-HT release, which may interact with all 5-HT receptor subsets, both pre- and postsynaptically. It has been suggested though that the neuroendocrine effects of 5-HTP are mediated through $5\text{-HT}_{2A}/5\text{-HT}_{2C}$ receptors, since ritanserin, a $5\text{-HT}_{2A}/5\text{-HT}_{2C}$ antagonist, is able to inhibit the 5-HTP-induced cortisol secretion (Lee et al., 1991). The failure of 5-HTP to increase plasma MHPG suggests that central NE-ergic activity was not affected by 5-HTP administration (Westenberg and Den Boer, 1989; Den Boer and Westenberg, 1990b).

In summary, the mCPP and fenfluramine findings are intriguing and putatively indicative of an impaired 5-HT function in PD patients. They suggest that an increase in 5-HT activity is positively correlated to anxiety. However, the data cited above do not permit any definite conclusion, because the effects are not unequivocal and were elicited by rather non-selective agents. The data beg for further clinical investigations with more selective 5-HT agonists and antagonists.

BLOOD PLATELETS IN PANIC DISORDER

Inferences about 5-HT functions in the brain may also be based on measurements in readily accessible biological fluids, such as blood, urine and cerebrospinal fluid (CSF). Blood platelets are considered as peripheral markers for some functions of the 5-HT neurons. They share with 5-HT neurons the ability to store and release 5-HT. In contrast to neurons, 5-HT is not synthesized in platelets, but derived from blood. It is taken up into the platelets by a 5-HT-specific transporter which resembles the transporter in the brain. Platelets also contain other constituents that are found in the brain. Thus, specific high-affinity binding sites for [³H]imipramine or [³H]paroxetine have been found in brain and platelet membranes (Paul *et al.*, 1980). There is circumstantial evidence that these sites are associated with, but not identical to, the 5-HT uptake mechanism in both platelets and neurons (Langer *et al.*, 1980). It has been suggested, therefore, that [³H]imipramine binding labels a physiological relevant site that modulates 5-HT reuptake. A reduction in the maximum concentration or density of platelet [³H]imipramine binding sites has been reported in depressed patients by many investigators (Paul *et al.*, 1981; Raisman *et al.*, 1981; Roy *et al.*, 1987; Innis *et al.*, 1987).

Studies conducted so far in patients with PD do not reveal abnormal [³H]imipramine binding characteristics (Norman *et al.*, 1986; Innis *et al.*, 1987; Nutt and Fraser, 1987; Schneider *et al.*, 1987; Uhde *et al.*, 1987; Norman *et al.*, 1989). In spite of the fact that the number of subjects was relatively small in most studies, it can be concluded that [₃H]imipramine binding in PD patients is normal, thus pointing to a different pathogenesis of PD as opposed to depression (for review of pathogenetic differences and similarities between depression and anxiety disorders, see Den Boer and Sitsen, 1994). Platelet 5-HT uptake is also considered to share several properties with the presynaptic terminal of 5-HT-containing fibers and are therefore used as a peripheral marker of the presynaptic 5-HT function in the brain (Stahl *et al.*, 1982). Platelet 5-HT uptake has been reported to be lowered among depressed patients (Tuomisto and Tukiainen, 1976; Meltzer *et al.*, 1984). In two studies an augmented maximal uptake rate (V_{max}) and a similar affinity for uptake (K_m) was found in patients with PD relative to healthy controls (Norman *et al.*, 1986, 1989). In contrast, Pecknold *et al.* (1988) found a reduced V_{max} in patients with PD, whereas Den Boer and Westenberg (1990a) found no difference in the platelet kinetics between patients with PD and healthy controls. Another similarity between platelets and the 5-HT system is that they contain 5-HT$_{2A}$ binding sites. Studying peripheral markers of 5-HT activity in PD patients, Butler *et al.* (1992) found that the density of 5-HT$_{2A}$ binding sites on platelets is elevated and that it remained increased after successful treatment, suggesting that it is a trait marker rather than a state marker in PD. In contrast, a decrease in [³H]LSD binding, which among others also labels the 5-HT$_{2A}$ sites, on platelets of PD patients was found by Norman *et al.* (1990).

CEREBROSPINAL FLUID

Measuring 5-hydroxy-indoleacetic acid (5-HIAA), the major metabolite of 5-HT, in cerebrospinal fluid (CSF) has also been used to evaluate brain 5-HT turnover. A number of studies has used lumbar CSF 5-HIAA as marker for 5-HT turnover. Studies in depression have revealed a decrease in CSF 5-HIAA levels in a subgroup of patients (Westenberg and Verhoeven, 1988). There is only one report on CSF 5-HIAA concentrations in PD patients (Eriksson *et al.*, 1991). In this study PD patients did not differ significantly from age- and sex-matched normal controls. Taking these data together, one may tentatively conclude that these peripheral indices of 5-HT function do not consistently disclose a 5-HT abnormality in PD. They might point, however, to a neurobiological difference between PD and depression.

In summary, peripheral markers as well as CSF data do not reveal a coherent picture with respect to the 5-HT function in anxiety disorders.

SUMMARY

TREATMENT STUDIES

1. 5-HT reuptake inhibitors are effective in the treatment of PD.
2. Partial 5-HT$_{1A}$, agonists like buspirone, ipsapirone and gepirone have been insufficiently investigated to justify a clear statement concerning their efficacy in PD, but available evidence suggests that they are not effective in reducing the number of panic attacks, nor do they diminish avoidance behavior.
3. The full 5-HT$_{1A}$ agonist flesinoxan was found to be anxiogenic in PD in one study. It is unknown whether this effect is mediated pre- or postsynaptically. Irrespective of this, it raises the possibility that 5-HT$_{1A}$ *antagonists* are effective anxiolytics or antipanic agents.
4. The 5-HT$_2$ receptor antagonist ritanserin is ineffective in PD suggesting that this receptor is not critically altered. This finding does not support the hypothesis of an increased sensitivity of this receptor subtype in PD.
5. So far the efficacy of 5-HT$_3$ antagonists in PD has hardly been investigated. Preliminary evidence suggests anxiolytic effects for ondansetron and tropisetron in GAD. The role of this receptor subtype in PD remains to be elucidated.

CHALLENGE STUDIES

6. 5-HTP is not anxiogenic in PD in dosages of 10, 20, 40 or 60 mg, adminis-

tered intravenously. In a recent study it has been found that administration of 40 mg of 5-HTP leads to an augmented cortisol response in PD compared to controls, thus supporting the idea that there exists a supersensitivity of post-synaptic 5-HT receptors PD.
7. Fenfluramine has been shown to increase anxiety in one study. Augmented cortisol and prolactin response during administration of fenfluramine in PD compared to normal controls suggests increased sensitivity of a subset of 5-HT receptors, possibly 5-HT$_{2C}$ receptors.
8. Data on mCPP are conflicting, possibly depending on differences in dose schedule and route of administration.
9. Challenge with the 5-HT$_{1A}$ agonist ipsapirone in PD is without effect on anxiety and reduces the release of ACTH and cortisol in PD compared to controls. This may hint at a presynaptic effect of ipsapirone, which is in contrast to behavioral findings in animal experiments, suggesting postsynaptic effects of ipsapirone.

DISCUSSION

In this chapter clinical findings regarding the role of 5-HT in PD have been critically reviewed. The advent of 5-HT selective drugs and the recent progress in the field of the molecular biology of 5-HT receptors have given strong impetus to research linking 5-HT to psychiatric conditions such as anxiety. The concept that 5-HT might play a role in anxiety is supported by neuroanatomical, neuro-chemical, electrophysiological and behavioral findings. Generally, the results from animal and clinical research converge to suggest a role for 5-HT in anxiety, but this overly broad generalization does not take into account the differences in results between animal models of anxiety and clinical trials, nor does it account for the differential effects of these drugs in different forms of anxiety in man. It is interesting to note that 5-HT$_{1A}$ agonists are effective in GAD, but not effective or even anxiogenic (flesinoxan) in PD. Similar differences in response have been reported for the 5-HT$_{2A,2C}$ antagonist, ritanserin.

The paucity of information on clinical effects of specific 5-HT agents makes it impossible to draw firm conclusions as to the role of specific 5-HT receptor subtypes in humans. Disturbances in the balance between the opposing effects of 5-HT receptors should also be considered as an important element. Gender differences found in clinical studies may be another confounding factor. This phenomenon requires further investigation, since it may be a clue to observed differences in vulnerability between males and females. It is also important to stress at this point that a variety of neurotransmitters have already been shown to play a role in anxiety. Because it is unlikely that any one system is crucial in this respect, any theory on the neurobiology of anxiety must take into account complex neuronal interaction. In OCD and PD, the most pertinent finding to emerge from the clinical studies relating 5-HT to anxiety is the effect of SSRIs. Although originally developed as antidepressants, these drugs have received

equal attention for their potential use in anxiety disorders. SSRIs have been
shown to exert beneficial effects in PD, OCD and social phobia, and although
their efficacy in GAD has not been tested yet, it is plausible to assume efficacy
in this condition as well. The picture that emerges from these findings is that
SSRIs are globally anxiolytic, irrespective of the syndromal background.
Studies relating the effects of selective 5-HT agonists and antagonists may help
to dissect the various effects of SSRIs. Whether such an undertaking would also
shed light on the pathogenesis of anxiety remains to be seen, since the efficacy
of 5-HT-specific drugs in a particular syndrome does not necessarily imply that
it must correct a specific psychopathological dysfunction in that syndrome.
Compensatory effects through other pathways, or processes beyond the 5-HT
system, must also be considered when pharmacological approaches are being
used in the search for pathogenetic factors involved in pathological anxiety. The
negative findings of some challenge studies and surrogate measures, although
by no means conclusive, urge restraint in drawing explicit conclusions. In the
meantime a large number of 5-HT receptor subtypes have been identified and
cloned (e.g. 5-HT_4, 5-HT_5, 5-HT_6, and 5-HT_7 receptors) of which the localization and function at present are totally unclear, let alone their significance for
the pathogenesis of different anxiety disorders. In the near future it is likely that
their function will be elucidated and it is possible that a decade from today the
pathogenesis of PD will be linked to these receptor subtypes. The problem in
the years ahead will be that of establishing meaning in the overwhelming and
sometimes conflicting neurobiological data and theories that will wash over us.

REFERENCES

American Psychiatric Association (1980). *Diagnostic and Statistical Manual of Mental Disorders*, 3rd edn. APA Press, Washington, DC.
American Psychiatric Association (1987). *Diagnostic and Statistical Manual of Mental Disorders*, 3rd edn, revised. APA Press, Washington, DC.
Andrade, R., Malenka R. C. and Nicoll, R. A. (1986). A G protein couples serotonin and GABA_B receptors to the same channels in hippocampus. *Science*, **234**, 1261–1265.
Apostolopoulos, M., Judd, F. K., Burrows, G. D. and Norman, T. R. (1993) Prolactin response to *dl*-fenfluramine in panic disorder. *Psychoneuroendocrinology*, **18** (5/6), 337–342.
Apud, J. A. (1993). The 5-HT3 receptor in mammalian brain: a new target for the develop-ment of antipsychotic drugs? *Neuropsychopharmacology*, **8**, 117–130.
Artigas, F., Adell, A., Celada, P. and Bel, N. (1992). The raphe nuclei as a preferential target for antidepressant drugs acting on the 5-HT system: in vivo microdialysis studies in freely-moving rats. *Eur. Neuropharmacol.*, **2**, 276–284.
Asnis, G., Brown, S., Black, D. *et al.* (1994). Fluvoxamine in the treatment of panic disorder: a multicentre double-blind, placebo-controlled study in outpatients. Submitted.
Bakish, D., Filteau, M. J., Charbonneau, Y. *et al.* (1994). A double blind placebo controlled trial comparing fluvoxamine and imipramine in the treatment of panic disorder with or without agoraphobia. Submitted.
Baraban, F. M. and Aghajanian, G. K. (1980). Suppression of firing activity of 5-HT neurons in the dorsal raphe by alpha-adrenoreceptor antagonists. *Neuropharmacology*, **19**, 355–363.

Black, D. W., Wesner, R., Bowers, W. and Gabel, J. (1993). A comparison of fluvoxamine, cognitive therapy and placebo in the treatment of panic disorder. *Arch. Gen. Psychiatry*, **50**, 44–50.

Blier, P. and De Montigny, C. (1987). Modification of 5-HT neuron properties by sustained administration of the 5-HT$_{1A}$ agonist gepirone: electrophysiological studies in the rat brain. *Synapse*, **1**, 470–480.

Blier, P. and De Montigny, C. (1990). Differential effects of gepirone on presynaptic and postsynaptic serotonin receptors: single-cell recording studies. *J. Clin. Psychopharmacol.*, **10**, 13S–20S.

Blier, P., De Montigny, C. and Chaput, Y. (1988). Electrophysiological assessment of the effects of antidepressant treatments on the efficacy of 5-HT neurotransmission. *Clin. Neuropharmacol.*, **11**, 1S–10S.

Bockaert, J., Demuis, A., Bouhelal, R. *et al.* (1987). Piperazine derivatives including the putative anxiolytic drugs, buspirone and ipsapirone, are agonists at 5-HT$_{1A}$ receptors negatively coupled with adenylcyclase in hippocampal neurons. *Naunyn Schmiedebergs Arch. Pharmacol.*, **335**, 588–592.

Böhm, C., Placchi, M., Stallone, F. *et al.* (1990). A double-blind comparison of buspirone, clobazam, and placebo in patients with anxiety treated in a general practice setting. *J. Clin. Psychopharmacol.*, **10**, 38S–42S.

Bonvento, G., Scatton, B., Claustre, Y. and Rouquier, L. (1992). Effects of local injection of 8-OH-DPAT into the dorsal or median raphe nuclei on the extracellular levels of serotonin in serotonergic projection areas in the rat brain. *Neurosci. Lett.*, **137**, 101–104.

Borison, R. L., Albrecht, J. W. and Diamond, B. I. (1990). Efficacy and safety of a putative anxiolytic agent: ipsapirone. *Psychopharmacol. Bull.*, **26**, 207–210.

Bruinvels, A. T. (1993) 5-HT$_{1D}$ receptors reconsidered, radioligand binding assays, receptor autoradiography and in situ hybridisation histochemistry in the mammalian nervous system. Academic thesis, University of Utrecht.

Butler, J., O'Halloran, A. and Leonard, B. E. (1992). The Galway study of panic disorder II: Changes in some peripheral markers of noradrenergic and serotonergic function in DSM-III-R panic disorder. *J. Affect. Disord.*, **26**, 89–100.

Ceulemans, D. L. S., Hoppenbrouwers, M. L. J. A., Gelders, Y. G. and Reyntjens, A. J. M. (1985). The influence of ritanserin, a serotonergic antagonist, in anxiety disorders: a double-blind placebo-controlled study versus lorazepam. *Pharmacopsychiatry*, **8**, 303–305.

Chaput, Y., Blier, P. and De Montigny, C. (1988). Acute and long-terms effects of antidepressant serotonin (5-HT) uptake blockers on the efficacy of 5-HT neurotransmission: electrophysiological studies in the rat central nervous system. *Adv. Biol. Psychiatry*, **17**, 1–17.

Charney, D. S. and Heninger, G. R. (1986). Serotonin function in panic disorders. *Arch. Gen. Psychiatry*, **43**, 1059–1065.

Charney, D. S., Woods, S. W., Goodman, W. K. and Heninger, G. R. (1987). Serotonin function in anxiety. *Psychopharmacology*, **92**, 14–24.

Charney, D. S., Delgado, P. L., Price, L. H. and Heninger, G. R. (1991). The receptor sensitivity hypothesis of antidepressant action: a review of antidepressant effects on serotonin function. In *The Role of Serotonin in Psychiatric Disorders* (eds S. L. Brown and H. M. van Praag), p. 27. Brunner/Mazel, New York.

Charney, D. S., Krystal, J. H., Southwick, S. M. and Delgado, P. L. (1994). The role of noradrenaline in anxiety disorders. In *Handbook of Depression and Anxiety: A Biological Approach* (eds J. A. Den Boer and J. M. A. Sitsen). Marcel Dekker, New York 473–495.

Clark, D. M. (1986). A cognitive approach to panic. *Behav. Res. Ther.*, **24**, 461–470.

Clomipramine Collaborative Study Group (1991). Clomipramine in the treatment of patients with obsessive-compulsive disorder. *Arch. Gen. Psychiatry*, **48**, 730–738.

Costall, B., Kelly, M. E., Naylor, R. J. and Onaivi, E. S. (1988). Actions of buspirone in a putative model of anxiety in the mouse. *J. Pharm. Pharmacol.* **40**, 494–500.

Costall, B., Domeney, A. M., Gerrard, P. A. *et al.* (1989a). The anxiolytic activities of the 5-

HT₃ receptor antagonists GR38032F, ICS-930 and BRL 43694. *Behav. Pharmacol. 5-HT*, **35**, 383–387.

Cottraux, J., Mollard, E., Bouvard, M. *et al.* (1990). A controlled study of fluvoxamine and exposure in obsessive-compulsive disorder. *Int. Clin. Psychopharmacol.*, **5**, 17–30.

De Montigny, C. and Aghajanian, G. K. (1978). Tricyclic antidepressants: long-term treatment increases responsivity of rat forebrain neurons to serotonin. *Science*, **202**, 1303–1306.

Den Boer, J. A. and Sitsen, J. M. A. (eds) (1994). *Handbook of Depression and Anxiety: A Biological Approach*. Marcel Dekker, New York.

Den Boer, J. A. and Westenberg, H. G. M. (1988). Effect of a serotonin and noradrenaline uptake inhibitor in panic disorder, a double-blind comparative study with fluvoxamine and maprotiline. *Int. Clin. Psychopharmacol.*, **3**, 59–74.

Den Boer, J. A. and Westenberg, H. G. M. (1990a). Serotonin function in panic disorder: a double blind placebo controlled study with fluvoxamine and ritanserin. *Psychopharmacology*, **102**, 85–94.

Den Boer, J. A. and Westenberg, H. G. M. (1990b). Behavioral, neuroendocrine and biochemical effects of 5-hydroxytryptophan administration in panic disorders. *Psychiatry Res.*, **31**, 267–278.

Den Boer, J. A. and Westenberg, H. G. M. (1991). Do panic attacks reflect an abnormality in serotonin receptor subtypes? *Hum. Psychopharmacol.*, **6**, S25–30.

Den Boer, J. A. and Westenberg, H. G. M. (1993) Critical notes on the locus coeruleus hypothesis of panic disorder (Dutch). *Acta Neuropsychiatr.,* **3**, 48–54.

Den Boer, J. A., Westenberg, H. G. M., Kamerbeek, W. D. J. *et al.* (1987). Effect of serotonin uptake inhibitors in anxiety disorders: a double-blind comparison of clomipramine and fluvoxamine. *Int. Clin. Psychopharmacol.*, **2**, 21–32.

Den Boer, J. A. Westenberg, H. G. M., Klompmakers, A. A. and van Lint, E. M. (1989). Behavioral biochemical and neuroendocrine concomitants of lactate-induced panic anxiety. *Biol. Psychiatry*, **26**, 612–622.

Den Boer, J. A., Van Vliet, I. M. and Westenberg, H. G. M. (1992). A double-blind placebo controlled study of fluvoxamine in social phobia. *Clin. Neuropharmacol.*, **15** (Suppl. 1b), 615.

Descarrier, L. and Léger, L. (1978). Serotonin nerve terminals in the locus coeruleus of the adult rat. In *Interactions Between Putative Neurotransmitters in the Brain*, (eds S. Garattini, S., J. F. Pujol and R. Samanin), pp. 355–367. Raven Press, New York.

Dumuis, A., Bouhelal, R., Sebben, M. *et al,* (1988). A non-classical 5-hydroxytryptamine receptor positively coupled with adenylate cyclase in the central nervous system. *Mol. Pharmacol.*, **34**, 880–887.

Dwoskin, L. P., Neal, B. B. and Sparber, S. B. (1988). Evidence for antiserotonergic properties of yohimbine. *Pharmacol. Biochem. Behav.*, **31**, 321–326.

Eison, A. S. and Yocca, F. D. (1985). Reduction in cortical 5HT₂ receptor sensitivity after continuous gepirone treatment. *Eur. J. Pharmacol.*, **111**, 389–392.

Eriksson, E., Westberg, P., Alling, C. *et al.* (1991). Cerebrospinal fluid levels of monoamine metabolites in panic disorder. *Psychiatr. Res.*, **36**, 243–251.

Erlander, M. G., Lovenberg, T. W., Baron, B. M. *et al.* (1993). Two members of a distinct subfamily of 5-hydroxytryptamine receptors differentially expressed in rat brain. *Proc. Natl Acad. Sci. USA*, **90**, 3452–3456.

Erzegovesi, S., Ronchi, P. and Smeraldi, E. (1992). 5-HT-2 receptor and fluvoxamine effect in obsessive-compulsive disorder. *Hum. Psychopharmacol.*, **7**, 287–289.

Evans, L., Moore, G. and Cox, J. (1980). Zimeldine—a serotonin uptake blocker—in the treatment of phobic anxiety. *Progr. Neuro-Psychopharmacol. Biol. Psychiatry*, **4**, 75–79.

Evans, L., Kenardy, P. and Hoey, H. (1986). Effect of a selective serotonin uptake inhibitor in agoraphobia with panic attacks. *Acta Psychiatr. Scand.*, **73**, 40–53.

Fanelli, R. J. and McMonagle-Strucko, K. (1992). Alteration of 5-HT₁A receptor binding sites following chronic treatment with ipsapirone measured by quantitative autoradiography. *Synapse*, **12**, 75–81.

Fawcett, J., Hoehn-Saric, R., Munjack, D. and Roy-Byrne, P. (1994). Fluvoxamine in the treatment of panic disorder: a multicentre double blind placebo controlled study in outpatients. Submitted.

Feighner, J. P. (1987). Buspirone in the long-term treatment of generalized anxiety disorder. *J. Clin. Psychiatry*, **48** (Suppl.), 3–6.

Fernandez-Guasti, A., Lopez-Rubalcava, C., Perex-Urizar, J. and Castaneda-Hernandez, G. (1992). Evidence for a postsynaptic action of the serotonergic anxiolytics: ipsapirone, indorenate and buspirone. *Brain Res. Bull.*, **28**, 497–501.

Feuerstein, T. J., Hertig, G. and Jackisch, R. (1985). Endogenous noradrenaline as modulator of hippocampal serotonin (5-HT)-release: dual effects of yohimbine, rauwolscine and corynanthine as α-adrenoceptor antagonists and 5-HT-receptor agonists. *Naunyn Schiedebergs Arch. Pharmacol*, **329**, 216–221.

Fineberg, N. A., Bullock, T., Montgomery, D. B. and Montgomery, S. A. (1992). Serotonin reuptake inhibitors are the treatment of choice in obsessive compulsive disorder. *Int. Clin. Psychopharmacol.*, **7** (Suppl. 1), 43–47.

Fletcher, A., Bill, D. J., Bill, S. J. *et al.* (1993). WAY 100135: a novel selective antagonist at presynaptic and postsynaptic 5-HT1A receptors. *Eur. J. Pharmacol.*, **237**, 283–291.

Fuller, R. W., Snoddy, H. D., Mason, N. R. and Owen, J. E. (1981). Disposition and pharmacological effects of mCPP. *Neuropharmacology*, **20**, 155–162.

Fuller, W. (1990). Serotonin receptors and neuroendocrine responses. *Neuropsychopharmacology*, **3**, 495–502.

Gillespie, D. D., Manier, D. H., Sanders-Bush, E. and Sulser, F. (1988). The serotonin/norepinephrine-link in brain. II. Role of serotonin in the regulation of beta adrenoceptors in the low agonist affinity conformation. *J. Pharmacol. Exp. Ther.*, **244**, 154–159.

Glennon, R. A., Darmani, N. A. and Martin, B. R. (1991). Multiple populations of serotonin receptors may modulate the behavioral effects of serotonergic agents. *Life Sci.*, **48**, 2493–2498.

Gloger, S., Grunhaus, L., Birmacher, B. and Troudart, T. (1981). Treatment of spontaneous panic attacks with clomipramine. *Am. J. Psychiatry*, **138**, 1215–1217.

Goddard, A. W., Woods, S. W., Sholomskas, D. E. *et al.* (1993). Effects of the serotonin reuptake inhibitor fluvoxamine on yohimbine-induced anxiety in panic disorder. *Psychiatr. Res.*, **48**, 119–133.

Goldberg, H. L., and Finnerty, R. J. (1987). The comparative efficacy of buspirone and diazepam in the treatment of anxiety. *Am. J. Psychiatry*, **136**, 1184–1187.

Goodall, E. M., Cowen, P. J., Franklin, M. and Silverstone, T. (1993). Ritanserin attenuates anorectic endocrine and thermic responses to d-fenfluramine in human volunteers. *Psychopharmacology*, **112**, 461–466.

Goodman, W. K., Price, L. H., Rasmussen, S. A. *et al.* (1989). The efficacy of fluvoxamine in obsessive compulsive disorder: a double-blind comparison with placebo. *Arch. Gen. Psychiatry*, **46**, 36–42.

Goodman, W. K., Delgado, P. L. and Price, L. H. (1990). Specificity of serotonin reuptake inhibitors in the treatment of obsessive-compulsive disorder: comparison of fluvoxamine and desimipramine. *Arch. Gen. Psychiatry*, **47**, 577–585.

Gorman, J. M., Liebowitz, M. R., Feyer, A. J. *et al.* (1987). An open trial of fluoxetine in the treatment of panic attacks. *J. Clin. Psychopharmacol.*, **7**, 329–332.

Grunhaus, L., Gloger, S. and Birmacher, B. (1984). Clomipramine treatment for panic attacks in patients with mitral valve prolapse. *J. Clin. Psychiatry*, **45**, 25–27.

Hamik, A. and Peroutka, S. J. (1989). 1 (m-Chlorophenyl)piperazine (mCPP) interactions with neurotransmitter receptors in the human brain. *Biol. Psychiatry*, **25**, 569–575.

Hamon, M., Lanfumey, L., Mestikawy, S. E. *et al.* (1990). The main features of central 5-HT$_1$ receptors. *Neuropsychopharmacology*, **3**, 349–360.

Harrington, M. A., Zhong, P., Garlow, S. J. and Ciaranello, R. D. (1992). Molecular biology of serotonin receptors. *J. Clin. Psychiatry*, **53** (Suppl.), 8–27.

Hartig, P. R. (1992). Molecular biology of 5-HT$_{1D}$ receptors. *Abstracts of the 2nd International Symposium on Serotonin*, Houston, p. 1.

Harto, N. E., Branconnier, R. J., Spera, K. F. and Dessain, E. C. (1988). Clinical profile of gepirone, a nonbenzodiazepine anxiolytic. *Psychopharmacol. Bull.*, **24**, 154–160.

Higgins, G. A., Bradbury, A. J., Jones, B. J. and Okley, N. R. (1988). Behavioral and biochemical consequences following activation of 5-HT$_1$-like and GABA receptors in the dorsal raphe nucleus of the rat. *Neuropharmacology*, **27**, 993.

Hoehn Saric, R., McLeod, D. R. and Hipsley, A. (1993). Effect of fluvoxamine on panic disorder. *J. Clin. Psychopharmacol.*, **5**, 321–326.

Hoyer, D. (1988). Functional correlates of serotonin 5-HT$_1$ recognition sites. *J. Recept. Res.*, **8**, 59–81.

Hoyer, D. and Middlemiss, D. N. (1989). Species differences in the pharmacology of terminal 5-HT autoreceptors in mammalian brain. *Trends Pharmacol. Sci.*, **10**, 130–132.

Humphrey, P. P. A., Hartig, P. and Hoyer, D. (1993). A proposed new nomenclature for 5-HT receptors. *Trends Pharmacol. Sci.*, **14**, 233–236.

Innis, R. B., Charney D. S. and Heninger, G. R. (1987). Differential ^{3}H-imipramine platelet binding in patients with panic disorder and depression. *Psychiatry Res.*, **21**, 33–41.

Jacobson, A. F., Dominguez, R. A., Goldstein, B. J. and Steinbook, R. M. (1985). Comparison of buspirone and diazepam in generalized anxiety disorder. *Pharmacotherapy*, **5**, 290–296.

Jenike, M. A., Hyman, S., Baer, L. *et al.* (1990). A controlled trial of fluvoxamine in obsessive compulsive disorder: implication for a serotonergic theory. *Am. J. Psychiatry*, **147**, 1209–1215.

Julius, D. (1991). Molecular biology of serotonin receptors. *Annu. Rev. Neurosci.*, **14**, 335–360

Jones, B. J., Costall, B., Domeney, A. Q. M. *et al.* (1988). The potential anxiolytic activity of GR38032 F, a 5-HT$_3$-receptor antagonist. *Br. J. Pharmacol.*, **93**, 985–993.

Kahn, R. S. and Wetzler, S. (1991). m-Chlorophenylpiperazine as a probe of serotonin function. *Biol. Psychiatry*, **30**, 1139–1166.

Kahn, R. S., Westenberg, H. G. M., Verhoeven, W. M. A. and Gispen de Wied, C. C. (1987). Effect of a serotonin precursor and uptake inhibitor in anxiety disorders: a double blind comparison of 5-hydroxytryptophan, clomipramine and placebo. *Int. Clin. Psychopharmacol.*, **2**, 33–45.

Kahn, R. S., Asnis, G. M., Wetzler, S. and Van Praag, H. M. (1988a). Neuroendocrine evidence for serotonin hypersensitivity in panic disorder. *Psychopharmacology*, **96**, 360–364.

Kahn, R. S., Wetzler, S., Van Praag, H. M. and Asnis, G. M. (1988b). Behavioral indications for serotonin receptor hypersensitivity in panic disorder. *Psychiatry Res.*, **25**, 101–104.

Kelly, D., Guirguis, W. and Frommer, E. (1970). Treatment of phobic states with antidepressants. *Br. J. Psychiatry*, **116**, 387–408.

Kilpatrick, G. J., Jones, B. J. and Tyers, M. B. (1987). Identification and distribution of 5-HT$_3$ receptors in rat brain using radioligand binding. *Nature*, **330**, 746–748.

Klein, D. F. (1964). Delineation of two drug-responsive anxiety syndromes. *Psychopharmacologia*, **5**, 397–408.

Klein, D. F. (1967). The importance of psychiatric diagnosis in prediction of clinical drug effects. *Arch. Gen. Psychiatry*, **16**, 118–126.

Klein, D. F. and Fink, M. (1962). Psychiatric reaction patterns to imipramine. *Am. J. Psychiatry*, **119**, 432–438.

Klein, E., Zohar J., Geraci, F. *et al.* (1991). Anxiogenic effects of mCPP in patients with panic disorder: comparison to caffeine's anxiogenic effects. *Biol, Psychiatry*, **30**, 973–984.

Koczkas, S. and Weissman, A. (1981). A pilot study of the effect of the 5-HT-uptake inhibitor, zimeldine, on phobic anxiety. *Acta Psychiatr. Scand.*, **290**, 328–341.

Lader, M. H. (1991). Ondansetron in the treatment of anxiety. In *Biological Psychiatry* (eds G. Racagni, N. Brunello and T. Fukuda) vol. 2, p. 885. Excerpta Medica, Amsterdam.

Langer, S. Z., Moret, C. and Raisman, R. (1980). High affinity ^{3}H-imipramine binding in rat hypothalamus: association with uptake of serotonin but not norepinephrine. *Science*, **210**, 1133–1135.

Lecrubier, Y., Puech, A. J., Azcona, A. *et al.* (1993). A randomized double blind placebo controlled study of tropisetron in the treatment of generalized anxiety disorder. *Psychopharmacology*, **112**, 129–133.

Lee, M. A., Nash, J. F., Barnes, M. and Meltzer, H. Y. (1991). Inhibitory effect of ritanserin on the 5-hydroxytryptophan-mediated cortisol, ACTH and prolactin secretion in humans. *Psychopharmacology*, **103**, 258–264.

Lesch, K. P., Mayer, S., Disslekamp-Tietze, J. *et al.* (1990). 5-HT$_{1A}$ receptor responsivity in unipolar depression: evaluation of ipsaspirone-induced ACTH and cortisol secretion in patients and controls. *Biol. Psychiatry*, **28**, 620–628.

Leysen, J. E. (1985). Characterization of serotonin receptor binding sites. In *Neuropharmacology of Serotonin* (ed. A. R. Green,), pp. 79–214. Oxford University Press, Oxford.

Lichtenberg, P., Shapiro, B., Blacker, M. *et al.* (1992) Effect of fenfluramine on mood: a double blind placebo controlled trial. *Biol. Psychiatry*, **31**, 351–356.

Lydiard, R., Morton, A. W., Emmanuel, N. P. *et al.* (1993). Preliminary report: placebo controlled double blind study of the clinical and metabolic effects of desimipramine in panic disorder. *Psychopharmacol. Bull.*, **29**(2), 183–188.

Manoumas, L. A. and Molliven, M. E. (1988). Evidence for dual serotonergic projections to neocortex: axons from the dorsal and median raphe nuclei are differentially vulnerable to the neurotoxin p-chloramphetamine (PCA). *Exp. Neurol.*, **102**, 23–32.

Matthes, H., Boschert, U., Amlaiky, N. *et al.* (1993). Mouse 5-hydroxytryptamine$_{2A}$ and 5-hydroxytryptamine$_{5B}$ define a new family of serotonin receptors: cloning, functional expression, and chromosomal localization. *Mol. Pharmacol.*, **129**, 333–337.

Mavissakalian, M. and Perel, J. M. (1989). Imipramine dose–response relationship in panic disorder with agoraphobia. *Arch. Gen. Psychiatry*, **46**, 127–131.

Meert, T. F. and Janssen, P. A. (1989). Psychopharmacology of ritanserin: comparison with chlordiazepoxide. *Drug Dev. Res.*, **18**, 119–144.

Meltzer, H. Y., Lowy, M., Robertson, A. *et al.* (1984). Effect of 5-hydroxytryptophan on serum cortisol level in major affective disorders. *Arch. Gen. Psychiatry*, **41**, 391–397.

Modigh, K. (1987). Antidepressant drugs in anxiety disorders. *Acta Psychiatr. Scand.*, **76** (Suppl. 335), 57–71.

Molineaux, S. M., Jessel, T. M., Axel, R. and Julius, D. (1989). 5-HT$_{1C}$ receptor is a prominent receptor subtype in the central nervous system. *Proc. Natl Acad. Sci. USA*, **86**, 6793–6797.

Monsma, F. J., Shen, Y., Ward, R. P. *et al.* (1993) Cloning and expression of a novel serotonin receptor with high affinity for tricyclics psychotropic drugs. *Mol. Pharmacol.*, **43**, 320–327.

Montgomery, S. A. (1992). OCD floats free of anxiety. *Eur. Neuropsychopharmacol.*, **2**, 217–218.

Montgomery, S. A., Montgomery, D. B. and Fineberg, N. (1990). Early response with clomipramine in obsessive compulsive disorder: a placebo controlled study. *Prog. Neuropsychopharmacol. Biol. Psychiatry*, **14**, 719–727.

Moret, C. and Briley, M. (1990). Serotonin autoreceptor subsensitivity and antidepressant activity. *Eur. J. Pharmacol.*, **180**, 351–356.

Morgane, P. J. and Jacobs, M. S. (1979). Raphe projections to the locus coeruleus in the rat. *Brain Res. Bull.*, **4**, 519–534.

Murphy, D. L., Mueller, E. A., Hill, J. L. *et al.* (1989). Comparative anxiogenic, neuroendocrine, and other physiologic effects of m-chlorophenylpiperazine given intravenously or orally to healthy volunteers. *Psychopharmacology*, **98**, 275–282.

Norman, T. R., Judd, F. K., Gregory, M. *et al.* (1986). Platelet serotonin uptake in panic disorder. *J. Affect. Disord.*, **11**, 69–72.

Norman, T. R., Sartor, D. M., Judd, F. K. *et al.* (1989). Platelet serotonin uptake and ³H-imipramine binding in panic disorder. *J. Affect. Disord.*, **17**, 77–81.

Norman, T. R., Judd, F. K., Staikos, V. *et al.* (1990). High-affinity platelet [³H]LSD binding is decreased in panic disorder. *J. Affect. Disord.*, **19**, 119–123.

Nutt, D. J. and Fraser, S. (1987). Platelet binding studies in panic disorder. *J. Affect. Disord.*, **12**, 7–11.

Olajide, D. and Lader, M. (1987). A comparison of buspirone, diazepam and placebo in patients with chronic anxiety state. *J. Clin. Psychiatry*, **7**, 148–152.

Palacios, J. M., Pazos, A. and Hoyer, D. (1987). Characterization and mapping of 5-HT$_{1A}$ sites in the brain of animals and man. In *Brain 5-HT$_{1A}$ Receptors* (eds C. T. Dourish, S. Ahlenius and P. H. Hutson), pp. 67–81. Ellis Horwood, Chichester.

Papeschi, R. and Theiss, P. (1975). The effect of yohimbine on the turnover of brain catecholamines and serotonin. *Eur. J. Pharmacol.*, **33**, 1–12.

Papp, M. and Przegalinski, E. (1989). The 5-HT$_3$ receptor antagonists ICS 205–930 and GR 38032F, putative anxiolytic drugs, differ from diazepam in their pharmacological profile. *J. Psychopharmacol.*, **3**, 14–20.

Paul, S. M., Rehavi, M., Skolnick, P. and Goodwin, F. K. (1980). Demonstration of high-affinity binding sites for ³H-imipramine on human platelets. *Life Sci.*, **26**, 953–959.

Paul, S. M., Rehavi, M., Skolnick, K. P. *et al.* (1981). Depressed patients have decreased binding of tritiated imipramine to platelet serotonin transporter. *Arch. Gen. Psychiatry*, **38**, 1315–1317.

Pazos, A. and Palacios, J. M. (1985). Quantitative autoradiographic mapping of serotonin receptors in rat brain. I. serotonin-I receptors. *Brain Res.*, **346**, 205–230.

Pazos, A., Probst, A. and Palacios, J. M. (1986). Serotonin receptors in the human brain, III: autoradiographic mapping of serotonin-I receptors. *Neuroscience*, **21**, 97–122.

Pazos, A., Probst, A. and Palacios, J. M. (1987). Serotonin receptors in the human brain, IV: autoradiographic mapping of serotonin-2 receptors. *Neuroscience*, **21**, 123–139.

Pecknold, J. C., Suranyi-Cadotte, B., Chang, H. and Nair, N. P. V. (1988). Serotonin uptake in panic disorder and agoraphobia. *Neuropsychopharmacology*, **39**, 917–928.

Pecknold, J. C., Luthe, L., Scott-Fleurie, M. H. and Jenkins, S. (1993). Gepirone in the treatment of panic disorder: an open study. *J. Clin. Psychopharmacol.*, **13**, 145–149.

Perse, T. L., Greist, J. H., Jefferson, J. W. *et al.* (1987). Fluvoxamine treatment of obsessive-compulsive disorder. *Am. J. Psychiatry*, **144**, 1543–1548.

Plassat, J. L., Boschert, U., Amlaiky, N. and Hen, R. (1992). The mouse 5-HT$_5$ receptor reveals a remarkable heterogeneity within the 5-HT$_{1D}$ receptor family. *EMBO J.*, **11**, 4779–4786.

Pohl, R., Balon, R., Yeragani, V. K. and Gershon, S. (1989). Serotonergic anxiolytics in the treatment of panic disorder: a controlled study with buspirone. *Psychopathology*, **22** (Suppl. 1), 60–67.

Pols, H. J., Griez, E. J. and Verburg, C. (1993). Fluvoxamine–ritanserin combination in the treatment of panic anxiety with avoidance behavior. *Neuropsychopharmacology*, (S), **3** (3), 377.

Raisman, R., Sechter, D. and Briley, M. S. (1981). High affinity ³H-imipramine binding in platelets form untreated and treated depressed patients compared to healthy controls. *Psychopharmacology*, **75**, 368–371.

Ramos, R. T., Gentil, V. and Gorenstein, C. (1993). Clomipramine and initial worsening in panic disorder: beyond the jitteriness syndrome. *J. Psychopharmacol.*, **7**(3), 265–269.

Rausch, J. L., Stahl, S. M. and Hauger, R. (1990). Cortisol and growth hormone responses to the 5-HT$_{1A}$ agonist gepirone in depressed patients. *Biol. Psychiatry*, **28**, 73–78.

Rickels, K., Weisman, K., Norstad, N. *et al.* (1982). Buspirone and diazepam in anxiety: a controlled study. *J. Clin. Psychiatry*, **43**, 81–86.

Robinson, D. R., Shrotriya, R. C., Alms, D. R. *et al.* (1989). Treatment of panic disorder: nonbenzodiazepine anxiolytics, including buspirone. *Psychopharmacol. Bull.*, **25**, 21–26.

Routledge, C., Gurling, J., Wright, I. K. and Dourish, C. T. (1993). Neurochemical profile of the selective and silent 5-HT1A receptor antagonist WAY 100135: an in vivo microdialysis study. *Eur. J. Pharmacol.*, **239**, 195–202.

Roy, A., Everett, D., Pickar, D. and Paul, S. M. (1987). Platelet tritiated imipramine binding and serotonin uptake in depressed patients and controls: relationship between plasma cortisol levels before and after dexamethasone administration. *Arch. Gen. Psychiatry*, **44**, 320–327.

Schneider, L. S., Munjack, D., Severson, J. A. and Palmer, R. (1987). Platelet [^{3}H]imipramine binding in generalized anxiety disorder, panic disorder and agoraphobia with panic attacks. *Biol. Psychiatry*, **22**, 59–66.

Schneier, F. R., Liebowitz, M. R., Davies, S. O. *et al.* (1990). Fluoxetine in panic disorder. *J. Clin. Psychopharmacol.*, **10**, 119–121.

Schoeffler, P. H. and Hoyer, D. (1989). Interaction of arylpiperazines with $5HT_{1a}$, $5HT_{1b}$, $5HT_{1c}$, and $5HT_{1d}$ receptors: do discriminatory $5HT_{1d}$ receptor ligands exist? *Naunyn Schmiedebergs Arch. Pharmacol.*, **339**, 675–683.

Schweizer, E. and Rickels, K. (1988). Buspirone in the treatment of panic disorder: a controlled pilot comparison with clorazepate. *J. Clin. Psychopharmacol.*, **8**, 303.

Segal, M., (1979). Serotonergic innervation of the locus coeruleus from the dorsal raphe and its action on responses to noxious stimuli. *J. Physiol. (Lond.)*, **286**, 401–405.

Segal, M., Azmitia, E. C. and Whitaker-Azmitia, P. M. (1989). Physiological effects of selective $5-HT_{1A}$ and $5-HT_{1B}$ ligands in rat hippocampus: comparison to 5-HT. *Brain Res.*, **502**, 67–74.

Seibyl, J. P., Krystal, J. H., Price, L. H. *et al.* (1991). Effects of ritanserin on the behavioral, neuroendocrine and cardiovascular responses to meta-chlorphenylpiperazine in healthy subjects. *Psych. Res.*, **38**, 227–236.

Sharp, T., Bramwell, S. R. and Grahame-Smith, D. G. (1989). $5-HT_1$ agonists reduce 5-hydroxytryptamine release in rat hippocampus in vivo as determined by brain microdialysis. *Br. J. Pharmacol.*, **96**, 283–290.

Sheehan, D. V., Raj, A. B., Sheehan, K. H. and Soto, S. (1988). The relative efficacy of buspirone, imipramine and placebo in panic disorder: a preliminary report. *Pharmacol. Biochem. Behav.*, **29**, 815–817.

Sprouse, J. S. and Aghajanian, G. K. (1988). Responses of hippocampal pyramidal cells to putative serotonin $5-HT_a$ and $5-HT_b$ agonists: a comparative study with dorsal raphe neurons. *Neuropharmacology*, **27**, 707–715.

Stahl, S. M., Ciaranello, R. D. and Berger, P. A. (1982). Platelet serotonin in schizophrenia and depression. In *Serotonin in Biological Psychiatry* (ed. B. T. Ho), p. 182. Raven Press, New York.

Strand, M., Hetta, J., Rosen, A. *et al.* (1990). A double-blind, controlled trial in primary care patients with generalized anxiety: a comparison between buspirone and oxazepam. *J. Clin. Psychiatry*, **51** (Suppl.), 40–45.

Targum, S. D. and Marshall, L. E. (1989). Fenfluramine provocation of anxiety in patients with panic disorder. *Psychiatry Res.*, **28**, 295–306.

Traber, J. and Glaser, T. (1987). 5-HT1a receptor-related anxiolytics. *Trends Pharmacol. Sci.*, **8**, 432–437.

Tuomisto, J. and Tukiainen, E. (1976). Depressed uptake of 5-hydroxytryptamine in blood platelets from depressed patients. *Nature*, **262**, 596–598.

Tyers, M. B. (1989). A review of the evidence supporting the anxiolytic potential of $5-HT_3$ receptor antagonists. In *Behavioral Pharmacology of 5-HT* (eds. P. Bevans, A. R. Cools and T. Arder). Erlbaum, Hillsdale, NJ.

Tyrer, P., Candy, J. and Kelly, D. (1973). A study of the clinical effects of phenelzine and placebo in the treatment of phobic anxiety. *Psychopharmacology*, **32**, 237–254.

Tyrer, P., Iversen, S. A. and Green, S. A. (1979). A study of the clinical effects of phenelzine and placebo in the treatment of phobic anxiety. *Psychopharmacolologia*, **32**, 237–254.

Uhde, T. W., Berrettini, W. H., Boy-Byrne, P. P. *et al.* (1987). [³H]Imipramine binding in patients with panic disorder. *Biol. Psychiatry*, **22**, 52–58.

Van Praag, H. M., Lemus, C. and Kahn, R. S. (1987). Hormonal probes of central serotonergic activity: do they really exist? *Biol. Psychiatry*, **22**, 86–98.

Van Vliet, I. M., Den Boer, J. A. and Westenberg, H. G. M. (1996a) Serotonergic challenge in panic disorder; a dose-response study with L-5-HTP. *Eur. Neuropsychopharmacol* (in press).

Van Vliet, I. M., Den Boer, J. A. and Westenberg, H. G. M. (1996b). A double blind comparative study of brofaromine and fluvoxamine in panic disorder. *J. Clin. Psychopharmacol.* (in press).

Van Vliet, I. M., Den Boer, J. A. and Westenberg, H. G. M. (1996c). Psychopharmacological treatment of social phobia: a double blind placebo controlled study with fluvoxamine. *Psychopharmacology*, **115**, 128–134.

Welner, S. A., De Montigny, C., Desroches, J. *et al.* (1989). Autoradiographic quantification of serotonin (5-HT$_{1A}$) receptors following long-term antidepressant treatment. *Synapse*, **4**, 347–453.

Westenberg, H. G. M. and Den Boer, J. A. (1989). Serotonin function in panic disorder: effects of L-5-hydroxytryptophan in patients and controls. *Psychopharmacology*, **98**, 283–286.

Westenberg, H. G. M. and Den Boer, J. A. (1993). Serotonergic basis of panic disorder. In *Psychopharmacology of Panic* (ed. S. A. Montgomery), pp. 91–109. Oxford University Press, Oxford.

Westenberg, H. G. M. and Den Boer, J. A. (1994). The neuropharmacology of anxiety: a review on the role of serotonin. In *Handbook of Depression and Anxiety: A Biological Approach* (eds J. A. Den Boer and J. M. A. Sitsen), pp. 405–445, Marcel Dekker, New York.

Westenberg, H. G. M. and Verhoeven, W. M. A. (1988). CSF monoamine metabolites in patients and controls: support for a bimodal distribution in major affective disorders. *Acta Psychiatr. Scand.*, **78**, 541–549.

Westenberg, H. G. M., Van Vliet, I. M. and Den Boer, J. A. (1992). Flesinoxan, a selective 5-HT$_{1A}$ agonist, in the treatment of panic disorder. *Clin. Neuropharmacol.*, **15** (Suppl. 1b), 60.

Winter, J. C. and Rabin, R. A. (1992). Yohimbine as a serotonergic agent: evidence from receptor binding and drug discrimination. *J. Pharmacol. Exp. Ther.*, **263**(2), 682–689.

Yocca, F. D. (1990). Neurochemistry and neurophysiology of buspirone and gepirone: interactions at the presynaptic and postsynaptic 5-HT$_{1A}$ receptors. *J. Clin. Psychopharmacol.*, **10**, 6S–12S.

Zohar, J. and Insel, T. R. (1987). Obsessive-compulsive disorder: psychobiological approaches to diagnosis, treatment, and pathophysiology. *Biol. Psychiatry*, **22**, 667–687.

Zuardi, A. W. (1990). 5-HT-related drugs and human experimental anxiety. *Neurosci. Biobehav. Rev.*, **14**, 507–510.

8 Pharmacological Probes in Panic Disorder

JEREMY D. COPLAN AND DONALD F. KLEIN

Department of Psychiatry, Columbia University, New York, USA

INTRODUCTION AND CLASSIFICATION: TWO GROUPS OF PROBES

Recent research into panic disorder (PD) has utilized the strategy of eliciting psychological and pathophysiological differences between patient groups and healthy controls by acute administration of a variety of pharmacological probes. This approach has yielded two general classes of compounds. We have divided them into two distinct groups (see Table 1):

1. The "respiratory" panicogens which induce panic where dyspnea and smothering symptoms are prominent and whose effects in panic patients are blocked by imipramine (IMI). The mechanism(s) by which respiratory panicogens exert their effects remains obscure although interaction with ventilatory factors related to an aberrant perception of suffocation are considered a crucial component of their action (Klein, 1993). Respiratory panicogens, thus far, do not appear to specifically effect one neurochemical system but putatively act at peripheral and/or central sites to affect multiple biological systems (see Coplan *et al.*, 1992a, 1992b). The respiratory panicogens comprise racemic (D,L) sodium lactate (Liebowitz *et al.*, 1984), carbon dioxide (Gorman *et al.*, 1988; Woods *et al.*, 1986), bicarbonate (Gorman *et al.*, 1989a), and sodium D-lactate (Gorman *et al.*, 1990). An important clue to the action of this group of compounds is the curious and counterintuitive absence of hypothalamic–pituitary–adrenal (HPA) activation in the face of extreme terror. Isoproterenol (Rainey *et al.*, 1984), a β-agonist which crosses the blood–brain barrier poorly, also produces dyspnea-dominated panic which is blocked by IMI. We propose that administration of such compounds in PD patients models spontaneous panic attacks.
2. The second group are characterized by compounds that share the common property of inducing anxiety accompanied by significant HPA activation.

Advances in the Neurobiology of Anxiety Disorders. Edited by H. G. M. Westenberg, J. A. Den Boer and D. L. Murphy
©1996 John Wiley & Sons Ltd

Respiratory symptoms are unremarkable and diverse neurochemical systems are targeted as part of the anxiogenic process. Yohimbine augments activity of the locus coeruleus (LC)/norepinephrine (NE) neurons (Charney *et al.*, 1983, 1984). Fenfluramine (Targum and Marshall, 1989) and *M*-chlorophenylpiperazine (mCPP) (Kahn *et al.*, 1988a, 1988b) are indirect and direct serotonin agonists respectively. β-Carboline esters in general (Insel *et al.*, 1984) and flumazenil (Nutt *et al.*, 1990), specifically in PD patients, act at GABA-ergic receptor sites predominantly as inverse agonists. This cluster of compounds have been argued to model generalized or anticipatory anxiety (Carr *et al.*, 1986) but may also model fear-like situationally provoked panics. Such effects are posited to represent clinical features which predominate the later phases of the illness and are clinically distinct from spontaneous panic where respiratory symptoms dominate.

Cholecystokinin (CCK) administration, which induces short-lived panic (Bradwejn *et al.*, 1991), possibly related to its rapid intravenous administration, produces a very transient period of gasping respiratory stimulation, whereas robust corticoid responses are observed particularly in individuals who panic (Bradwejn, 1993). Although CCK will not be a focus of this chapter, this neuropeptide might represent a panicogen sharing attributes of both the respiratory and the HPA activating group. Although its effects are blocked by IMI, the brief duration of CCK-induced respiratory stimulation when compared to respiratory panicogens suggests a primary role for corticoid activation in its anxiogenic mechanisms. The reader is referred to Chapter 9, where CCK is dealt with in detail. The pentapeptide, pentagastrin, appears in preliminary work (Abelson *et al.*, 1994; Uhde *et al.*, 1993) to share many of the clinical features of CCK-induced panic. Although caffeine (Uhde, 1990; Uhde *et al.*, 1992), which interacts with the adenosine system, produces hyperventilation and an increase in lactate, the observation that dyspnea does not predominate its clinical effects. That HPA activation accompanies caffeine's panicogenic effects and non-blockade by IMI suggests inclusion in the second category of panicogens. Doxapram (Lee *et al.*, 1993), which acts at carotid chemoreceptors, induces panic and hyperventilation but information regarding degree of dyspnea and HPA axis status during doxapram-induced panic, as well as the effects of IMI treatment, is required before classification.

Studies which focus on the physiological and biochemical effects of "nonanxiogenic probes" selected on the basis of their putative receptor specificity are beyond the scope of this chapter. These include studies using the α_2-adrenoreceptor agonist, clonidine (Nutt, 1989; Charney and Heninger, 1986; Uhde *et al.*, 1992; Abelson *et al.*, 1992), the NE reuptake inhibitor, desipramine (Asnis *et al.*, 1992) and ipsapirone, a 5-HT$_{1A}$ partial agonist (Lesch *et al.*, 1992). Such pharmacological probe studies have provided important information regarding the neurobiology of PD although direct integration with data generated from administration of panicogens is lacking.

COGNITIVE BEHAVIORAL THEORIES AND PHARMACOLOGICAL PROBES

It is conceivable that panicogenic agents do not interact with specific biological abnormalities, but rather act to induce panic by the non-specific induction of unpleasant physical symptoms which are catastrophized by the patient to represent impending disaster. For instance, cognitive-behavioral investigators have posited that lactate causes panic by non-specific simulation of somatic cues similar to those associated with the patient's naturally occurring panic (Barlow, 1985; Barlow et al., 1985). Not all challenges, however, which produce acute somatic symptoms are panicogenic (e.g. ethylenediaminetetraacetic acid (EDTA), thyrotropin, physostigmine, tryptophan and insulin) (see Klein, 1993). Moreover, the propensity to catastrophization and misattribution cannot alone account for patient/control differences in response to non-anxiogenic probes. Certain basic physiological functions, such as pregnancy and parturition, induce a plethora of uncomfortable physical sensations in the context of heightened danger and rarely induce panic attacks (Klein, 1993). Moreover, the frequent occurrence of sleep panic attacks, which are observed during deepening non-REM sleep (Mellman and Uhde, 1990) suggests that panic attacks are not merely extensions of nightmares or sleep terror but a discrete, aberrant activation of a biological alarm mechanism.

THE "IDEAL" PANICOGEN

Before reviewing the work to date on pharmacological induction of panic, it would be useful to reiterate the attributes possessed by the ideal panicogenic agent elucidated by Gorman et al. (1987b):

1. The panic attack should combine physical symptoms of panic with a subjective sense of terror and a desire to flee and should be distinguished from states of anticipatory or generalized anxiety.
2. The provoked attack should be judged as symptomatically very similar to the patient's regularly occurring spontaneous panic attacks, particularly with respect to the co-occurrence of dyspnea.
3. The induction of panic should be specific to patients with a history of spontaneous attacks. This may be expressed in one of two ways. Either only patients with a history of panic attacks occurring spontaneously have panic attacks under provocation (absolute specificity) or such patients routinely panic at lower doses than other subjects (threshold specificity).
4. The agent, in the panicogenic dose, should be safe for routine administration to human subjects.
5. The effect of the agent provoking panic should be consistent in a given patient. If a desensitization effect to the panicogenic effects of an agent occurs, this should be predictable.

Table 1.

Panicogen	Dyspnea and smothering	Respiratory stimulation	HPA axis	LC/NE stimulation	IMI blockade	Alprazolam blockade	Diazepam blockade
Lactate	+	+	-	-	+	+	-
CO_2	+	+	-	-	+	+	?
Bicarbonate	+	+	-	-	?	?	?
D-Lactate	+	+	-	-	?	?	?
Isoproterenol	+	+	?	?	+	?	?
Doxapram	?	+	?	?	?	?	?
Caffeine	-	+	+	-	-	+	+
Cholecystokinin/ Pentagastrin	+	+(transient)	+	?	+	?	?
Yohimbine	-	-	+	+	-	+	+
mCPP	-	-	+	-	?	?	?
Fenfluramine	-	-	+	-	?	?	?
B Carboline	-	-	+	+	?	+	+
Flumazenil	-	-	?	+	+(?)	+	+

6. Drugs that block spontaneous panic attacks when given for prolonged periods, such as tricyclic antidepressants, monoamine oxidase inhibitors, and alprazolam, should also block the acute pharmacologically induced attack.
7. Agents that do not block clinical panic acutely or chronically should not block the pharmacologically induced panic.

A plethora of panicogenic agents have been described which to variable degrees satisfy the above criteria. Unfortunately, agents which most completely fulfill the above criteria, like sodium lactate, are not necessarily the best understood in terms of their central action. Attempts to create a unifying rubric from which to conceptualize the action of these agents becomes increasingly complex, as new and often discrepant data emerge in the literature.

"RESPIRATORY" PANICOGENS

SODIUM (D,L)-LACTATE

Historical overview

The sodium lactate infusion procedure stems from work begun by Cohen and White (1951), who noted that patients suffering from "neurocirculatory asthenia" were prone to discrete spells of anxiety and developed higher blood lactate levels on physical exertion than healthy controls. The presence of hyperlactatemia in PD has not, however, been replicated by our group (Stein et al., 1992). The authors hypothesized that a defect of anaerobic metabolism accounted for the disproportionate increase of blood lactate in exercised neurocirculatory asthenics. Reasoning that high blood lactate levels were responsible for pathological anxiety, Pitts and McClure (1967) infused sodium lactate into patients with "anxiety neurosis", whose symptoms approximated those observed in neurocirculatory asthenia. Sodium lactate, in contrast to an isosmotic infusion, provoked acute panic attacks in patients and not in healthy controls. The authors hypothesized that lactate-induced hypocalcemia was responsible for the panic responses (Pitts and McClure, 1967). Excluding the hypocalcemic hypothesis, Pitts and Allen (1969) induced hypocalcemia to tetanic levels by EDTA without producing panic responses. Further, in normal controls, Grosz and Farmer (1972) demonstrated that although sodium lactate infusions produced a metabolic alkalosis, reductions of serum calcium were modest. These results are of questionable relevance as they were not derived from patients.

Carr et al. (1986) suggested that cerebrovascular vasoconstriction in PD patients followed after lactate-induced systemic alkalosis. Subsequent ischemia of cerebral tissues would lead to anerobic glycolysis with an intracellular increase in the lactate:pyruvate ratio. In addition, the authors posited that penetration of lactate following infusion into medullary chemoreceptor zones located outside the blood–brain barrier lowered intracellular pH. An abnormal sensitivity to fluxes in acid–base status was postulated to antecede panic responses. Although, in general, metabolic alkalosis may result in an intracellular acidosis (Ritter *et al.*, 1990), direct and specific documentation of chemoreceptor neuronal sensitivity in PD has not, to our knowledge, been reported. Furthermore, Nutt and Lawson (1992), in an elegant review of the area, point out that hypoxia at levels producing coma or death without concomitant hypercarbia fail to elicit panic responses. This scenario occurs in the "no-panic syndrome" in divers. Such individuals prolong the duration of the dive by a preparatory voluntary hyperventilation which produces hyperoxia. If, however, hyperventilation-induced levels of hypocarbia are sufficient to lose respiratory drive, loss of consciousness secondary to hypoxia occurs without warning. Similarly, carbon monoxide poisoning produces hypoxia without hypercarbia and coma and death ensue without warning. Thus, to the extent that it occurs, lactate-induced hypoxemia appears insufficient by itself to account for panic responses. However, loss of consciousness may occur so abruptly as to prevent the development of dyspnea in these situations. Hypoxic challenges would be of interest.

Sensitivity and specificity of sodium lactate

The sodium lactate infusion model has been shown to induce panic attacks in approximately two-thirds of patients with panic disorder with or without agoraphobia (PD) but rarely in healthy volunteers (Liebowitz *et al.*, 1984). Sodium lactate, the most extensively studied panicogenic agent, has been shown to be specifically panicogenic to patients with a history of spontaneous panic attacks (see Gorman *et al.*, 1989b). Sodium lactate-induced panic closely resembles naturally occurring panic (Dillon *et al.*, 1987), and is effectively blocked following chronic, symptom-remitting, administration by agents known to block naturally occurring panic, i.e. tricyclic antidepressants (Rifkin *et al.*, 1981; Liebowitz *et al.*, 1985a), monoamine inhibitors (Kelly *et al.*, 1974), alprazolam (Carr *et al.*, 1986) and cognitive-behavioral therapy (Shear *et al.*, 1991). These data may simply mean that lactate panicogenesis is a state marker.

Lactate-induced panic is specific to patients with a history of panic attacks rather than the more restricted group that meet formal criteria for the diagnosis of PD. Patients with atypical depression, major depressive disorder, and generalized anxiety disorder who have a history of panic attacks may show panic responses to sodium lactate infusion (McGrath *et al.*, 1985). Conversely, patients with depression, generalized anxiety disorder (McGrath *et al.*, 1985; Cowley *et al.*, 1988), obsessive-compulsive disorder (Gorman *et al.*, 1985), and social phobia (Liebowitz *et al.*, 1985b) without a history of panic are lactate insensitive.

Of note, the only study contradicting the specificity of lactate demonstrated panic responses to lactate in panic-free patients with late luteal phase dysphoria (LLPD). Interestingly, panic responses occurred during both the asymptomatic follicular and symptomatic luteal phase of the disorder (Sandberg *et al.*, 1993). Halbreich *et al.* (1986) reported that women with the most severe cases of LLPD had the highest luteal progesterone production preceding onset of dysphoria and these patients also showed the greatest rate of progesterone decrement. Progesterone is a respiratory stimulant. Klein (1993) has posited that large and rapid decreases in progesterone results in a rapid build-up of carbon dioxide (CO_2) which activates a suffocation alarm in susceptible patients and renders them sensitive to respiratory panicogens. Combined with the observation of fluoxetine effectiveness for LLPD (Stone *et al.*, 1992), which parallels its antipanic effects, the study suggests that menstrually related anxiety disorders and PD may share a common underlying pathophysiology involving chronic CO_2 hypersensitivity.

Determinants of lactate-induced panic

To further delineate the pathophysiology of lactate-induced panic, studies have examined the antecedents of lactate-induced panic measured during the experimental 30 min baseline "placebo" infusion period. Liebowitz *et al.* (1984,1985) reported that the "fear in general" item of the Acute Panic Inventory (API) and the API total score (Dillon *et al.*, 1987) predicted lactate-induced panic. Margraf and associates (1986), arguing that lactate produced a non-specific additive intensification of baseline arousal, noted that increased baseline heart rate was associated with an increased rate of panic to lactate. In support of baseline hyperventilation predicting lactate-induced panic, Gorman *et al.* (1986) reported relatively low levels of phosphate (a consequence of respiratory alkalosis) in lactate-sensitive PD subjects. Further, measuring arterial samples in males, Papp *et al.* (1989) demonstrated that, at baseline, high carbon dioxide tension (pCO_2) and low pH predicted no subsequent panic to lactate. Also studying the Columbia sample, Hollander *et al.* (1989) reported that late panickers (patients who panicked during minutes 15–22 of a standard lactate infusion) had significantly higher cortisol levels than early panickers (patients who panicked during minutes 0–14 of the infusion). Based on the peculiar observation that cortisol levels fell in all subjects during lactate infusions, including those who panicked, the authors suggested that the relatively elevated baseline cortisol levels in late panickers suggested true anticipatory anxiety. Thus, induction of late panic entailed a complete transition from anticipatory anxiety to the panic attack. In contrast, early panickers, who showed relatively lower cortisol levels but higher levels of somatic symptoms on the API, were actually in the process of experiencing the early "rumblings" of a panic attack at the initiation of the lactate infusion.

Scanning studies using positron emission tomography (PET) by Reiman and colleagues (1989) have demonstrated an abnormal asymmetry in metabolic activity of the parahippocampal gyrus (right greater than left) as well as low pCO_2 in those patients who go on to panic to lactate. Consistent with the

Reiman *et al.* study, Nordahl *et al.* (1990) reported a similar parahippocampal asymmetry during a baseline period. Unfortunately, only a small number of PD subjects were then challenged with caffeine, which limits any inference regarding lactate vulnerability. A single-photon emission completed tomography (SPECT) study by De Cristofaro *et al.* (1993) reports hippocampal hypoperfusion bilaterally with significant right greater than left asymmetry of the inferior frontal cortex at baseline in lactate-sensitive subjects. Taken together, the scanning studies implicate limbic and frontal structures in the pathophysiology of panic disorder.

Antecedent HPA–ventilatory interaction and lactate panic

In an extension of the Columbia group lactate infusion studies cited above, we (Coplan *et al.*, 1993a) examined data from an extended sample collected during the 35 min experimental baseline "placebo" infusion period. One hundred and seventy PD patients (101 of whom panicked (59%)) and 43 normal volunteers (0 panic rate) were studied. Supporting findings of the earlier studies on smaller portions of the sample, at baseline, lactate-sensitive PD patients are distinguished from lactate-insensitive PD patients by degree of hyperventilation and fear scores. However, additional findings were noted. Baseline diastolic blood pressure was elevated in the group who would go on to panic. Moreover, antecedent HPA activation was also evident in the lactate-sensitive patient group versus the lactate-insensitive group, which suggested that HPA activation is not only confined to late panickers (Hollander *et al.*, 1989). Logistic regression analyses using panic/no panic as an outcome variable suggested that the strongest predictors of panic were fear and the combination of high cortisol and low pCO_2. When normal controls and the API item of fear were removed from the analysis, pre-lactate dyspnea predicted panic.

Multiple intercorrelations were noted specifically in the lactate-sensitive patient group. A significant negative correlation between baseline cortisol and pCO_2 was noted, and both variables correlated significantly—pCO_2 negatively and cortisol positively—with prelactate fear scores on the API. Thus, the data suggested that, prior to the infusion of lactate, fearful (and dyspneic) PD patients showing HPA activation and hyperventilation were likely to panic during the infusion.

Fear versus panic and pharmacological probes

In a theoretical treatise based primarily on preclinical studies, Deakin and Graeff (1991) have proposed that fear (or anticipatory anxiety) and panic are distinct entities and are mediated through different neuroanatomical substrates. The authors have suggested that "during anticipation of threat, 5-HT projections from the serotonergic dorsal raphe nucleus mediate or facilitate avoidance behavior and restrain or disconnect the fight/flight components of the proximal defense system." Thus, fear entails the appraisal of distant threat and facilitates freezing or avoidant responses. Such responses are mediated, following cortical input, by the "amygdalofugal" pathways (Gray, 1988).

Although direct implication of the serotonin (5-HT) system in the clinical setting is lacking, our study of the correlates of anticipatory anxiety implicate the amygdalofugal pathways as a potential common substrate for lactate sensitivity: (1) direct amygdaloid stimulation during surgery in humans has been shown to produce fear responses (see Graeff, 1990); (2) descending amygdalofugal fibers project to the paraventricular nucleus of the hypothalamus where corticotropin-releasing factor (CRF) is released, reflected in high serum cortisol levels; and (3) caudal projections also synapse at the brain stem nucleus brachialis (and other brain stem nuclei) (Davis, 1986), which may mediate increases of respiratory rate driven by amygdaloid neurons (Frysinger and Harper, 1989).

In contrast, spontaneous panic has been proposed by Graeff (1990) to be due to spontaneous activation of the flight component of the periaqueductal gray matter (PAG), following failure of serotonergic neurotransmission to restrain or inhibit its activation. Direct electrical stimulation of the PAG in humans (Nashold et al., 1974; Akil et al., 1978) results in symptoms and signs strikingly similar to panic—fear of dying, an overwhelming desire to flee and physiological activation such as hyperventilation and tachycardia. We have hypothesized that a further distinction between fear and panic is that only in the former instance do we observe HPA activation (Cannon, 1920; Selye, 1956). Unfortunately, we are not aware of studies which have explored the effects of *dorsal* PAG stimulation on HPA axis function. Studies by Akil and colleagues (1978) report minimal HPA activation during *ventral* PAG stimulation but the ventral aspect of the PAG appears to mediate antinociceptive effects, whereas dorsal stimulation is associated with the distress and flight responses reminiscent of clinical panic.

Ostensibly, panic responses to lactate appear dependent on anticipatory anxiety. For instance, using a panic attack frequency index, Targum (1990) demonstrated that change of API to sodium lactate correlated ($r = 0.6$) with recent panic attack frequency and suggested that heightened state of anticipatory anxiety (presumably influenced by recent spontaneous panic attacks) rather than "putative underlying trait factors" predicts panic response. It is important to note that panic responses to sodium lactate do not appear solely dependent on high anticipatory anxiety. Spontaneous panic attacks usually occur without warning or pre-existing perceived anxiety. In addition, Liebowitz et al. (in review) significantly reduced anticipatory anxiety with diazepam pretreatment of sodium lactate infusions in previously lactate-sensitive PD patients. Although diazepam significantly delayed the onset of panic, only three of 10 subjects experienced panic blockade when diazepam pretreated. Thus, the initial spontaneous panic attack may result from spontaneous loss of restraint of a primitive flight mechanism. This mechanism is postulated to be closely linked to the brain substrate responsible for the perception of asphyxic stimuli. Although certain sites within the PAG are potential candidates for such behavioral and physiological responses (Akil *et al.*, 1978), further studies are required to assess HPA function while these sites are stimulated before any analogies can be made to clinical panic.

CARBON DIOXIDE

Cohen and White (1951) first made the observation that "neurocirculatory asthenics" experienced panic-like symptoms during inhalation of small amounts (4%) of CO_2, but not during hyperventilation. Years later, Gorman *et al.* (1984) challenged PD patients and normal controls with inhalation of 5% CO_2.

Although normal controls did not panic under this condition, patients reacted with a mixture of physical and emotional symptoms similar to their naturally occurring panic attacks. Also, minute ventilation (i.e. the product of respiratory rate and tidal volume) increased more rapidly in patients who went on to panic than non-panicking patients and normal controls (Gorman *et al.*, 1988). Woods *et al.* (1986), using the Read rebreathing method, also did not replicate the finding of CO_2 sensitivity. Another measure of brain stem control of respiration, inspiratory drive, was found to parallel the rapid increase of minute ventilation in patients who panicked to 5% CO_2, and increased more rapidly in panicking patients than non-panicking patients (Carr *et al.*, 1987). Inspiratory drive is believed by respiratory physiologists to reflect brain stem control over respiration (Milc-Emil and Brunstein, 1976). Further studies are required to clarify the issue of CO_2 sensitivity.

In a test of the panicogenic effects of hypercarbia, Mathew *et al.* (1989) administered acetazolamide, an agent believed to cause central hypercarbia. The authors failed to detect any panic responses in patients with PD. In a follow-up study, Gorman *et al.* (1993) replicated the lack of panic responses to acetazolamide but noted an absence of respiratory stimulation, a regular concomitant of central hypercarbia. The failure of acetazolamide to induce panic or hyperventilation suggests that it is unlikely whether central hypercarbia is, in fact, induced by acetazolamide administration.

Alternatively, the hypercarbia produced by acetazolamide does not drive respiration because inhibition of carbonic anhydrase prevents build-up of H^+ ions.

Cortisol and CO_2-induced panic

Supporting the view that panic attacks are distinguishable from natural stressors and compounds which activate the HPA axis (Klein, 1993), cortisol levels regularly decrease during lactate-induced panic. We (Coplan *et al.*, unpublished data) have examined blood cortisol levels during CO_2 inhalation, where confounding volumetric factors are not a consideration. The means of cortisol values from 5% and 7% CO_2 inhalation procedures were used if both were available. Cortisol levels drawn prior to CO_2 inhalation compared to levels drawn at the point-of-panic in 10 PD subjects decreased significantly ($p<0.015$). No reductions were noted after 20 min of CO_2 inhalation in either eight normal controls or nine non-panicking PD patients. However, in eight non-PD anxiety disorder subjects, cortisol levels dropped significantly ($p< 0.0025$) following CO_2 inhalation without panic. A trend for voluntary (non-panicogenic) hyperventilation to increase cortisol in normal controls ($n=4$) and decrease cortisol in anxiety-disordered subjects ($n=8$) (interactive effect; $p< 0.005$) was also noted. Woods et al. (1988) report a trend increase in cortisol levels following 5% CO_2-induced panic to a level similar to the trend increase observed following 7.5% CO_2 inhalation in healthy controls, but the cortisol levels reported were drawn 15 min following cessation of a 15 min CO_2 inhalation epoch and may not accurately reflect HPA status during panic. A delayed increase in cortisol would be expected following corticoid reduction as the patient reverted back to a state of anticipatory anxiety. These data further support the view that activation of the suffocation alarm mechanism to the level of panic by CO_2, where hemodilution is not a factor, is nevertheless insufficient to activate the HPA axis.

SODIUM BICARBONATE

The usual pulmonary response to metabolic alkalosis is hypoventilation, as the body homeostatically keeps the pH normal by retaining CO_2. Peculiarly, Gorman and colleagues (1986) have noted that patients who panic during lactate infusion in fact hyperventilate, suggesting that metabolic alkalosis associated with the lactate infusion is insufficient to override the respiratory stimulation accompanying panic. Other investigations of lactate panicogenesis have focused on its metabolic fate. Conversion of infused lactate to pyruvate and ensuing metabolism via the tricarboxylic acid cycle produces bicarbonate on a mole-for-mole basis (Grosz and Farmer, 1972). Bicarbonate traverses the blood–brain barrier poorly (Whitwam et al., 1976) but could theoretically be peripherally converted back to carbonic acid and then to CO_2, which does penetrate the blood–brain barrier, and water by the enzyme carbonic anhydrase. This latter view, initially proposed by our group, appears unlikely as studies in non-human primates, using different methodologies (Dager et al., 1990; Coplan et al., 1992b) failed to detect an increase in cisternal pCO_2 following large increases in serum lactate levels during lactate infusions.

To test the panic-provoking properties of bicarbonate and metabolic alkalosis, Gorman et al. (1989a) compared sodium bicarbonate infusions to sodium lactate infusions in PD patients. Bicarbonate infusion only caused panic in PD subjects with comorbid agoraphobia, but rates of panic responses for the two panicogens were not significantly different. Bicarbonate-induced panic was associated with reductions in arterial CO_2 pressure, suggesting that respiratory stimulation associated with the panic process overrode the expected homeostatic response to metabolic alkalosis. In contrast, PD patients who did not panic to bicarbonate responded with the expected homeostatic mechanism and showed increases in arterial CO_2 levels. Again, the paradoxical ventilatory response despite metabolic alkalosis evident in the bicarbonate-panickers suggested the presence of a hypersensitive suffocation alarm mechanism.

SODIUM D-LACTATE

The premise of most theories involving lactate panic provocation by bicarbonate and CO_2 are dependent on its metabolism. The standard sodium lactate infusion entails administration of the racemic compound which contains both the "D" and "L" stereoisomeric forms in approximately equal amounts. Although the "L" isomeric form is metabolically active, the "D" form, as far as is known, is metabolically inactive (Alpert and Root, 1954). To test the hypothesis that the effects of sodium lactate are dependent on its metabolism, Gorman et al. (1990) administered D-lactate and racemic lactate to PD patients. If metabolism of lactate is a prerequisite for panic induction, D-lactate should be devoid of panicogenic properties. In fact D-lactate provoked panic at similar rates to the racemic form. D-Lactate, like other respiratory panicogens, caused alkalosis and hypocapnia, indicating hyperventilation. Thus, it may be that PD subjects "recognize" the lactate molecule in its unmetabolized form, and, because of a hypersensitive suffocation alarm mechanism, interpret its increasing presence as a signal of asphyxiation.

Lactate and the blood–brain barrier

Based on the above studies, where is lactate, in its pure state, detected by the body? Conflicting data exist as to whether lactate crosses the blood–brain barrier. Coplan et al. (1992b) reported an absence of increase in cisternal lactate in macaques whereas Dager et al. (1990) reported increases in cisternal lactate in baboons, following sodium lactate infusions. Dager et al. (in press) followed up these studies by assessing brain lactate levels in human subjects using proton magnetic resonance spectroscopy (MRS). Brain lactate levels increased in all subjects following lactate infusions, suggesting penetration of the blood–brain barrier. These findings were complicated by the observation that PD patients who went on to panic showed higher initial blood lactate levels as well as an increase in brain lactate levels even after blood lactate levels had decreased following the infusion. Maddock and Carter (1991) and our group (Gorman et al., 1984) have also noted that blood lactate levels increase to a greater extent in patients who panic versus non-panicking subjects. In addition, voluntary hyperventilation produces increases in blood lactate (Maddock and Carter, 1991). Thus, hyperventilation itself produces an increase in blood and brain lactate levels, possibly by cerebral vasoconstriction in the brain in the latter instance (Carr et al., 1986) and/or alkalotic inhibition of the metabolic conversion of lactate to pyruvate in the periphery and brain. It is also important to note, as mentioned previously, that ventral medullary chemoreceptors are located outside the blood–brain barrier, where lactate may be detected in the systemic circulation.

DOXAPRAM AND ISOPROTERENOL

Further negating the putative necessity for panicogens to cross the blood–brain barrier are studies involving doxapram and isoproterenol. Both of these compounds induce panic responses accompanied by hyperventilation (Rainey et al., 1984; Lee et al., 1993), but, curiously, appear to have virtually exclusive peripheral effects.

Doxapram derives its respiratory stimulant properties from its effect on the carotid chemoreceptors (Calverley et al., 1983) based on the observation that elimination of its ventilatory effects occurred in cats who had undergone sectioning of their carotid sinus nerves. Isoproterenol, a cardiac stimulant, is a β-agonist which crosses the blood–brain barrier poorly (Rainey et al., 1984). Conduction of afferent cardiorespiratory stimuli via vagus and glossopharyngeus to the nucleus tractus solitarius (NTS) may be an initial step in this panic cascade. Hsiao and Potter (1990) and Gorman et al. (1989b) have proposed that peripheral stimuli relayed by the NTS are then processed by the medullary nucleus paragigantocellularis which projects to the pontine LC, which in turn projects to limbic forebrain structures (Aston-Jones et al., 1986). Another important and neglected route for relaying viscerosensory information to limbic sites involves NTS projections to the nucleus brachialis and from there to the hypothalamus and amygdala (Berkley and Scofield, 1990). It is unclear if the latter route involves HPA activation, whereas the former route, which includes LC activation, is clearly associated with HPA activation.

A similar panicogenic process that occurs for doxapram and isoproterenol appears to occur during hypertonic saline infusion (Jensen et al., 1991), although a very small number of subjects were studied and replication is required. These authors note that the hyperosmolar infusions performed by Pitts and McClure were glucose solutions, which, in contrast to osmotic stimuli such as sodium lactate and hypertonic saline, is ineffective in induction of arginine vasopressin release (AVP). AVP is permissive of CRF release (Rittmaster et al., 1987); thus the hypothesis that stimulation of AVP release is an important factor in panicogenesis is contradicted by the lack of corticoid response to lactate, which would be associated with no AVP release. AVP levels during lactate infusion have not, to our knowledge, been measured nor have cortisol levels during doxapram or isoproterenol infusion been examined.

NORADRENERGIC PHARMACOLOGICAL PROBES

Potential abnormalities within the noradrenergic (NE) system in PD have been extensively studied (Charney and Heninger, 1986; Nutt, 1989; Uhde et al.,

1992; Cameron *et al.*, 1990; see Abelson *et al.*, 1992, for review). Although this subject is dealt with in Chapter 6, we will highlight the differences between adrenergic versus respiratory related panic.

In general, PD patients develop more frequent panic attacks than normal subjects following oral yohimbine ingestion (Gurguis and Uhde, 1990; Charney *et al.*, 1984), although this effect is not consistent (see Albus *et al.*, 1992). Furthermore, questions regarding the definition and clinical relevance of yohimbine-induced panic have been raised (Klein, 1993). Yohimbine, an α_2-antagonist (Svensson and Usdin, 1978), stimulates firing of the LC (Redmond, 1977), which contains the majority of central noradrenergic cell bodies. LC stimulation by yohimbine is mediated by interruption of an autoreceptor negative feedback mechanism.

Yohimbine-induced anxiety has been positively correlated with serum increases of the principal noradrenergic metabolite, 3-methoxy-4-hydroxy-phenethyleneglycol (MHPG) (Charney and Heninger, 1986; Gurguis and Uhde, 1990). Panic responses to yohimbine appear specific to PD, with an absence of yohimbine-induced panic response in patients with depression, schizophrenia, generalized anxiety disorder, and obsessive-compulsive disorder (Heninger *et al.*, 1988). Of note, patients with post-traumatic stress disorder also respond to yohimbine with panic and flashbacks (Southwick *et al.*, 1993) and yohimbine, unlike lactate, also induces anxiety in normal controls (Charney *et al.*, 1983). Chronic administration of the drugs most often associated with clinical utility in the blockade of panic—IMI and desipramine—reduce central noradrenergic turnover and LC firing rate (Svensson and Usdin, 1978). Nevertheless, IMI has no effect on yohimbine-induced anxiety (Charney and *et al.*, 1985) and may in fact worsen yohimbine anxiogenesis (Garfield *et al.*, 1967).

In contrast to yohimbine-induced anxiety, panic attacks provoked by lactate infusion (Carr *et al.*, 1986), CO_2 inhalation (Woods *et al.*, 1986), or naturalistic exposure to predisposing phobic stimuli (Woods *et al.*, 1987) do not increase serum MHPG. Intravenous clonidine pretreatment failed to block lactate-induced panic in six of 10 patients who had previously panicked to lactate (Coplan *et al.*, 1992a), suggesting that activation of the LC may not be critical for lactate-induced panic. Moreover, corticoid responses are regularly observed during yohimbine-induced panic (Charney *et al.*, 1984). When considering the "fear versus panic" model proposed by Deakin and Graeff (1991), it is noteworthy that NE in fact inhibits the PAG area whereas LC efferents to the amygdala and hypothalamus may be stimulatory (Gray, 1988). In fact, Garvey *et al.* (1990) has noted that high urinary MHPG excretion is associated with lower rates of panic. In a similar vein, we (Coplan *et al.*, 1993b) have noted that PD patients who showed the largest decrements of serum MHPG to clonidine (largely reflective of high baseline serum MHPG levels) showed a lower frequency of clinical panic in the week preceding the challenge. Chronic noradrenergic overdrive may therefore bear a relationship to chronic anticipatory or generalized anxiety and may represent a partially adaptive compensatory mechanism attempting to reduce an elevated rate of spontaneous panic, a pattern most evident later in the illness. The compensatory effects of noradrenergic overdrive appear insufficient to cope with certain panicogenic stimuli, such as the asphyxic stimuli associated with lactate infusions, as *increased* anticipatory or generalized anxiety is associated with an *increased* rate of lactate-induced panic (Coplan *et al.*, 1993a). This puzzling relationship between noradrenergic overdrive, anticipatory anxiety and lactate vulnerability may be explained by the untested hypothesis that it is those subjects who are in most dire danger for losing restraint (or "control") of a primitive flight/alarm mechanism that show the highest compensatory noradrenergic overdrive, which correlates with high anticipatory anxiety and lactate vulnerability. Taken together, these data highlight critical differences between yohimbine and respiratory panicogens, which are not readily reconcilable.

SEROTONIN SYSTEM

Several lines of evidence have suggested an important role for 5-HT-related function in PD (see Chapter 6; for review, see Coplan *et al.*, 1992c). The strongest evidence for an important role for 5-HT in PD derives from the clinical efficacy of a range of selective serotonin reuptake inhibitors (SSRIs) (e.g. fluoxetine (Gorman *et al.*, 1987a; Schneier *et al.*, 1990), fluvoxamine (Den Boer and Westenberg, 1988), zimelidine (Evans *et al.*, 1986), and paroxetine (Christiansen *et al.*, 1992)). Clomipramine (CMI), a tricyclic with potent 5-HT reuptake properties, may be effective in PD at lower than standard tricyclic doses (Gloger *et al.*, 1989) and, in one study, showed superiority to IMI, a less potent 5-HT reuptake inhibitor, on several measures (Modigh *et al.*, 1990). The current view is that the long-term administration of these drugs enhances serotonergic neurotransmission (Blier *et al.*, 1987). A regular phenomenon early in the treatment of PD patients with SSRIs is the emergence of a jitteriness syndrome, characterized by motor restlessness, insomnia, diarrhea, heightened anxiety (without an increase in panic) and a "jumping out of the skin feeling." If patients are able to tolerate these symptoms, panic blockade ensues in a few weeks.

Unfortunately, limited data is available on the jitteriness syndrome, but it occurs frequently with desipramine (Pohl *et al.*, 1988) and IMI (Zitrin *et al.*, 1983). Challenge studies using 5-HT agonists may bear a time-limited similarity to the jitteriness syndrome. 5-HT agonists represent typical "corticoid-activating" panicogens. Challenges using oral mCPP (Kahn *et al.*, 1988b; Klein *et al.*, 1991) and fenfluramine (Targum and Marshall, 1989), direct and indirect 5-HT agonists respectively, produce increased rates of anxiety, but not panic responses, HPA activation, particularly in PD patients, and a minimum of ventilatory effects. Of note, differential responses to mCPP relative to normal controls are not observed in intravenous studies (Charney *et al.*, 1987). Fenfluramine induces presynaptic release of 5-HT and blocks its reuptake whereas mCPP does not functionally interact with 5-HT_{1A} receptor sites in rodent studies, but acts as a 5-HT_{1C} and 5-HT_2 agonist (Winslow and Insel, 1991).

Such exaggerated responses to 5-HT agonists have been interpreted to reflect deafferentation 5-HT receptor hypersensitivity in some patients with PD (Gorman et al., 1987a; Kahn et al., 1988a). An absence of anxiogenic response to 5-hydroxytryptophan (Westenberg and Den Boer, 1989) has complicated this view. In fact, the enhanced sensitivity to 5-HT agonism (SSRIs, fenfluramine and mCPP) may in fact reflect increased activity of the dorsal raphe projection to the amygdala and hypothalamus which manifests as generalized or anticipatory anxiety. Moreover, 5-HT agonists exert restraining effects on the PAG, which would counteract the development of panic. This view is supported by studies using ritanserin, a $5\text{-HT}_{1C}/5\text{HT}_2$ antagonist, in anxiety disorder patients. The drug is effective in generalized anxiety disorder (Bressa et al., 1987) (by reduction of serotonergic neurotransmission arising from the dorsal raphe) but has no effect on panic attacks (Den Boer and Westenberg, 1990), where enhanced 5-HT neurotransmission appears to be necessary for therapeutic response. In a test of the effects of acute reduction of 5-HT neurotransmission on the occurrence of panic attacks, Goddard et al. (1992) report no anxiogenic effects following administration of a tryptophan-depleted solution which reduces central 5-HT levels. Thus, further studies are required to delineate the paradoxical role of 5-HT-related function in anticipatory and generalized anxiety and panic.

More recently, an important role for 5-HT is emerging in respiratory control although interpretation of these preclinical studies are complex. In rat studies, systemic administration of 5-OH-tryptophan, the 5-HT precursor, produces a decrease in CO_2 sensitivity (Lundberg et al., 1980), whereas parachlorophenylanaline (PCPA), which depletes 5-HT, produces hyperventilation (Olson et al., 1979). However, bull-dog studies (Kubin et al., 1992), investigating the pathophysiology of sleep apnea, indicate an important role for brain stem 5-HT neurotransmission at cranial nerve nuclei in the maintenance of muscular tone in the upper airways. The amygdalohippocampus, a site rich in inhibitory 5-HT receptors (see Edwards et al., 1990), possesses neurons that fire in synchrony with the cardiorespiratory cycle (Frysinger and Harper, 1989). A serotonergic deficit state may therefore result in respiratory stimulation at amygdalohippocampal sites but hypotonia in upper airway musculature. This intriguing link between 5-HT function and respiration requires further exploration in PD patients.

Animal studies suggest a modulatory role for 5-HT in behaviors potentially linked to human panic–anxiety. These include infant separation protest responses (Panksepp et al., 1980) and conditioned inhibition (see Deakin and Graeff, 1991). Lingjaerde (1985) demonstrated rapid influx of 5-HT into human platelets following in vitro exposure to sodium lactate, although this provocative hypothesis has not been explored further.

GABA-RELATED PROBES

More recently, high-potency benzodiazepines, such as the triazolobenzodiazepine derivative, alprazolam and clonazepam, have been found highly effective in blocking panic attacks (Ballenger *et al.*, 1988; Spier *et al.*, 1986). The initial impression in trials using conventional low-potency benzodiazepines, such as diazepam, suggested efficacy for anticipatory anxiety but not panic attacks, whereas imipramine treatment was viewed as helpful for blocking panic but not anticipatory anxiety (Klein, 1964). Promising results with lorazepam (Schweizer *et al.*, 1990) have also been reported, although efficacy has been most consistent for the high-potency benzodiazepines.

With respect to pharmacological probes, Nutt *et al.* (1990) demonstrated panic responses in patients with PD compared to no responses in healthy controls following intravenous administration of the benzodiazepine antagonist RO 15–1788 (flumazenil). The authors concluded that PD patients may be in a state of agonist subsensitivity and inverse agonist supersensitivity and therefore flumazenil acted as an inverse agonist and not a neutral antagonist in PD patients. Their conclusion suggested a change in the equilibrium between conformational states of the receptor, rather than number of receptors in PD patients.

Klein had predicted to Nutt (personal communication) that flumazenil would produce a non-dyspneic behavioral profile since inverse agonists were HPA activators. Administration of benzodiazepine inverse agonists such as β-carboline-3-carboxylic acid (BCCE) to non-human primates induced responses characteristic of marked fear along with increases in blood pressure, heart rate, cortisol and catecholamines (Insel *et al.*, 1984). The latter two features are in contrast to panic produced by sodium lactate (Hollander *et al.*, 1987), CO_2 (Woods *et al.*, 1988) or naturalistic phobic exposure (Woods *et al.*, 1987). The effects of BCCE were blocked by diazepam (Insel *et al.*, 1984), an effect not observed for lactate-panic in PD patients (Liebowitz *et al.*,1995). Confirming Klein's predictions, Nutt *et al.* (1990) observed a paucity of dyspnea during flumazenil-induced panic. Flumazenil also induces increases in serum MHPG. However, flumazenil-induced panic was blocked by symptom-remitting IMI treatment (Nutt, personal communication), which requires further consideration.

ADENOSINE SYSTEM

Caffeine also possesses panicogenic properties (Uhde, 1990). Theories accounting for its panicogenic effect include antagonism of the adenosine system, and the observation that caffeine increases lactate levels (Uhde, 1990). However, like yohimbine, mCPP and fenfluramine, caffeine-induced panic is associated with a rise in cortisol, although this effect is reduced by repeated administration (Uhde, 1990). Alprazolam blocks caffeine-induced panic consistently but its effects are not blocked by IMI (Uhde, 1990). Although caffeine is a respiratory stimulant (Uhde, 1990), it does not produce prominent levels of dyspnea. The lack of dyspnea-inducing effects during caffeine-induced panic, the presence of corticoid activation and the lack of IMI blockade suggest poor modeling of spontaneous panics and similarity to the effects of yohimbine and mCPP.

CONCLUSION

Despite the emerging complexity of data derived from studies using pharmacological probes, several key points point to future directions of study:

1. There appear to be at least two forms of panic induced by pharmacological probes; the first entails prominent dyspnea and smothering symptoms, an increase in tidal volume, no HPA activation and models spontaneous panic. Panicogens belonging to the first group do not induce anxiety in normals and are blocked by IMI. The second entails "direct" action on neurotransmitter sites, produces HPA activation and produces minimal respiratory symptoms and models anticipatory or generalized anxiety. Panicogens belonging to the second group tend to affect normals and their effects, to the extent studied, are not blocked by imipramine.
2. Lacate-induced panic was predicted by fear and the baseline combination of high cortisol and low pCO_2. The observation that HPA activation predicted panic points to involvement of amygdaloid–hypothalamic sites of activation—the amygdalofugal pathways—in the pathophysiology of anticipatory anxiety. Study of the factors linking fear, ventilation and the HPA axis (e.g. 5-HT) are warranted.
3. The panic attack induced by respiratory panicogens may involve failure of restraint of a suffocation alarm mechanism (the dorsal PAG?), which is characterized by further increases in hyperventilation and subjective dyspnea. This response is elicited only by the first group of panicogens. Study of the possible mechanisms whereby inhibitory effects on the suffocation alarm are disrupted are warranted.
4. The panic attack induced by respiratory panicogens is characterized by the absence of HPA axis activation. Given the usual response of the body to natural fearful stressors of HPA activation, this observation suggests direct restraint of the HPA axis during panic. Investigations of mechanisms for this counterintuitive phenomenon may provide clues to the mechanisms of panic dominated by dyspnea. Preclinical studies which address the effects of dorsal PAG stimulation on the HPA axis are indicated.

REFERENCES

Abelson, J. L., Glitz, D., Cameron, O. G. *et al.* (1992). Endocrine, cardiovascular and behavioral responses to clonidine in patients with panic disorder. *Biol. Psychiatry*, **32**, 18–25.

Abelson, J. L., Nesse, R. M. and Vinik, A. I. (1994). Pentagastrin infusions in patients with panic disorder. II. Neuroendocrinology. *Biol. Psychiatry*, **36**, 84–96.

Akil, H., Richardson, D. E., Hughes, J. *et al.* (1978). Enkephalin-like material elevated in ventricular cerebrospinal fluid of pain patients after analgetic focal stimulation. *Science*, **201**, 463–465.

Albus, M., Zahn, T. P. and Breier, A. (1992). Anxiogenic properties of yohimbine. I. Behavioral, physiological and biochemical measures. *Eur. Arch. Psychiatry Clin. Neurosci.*, **241**, 337–344.

Alpert, N. R. and Root, W. S. (1954). Relationship between excess respiratory metabolism and utilization of intravenously infused sodium racemic lactate and sodium L(–)lactate. *Am. J. Physiol.*, **177**, 455–462.

Asnis, G. M., Wetzler, S., Sanderson, W. *et al.* (1992). Functional interrelationship of serotonin and norepinephrine: cortisol response to MCPP and DMI in patients with panic disorder, patients with depression, and normal control subjects. *Psychiatr. Res.*, **43**, 65–76.

Aston-Jones, G., Ennis, M., Pieribone, V. A., *et al.* (1986). The brain nucleus locus ceruleus: restricted afferent control of a broad efferent network. *Science*, **234**, 734–737.

Ballenger, J. C., Burrows, G. D., Dupont, R. L. *et al.* (1988). Alprazolam in panic disorder and agoraphobia: results from a multicenter trial. *Arch. Gen. Psychiatry*, **45** (5), 413–422.

Barlow, D. H. (1985). The dimensions of anxiety disorders. In *Anxiety and Anxiety Disorders* (eds A. H. Tuma and J. D. Maser), pp. 479–500. Erlbaum, Hillsdale, NJ.

Barlow, D. H., Vermilyea, J. A., Blanchard, E. B. *et al.* (1985). The phenomenon of panic. *J. Abnorm. Psychol.,* **94**, 320–328.

Berkley, K. J. and Scofield, S. L. (1990). Relays from the spinal cord and solitary nucleus through the parabrachial nucleus to the forebrain of the cat. *Brain Res.,* **529** (1–2), 333–338.

Blier, P., de Montigny, C. and Chaput Y. (1987). Modifications of the serotonin system by antidepressant treatments: implications for the therapeutic response in major depression. *J. Clin. Psychopharmacol.*, **7**(6s), 24s–35s.

Bradwejn, J. (1993). C C K and panic disorder: a review of clinical and animal data. American College of Neuropsychopharmacology 32nd Annual Meeting, Honolulu.

Bradwejn, J. Koszycki, and Shriqui, C. (1991). Enhanced sensitivity to cholecystokinin tetrapeptide in panic disorder: clinical and behavioral findings. *Arch. Gen. Psychiatry*, **48** (7), 603–610).

Bressa, G. M., Marini, S. and Gregori, S. (1987). Serotonin S2 receptors blockage and generalized anxiety disorders: a double-blind study on ritanserin and lorazepam. *Int. J. Clin. Pharmacol. Res.*, **7**(2), 111–119.

Calverley, P. M. A., Robson, R. H. Wraith, P. K. *et al.* (1983). The ventilatory effects of doxapram in normal man. *Clin. Sci.*, **65**, 65–69.

Cameron, O. G., Smith, C. B., Lee, M. A. *et al.* (1990). Adrenergic status in anxiety disorders: platelet alpha-2-adrenergic receptor binding, blood pressure, pulse and plasma catecholamines in panic and generalized anxiety disorder patients and in normal subjects. *Biol. Psychiatry*, **28**, 3–20.

Cannon, W. B. (1920). Bodily changes. In *Pain, Fear, Hunger and Rage*. Appleton, New York.

Charney, D. S., and Heninger, G. R. (1985). Noradrenergic function and the mechanism of action of antianxiety treatment, 11: the effect of long-term imipramine treatment. *Arch Gen. Psychiatry,* **42**, 475–481.

Charney, D. S. and Heninger, G. R. (1986). Abnormal regulation of noradrenergic function in panic disorders: effects of clonidine in healthy subjects and patients with agoraphobia and panic disorder. *Arch. Gen. Psychiatry*, **43**, 1042–1055.

Charney, D. S., Heninger, G. R. and Redmond, D. E. (1983). Yohimbine induced anxiety and increased noradrenergic function in humans: effects of diazepam and clonidine. *Life Sci.,* **33**, 19–29.

Charney, D. S., Heninger, G. R. and Breier, A. (1984). Noradrenergic function in panic anxiety: effects of yohimbine in healthy subjects and patients with agoraphobia and panic disorder. *Arch. Gen. Psychiatry.,* **41**, 751–763.

Charney, D. S., Woods, S. W., Goodman, W. K. *et al.* (1987). Serotonin function in anxiety, 11: effects of the serotonin agonist mCPP in panic disorder patients and healthy controls. *Psychopharmacology (Berlin)*, **92**, 14–24.

Christiansen, P. E., Judge, R. and Ohrstrom, J. (1992). A double-blind, randomized, multicenter, placebo controlled parallel group study of paroxetine in combination with psychotherapy in treatment of patients with panic disorder (DSM–III-R). Annual Neuropsychopharmacology Meeting, San Juan, Puerto Rico.

Cohen, M. E. and White, P. D. (1951). Life situations, emotions and neurocirculatory asthenia. *Psychosom. Med.,* **13**, 335–357.

Coplan, J. D., Liebowitz, M. R., Gorman, J. M. *et al.* (1992a). Noradrenergic function in panic disorder: clonidine pretreatment of sodium lactate infusions. *Biol. Psychiatry*, **31**, 135–146.

Coplan, J. D., Rosenblum, L. A., Friedman, J. M. *et al.* (1992b). Cerebrospinal fluid lactate and CO_2 levels during sodium lactate infusion in nonhuman primates. *Am. J. Psychiatry*, **149**(10), 1369–1373.

Coplan, J. D., Gorman, J. M. and Klein, D. F. (1992c). Serotonin-related function in panic disorder; a critical overview. *Neuropsychopharmacology*, **6**(3), 189–200.

Coplan, J. D., Goetz R., Klein, D. F. *et al.* (1993a). Determinants of lactate-induced panic: an extended sample review. New Research Program, American Psychiatric Association, San Francisco.

Coplan, J. D., Papp, L. A., Martinez J. *et al.* (1993b). Persistence of noradrenergic–related dysregulation in panic disorder following chronic serotonin reuptake blockade with fluoxetine: a preliminary report. American College of Neuropsychopharmacology 32nd Annual Meeting, Honolulu.

Cowley, D. S., Dager, S. R. and Dunner, D. L. (1986). Lactate induced panic in primary affective disorder. *Am. J. Psychiatry*, **143**, 646–648.

Dager, S. R., Rainey, J. M., Kenny, M. A. *et al.* (1990). Central nervous system effects of lactate infusion in primates. *Biol. Psychiatry*, **27**(2), 193–204.

Dager, S. R., Strauss, W. L., Marro, K. I. *et al.* (1995), Proton magnetic response spectroscopy investigation of hyperventilation in subjects with panic disorder and comparison subjects. *Am. J. Psychiatry,* **152**, 666–672.

Davis, M. (1986) Pharmacological and anatomical analysis of fear conditioning using the fear-potentiated startle paradigm. *Behav. Neurosci.,* **100**, 814–824.

Deakin, J. F. W. and Graeff, F. G. (1991). 5–HT and mechanisms of defence. *J. Psychopharmacol.,* **5**(4), 305–315.

De Cristofaro, M. T. R., Sessarego, A., Pupi, A. *et al.* (1993). Brain perfusion abnormalities in drug-naive lactate-sensitive panic patients: a SPECT study. *Biol. Psychiatry*, **33**, 505–512.

Den Boer, J. A. and Westenberg, H. G. (1988). Effect of a serotonin and noradrenaline uptake inhibitor in panic disorder: a double-blind comparative study with fluvoxamine and maprotiline. *Int. Clin. Psychopharmacol.,* **3**(1), 59–74.

Den Boer, J. A. and Westenberg, H. G. (1990). Serotonin function in panic disorder: a double blind placebo controlled study with fluvoxamine and ritanserin. *Psychopharmacol. Berl.,* **102**(1), 85–94.

Dillon, D. J., Gorman, J. M., Liebowitz, M. R. *et al.* (1987). The measurement of lactate-induced panic and anxiety. *Psychiatry Res.,* **20**, 97–105.

Edwards, E., Whitaker-Azmitia, P. M. and Harkins, K. (1990). 5HT1a and 5HT1b agonists play a differential role on the respiratory frequency in rats. *Neuropsychopharmacology*, **3**(2), 129–136.

Evans, L., Kenardy, J., Schneider, P. *et al.* (1986). Effect of a selective serotonin uptake inhibitor in agoraphobia with panic attacks. *Acta Psychiatr. Scand.,* **73**, 49–53.

Fishman, S. M., Carr, D. B., Beckett, A and Rosenbaum, J. F. (1994). Hypercapneic ventilatory response in patients with panic disorder before and after alprazolam treatment and in pre- and postmenstrual women. *J. Psychiatr. Res.*, **28**, 165–170.

Frysinger, R. C. and Harper, R. M. (1989). Cardiac and respiratory correlations with unit discharge in human amygdala and hippocampus. *Electroencenphalogr. Clin. Neurophysiol.*, **72**(6), 463–470.

Garfield, S., Gershon, S. and Sletten, I. (1967). Chemically induced anxiety. *Int. J. Neuropsychiatr.* **3**, 426–433.

Garvey, M., Noyes, R. and Cook B. (1990). Comparison of panic disordered patients with high versus low MHPG. *J. Affect. Disord.*, **20**, 7–12.

Gloger, S., Grunhaus, L., Gladic, D. *et al.* (1989). Panic attacks and agoraphobia: low dose clomipramine treatment. *J. Clin. Psychopharmacol.*, **9**(1), 28–32.

Goddard, A. W., Goodman, W. K., Woods, S. W. *et al.* (1992). Effects of tryptophan depletion on panic anxiety (abstract). American College of Neuropsychopharmacology 31st Annual Meeting, Puerto Rico.

Gorman, J. M., Askanazi, J., Liebowitz, M. R. *et al.* (1984). Response to hyperventilation in a group of patients with panic disorder: *Am. J. Psychiatry*, **141**, 857–861.

Gorman, J. M., Liebowitz, M. R., Fyer, A. J. *et al.* (1985). Lactate infusions in obsessive-compulsive disorder. *Am. J. Psychiatry*, **142**(7), 864–866.

Gorman, J. M., Cohen, B. S., Liebowitz, M. R. *et al.* (1986). Blood gas changes and hypophosphatemia in lactate induced panic. *Arch. Gen. Psychiatry.*, **43**, 1067–1075.

Gorman, J. M., Liebowitz, M. R., Fyer, A. J. *et al.* (1987a). An open trial of fluoxetine in the treatment of panic attacks. *J. Clin. Psychopharmacol.*, **7**, 329–332.

Gorman, J. M., Fyer, M. R., Liebowitz, M. R. *et al.* (1987b). Pharmacological provocation of panic attacks. *Psychopharmacology: The Third Generation of Progress* (ed. H. Y. Meltzer), pp. 985–993. Raven Press, New York.

Gorman, J. M., Fyer, M. R., Goetz, R. *et al.* (1988). Ventilatory challenge studies of patients with panic disorder. *Arch. Gen. Psychiatry*, **45**(1), 31–39.

Gorman, J. M., Battista, D., Goetz, R. R. *et al.* (1989a). A comparison of sodium bicarbonate and sodium lactate infusion in the induction of panic attacks. *Arch. Gen. Psychiatry*, **46**, 145–150.

Gorman, J. M., Liebowitz, M. R., Fyer, A. F. *et al.* (1989b). A neuroanatomical hypothesis for panic disorder. *Am. J. Psychiatry.* **146**(2), 148–161.

Gorman, J. M., Goetz, R. R., Dillon, D. *et al.* (1990). Sodium D-lactate infusion of panic disorder patients. *Neuropsychopharmacology*, **3**(3), 181–189.

Gorman, J. M., Papp, L. A., Coplan, J. D. *et al.* (1993). The effect of acetazolamide on ventilation in panic disorder patients. *Am. J. Psychiatry*, **150**, 1480–1484.

Graeff, F. G. (1990). Brain defence systems and anxiety. In *Handbook of Anxiety,* Vol. 3 (eds M. Roth, G. D. Burrows and R. Noyes), pp. 307–354. Elsevier, Amsterdam.

Gray, J. A. (1988). The neuropsychological basis of anxiety. In *Handbook of Anxiety Disorders* (eds. G. C. Last and M. Hersen), pp. 10–40. Pergamon Press, New York.

Grosz, H. J. and Farmer, B. B. (1972). Pitts' and McClure's lactate anxiety study revisited. *Br. J. Psychiatry*, **120**, 415–418.

Gurguis, G. N. M. and Uhde, T. W. (1989). Plasma 3-methoxy-4-hydroxyphenylethylene glycol (MHPG) and growth hormone responses to yohimbine in panic disorder patients and normal controls. *Psychoneuroendocrinology*, **15**(3), 217–224.

Halbreich, U., Endicott, J., Goldstein, S. *et al.* (1986). Premenstrual changes and changes in gonadal hormones. *Acta Psychiatr. Scand.*, **74**, 576–586.

Heninger, G.R., Charney, D. S. and Price, L. H. (1988). Alpha-2 adrenergic receptor sensitivity in depression. *Arch. Gen. Psychiatry,* **45**, 718–726.

Hollander, E., Liebowitz, M. R., Gorman, J. M. *et al.* (1989). Cortisol and sodium lactate-induced panic. *Arch. Gen. Psychiatry*, **46**, 135–140.

Hsiao, J. K. and Potter, W. Z. (1990). Mechanisms of action of antipanic drugs. In *Clinical Aspects of Panic Disorder* (ed. J. C. Ballenger). Liss, New York.

Insel, T. R., Ninan P. T., Aloi, J. et al. (1984). A benzodiazepine receptor-mediated model of anxiety. Arch. Gen. Psychiatry, 41, 741–750.

Jensen, C. F., Peskind, E. R., Veith, R. C. et al. (1991). Hypertonic saline-infusion induces panic in patients with panic disorder. Biol. Psychiatry, 30, 628–630.

Kahn, R. S., Wetzler, S., Van Praag, H. M. et al. (1988a). Behavioral indication of serotonergic supersensitivity in panic disorder. Psychiatry Res., 25, 101–104.

Kahn, R. S., Asnis, G. M., Wetzler, S. and Van Praag, H. M. (1988b). Neuroendocrine evidence for a serotonin receptor supersensitivity in panic disorder. Psychopharmacology, 96, 360–364.

Kelly, D., Mitchell-Heggs, N., and Shean, D. (1974). Anxiety and the effects of sodium lactate assessed clinically and physiologically. Br. J. Psychiatry, 119, 129–141.

Klein, D. F. (1964). Delineation of two drug responsive anxiety syndromes. Psychopharmacology, 5, 397–408.

Klein, D. F. (1993). False suffocation alarms, spontaneous panics, and related conditions: an integrative hypothesis. Arch. Gen. Psychiatry, 50(4), 306–318.

Klein, E., Zohar, J., Geraci, M. F. et al. (1991). Anxiogenic effects of m-CPP in patients with panic-disorder: comparison to caffeine's anxiogenic effects. Biol. Psychiatry, 30, 973–984.

Kubin, L., Tojima, H., Davies, R. O. et al. (1992). Serotonergic excitatory drive to hypoglossal motoneurons in the decerebrate cat. Neurosci. Lett., 139, 243–248.

Lee, Y. J., Curtis, G. C., Weg, J. G. et al. (1993). Panic attacks induced by doxapram. Biol. Psychiatry, 33, 295–297.

Lesch, K. P., Wiesmann, M., Hoh, A. et al. (1992). 5-HT$_{1A}$ receptor–effector system responsivity in panic disorder. Psychopharmacol. Berl., 106(1), 111–117.

Liebowitz, M. R., Fyer, A. J. and Gorman, J. M. (1984). Lactate provocation of panic attacks: 1 Clinical and behavioral findings. Arch. Gen. Psychiatry, 41, 764–770.

Liebowitz, M. R., Gorman, J. M., Fyer, A. J. et al. (1985a). Lactate provocation of panic attacks. Arch. Gen. Psychiatry, 42, 709–719.

Liebowitz, M. R., Fyer, A. J., Gorman, J. M. et al. (1985b). Specificity of lactate infusions in social phobia versus panic disorder. Am. J. Psychiatry, 142(8), 947–950.

Liebowitz, M. R., Coplan, J. D., Gorman, J. M. et al. (1995). Diazepam pretreatment of sodium lactate infusion in panic disorder. Psychiatry Res., 58, 127–138.

Lingjaerde, O. (1985). Lactate-induced panic attacks: possible involvement of serotonin reuptake stimulation. Acta Psychiatr. Scand., 72, 206–208.

Lundberg, D. B. A., Mueller, R. A. and Breese, G. R. (1980). An evaluation of the mechanism by which serotonergic activation depresses respiration. J. Pharmacol. Exp. Ther., 212(3), 397–404.

Maddock, R. J. and Carter, C. S. (1991). Hyperventilation-induced panic attacks in panic disorder with agoraphobia. Biol. Psychiatry, 29, 843–854.

Margraf, J., Ehlers, A. and Roth, W. T. (1986). Sodium lactate infusions and panic attacks: a review and critique. Psychosom. Med., 48, 23–51.

Mathew, R. J., Wilson, W. H. and Tant, S. (1989). Responses to hypercarbia induced by acetazolamide in panic disorder patients. Am. J. Psychiatry, 146, 996–1000.

McGrath, P. J., Stewart, J. W., Harrison, W. M. et al. (1985). Lactate infusion in patients with depression and anxiety. Psychopharmacol. Bull., 21(3), 555–557.

Mellman, T. A. and Uhde, T. W. (1990). Sleep in panic and generalized anxiety disorders. In Neurobiology of Panic Disorders (ed. J. C. Ballenger), pp. 365–376. Liss, New York.

Milc-Emil, J. and Brunstein, M. M. (1976). Drive and timing components of ventilation. Chest, 70 (1 Suppl.), 131–133.

Modigh, K., Westberg, P. and Eriksson, E. (1990). Superiority of clomipramine over imipramine in the treatment of panic disorder: a placebo-controlled trial. 17th Congress of Collegium Internationale Neuropsychopharmacologicum, Kyoto, Japan.

Nashold, B. S., Jr, Wilson, N. P. and Slaughter, G. S. (1974). The midbrain and pain. In *Advances in Neurology*, Vol. 4 (ed. J. J. Bonica), pp. 191–196. International symposium on Pain, Raven Press, New York.

Nordahl, T. E., Semple, W. E., Gross, M. *et al.* (1990). Cerebral glucose metabolic differences in patients with panic disorders. *Neuropsychopharmacology*, **3**, 261–272.

Nutt, D. J. (1989). Altered central alpha-2 sensitivity in panic disorder. *Arch. Gen. Psychiatry*, **46**, 165–169.

Nutt, D. J., and Lawson, C. (1992). Panic attacks: a neurochemical overview of models and mechanisms. *Br. J. Psychiatry*, **160**, 165–178.

Nutt, D. J., Glue, P., Lawson, C. and Wilson, S. (1990). Flumazenil provocation of panic attacks: evidence for altered benzodiazepine sensitivity in panic disorder. *Arch. Gen. Psychiatry*, **47**, 917–925.

Olson, E. B., Dempsey, J. A. and McCrimmon, D. R. (1979). Serotonin and the control of ventilation in the awake rats. *J. Clin. Invest.*, **64**, 689–693.

Panksepp, J., Meeker, R. and Bean, N. J. (1980). The neurochemical control of crying. *Pharmacol. Biochem. Behav.*, **12**(3), 437–443.

Papp, L. A., Martinez, J. M. and Klein, D. F. (1989). Arterial blood gas changes during lactate-induced panic. *Psychiatry Res.*, **28**, 171–180.

Pitts, F. N. and Allen, R. E. (1979). In *Biochemical Induction of Anxiety* (eds W. E. Fann, I. Karacan, A. D. Pokorny and I. Williams), pp. 125–140. SP Medical & Scientific, New York.

Pitts, F. N. and McClure, J. N. (1967). Lactate metabolism in anxiety neurosis. *N. Engl. J. Med.*, **277**, 1329–1336.

Pohl, R., Yeragani, V. K., Balon, R. *et al.* (1988). The jitteriness syndrome in panic disorder patients treated with antidepressants. *J. Clin. Psychiatry*, **49** 100–104.

Rainey, J. M., Jr, Pohl, R. B., Williams, M. *et al.* (1984). A comparison of lactate and isoproterenol anxiety states. *Psychopathology*, **17** (Suppl. 1), 74–82.

Redmond, D. E. (1977). Alterations in the function of the nucleus locus ceruleus: a possible model for studies of anxiety. In *Animal Models in Psychiatry and Neurology* (eds I. Hanin and E. Usdin). Pergamon Press, New York.

Reiman, E. M., Raichle, M. E., Robins, E. *et al.* (1989). Neuroanatomical correlates of a lactate-induced anxiety attack. *Arch. Gen. Psychiatry*, **46**, 493–510.

Rifkin, A., Klein, D. F., Dillon, D. *et al.* (1981). Blockade by imipramine or desipramine of panic induced by sodium lactate. *Am. J. Psychiatry*, **138**, 676–677.

Ritter, J. M., Dokoter, H. S. and Benjamin, N. (1990). Paradoxical effect of bicarbonate on cytoplasmic pH. *Lancet*, **335**, 1243–1246.

Rittmaster, R. S., Cutler, G. B., Gold, P. W. *et al.* (1987). The relationship of saline-induced changes in vasopressin secretion to basal and corticotrophin-releasing hormone stimulated adrenocorticotrophin and cortisol secretion in man. *J. Clin. Endocrinol. Metab.*, **64**, 371–376.

Sandberg, D., Endicott, J., Harrison, W. *et al.* (1993). Sodium lactate infusion in late luteal phase dysphoric disorder. *Psychiatry Res.*, **46**, 79–88.

Schneier, F. R., Liebowitz, M. R., Davies, S. O. *et al.* (1990). Fluoxetine in panic disorder. *J. Clin. Psychopharmacol.*, **10** (2), 119–121.

Schweizer, E., Pohl, R., Balon, R. *et al.* (1990). Lorazepam vs. alprazolam in the treatment of panic disorder. *Pharmacopsychiatry*, **23**, 90–93.

Selye, H. (1956). *The Stress of Life*. McGraw-Hill, New York.

Shear, M. K., Fyer, A. J., Ball, G. *et al.* (1991). Vulnerability to sodium lactate in panic disorder patients given cognitive-behavioral therapy. *Am. J. Psychiatry*, **148**(6), 795–797.

Southwick, S. M., Krystal, J. H., Morgan, C. A. *et al.* (1993). Abnormal noradrenergic function in posttraumatic stress disorder. *Arch. Gen. Psychiatry*, **50**(4), 266–274.

Spier, S. A., Tesar, G. E., Rosenbaum, J. F. *et al.* (1986). Treatment of panic disorder with clonazepam. *J. Clin. Psychiatry*, **47**, 238–242.

Stein, J. M., Papp, L. A., Klein, D. F. *et al.* (1992). Exercise tolerance in panic disorder patients. *Biol. Psychiatry*, **32**, 281–287.

Stone, A. B., Pearlstein, T. B. and Brown, W. A. (1992). Fluoxetine in the treatment of late luteal phase dysphoric disorder. *J. Clin. Psychiatry*, **52**, 290–293.

Svensson, T. H. and Usdin, T. (1978). Feedback inhibition of brain noradrenaline neurons by tricyclic antidepressants: alpha-receptor mediation. *Science,* **202**, 1089–1091.

Targum, S. D. (1991). Panic attack frequency and vulnerability to anxiogenic challenge studies. *Psychiatry Res.*, **36**, 75–83.

Targum, S. D. and Marshall, L. E. (1988). Fenfluramine provocation of anxiety in patients with panic disorder. *Psychiatry Res.*, **28**, 295–306.

Uhde, T. W. (1990). Caffeine provocation of panic: a focus on biological mechanisms. In *Neurobiological Aspects of Panic Disorder* (ed. J. D. Ballenger), pp. 219–242. Liss, New York.

Uhde, T. W., Tancer, M. E., Rubinow, D. R. *et al.* (1992). Evidence for hypothalamo-growth hormone dysfunction in panic disorder: profile of growth hormone responses to clonidine, yohimbine, caffeine, glucose, GRF and TRH in panic disorder patients versus healthy volunteers. *Neuropsychopharmacology*, **6**(2), 101–118.

Uhde, T. W., Roscow Terril, D., Chambless, D. L. *et al.* (1993). Pentagastrin model of anxiety in humans. American College of Neuropsychopharmacology 32nd Annual Meeting, Honolulu.

Westenberg, H. G. M. and Den Boer, J. A. (1989). Serotonin function in panic disorder: effect of 1–5-hydroxytryptophan in patients and controls. *Psychopharmacology*, **98**, 283–285.

Whitwam, J. G., Doffin, J., Triscott, A. *et al.* (1976). Stimulation of the peripheral chemoreceptors with sodium bicarbonate. *Br. J. Aaesth.*, **48**, 853–857.

Winslow, J. T. and Insel, T. R. (1990). Serotonergic and catecholaminergic reuptake inhibitors have opposite effects on the ultrasonic isolation calls of rat pups. *Neuropsychopharmacology*, **3**(1), 51–59.

Woods, S. W., Charney, D. S., Lake, J. *et al.* (1986). Carbon dioxide sensitivity in panic anxiety. *Arch. Gen. Psychiatry*, **43**, 900–909.

Woods, S. W., Charney, D. S., McPherson, C. A. *et al.* (1987). Situational panic attacks: behavioral, physiological and biochemical characterization. *Arch. Gen. Psychiatry*, **44**, 365–375.

Woods, S. W., Charney, D. S., Goodman, W. K. *et al.* (1988). Carbon dioxide-induced anxiety. *Arch. Gen. Psychiatry*, **45**, 43–52.

Zitrin, C. M., Klein, D. F., Woerner, M. G. *et al.* (1983). Treatment of phobias. I. Comparison of imipramine hydrochloride and placebo. *Arch. Gen. Psychiatry*, **40**, 125–138.

9 Cholecystokinin in Panic Disorder

HAROLD J. G. M. VAN MEGEN, HERMAN G. M. WESTENBERG,
JOHAN A. DEN BOER AND RENÉ S. KAHN
*Department of Psychiatry, University Hospital Utrecht,
Utrecht, The Netherlands*

INTRODUCTION

Ivy and Oldberg (1928) were the first to describe a "substance that was released from the upper intestine and produced gallbladder contraction". They suggested that this hormone be named *cholecystokinin* (CCK; "the gallbladder mover"). Others (Harper and Vass, 1941; Harper and Raper, 1943) discovered a substance from the duodenal mucosa of the pig, which stimulated pancreatic enzyme secretion. They called this hormone pancreozymin (PZ). Originally CCK and PZ were thought to be different hormones, but after purification and characterization they proved to be identical (Mutt and Jorpes, 1971). CCK is a peptide characterized by an α-aminated terminus Trp-Met-Asp-Phe-NH$_2$ amino acid sequence and initially identified as a 33 amino acid peptide (CCK$_{33}$; Ivy and Oldberg, 1928; Mutt and Jorpes, 1971). Subsequent studies revealed the existence of multiple forms of CCK (Eysselein *et al.*, 1986). CCK was found to be derived from the primary prepro-CCK polypeptide of 115 residues. After transcription, enzymatic cleavage produces several different CCK fractions (i.e. CCK$_{58}$, CCK$_{39}$, CCK$_{33}$, CCK$_{22}$, CCK$_{8s}$, (sulphated), CCK$_8$ (non-sulphated), CCK$_7$, CCK$_5$, and CCK$_4$), all with biological activity (Deschodt-Lanckman *et al.*, 1984; Rehfeld and Hansen, 1986; Lindefors *et al.*, 1993). The CCK family extends to two other peptides, the synthetic peptide pentagastrin (Pentavlon®) and caerulein, which is isolated from frog skin. Both peptides share the characteristic CCK amino acid sequence and are frequently used in studies investigating the role of CCK (see Table 1).

In the 1960s Pearse (1966) postulated that endocrine polypeptide-producing cells originating from the embryonic neural chest were of neuronal origin. Following this idea Vanderhaegen *et al.* (1975) discovered a small peptide with gastrin-like immunoreactivity in the mammalian brain, which was evidently not gastrin. This so-called brain gastrin immunoassayable peptide (BGP) was identified as the sulphated C-terminal octapeptide of CCK (Asp-Tyr(SO$_3$)-Met-Gly-

Advances in the Neurobiology of Anxiety Disorders. Edited by H. G. M. Westenberg, J. A. Den Boer and D. L. Murphy
©1996 John Wiley & Sons Ltd

Table 1. Amino acid sequences of CCK fragments and CCK-related peptides

CCK(17–33)	R-Tyr(SO$_3$H)-MET-**Gly-Trp-Met-Asp-Phe-NH$_2$**
Gastrin	(pyro)-R-Tyr(SO$_3$H)-**Gly-Trp-Met-Asp-Phe-NH$_2$**
Caerulein	(pyro)-R-Tyr(SO$_3$H)-Thr-**Gly-Trp-Met-Asp-Phe-NH$_2$**
Pentagastrin	C-Ala-**Trp-Met-Asp-Phe-NH$_2$**

Trp-Met-Asp-Phe-NH$_2$) (CCK$_{8s}$). CCK$_{8s}$ appeared to be the most abundant CCK fraction in the mammalian brain (Dockray, 1976; Beinfeld and Palkovits, 1981). Presently, CCK is recognized as the most widely distributed neuropeptide in the brain. CCK-like immunoreactivity has been demonstrated in the cerebral cortex, olfactory bulb, hypothalamus, amygdala, hippocampus, striatum and spinal cord (Emson et al., 1982).

The functional role of CCK in the CNS has been an area of intensive investigation over the past 20 years. As a result of these investigations, a role for neuronal CCK has been proposed, e.g. in feeding and satiety (for review see Morley, 1990), pain perception (for review see Wang et al., 1990) and psychiatric diseases like schizophrenia (for review see Nair et al., 1986) and anxiety disorders (for review see Van Megen et al., 1994d). Although this might imply a single role for CCK in these domains, more likely the involvement in such an array of behaviors suggests an interaction with other neurotransmitters systems. Indeed, evidence has been found for interactions between CCK and dopamine (DA), γ-aminobutyric acid (GABA), serotonin (5-HT), norepinephrine (NE), excitatory amino acids (EAAs) and opioid peptides. In addition, CCK is colocalized with several of these neurotransmitters (Fuxe et al., 1980; Somogyi et al., 1984; Bradwejn and De Montigny, 1984; Mantyh and Hunt, 1984; Stengaard-Peterson and Larsson, 1984; Hökfelt et al., 1985; Pittaway and Hill, 1987; Yaksh et al., 1987; Boden et al., 1991; Harro et al., 1992). This paper reviews the CCK neuronal system and its colocalizations and interactions with GABA and 5-HT neuronal systems. In addition, findings in animal and human studies in relation to its possible role in anxiety will be discussed.

PHARMACOLOGY OF CHOLECYSTOKININ

CHOLECYSTOKININ DISTRIBUTION IN THE HUMAN BRAIN

CCK has been found to be the most abundant neuropeptide in the human brain; it is distributed heterogeneously (Rehfeld, 1978). Highest levels of CCK immunoreactivity are found in the (temporal and frontal) cortex, caudate nucleus, putamen, and in hippocampus and subiculum; intermediate levels are found in the nucleus accumbens, septum, ventromedial thalamus, periaqueductal gray and substantia nigra pars compacta, and low amounts are found in globus pallidus, lateral thalamic nuclei and other meso- and metencephalic nuclei (Emson *et al.*, 1982; Cross *et al.*, 1988).

Most CCK immunoreactivity is found in cell bodies and fibers of non-pyramidal neurons. Glia cells do not contain CCK. The highest density of CCK receptor binding sites are found in the olfactory bulb, amygdala, neocortex, cerebellum, efferents of the nucleus vagus and nucleus tractus solitarius (NTS) and solitary complex (SC). Intermediate densities of binding sites are found in hippocampus, the inferior olives and the substantia gelatinosa of the cervical and thoracic spinal cord (Dietl *et al.*, 1987).

In contrast to CCK immunoreactivity and CCK binding sites, the distribution of the CCK pathways have not yet been resolved. Neuropeptides are synthesized in the perikaryon of the cell and transported along the axon to the nerve terminal. High CCK immunoreactivity in the presence of low CCK binding suggests the presence of CCK cell bodies. Following this idea, the most recent view is that that CCK is synthesized in the cortex, hippocampus and substantia nigra. From here CCK may be distributed to other brain regions (Hökfelt *et al.*, 1991; Schalling *et al.*, 1990; Lindefors *et al.*, 1993).

CHOLECYSTOKININ RECEPTORS

The various CCK fractions show different affinity for CCK binding sites in the periphery and brain. CCK_{8s} is the shortest CCK sequence with biological activity in the periphery. In contrast, smaller sequences and non-sulphated fractions of CCK, e.g. CCK_{8ns} and CCK_4, possess biological activity in the brain. Based on these differences in binding affinity, CCK binding sites were divided into CCK_A (alimentary tract) receptors, mainly found in the periphery, and CCK_B (brain) receptors exclusively found in the brain, although more recent studies suggest that the CCK_B receptor may be homologous with the gastrin receptor. The development of selective CCK antagonists enabled mapping of the distribution pattern of these different receptors (Kubota *et al.*, 1989; Woodruff *et al.*, 1991; Dethloff *et al.*, 1992). In humans, CCK_A receptors are found in the alimentary tract and discrete areas of the brain like the area postrema and nucleus solitarius, dorsal horn of the spinal cord, vagus nerve complex, hypothalamus, interpeduncular nucleus and substantia nigra (primates). CCK_B receptors are more widely distributed in the central nervous system (CNS) and have been discovered in the cortex, olfactory bulb, nucleus accumbens, amygdala, hippocampus, caudate nucleus, cerebellum and hypothalamus.

CHOLECYSTOKININ RECEPTOR ANTAGONISTS

The CCK receptor antagonists can be divided into six categories (see Table 2): The first group of CCK receptor antagonists are the cyclic nucleotide derivatives, like dibutyryl cyclic guanosine monophosphate (Bt_2cGMP), which have the highest affinity for the CCK_A receptor.

A second group consists of amino acid derivatives. The most important members of this group are benzotript, proglumide, lorgumide (=CR 1409), loxiglumide (=CR 1505) and CR 1392. They possess the same specific affinity for the CCK_A receptor as the cyclic nucleotide derivates. However, in contrast to Bt_2cGMP, they are more potent and can be administered orally.

A third class of CCK receptor antagonists consists of a group of modified CCK peptides like the COOH-terminal heptapeptide of CCK (CCK-JMV-180). Although this peptide is of great scientific interest, because it can distinguish between high- and low-affinity CCK_A receptors, its therapeutic role is limited because of its poor bioavailability after oral administration.

The benzodiazepine derivates constitute a fourth class of CCK antagonist. The finding that benzodiazepines can antagonize the effect of iontophoric administered CCK on hippocampal neurons (Bradwejn and de Montigny, 1984) led this class of CCK receptor antagonists. Initially, benzodiazepine derivatives were derived from the naturally occurring benzodiazepine asperlicin. Two representatives of this group are of major interest since they show high CCK receptor affinity with sufficient bioavailability after oral administration. The first one is L-364,718 also known as MK-329 or devazepide (Chang and Lotti, 1986; Lotti *et al.*, 1987). L-364,718 is a very potent CCK_A receptor antagonist and is two orders of magnitude more potent than most selective CCK_A receptor antagonists. On the other hand, its selectivity for the CCK_A is low since it is also a strong CCK_B receptor antagonist. The second compound, L-365,260, is a highly selective CCK_B receptor antagonist showing low affinity for the CCK_A receptor.

More recently a fifth group of CCK receptor antagonists, the peptoids, have been described (Woodruff *et al.*, 1991). The members of this family that have been most extensively investigated are CI-988 (= PD 134,308; Horwell, 1991) and PD 135,158. They are both CCK_4 structural derivates and are highly selective for the CCK_B receptor (1600 and 400-fold selectivity respectively; Hughes *et al.*, 1990). Actually, they are the most selective CCK_B receptor antagonists. In comparison with the benzodiazepine derivative L-365,260 they show an approximately 30-fold greater selectivity ratio.

The pyrazolidinone derivates are the sixth group of CCK_B receptor antagonists. The major representatives of this group are LY 262,691 and LY 288,513. These compounds are approximately 300-fold more potent at the CCK_B receptor as compared to the CCK_B receptor; their selectivity ratio is comparable with that of the benzodiazepine derivate L-365,260 (Howbert *et al.*, 1992; Dethloff and de la Iglesia, 1992).

CHOLECYSTOKININ: A NEUROTRANSMITTER?

Neurotransmitters are chemicals released by nerve endings that can change or alter the activity of adjacent neurons or organs by acting on a specific receptor site and are then rapidly deactivated by a reuptake mechanism, degradation or both.

CCK_8 meets most criteria for a neurotransmitter:

1. It is localized within neurons (Crawley, 1985).

Table 2. Affinity of different CCK (ant)agonists for the CCK_A and CCK_B receptors

Agent	CCK_B receptor	CCK_A receptor	Effect
CCK_{8s}[1]	++	++	(n.r.)
CCK_8	+	±	n.r.
CCK_4	++	−	Anxiogenic
Caerulein[2]	+	++	Anxiogenic
Pentagastrin[3]	++	±	Anxiogenic
A 68552[7]	++	++	n.r
A 65168[8]	?	++	n.r
Amino acid derivatives			
Benzotript	±	±	n.r.
Proglumide[4]	+	++	Acid production ↓
Lorgumide[4] (=CR 1409)	±	++	Gallbladder contraction ↓
Loxiglumide[4] (=CR 1505)	±	++	Gallbladder contraction ↓
CR 1392[4]	±	++	Pancreas secretion ↓
Benzodiazepine derivatives			
Asperlicin	−	+	None
Anthramycin[6]	+	±	Antibiotic
L-364,718[4]	+	++	Gallbladder
(=devazepine)			contraction ↓
(=MK-329)			Pain perception
L-365,260[5]	++	+	Anxiolytic appetite ↑
Peptoids			
PD 134,308[5] (=CI-988)	++	−	Anxiolytic
			Pain perception
PD 135,158[5]	++	−	Anxiolytic
Diphenylpyrazondinone			
LY 262,691[5]	++	−	n.r.
LY 288,513[5]	++	−	Anxiolytic
LY 219,057[6]	+	++	n.r.

[1] Sulphated octapeptide; [2] CCK_8 analogon; [3] CCK_B agonist; [4] CCK_A agonist; [5] CCK_B antagonist; [6] $CCK_{A/B}$ antagonist; [7] $CCK_{A/B}$ agonist; [8] CCK_A agonist; n.r. not reported.

2. CCK is synthesized in nervous tissue, probably as a pro-CCK peptide which undergoes proteolytic cleavage (Deschenes *et al.*, 1984; Turkelson *et al.*, 1990; Blanke *et al.*, 1993).

3. Two different CCK receptors, CCK_A and CCK_B, have been identified in the brain. These receptors can be stimulated and inhibited by an agonist and antagonist, respectively (Hill *et al.*, 1990; Woodruff *et al.*, 1991).

4. In accordance with the mechanism found for other neurotransmitters, *in vitro* and *in vivo* studies have shown that depolarization by high potassium levels releases neuronal CCK immunoreactivity in a Ca^{2+}-dependent way (Raiteri *et al.*, 1993b). In addition, CCK is rapidly inactivated by the mem-

brane-bound neuropeptidase serine (Deschodt-Lanckman and Bui, 1981; Rose et al., 1989). In contrast to neurotransmitters like glutamate and GABA which are completely adenosin triphosphate (ATP) dependent, CCK release is only attenuated, not blocked after cellular ATP depletion (Verhage et al., 1991).

5. CCK is a potent neuronal excitant in many regions of the brain, including the spinal cord (Jeftinija et al., 1981; Bradwejn and de Montigny, 1984; Dahl, 1987), and an inhibitory effect has been demonstrated in the NTS (Morin-Surun et al., 1983).

INTERACTIONS BETWEEN CHOLECYSTOKININ AND THE NEUROTRANSMITTERS GABA AND SEROTONIN

Cholecystokinin and GABA

The first evidence for a possible interaction of CCK and GABA was derived from immunohistochemical studies in rodents. Several studies reported that GABA-ergic neurons in the cortex and hippocampus contain CCK. In fact, almost all CCK-containing neurons are colocalized with GABA, while only 10% of the GABA-ergic neurons contain CCK (Somogyi et al., 1984; Hendry et al., 1990; Kosaka et al., 1987; Gulyás et al., 1991).

Electrophysiological studies in rodents

Because of high density of both CCK immunoreactivity and CCK receptors in the hippocampus and the extensive colocalization of CCK and GABA in this brain region, the effect of CCK and the interaction of the CCK- and GABA-containing neurons have been investigated particularly in this brain area. The effect of CCK on the hippocampal neurons has been studied in in vivo and in vitro experiments, following local and systematic application. Of all CCK fractions tested, CCK_{8s} displayed the most powerful excitatory effect on hippocampal pyramidal and non-pyramidal neurons (Dahl, 1987; Dahl and Sinton, 1978; Brooks and Kelly, 1985; Bradwejn and de Montigny, 1984, 1985a, 1985b; Böhme et al., 1988). There is evidence that the GABA-ergic system can influence CCK neuronal functioning and alter its effect in at least four different ways:

1. GABA can change the CCK effect on the neuronal level: CCK-induced excitation of hippocampal neurons was found to be antagonized by application of both full (benzodiazepines, BZDs) and partial (PK8165) GABA agonists (Bradwejn and de Montigny, 1984, 1985a, 1985b; Bouthillier and de Montigny, 1988).
2. GABA seems to alter CCK transcription: CCK mRNA in cortex and hippocampus was found to be increased after a single BZD injection and 24 h after BZD withdrawal (Rattray et al., 1993).
3. GABA displays an effect on CCK release: in an in vitro study, using a corti-

cal superfusion paradigm in rats, GABA agonist (i.e. GABA and diazepam) attenuated, whereas GABA antagonist (i.e. picrotoxin and biculline) increased CCK release (Yaksh et al., 1987).

4. GABA shows an effect on CCK receptor density: cessation of chronic BZD treatment was found to be followed by an increase in CCK receptors in the frontal cortex and certain hippocampal areas (e.g. CA_1) (Harro et al., 1990a).

The interaction between CCK and GABA seems to be reciprocal. In vitro, CCK_8 significantly enhanced K^+-stimulated GABA release in the caudate putamen, substantia nigra, the parietofrontal cortex and in the hippocampal formation (De la Mora et al., 1993). The effect of CCK on GABA is probably mediated through CCK_B receptors since the stimulated GABA release could be abolished by CCK_B receptor antagonists like PD 135,158 and L-365,260. In line with this assumption, CCK_B receptor antagonists L-365,260 and CI-988 enhanced GABA-ergic inhibition of postsynaptic NTS or preganglionic vagal neurons in rat brain stem slices, while the CCK_A receptor antagonist devazepine showed no effect (Branchereau et al., 1992).

In summary, findings from electrophysiologic studies suggest a reciprocal interaction between the CCK-ergic and GABA-ergic neuronal systems. Since the role of GABA in the regulation of anxiety is well established (Haefely, 1994), these findings hint at a possible involvement of CCK in the neurobiology of anxiety.

Cholecystokinin and serotonin

Apart from the well-established role of the GABA-ergic system in modulating anxiety, brain 5-HT is considered to be involved in anxiety too (Westenberg and Den Boer, 1994). For this reason, studying the possible interaction of 5-HT and CCK is of great interest and might shed more light on the regulation of anxiety.

The brain stem dorsal raphe is an important serotonergic nucleus with ascending projections to, for example, the hippocampus and caudate nucleus. In this nucleus, CCK immunoreactivity is found in cell bodies both rostrally and caudally to 5-HT-immunoreactive cell bodies. No evidence was found for coexistence of peptide and monoamine in the same cell (Van der Kooy et al., 1981). On the other hand CCK-containing neurons descending from dorsal raphe nucleus (DRN) to the spinal cord and ascending from the DRN to the forebrain regions were found to be colocalized with 5-HT (Mantyh and Hunt, 1984; Fallon and Seroogy, 1985). These neuroanatomic findings provide putative evidence that a 5-HT/CCK interaction may exist.

In the DRN, using electrophysiologic measurements, two different neuronal populations could be discerned: one group of neurons which is 5-HT-sensitive, and another which is not (Boden et al., 1991). The non-serotonergic neurons showed no response to CCK application. In contrast, intracellular recordings from 5-HT neurons in the DRN slices showed an excitatory effect of the mixed $CCK_{A/B}$ receptor agonist CCK_{8s}. CCK effects in DRN are probably mediated through the CCK_A receptors, because the CCK_A receptor antagonist L-364,718 blocked this CCK_{8s}-induced excitation, whereas the CCK_B receptor agonist pentagastrin and the CCK_B receptor antagonist CI-988 showed no effect (Boden et al., 1991; Hughes et al., 1990; Pinnock et al., 1990).

The CCK interaction with 5-HT is not limited to the DRN. In rats, intracerebroventricular (i.c.v.) injections of CCK_8 significantly decreased 5-HT content in the hypothalamus, the mesencephalon and striatum (Fekete et al., 1981). Intraperitoneally (i.p) administered CCK_{8s} reduced the 5-HT metabolite 5-hydroxyindoleacetic acid (5-HIAA) levels in the hippocampus, suggesting it decreases 5-HT turnover (Rybarczyk et al., 1990). In contrast, CCK_4 (i.c.v. administered) decreased 5-HT content, while at the same time increasing the 5-HIAA content in cerebral cortex, septum, thalamus, hypothalamus, midbrain and the medulla oblongata (Itoh et al., 1988). Using brain microdialysis, we found that local administration of CCK_4 into the raphe region decreased the extracellular 5-HT content in both the raphe and dorsal hippocampus. This effect could be completely blocked by pretreating the animals with the CCK_B antagonist L-365,260 (unpublished observations). These results suggest that CCK_4 reduces 5-HT neurotransmission in the brain by attenuating cell firing. Taken together, these findings suggest a CCK/5-HT interaction with various CCK fractions practicing differential effects on the 5-HT system.

Electrophysiological studies of the modulatory role of serotonin on the cholecystokinergic system

In addition to the effect of CCK on serotonergic systems, there is some evidence for a reciprocal interaction between 5-HT- and CCK-containing neural systems. In vitro studies revealed that 5-HT increased the calcium-dependent K^+-evoked CCK release in rat cerebral cortex and nucleus accumbens synaptosomes. This effect could be blocked by the $5-HT_3$ receptor antagonists ICS 205–930, MDL 72222 and ondansetron, while the $5-HT_1/5-HT_2$ receptor antagonist methiothepine was ineffective. Moreover, the $5-HT_3$ receptor agonist 1-phenylbiguanide enhanced CCK release in the cerebral cortex comparable to 5-HT (Paudice and Raiteri, 1991; Raiteri et al., 1993a). These findings suggest that 5-HT acts as a potent CCK releaser through $5-HT_3$ receptors on CCK-releasing terminals. However, neither 5-HT nor 1-phenylbiguanide influenced CCK release under basal conditions. Apparently, depolarization is required to permit modulation of release through $5-HT_3$ receptors. Using microdialysis in rat frontal cortex, Raiteri and coworkers (1993a) have demonstrated an effect of $5-HT_3$ receptor antagonists on CCK release. The antagonists ondansetron and tropisetron both decreased drug-evoked efflux of CCK. From these findings, the following model was proposed: depolarization causes the release of CCK as well as 5-HT; endogenous 5-HT potentiates the drug-induced release of CCK through $5-HT_3$ receptor sites on CCK-containing neurons. Infusion of $5-HT_3$ receptor antagonists prevents the effect of endogenous 5-HT, causing a decrease of CCK release.

In summary, electrophysiological studies on the interaction between the CCK and 5-HT neuronal system suggest that they interact reciprocally. There is some evidence that the effect of the 5-HT system on CCK might be mediated through the 5-HT$_3$ receptor.

CHOLECYSTOKININ IN ANXIETY

CHOLECYSTOKININ IN ANIMAL MODELS OF ANXIETY

A summary of studies on the effects of CCK related substances in animal models of anxiety is given in Table 3. Harro et al., (1990a), using the elevated plus-maze paradigm, reported that rats exhibiting low levels of exploratory activity in the open arms, referred to as "anxious" rats, had a significantly higher number of CCK receptors in the frontal cortex as compared to "non-anxious" animals. Furthermore, cessation of chronic administration of diazepam (5 mg/kg per day) resulted in an increase in the number of CCK_{8s} binding sites in frontal cortex and hippocampus along with an apparent withdrawal anxiety (Harro et al., 1990b). CCK_8 and two structural analogs of CCK_8, caerulein and $Boc[Nle^{28},Nle^{31}]CCK_{27-33}$ (BDNL), have been found to display anxiogenic-like properties (decrease in time spent in open arms and decrease in line-crossing) in the elevated plus-maze after systemic administration (Harro et al., 1990b; Vasar et al., 1993, 1994; Chopin and Briley, 1993; Derrien et al., 1994). The effects of caerulein could be completely abolished by pretreatment with proglumide (a CCK_A receptor antagonist). In contrast, pretreatment with proglumide potentiated the effect of CCK_8. In the open field test a combination of CCK_8 and proglumide decreased the motor activity. This could suggest that the potentiating effect of proglumide in the plus-maze should merely be interpreted as an effect on locomotion rather than as an increase in anxiety (Vasar et al., 1994). Both the CCK_B receptor antagonist CI-988 (PD 134,308) and the non-specific CCK receptor antagonist L-364,718 were found to antagonize the anxiogenic-like effect of BDNL. L-364,718 displayed its effect at a dose 10-fold higher than CI-988, suggesting an involvement of CCK_B receptors in the induction of an anxiogenic-like behavior. In contrast to the anxiogenic-like responses of CCK_8 in the elevated plus-maze, Cohen et al. (1983) found a decreased avoidance response using the free operant (Sidman) avoidance paradigm in rats, suggesting an anxiolytic rather than an anxiogenic effect of CCK_8. Comparable results were reported by Hsiao et al. (1984), who have found that CCK_4 increased exploratory behavior in the open field.

The elevated plus-maze test has also been used to investigate the more specific CCK_B receptor agonists like CCK_4, pentagastrin, BC261 and BC197 (Harro and Vasar, 1991, Singh et al., 1991; Rex et al., 1994a, 1994b; Derrien et al., 1994). With the exception of BC261, these CCK_B receptor agonists showed an anxiogenic-like response without altering the motor activity. The effects of

CCK_4 were antagonized by several CCK_A and CCK_B receptor antagonists. The CCK_B receptor antagonist L-365,260 attenuated the CCK_4 effect at low doses (10 μg/kg), and lost this antagonism at higher dosages (Harro and Vasar, 1991; Rex et al., 1994a). CI-988 antagonized the effect of pentagastrin and BC197, while the CCK_A receptor antagonists devazepide and L-364,718 revealed no attenuating effects (Singh et al., 1991; Derrien et al., 1994).

Csonka and coworkers (1988), using the defensive burying paradigm, found that systemic and central administration of CCK_8 and CCK_{8s} dose-dependently increased the defensive motivated burying behavior (modeling an anxiogenic response); BZDs were found to have an opposite effect, which could be blocked by CCK_8 (Csonka et al., 1988). The effects of CCK fragments have not only been studied in rodents; Palmour et al. (1992) investigated the effect of intravenously injected CCK_4 in African green monkeys and found a series of behaviors associated with fear and defence, in addition to the fact that uptight monkeys (according to the criteria of Suomi; Novak and Suomi, 1988) appeared to be more vulnerable to the anxiogenic effects of CCK_4. Another CCK_B receptor agonist, pentagastrin, was without any effect in a behavioral evaluation in rhesus monkeys (Rupniak et al., 1993).

More recently, Charrier et al. (1995) studied the effects of CCK_4 in an operant conflict paradigm in rats. This paradigm is sensitive to both anxiolytic and anxiogenic compounds. There was no significant alteration in responding, indicating that in this test CCK_4 had no anxiogenic properties in the rat.

The auditory startle reflex has been used to study the effects of the CCK_B receptor antagonist LY 288,513. LY 288,513 was found to partially reduce the effects of BZD withdrawal, suggesting a possible anxiolytic effect (Rasmussen et al., 1993).

The effects of PD 134,308 (CI-988), a selective CCK_B receptor antagonist, has also been investigated in various animal models of anxiety. Hughes et al. (1990), Singh et al. (1991) and Costall et al. (1991) studied the effect of CI-988 in the elevated plus-maze, the social interaction test, human treat model and in the light/dark box. In these models CI-988 showed anxiolytic-like effects comparable with those of the BZDs, hinting at intrinsic anxiolytic properties. Others (Belzung et al., 1994) confirmed these findings using the light/dark box model, but failed when using the free exploratory paradigm. The effect of CI-988 has also been studied in two conditioned anxiety models. In the conflict model in monkeys and in the conflict model in mice CI-988 increased the shocks taken, a behavioral response which suggests anxiolysis (Powell and Barrett, 1991; Dooley and Klamt, 1993). At variance with these data, CI-988 was found to be ineffective in a safety signal withdrawal paradigm, which has been shown to be sensitive not only to BZDs but also to anxiolytics like buspirone. In another study CI-988 also failed to show anxiolytic effects in three different models of anxiety, viz. the elevated plus-maze, the conditioned suppression of drinking and the conditioned emotional response (Dawson et al., 1995).

The data on the CCK_B receptor antagonist L-365,260 are also not unequivocal. L-365,260 was able to antagonize the CCK_4-induced anxiogenic-like behavior in the elevated plus-maze (Harro and Vasar, 1991; Rex et al., 1994a), but failed to block this behavior elicited by BC197 and BDNL (Derrien et al., 1994). Moreover, it failed to show an anxiolytic-like response in both the light/dark and zero-maze test (Hendrie et al., 1993; Bickerdike et al., 1994). Lack of effect of L-365,260 was also reported by two other groups using different models of anxiety (Charrier et al., 1995; Dawson et al., 1995). A study with L-740,093, a new compound with improved bioavailability and brain penetration, also failed to induce an anxiolytic-like effect in either ethological or classical operant animal screens for anxiolytic agents.

Following the findings from electrophysiological studies, in which putative evidence was found for an interaction between the CCK and 5-HT neuronal system, animal models have been used to further substantiate this interaction. In guinea-pigs exposed to the elevated plus-maze, an increase of extracellular 5-HT in lateral prefrontal cortex was found. This increase was potentiated by the CCK_B receptor agonist BOC-CCK-4 (Rex et al., 1994a). Pretreatment with the CCK_B receptor antagonist L-365,260 antagonized the anxiogenic effect, but also prevented the increase of extracellular 5-HT. In the four-plate test both the CCK_B receptor antagonist CI-988 and the $5-HT_3$ antagonist ondansetron showed similar anxiolytic effects, whereas in the elevated plus-maze ondansetron was able to block the caerulein (mixed $CCK_{A/B}$ receptor agonist)-induced anxiogenic effects (Dooley and Klamt, 1993; Vasar et al., 1993). Recently, Bickerdike (1994) confirmed the involvement of both 5-HT and CCK in anxiety. In rodents, using the zero-maze test, the CCK_A receptor antagonist Devazepide and the CCK_B receptor antagonist CI-988 showed anxiolytic properties—effects which could be attenuated or blocked by giving a selective serotonin reuptake inhibitor (SSRI) (zimelidine or Wy-27587) at the same time (acute treatment).

In summary, the results of animal studies with CCK receptor agonists and antagonists vary considerably. Depending on the experimental situation, both positive and negative findings have been reported for each category of compounds. It is possible, however, that some models would be less relevant in examining panic-related phenomena in animals and the effects of CCK receptors ligands thereon. Furthermore, evidence has been found hinting at the existence of a close functional relationship between the serotonergic system and the CCK-ergic system.

CHOLECYSTOKININ IN HUMAN ANXIETY STUDIES

Cholecystokinin challenge as a human panic model

According to the DSM-IV criteria, panic attacks are defined by a crescendo of extreme fear or apprehension concomitant with at least four out of 12 somatic symptoms (American Psychiatric Association, 1994). Panic attacks do not

Table 3. Cholecystokinin in animal models of anxiety

Reference	Anxiety model/species	Agent/route of administration	Effect
Cohen *et al.* (1983)	Free operant avoidance paradigm in rats	Acute CCK_8 injection i.p.	Depression of avoidance
		Long-term CCK_8 i.p.	Neutralize acute CCK_8 effect
Csonka *et al.* (1988)	Defensive burying in rats	Diazepam i.c.v. and i.c. Chlordiazepoxide i.c.v. and i.c.	Decreased burying
		CCK_8 CCK_{8s} i.c.v. and s.c.	Blocks effect of diazepam/chlordiazepoxide
Harro *et al.* (1990b)	Plus-maze in mice Open field in mice	Caerulein[1] i.p.	Reduction of exploratory activity, no change in locomotion
		Proglumide[2] i.p.	Blocks effect of caerulein
Hsiao *et al.* (1984)	Open field in rats	CCK_4 i.c.v.	Increased locomotion and rearing
		Proglumide i.c.v.	Enhances CCK_4 effect
Hughes *et al.* (1990)	Plus-maze Social interaction Marmoset human threat test	PD 134,308[3] (=CI-988) PD 135,158[3]	Anxiolytic and suppress BZD withdrawal anxiety
Harro and Vasar (1991)	Plus-maze in rats	CCK_4 i.p.	Reduction of exploratory activity, no change in locomotion
		Proglumide i.p. Lorgumide[4] i.p. L-365,260[3] i.p. Devazepide[4] i.p.	All able to reduce effect of CCK_4
Powell and Barratt (1991)	Conflict test in monkeys	CI-988 i.m.	Increase of punished responding, no effect on non-punished responding
Singh *et al.* (1991)	Plus-maze in rats Social interaction in rats Light/dark box in mice	CI-988 i.p. or p.o.	Increase in: time spent in open arms, no effect on locomotion/time spent in light compartment/social interaction. Blocks the effect of pentagastrin
		Devazepide i.p. Pentagastrin[5] i.p.	No effect Reduced time spent in open arms, no effect on locomotion
Costall *et al.* (1991)	Light/dark box in mice Social interaction in rats Plus-maze in rats Human treat model in rats	CI-988 s.c. and i.p.	Increase in time spent in light section/social interaction/decrease in number of postures. No effect on locomotion
		PD 135,158 s.c. and i.p. Diazepam i.p.	Same effect Same effect. High dosages reduced locomotion
Palmour *et al.* (1992)	Social observation in African green monkeys	CCK_4 i.v.	Behavior associated with fear and defense

Table 3 (*continued*)

Reference	Anxiety model/species	Agent/route of administration	Effect
Dooley and Klamt (1993)	Four-plate test in mice	Diazepam p.o.	Increase of shocks taken/dose dependently
		CI-988 p.o.	Increase of shocks taken/no dose–response
		Ondansetron[6] p.o.	Similar effect as CI-988
Rupniak et al. (1993)	Behavioral evaluation in rhesus monkeys	Pentagastrin i.v.	No effect
Hendrie et al. (1993)	Light/dark box in mice	Devazepide i.v.	Increased line-crossing
		L-365,031[4] i.v.	Similar effect but less potent
		L-365,260	No effect
Vasar et al. (1993)	Plus-maze in rats	Caerulein s.c.	Decrease in line-crossing/ arm entries. No effect on locomotion
		Ondansetron i.p.	Reversion of caerulein's anti-exploratory effect
Rasmussen et al. (1993)	Auditory startle response	Diazepam	Blocks BZD withdrawal effect
		LY 288,513[5]	Blocks BZD withdrawal effect
Chopin and Briley (1993)	Plus-maze in rats	CCK-8 i.p.	Decrease in open-arm entries
		Devazepide i.p. L-365,260 i.p.	Increase in open-arm entries
Rex et al. (1994b)	Plus-maze in rats Light/dark box in rats Ultrasonic distress vocalizations in rats	BOC-CCK-4 i.p.	Decrease in open-arm entries, no effect on locomotion/decrease in line-crossing and time spent in light/increase in vocalization
		CCK_{8s} i.p.	No effect in plus-maze/ increase in line-crossing and time spent in light/ no effect on vocalizations
Rex et al. (1994a)	Elevated plus-maze in guinea-pigs	Plus-maze alone	Increases 5-HT content in lateral prefrontal cortex
		BOC-CCK-4 i.p.	Decrease in time spent in open arms and entries/ potentiation of 5-HT increase/no effect on locomotion
		L-365,260 i.p.	Antagonizes BOC-CCK-4 induced behavioral and neuro-chemical effects cortex
Belzung et al. (1994)	Free exploratory paradigm in mice	PD 135,158 s.c.	No significant changes

Table 3 (*continued*)

Author	Anxiety model/species	Agent/route of administration	Effect
	Light/dark box in mice	PD 135,158 s.c.	Increase in time spent in light compartment and in transitions
Derrien *et al.* (1994)	Elevated plus-maze in rats	BC261[5] i.p.	No change
		BC197[5] i.p.	Decrease in % time spent in open arm
		BDNL[7] i.p.	Decrease in % time spent in open arm
		L-365,260 i.p.	No effect on behavior response induced by BC264, BC197, BDNL
		CI-988 i.p.	Blocks BC197 BDNL effect
		L-364,718 i.p.	Blocks BDNL effect
Vasar *et al.* (1994)	Elevated plus-maze in mice Open field test in mice	CCK-8 s.c.	Decrease in line-crossing and rearings time spent in open arm
		L-365,260 i.p.	Potentiation of CCK-8 effect/locomotion suppressed when given in combination with CCK_8
		Proglumide i.p.	Same effect as with L-365,260
		Devazepide i.p.	Trend to potentiate CCK-8 effect/no effect on locomotion
Bickerdike *et al.* (1994)	Zero-maze in rats	CI-988 s.c. Devazepide s.c.	Increase in exploratory head dips and stretched-attend postures
		L-365,260 s.c.	No effect
		Zimelidine or Wy-2758[8] s.c.	Attenuates or blocks effects of CI-988/devazepide
Dawson *et al.* (1995)	Elevated plus-maze Conditioned suppressed drinking Conditioned emotional response	L-365,260 L-740,093 CI-988	No significant effects
Charrier *et al.*, (1995)	Conflict paradigm	CI-988 L-365,260 LY 7262,691 CCK	No significant behavioral alterations

[1]CCK_8 analog; [2]mixed $CCK_{A/B}$ antagonist; [3]CCK_B antagonist; [4] CCK_A antagonist; [5]selective CCK_B agonist; [6]5-HT_3 antagonist; [7]mixed $CCK_{A/B}$ agonist; [8]selective serotonin reuptake inhibitor.

exclusively occur in the course of panic disorder (PD), but are found in other anxiety disorders (i.e. simple phobia, social phobia and obsessive-compulsive disorder according to DSM-IV) as well. Panic attacks can also be provoked by a number of challenge agents, like m-chlorophenylpiperazine (mCPP), yohimbine, carbon dioxide inhalation and sodium lactate infusion (Liebowitz et al., 1984, 1985, 1986; Van den Hout and Griez, 1984; Griez et al., 1987; Den Boer and Westenberg, 1990; Kahn and Wetzler, 1991; Zandbergen et al., 1991; Klein et al., 1991; Charney et al., 1992; Albus et al., 1992). The use of pharmacological agents to probe biological aspects of PD is a promising strategy to elucidate the neurobiological underpinnings of panic. Guttmacher et al. (1983) suggested that a valid experimental model for PD should satisfy several criteria:

1. The panic attack induced by a challenge agent should combine physical symptoms of panic with a subjective sense of terror and a desire to flee, and PD patients should equate these attacks with their usual attacks.
2. It reliably reproduces the emotional and somatic symptoms that accompany panic attacks.
3. The challenge agent is safe for use in humans.
4. The effects of the challenge agent are consistent and reproducible and behave in a dose-dependent manner.
5. PD patients show an enhanced sensitivity to this panicogenic effect (threshold specificity).
6. Clinically effective antipanic agents are able to antagonize the panicogenic effect.
7. Drugs which are clinically ineffective against panic are unable to block panic elicited by a challenge agent.

Results from animal behavioral studies suggest that CCK receptor agonists possess anxiogenic properties. These results have prompted others to study the effects of CCK in man and in addition evaluate whether a CCK-challenge fulfills the criteria for an "ideal" panic-agent.

The anxiogenic effects of CCK_4 in humans were first reported by J. F. Rehfeld, who experienced "a very unpleasant anxiety as if the world was sliding away" after an intravenous injection of 70 µg CCK_4 (see De Montigny, 1989; personal communication). Rehfeld's report together with results from animal studies inspired De Montigny (1989) to study the effects of CCK in humans. In an open label study, he found that the CCK_B receptor agonist CCK_4, in doses ranging from 20 to 150 µg, elicited panic-like symptoms in seven out of 10 healthy volunteers. In contrast, administration of the mixed $CCK_{A/B}$ receptor agonist CCK_8 to two subjects induced gastrointestinal complaints, but no anxiety, suggesting that CCK_B rather than CCK_A receptors are involved in the mechanism underlying CCK induced anxiety (see Table 4). In the same study, De Montigny investigated the effect of BZD (lorazepam 3 mg on the day before the test, 1 mg 1 h prior to the test) treatment on the CCK_4-induced attacks. Lorazepam treatment was able to antagonize the panic-like attack in subjects who were found to be susceptible to the CCK_4 effect on an earlier occasion.

To further elucidate the putative role of CCK_4 as an panicogenic agent, others

Table 4. Cholecystokinin challenge in humans

Reference	Design/compound	N/diagnosis	Dose/panic rate				
De Montigny (1989)	Open CCK$_4$	10 volunteers	20–100 µg 70%				
Bradwejn et al. (1990)	Double-blind CCK$_4$	11 PD	0 0%	50 µg 100%			
Abelson and Nesse (1990)	Open Pentagastrin	4 PD 4 controls	0.6 µg 60–80% 0–25%				
Bradwejn et al. (1991)	Double-blind CCK$_4$	12 PD 15 controls	0 µg 9% 0%	25 µg 91% 17%	50 µg 100% 47%		
Bradwejn et al. (1991)	Double-blind CCK$_4$	29 PD	0 µg 0%	10 µg 17%	15 µg 64%	20 µg 75%	25 µg 75%
Van Megen et al. (1992)	Single-blind CCK$_4$	12 PD	0 µg 0%	25 µg 44%	50 µg 71%		
Van Megen et al. (1994a)	Double-blind Pentagastrin	0 µg 15 PD 15 controls	0.1 µg 0% 0%	0.3 µg 50% 0%	0.6 µg/kg 67% 0%	50% 13%	
Van Megen et al. (1994b)	Double-blind L-365,260–placebo 0.5 M/min/kg lactate infusion	24 PD	0 µg 50%	50 µg 25%			

Study	Design	Subjects	Pretreatment		Post-treatment	
Van Megen et al. (1994c)	Double-blind treatment Fluvoxamine–placebo CCK$_4$ challenge	26 PD	Placebo 67%	150 mg 76%	Placebo 56%	150m 29%
Bradwejn et al. (1994a)	Double-blind L-365,260 20 µg CCK$_4$	24 PD	Placebo 87%	10 mg 33%	50 mg L-365,260 0%	
Bradwejn et al. (1994b)	Double-blind Cross-over flumazenil 20 µg CCK$_4$	30 volunteers	0 mg 47%		20 mg 43%	
Bradwejn et al. (1994c)	Double-blind Placebo–saline 50 µg CCK$_4$ 100 mg CI-988	30 volunteers	Placebo — Saline 0%	Placebo — CCK$_4$ 53%	CI-988 — CCK$_4$ 27%	
Bradwejn and Koszycki (1994)	Treatment with 100–300 mg of imipramine Challenge with 20 µg CCK$_4$	11 PD patients	18% on treatment			
Abelson and Nesse (1994)	Single-blind Pentagastrin	10 PD / 9 controls	Saline 0% / 0%	0.6 µg 70% / 11%		

continued overleaf

Table 4 (*continued*)

Reference	Design/compound	N/diagnosis	Dose/panic rate	Group	a	b	c	d	e
Lines *et al.* (1995)	Double-blind five-period cross-over design a. Placebo–saline b. Placebo–pentagastrin 0.3 µg/kg c. L-365,260 10 mg–pentagastrin 0.3 µg/kg d. L-365,260 50 mg–pentagastrin 0.3 µg/kg e. L-365,260 50 mg–saline	15 volunteers		VAS score	16	123	39	16	14
				PSS score	1.1	19.3	7.0	3.0	0.6

investigated the effect of CCK_4 in PD patients. In a double-blind study, 11 PD patients were challenged with 50 μg CCK_4 and saline on two separate occasions (Bradwejn et al., 1990). All patients panicked with CCK_4, while none of the subjects panicked on saline. Patients judged CCK_4-induced symptomatology to their natural occurring panic attacks as identical but more abrupt in onset and more condensed in time. These findings have been confirmed in a single-blind placebo-controlled study, using an unbalanced incomplete block design in PD patients (Van Megen et al., 1992). In this study the panic rate with 50 μg CCK_4 was 71%; 25 μg CCK_4 induced a panic rate of 44%. Again none of the patients panicked on placebo. Bradwejn et al. (1992) conducted a dose-finding study in 29 PD patients, using 0, 10, 15, 20 and 25 μg CCK_4 as an intravenous bolus injection. They reported a panic rate of 0%, 17%, 64%, 75% and 75% respectively, suggesting a plateau in panic rate at dosages ranging from 20 μg and higher. In accordance with earlier studies, CCK_4 injection was found to be safe for use in man.

With the outcome of these studies (Bradwejn et al., 1990, 1992; Van Megen et al., 1992) the first four criteria for an "ideal" panicogenic agent seems to have been satisfied.

In a subsequent study, an enhanced sensitivity (criteria 5) of PD patients to CCK_4 was found (Bradwejn et al., 1991a). In this study, 10 out of 11 patients (91%) reported a panic attack following a 25 μg bolus injection of CCK_4, whereas only two out of 12 healthy controls (17%) experienced panic-like symptoms. The panic rate with 50 μg of CCK_4 was 100% for patients and 47% for controls.

Studies with the CCK_B receptor agonist pentagastrin, a synthetic analogue of CCK_4, have confirmed these observations (Abelson and Ness, 1990, 1994; Van Megen et al., 1994a). In an open study with 10 patients and nine healthy controls, Abelson and Nesse (1990, 1994) found that injection of 0.6 μg/kg of pentagastrin could provoke panic attacks in patients with PD and to a lesser extent in normal controls. Van Megen and collaborators (1994a) conducted a dose-finding study in 15 PD patients and 15 controls, using 0, 0.1, 0.3 and 0.6 μg/kg pentagastrin as intravenous bolus injection. Again, PD patients were found to be more sensitive to the panicogenic effects of pentagastrin. In patients, the mean panic rate with pentagastrin was about 55%, whereas in the control group only one subject panicked on the highest dosage used (5%). The results of these studies with pentagastrin suggest that CCK_4 and pentagastrin are interchangeable, in that both CCK_B, receptor agonists seem to satisfy the first five criteria for an ideal panic agent.

Treatment effects on CCK_4-induced panic

Bradwejn (1994d) reported that PD patients ($n = 30$) successfully treated with 100–300 mg imipramine showed a reduced sensitivity to the panicogenic effects of CCK_4. Only 18% had a panic attack after a 20 μg CCK_4 challenge.

Imipramine has consistently been found clinically effective in the treatment of PD (see for review: Liebowitz, 1985). Bradwejn's findings (1994d) suggest that a well-established antipanic agent such as imipramine is able to antagonize the panicogenic effects of CCK_4 (criteria 6). Bradwejn's open label study (1994d) has been confirmed by Van Megen et al. (1994c), who investigated the treatment effect of 150 mg fluvoxamine on CCK_4 induced panic attacks in PD patients. The reason for selecting fluvoxamine was that this drug has been found to be clinically effective in reducing both panic attacks and avoidance behavior (Den Boer et al., 1987; Den Boer and Westenberg, 1988, 1990; Hoehn Saric et al., 1993; Black et al., 1993). Before and after an eight-week double-blind placebo-controlled treatment phase, 26 PD patients were challenged with 50 μg CCK_4. In contrast to the patients treated with placebo, those patients receiving fluvoxamine showed a statistically significant decrease of the CCK_4-induced panic after treatment (the panic rate dropped from 76% before treatment to 29% after eight weeks of treatment). This effect was even more robust when comparing patients who responded to treatment versus those who did not. In the responder group the panic rate declined from 75% to 13%. In summary, so far, studies investigating the role of CCK_4 as a panic agent suggest that this challenge agent seems to be a valid human panic model, satisfying six out of the seven proposed criteria for an ideal panic agent. Criteria 7 has only been studied in healthy volunteers and was found to be negative (De Montigny, 1989).

Cholecystokinin and the pathophysiology of panic disorder

In addition to studies which investigated the anxiogenic properties of CCK_B receptor agonists in man, others attempted to further elaborate why PD patients seem to be more vulnerable to the effect of the CCK_B receptor agonists. One of the possible hypotheses to explain the enhanced sensitivity in PD patients for CCK_4 and pentagastrin is either an increased CNS CCK_4 neuronal activity or an enhanced CCK receptor sensitivity. Lydiard and coworkers (1992) found significantly reduced CNS cerebrospinal fluid (CSF) CCK_8 levels in PD patients. Taking into account the finding that CCK_4 can prevent CCK_8-induced neuronal firing, Denavit-Soubie et al. (1985) hypothesized that the enhanced sensitivity of PD patients is due to an increased CCK_4 activity in the brain. On the other hand, Tamminga et al. (1985) and Geracioti et al. (1993) suggest that those CCK levels do not reflect changes in neuropeptide functioning in the brain, which may question the validity of these findings. Following the findings from animal studies in which interaction and colocalization between CCK and GABA receptors were found, it has been suggested that the GABA receptor mediates the panicogenic effect of CCK_4. To further elaborate this possible interaction in man, Bradwejn et al. (1994b) studied the effect of the GABA antagonist flumazenil (2 mg) on CCK_4 panic in 30 healthy volunteers. Flumazenil was found to have no impact on panic elicited by CCK_4. This finding suggests that the anxiogenic effects of CCK_4 are not mediated through the GABA receptor.

Animal studies have shown that CCK_B receptor agonists induce anxiogenic responses and that CCK_B receptor antagonists can block these responses. Moreover, CCK_B receptor antagonists may have anxiolytic properties. Following the findings in animal studies, Bradwejn et al. (1994a) investigated the effect of a selective CCK_B receptor antagonist L-365,260 on CCK_4-induced panic attacks in PD patients. In this double-blind placebo-controlled study, 24 PD patients were treated with two different dosages of L-365,260 (0, 10, 50 mg) on two separate occasions and subsequently challenged with 20 μg CCK_4. Both L-365,260 dosages significantly reduced the likelihood of PD patients to respond to CCK_4 with a panic attack. Moreover, 50 mg L-365,260 was able to block the CCK_4-elicited panic attacks completely. Similarly, L-365,260 significantly reduced the number of somatic anxiety symptoms induced by CCK_4. These results are in line with those of Lines et al. (1995), who investigated the effect of L-365,260 (10 mg and 50 mg) or placebo on an intravenous bolus injection of pentagastrin (0.3 μg/kg) in 15 healthy volunteers. In accordance with the effect of L-365,260 in Bradwejn et al.'s study (1994a), 10 mg partially reversed the pentagastrin-induced symptoms, while 50 mg blocked the effects completely.

The effect of another CCK_B receptor antagonist, CI-988, on CCK_4 panic has been studied in 30 healthy volunteers, using a three-way cross-over design: (1) placebo/saline injection; (2) placebo/50 μg CCK injection; (3) 100 mg CI-988/50 μg CCK_4 injection (Bradwejn et al., 1994c). In this study CI-988 reduced the panic rate by 50%. In contrast, we were unable to block the CCK-induced panic in patients with PD by pretreatment with CI-988 (unpublished observations). This raises the question whether the effect of CCK_B receptor antagonists on CCK_4-induced panic can be generalized to panic induced by other panicogenic agents and, ultimately, to naturally occurring panic attacks. Clinically effective antipanic agents have been found to be able to antagonize sodium lactate-induced panic attacks. This was the main reasons for studying the effect of L-365,260 on sodium lactate-induced panic attacks (Van Megen et al., 1994b). Twenty-four PD patients participated in this double-blind placebo-controlled study. Patients pretreated with 50 mg L-365,260 experienced significantly less anxiety following the lactate infusion than those pretreated with placebo; L-365,260 treatment resulted in a 50% reduction of the panic rate; however, this reduction was not statistically significant. In contrast to the effect on fear and apprehension, L-365,260 was unable to block the physical symptoms elicited by lactate infusion. These data suggest that L-365,260 possesses anxiolytic but no antipanic properties.

To answer the question whether CCK_B receptor antagonists are clinically effective in treating naturally occurring panic attacks, one would need to study these compounds in PD patients. So far, only one clinical trial with L-365,260 has been performed. In this six-week multicenter placebo-controlled trial, the effect of L-365,260 (30 mg q.i.d.) has been tested in 88 PD patients (Kramer *et al.*, 1995). This study revealed no clinically significant differences between L-365,260 and placebo in global improvement ratings, Hamilton anxiety ratings, panic attack frequency and intensity or disability measurements. These results suggest L-365,260, at the dose tested, to be ineffective in treating PD. Although these preliminary findings with repeated dosing of L-365,260 are not encouraging, the formulation difficulties associated with the compound prevented a definitive evaluation of the therapeutic utility of this CCK_B antagonist. A more rigorous appraisal of the anxiolytic efficacy of these agents in man is awaited, using more suitable compounds. Interestingly, one site ($n=38$; Cutler *et al.*, 1994) reported a statistically significant anxiolytic effect measured by the inter-panic Hamilton Rating Scale of anxiety. This finding is in line with the findings in the study investigating the effect of L-365,260 on panic attacks elicited by sodium lactate (Van Megen *et al.*, 1994b), in that L-365,260 failed to reduce the panic rate but did reduce anxiety ratings and might suggest that L-365,260 possesses anxiolytic properties.

In summary, studies investigating the role of CCK in anxiolysis hint at an anxiolytic profile for the CCK_B antagonist, but fail in finding evidence for these compounds to have antipanic properties.

DISCUSSION

CCK is a neuropeptide characterized by an α-carboxyamidated tetrapeptide peptide, with multiple biologically active CCK fractions (Ivy and Oldberg, 1928; Mutt and Jorpes, 1971). CCK was first discovered in the alimentary tract as a hormone, producing gallbladder contraction (Harper and Raper, 1943). In addition, it proved to be abundantly present in the brain (Dockray, 1976; Beinfeld and Palkovits, 1981). In brain, CCK is heterogeneously distributed and functions as a neurotransmitter (Rehfeld, 1978). The main source of CCK synthesis appears to be in the cortex, hippocampus and substantia nigra (Hökfelt *et al.*, 1991; Schalling *et al.*, 1990; Lindefors *et al.*, 1993). So far, two different CCK receptor subtypes have been delineated, based on differences in binding affinity of the various CCK fractions (Dethloff and Iglesia, 1992). The CCK_A receptor subtype is present in the alimentary tract and in discrete parts of the CNS; the CCK_B receptor is exclusively found in the brain. The CCK neuronal system appears to interact with several other neuronal systems. For instance, a reciprocal relationship between the GABA-ergic system and CCK has been found (Dahl, 1987; De la Mora *et al.*, 1993). Most likely, the effect of CCK on the GABA-ergic neuronal system is mediated through the CCK_B receptor subtype (Branchereau *et al.*, 1992). In addition, there is evidence for a reciprocal CCK/5-HT interaction, with the serotonergic system interacting with the CCK-ergic system via the $5\text{-}HT_3$ receptor (Raiteri *et al.*, 1993a).

Behaviorally, animal studies suggest that stimulation of the CCK_B receptor generates an anxiogenic behavioral response (Harro *et al.*, 1990b; Vasar *et al.*, 1993, 1994). Moreover, CCK_B receptor antagonists display intrinsic anxiolytic properties in animals (Hughes *et al.*, 1990; Singh *et al.*, 1991; Costall *et al.*, 1991). However, a number of studies also failed to detect clear-cut effects of CCK receptor ligands in a variety of animal models of anxiety, including operant conflict procedures. It should also be emphasized that most animal models of anxiety predict efficacy for anxiolysis in patients with generalized anxiety disorders, since they are validated using BZDs. Thus far, no clinical data on the therapeutic efficacy of CCK_B receptor antagonists against symptoms in generalized anxiety disorders have been reported.

In humans, CCK_B receptor agonists, such as CCK_4 and pentagastrin, elicit panic-like reactions, reminiscent of naturally occurring panic attacks in both PD patients and healthy volunteers (De Montigny, 1989; Bradwejn *et al.*, 1990, 1991; Van Megen *et al.*, 1992). Indeed, patients show an enhanced sensitivity to the effect of CCK_4 and pentagastrin. These effects appear due to stimulation of the CCK_B receptor (Bradwejn *et al.*, 1994a). Clinically effective antipanic agents (i.e. imipramine and fluvoxamine) and the BZD lorazepam reduce the sensitivity to CCK_4 in PD patients (Bradwejn and Koszycki, 1994; Van Megen *et al.*, 1994c; De Montigny, 1989). Taken together, these findings may suggest a role for CCK in the neurobiology of PD. On the other hand, there is circumstantial evidence for involvement of several other neuronal systems, such as the serotonergic, noradrenergic and GABA-ergic systems, in the regulation of anxiety (Westenberg and Den Boer, 1994; Charney *et al.*, 1994; Haefely, 1994). The question emerges whether it is possible to explain the panic reaction, induced by CCK_4 and pentagastrin, solely by their single effect at the CCK_B receptor or by the interaction of the CCK-ergic system with other neurotransmitter systems. Were stimulation of the CCK_B receptor indeed the final common pathway leading to panic, CCK_B receptor antagonists would be expected to be clinically effective in treating PD. Moreover, since clinically effective antipanic agents have been found to block sodium lactate-induced panic attacks, one would expect CCK_B receptor antagonists to block sodium lactate-induced panic attacks as well (Keck *et al.*, 1993; Cowley *et al.*, 1991; Ortiz *et al.*, 1985; Rifkin *et al.*, 1981). However, L-365,260 does not block the sodium lactate-induced panic attacks (Van Megen *et al.*, 1994b). Moreover, in a separate treatment study, L-365,260 failed to reveal any efficacy in PD (Kramer *et al.*, 1995).

These findings make it unlikely that stimulation of the CCK_B receptor by itself is the final common pathway leading to panic, but rather suggests that CCK displays its effect on anxiety by interactions with other neuronal systems. Indeed, evidence.was found for a functional interaction between the CCK-ergic and serotonergic systems: treatment with fluvoxamine blocked CCK_4-induced panic attacks (Van Megen *et al.*, 1994c). A functional interaction between these two neurotransmitter systems is further upheld by an open study, in which treatment with the mixed 5-HT/NE reuptake inhibitor, imipramine, blocked the CCK_4-induced attacks (Bradwejn and Koszycki, 1994). As indicated, several animal studies confirm the 5-HT/CCK functional interaction.

It is also still unknown whether the induction of panic attacks in humans results from a direct action on the CNS, since it is not yet established whether CCK_4 or pentagastrin can easily cross the blood–brain barrier. Therefore it cannot be ruled out that panic attacks are triggered by peripheral CCK receptors or receptors at the level of brain regions not fully protected by the blood–brain barrier, such as the brain stem NTS. If this is the case, one may not expect CCK_B antagonists to reduce spontaneous panic attacks or attacks elicited by stimulation of higher brain regions. Therefore, it remains to be seen whether the CCK_4-induced panic attacks are a good human model of antipanic efficacy. The efficacy of CCK_B antagonists in generalized anxiety disorder needs to be assessed to prove general anxiolytic effects. In summary, although the question whether stimulation of the CCK_B receptor is the final common pathway leading to panic cannot be fully answered yet, it appears likely that the role of CCK in anxiety is through its interaction with other neurotransmitter systems. Indeed, putative evidence exists that the role of CCK in anxiety is mediated by its interaction with the serotonergic neuronal system.

REFERENCES

Abelson, P. L. and Nesse, R. M. (1990). Cholecystokinin-4 and panic. *Arch. Gen.* etc. *Psychiatry*, **47**, 395.

Abelson, P. L. and Nesse, R. M. (1994). Pentagastrin infusion in patients with panic disorder. I. Symptoms and cardiovascular responses. *Biol. Psychiatry*, **36**, 73–83.

Albus, M., Zahn, T. P. and Breier, A. (1992). Anxiogenic effects of yohimbine. I. Behavioral, physiological and biochemical measures. *Eur. Arch. Psychiatry*, **241**, 337–344.

American Psychiatric Association (1994). *Diagnostic and Statistical Manual of Mental Disorders* (DSM-IV). American Psychiatric Association, Washington, DC.

Beinfeld, M. C. and Palkovits, M. (1981). Distribution of cholecystokinin in the hypothalamus and the limbic system of the rat. *Neuropeptides*, **2**, 123–129.

Belzung, C., Pineau, N., Beuzen, A. and Misslin, R. (1994). PD135158, a CCK-B antagonist, reduces "state," but not "trait" anxiety in mice. *Pharmacol. Biochem. Behav.*, **49**, 433–436.

Bickerdike, M. J., Marsden, C. A., Dourish, C. T. and Fletcher, A. (1994). CCK antagonist effects in the rat elevated zero-maze model of anxiety: influence of 5-HT re-uptake blockade. *Eur. J. Pharmacol.*, **271**, 403–411.

Black, D. W., Wesner, R., Bowers, W. and Gabel, J. (1993). A comparison of fluvoxamine, cognitive therapy and placebo in the treatment of panic disorder. *Arch. Gen. Psychiatry*, **50**, 44–50.

Blanke, S. E., Johnsen, A. H. and Rehfeld, J. F. (1993). N-terminal fragments of intestinal cholecystokinin: evidence for release of CCK-8 by cleavage on the carboxyl side arg(74) of proCCK. *Regul. Peptides*, **46**, 575–582.

Boden, P. R., Woodruff, G. N. and Pinnock, R. D. (1991). Pharmacology of a chlolecystokinin receptor on 5-hydroxytryptamine neurones in the dorsal raphe of the rat brain. *Br. J. Pharmacol.*, **102**, 635–638.

Böhme, G. A., Stuzmann, J. M. and Blanchard, J. C. (1988). Excitatory effects of cholecystokinin in rat hippocampus: pharmacological response compatible with "central" or B-type CCK receptors. *Brain Res.*, **451**, 309–318.

Bouthillier, A. and Montigny de, C. (1988). Long-term benzodiazepine treatment reduces neuronal responsiveness to cholecystokinin: an electrophysiological study in the rat. *Eur. J. Pharmacol.*, **151**, 135–138.

Bradwejn, J. and Koszycki, D. (1994). Imipramine antagonism of the panicogenic effects of cholecystokinin tetrapeptide in panic disorder patients. *Am. J. Psychiatry*, **151**, 261–263.

Bradwejn, J. and De Montigny, C. (1984). Benzodiazepines antagonize cholecystokinin-induced activation of rat hippocampal neurones. *Nature*, **312**, 363–364.

Bradwejn, J. and De Montigny, C. (1985a). Antagonism of cholecystokinin-induced activation by benzodiazepine receptor agonists. *Ann. NY Acad. Sci.*, **448**, 575–581.

Bradwejn, J. and De Montigny, C. (1985b). Effects of PK 8165, a partial benzodiazepine receptor agonist, on cholecystokinin-induced activation of hippocampal pyramidal neurons: a microiontophoretic study in the rat. *Eur. J. Pharmacol.*, **112**, 415–418.

Bradwejn, J., Koszycki, D. and Meterissian, G. (1990). Cholecystokinin tetrapeptide induces panic attacks in patients with panic disorder. *Can. J. Psychiatry*, **35**, 83–85.

Bradwejn, J., Koszycki, D. and Shriqui, C. (1991). Enhanced sensitivity to cholecystokinin tetrapeptide in panic disorder. *Arch. Gen. Psychiatry*, **48**, 603–610.

Bradwejn, J., Koszycki, D., Annable, L. *et al.* (1992). A dose-ranging study of the behavioural and cardiovascular effects of CCK-tetrapeptide in panic disorder. *Biol. Psychiatry*, **32**, 903–912.

Bradwejn, J., Koszycki, D., Couetoux du tertre, A. *et al.* (1994a). The panicogenic effects of cholecystokinin tetrapeptide are antagonized by L-365,260, a central cholecystokinin receptor antagonist in patients with panic disorder. *Arch. Gen. Psychiatry*, **51**, 486–493.

Bradwejn, J., Koszycki, D., Annable, L. *et al.* (1994b). Effects of flumazenil on cholecystokinin-tetrapeptide-induced panic symptoms in healthy volunteers. *Psychopharmacology*, **114**, 257–261.

Bradwejn, J., Paradis, M., Koszycki, D. *et al.* (1994c). The effects of CI-988 on CCK-4 panic in healthy volunteers. *Neuropsychopharmacology*, **10**, 27–42.

Branchereau, P., Champagnat, J., Roques, B. P. and Denavit-Saubie, M. (1992). CCK modulates inhibitory synaptic transmission in the solitary complex through CCK_B sites. *Neuroreport*, **3**, 909–912.

Broekkamp, C. L., Rijk, H. W., Joly-Gelouin, D. and Lloyd, K. L. (1986). *Eur. J. Pharmacol.*, **126**, 223–229.

Brooks, P. A. and Kelly, J. S. (1985). Cholecystokinin as a potent excitant of neurons of the dentate gyrus in rats. In *Neuronal Cholecystokinin* (eds J. J. Vanderhaegen and J. N. Crawley). *Ann. NY Acad. Sci.*, **448**, 123.

Chang, R. S. L. and Lotti, V. L. (1986). Biochemical and pharmacological characterization of an extremely potent and selective nonpeptide cholecystokinin antagonist. *Proc. Natl Acad. Sci. USA*, **83**, 4923–2926.

Charney, D. S., Woods, S. W., Krystal, J. H. *et al.* (1992). Noradrenergic neuronal dysregulation in panic disorder: the effects of intravenous yohimbine and clonidine in panic disorder. *Acta Psychiatr. Scand.*, **86**, 273–282.

Charney, D. S., Krystal, J. H., Southwick, S. M. and Delgado, P. L. (1994). The role of noradrenergic functioning in human anxiety and depression. In *Handbook of Depression and Anxiety* (eds J. A. Den Boer and J. M. A. Sitsen) pp. 473–497. Marcel Dekker, New York.

Charrier, D., Dangoumau, L., Puech, A. J. *et al.* (1995). Failure of CCK receptor ligands to modify anxiety-related behavioural suppression in an operant conflict paradigm in rats. *Psychopharmacology*, **121**, 127–134.

Chopin, Ph. and Briley, M. (1993). The benzodiazepine antagonist flumazenil blocks the effects of CCK receptor agonists and antagonists in the elevated plus-maze. *Psychopharmacology*, **110**, 409–414.

Cohen, S. L., Knight, M., Tamminga, C. A. and Chase, T. N. (1983). Tolerance to the anti-avoidance properties of cholecystokinin-octapeptide. *Peptides*, **4**, 67–70.

Costall, B., Kelly, M. E., Naylor, R. J. *et al.* (1989). Neuroanatomical sites of action of 5-HT_3 receptor agonist and antagonists for alteration of aversive behaviour in the mouse.

Br. J. Pharmacol., **96**, 325–332.

Costall, B., Domeney, A. M., Hughes, J. *et al.* (1991). Anxiolytic effects of CCK B antagonists. *Neuropeptides*, **19** (Suppl.), 65–73.

Cowley, D. S., Dager, S. R., Roy-Byrne, P. P. *et al.* (1991). Lactate vulnerability after alprazolan versus placebo treatment of panic disorder. *Biol. Psychiatry*, **30**, 49–56.

Crawley, J. N. (1985). Neurochemical investigation of the afferent pathway from the vagus nerve to the nucleus tractus solitarius in mediating the "satiety syndrome" induced by systemic cholecystokinin. *Peptides*, **6**, 133–137.

Cross, A. J., Slater, P. and Skan, W. (1988). Characteristics of ^{125}I-Bolton–Hunter Labelled Cholecystokinin Binding in Human Brain. *Neuropeptides*, **11**, 73–76.

Csonka, E., Fekete, M., Nagy, G. *et al.* (1988). Anxiogenic effect of cholecystokinin in rats. *Peptides*, **9**, 249–252.

Cutler, N. R., Sramek, J. J., Kramer, M. S. and Reines, S. A. (1994). Pilot study of a CCK-B antagonist in panic disorder. NCDEU 34th annual meeting, Marco Island, FL.

Dahl, D. (1987). Systemically administered cholescystokinin affects an evoked potential in the hippocampus dentate gyrus. *Neuropeptides*, **10**, 165–173.

Dahl, D. and Sinton, C. M. (1978). The action of cholecystokinin in the dentate gyrus: stimulation of the locus coeruleus. *Exp. Brain Res.*, **59**, 491–496.

Dawson, G. R., Rupnial, N. M. J., Iversen, S. D. *et al.* (1995). Lack of effect of CCK$_B$ receptor antagonists in ethological and conditioned animal screens for anxiolytic drugs. *Psychopharmacology*, **121**, 109–117.

De la Mora, M. P., Hernandez-Gómez, A. M., Méndez-Franco, J. and Fuxe, K. (1993). Cholecystokinin-8 increases K$^+$-evoked [^{3}H] γ-aminobutyric acid release in slices from rat brain areas. *Eur. J. Pharmacol.*, **250**, 423–430.

De Montigny, C. (1989). Cholecystokinin tetrapeptide induces panic like attacks in healthy volunteers. *Arch. Gen. Psychiatry*, **46**, 511–517.

Den Boer, J. A. and Westenberg, H. G. M. (1988). Effect of a serotonin and noradrenaline uptake inhibitor in panic disorders: a double blind study with fluvoxamine and maprotiline. *Int. Clin. Psychopharmacol.*, **3**, 59–74.

Den Boer, J. A. and Westenberg, H. G. M. (1990). Serotonin function in panic disorder: a double blind placebo controlled study with fluvoxamine and ritanserin. *Psychopharmacology*, **102**, 85–94.

Den Boer, J. A., Westenberg, H. G. M., Kamerbeek, W. D. J. *et al.* (1987). Effect of serotonin uptake inhibitors in anxiety disorders, a double-blind comparison of clomipramine and fluvoxamine. *Int. Clin. Psychopharmacol.*, **2**, 21–32.

Denavit-Soubie, M., Hurle, M. A., Morin-Suryn, M. P. *et al.* (1985). The effect of cholecystokinin-8 on the nucleus tractus solitarius. *Ann. NY Acad. Sci.*, **448**, 375–384.

Derrien, M., Durieux, C., Daugé, V. and Roques, B. P. (1993). Involvement of D$_2$-dopaminergic receptors in the emotional and motivational responses induced by injection of CCK-8 in the posterior part of the rat nucleus accumbens. *Brain Res.*, **617**, 181–188.

Derrien, M., McCort-Tranchepain, I., Ducos, B. *et al.* (1994). Heterogeneity of CCK-B receptors involved in animal models of anxiety. *Pharmacol. Biochem. Behav.*, **49**, 133–141.

Deschenes, R. J., Lorenz, L. J., Haun, R. S. *et al.* (1984). Cloning and sequence analysis of a cDNA encoding rat preprocholecystokinin. *Proc. Natl Acad. Sci. USA*, **81**, 726–730.

Deschodt-Lanckman, M. and Bui, N. D. (1981). Cholecystokinin octa- and tetrapeptide degradation by synaptic membranes. I. Evidence for competition with enkephalins for in vitro common degradation pathways. *Peptides*, **2**, 113–118.

Deschodt-Lanckman, M., Koulischer, D., Przedborski, S. and Lauwereys, M. (1984). Cholecystokinin octa- and tetrapeptide degradation by synaptic membranes. III. Inactivation of CCK-8 by a phosphoramidon-sensitive endopeptidase. *Peptides*, **5**, 649–651.

Dethloff, L. A. and Iglesia de la, F. A. (1992). Cholecystokinin antagonists: a toxicologic perspective. *Drug Metab. Rev.*, **24**, 267–293.

Dietl, M. M., Probst, A. and Palacios, J. M. (1987). On the distribution of cholecystokinin receptor binding sites in the human brain: an autoradiographic study. *Synapse*, **1**, 169–183.

Dockray, G. J. (1976). Immunochemical evidence of cholecystokinin-like peptides in brain. *Nature*, **264**, 568–570.

Dooley, D. J. and Klamt, I. (1993). Differential profile of the CCK-B receptor antagonist CI-988 and diazepam in the four-plate test. *Psychopharmacology*, **112**, 452–454.

Emson, P. C., Rehfeld, J. F. and Rossor, M. N. (1982). Distribution of cholecystokinin in the human brain. *J. Neurochem.*, **38**, 1177–1179.

Eysselein, V. E., Reeve, J. R. and Eberlein, G. (1986). Cholecystokinin gene structure, and molecular forms in tissue and blood. *Gastroenterology*, **24**, 645–659.

Fallon, J. H. and Seroogy, K. B. (1985). The distribution and some connections of cholecystokinin neurons in the rat brain. *Ann. NY Acad. Sci.*, **448**, 121.

Fekete, M., Varszegi, M., Kadar, T. *et al.* (1981). Effect of cholecystokinin octopeptide sulphate ester on brain monoamines in the rat. *Acta Physiol. Acad. Sci. Hung.*, **57**, 37–46.

Fuxe, K., Anderson, K., Locatelli, V. *et al.* (1980). Cholecystokinin peptides produce marked reduction of dopamine turnover in discrete areas in the rat brain following intraventricular injection. *Eur. J. Pharmacol.*, **67**, 325–331.

Geracioti, T. D., Jr, Nickelson, W. E., Orth, D. N. *et al.* (1993). Cholecystokinin in human cerebrospinal fluid: concentrations, dynamics, molecular forms and relationship to fasting and feeding in health, depression and alcoholism. *Brain Res.*, **629**, 260–268.

Griez, E. J., Lousberg, H., Van den Hout, M. A. and van der Molen, G. M. (1987). CO_2 vulnerability in panic disorder. *Psychiatr. Res.*, **20**, 87–95.

Gulyás, A. I., Tóth, K., Danos, P. and Freund, T. F. (1991). Subpopulations of GABAergic neurons containing parvalbumin, calbindin D28k, and cholecystokinin in the rat hippocampus. *J. Comp. Neurol.*, **312**, 371–378.

Guttmacher, L. B., Murphy, D. L. and Insel, T. R. (1983). Pharmacologic models of anxiety. *Compr. Psychiatry*, **24**, 312–326.

Haefely, W. (1994). Benzodiazepines, benzodiazepine receptors, and endogenous ligands. In *Handbook of Depression and Anxiety* (eds J. A. Den Boer and J. M. A. Sitsen), pp. 573–609. Marcel Dekker, New York.

Harper, A. A. and Raper, H. S. (1943). Pancreoenzymin, a stimulant of the secretion of pancreatic enzymes in extracts of the small intestine. *J. Physiol. (Lond.)*, **180**, 77–83.

Harper, A. A. and Vass, C. C. N. (1941). *J. Physiol. (Lond.)*, **99**, 415–435.

Harro, J. and Vasar, E. (1991). Evidence that CCK_B receptors mediate the regulation of exploratory behaviour in the rat. *Eur. J. Pharmacol.*, **193**, 379–381.

Harro, J., Lang, A. and Vasar, E. (1990a). Long-term diazepam treatment produces changes in cholecystokinin receptor binding in rat brain. *Eur. J. Pharmacol.*, **180**, 77–83.

Harro, J., Pold, M. and Vasar, E. (1990b). Anxiogenic-like action of caerulein, a CCK-8 receptor antagonist, in the mouse: influence of acute and subchronic diazepam treatment. *Naunyn Schmiedebergs Arch. Pharmacol.*, **341**, 62–67.

Harro, J., Jossan, S. S. and Oreland, L. (1992). Changes in cholecystokinin receptor binding in rat brain after selective damage of the locus coeruleus projections by DSP-4 treatment. *Arch. Pharmacol.*, **364**, 425–431.

Hendrie, C. A., Neill, J. C., Shepherd, J. K. and Dourish, C. T. (1993). The effects of CCK_A and CCK_B antagonists on activity in the black/white exploration model of anxiety in mice. *Physiol. Behav.*, **54**, 689–693.

Hendry, S. H., Jones, E. G., De Felipe, J. *et al.* (1990). Neuropeptide-containing neurons of the cerebral cortex are also GABAergic. *Proc. Natl. Acad. Sci. USA*, **81**, 6526–6530.

Hill, D. R., Shaw, T. M., Graham, W. and Wiidryff, G. N. (1990). Autoradiographic detection of cholecystokinin-A receptors in primate brain using [125]Bolton Hunter CCK-8 and ^{3}H-MK-329. *J. Neurosci.*, **10**, 1070–1081.

Hoehn Saric, R., Mcleod, D. R. and Hipsley, A. (1993). Effect of fluvoxamine on panic disorder. *J. Clin. Psychopharmacol.*, **5**, 321–326

Hökfelt, T., Skirboll, L. and Everitt, B. (1985). Distribution of cholecystokinin-like immunoreactivity in the nervous system: co-existence with classical neurotransmitters and other neuropeptides. In *Neuronal Cholecystokinin*, Vol. 448 (eds J. N. Crawley and J. J. Vanderhaeghen), pp. 255–274. New York Academy of Sciences, New York.

Hökfelt, T., Cortes, R., Schalling, M. *et al.* (1991). Distribution pattern of CCK and CCK mRNA in some neuronal and non-neuronal tissues. *Neuropeptides*, **19** (Suppl.), 31–43.

Horwell, D. C. (1991). Development of CCK-B antagonists. *Neuropeptides*, **19** (Suppl.), 57–64.

Howbert, J. J., Lobb, K. L. and Brown, R. F. (1992). *A Novel Series of Nonpeptide CCK and Gastrin Antagonists*, pp. 28–37. Oxford Science Publishers, Oxford.

Hsiao, S., Katsuura, G. and Itoh, S. (1984). Cholecystokinin tetrapeptide proglumide and open-field behavior in rats. *Life Sci.*, **34**, 2165–2168.

Hughes J., Boden P., Costall B. *et al.* (1990). Development of a class of selective cholecystokinin type B receptor antagonists having potent anxiolytic activity. *Proc. Natl Acad. Sci. USA*, **87**, 6728–6732.

Itoh, S., Takahishima, A. and Katsuura, G. (1988). Effect of cholecystokinin tetrapeptide amide on the metabolism of 5-hydroxytryptamine in the rat brain. *Neuropharmacology*, **27**, 427–431.

Ivy, A. C. and Oldberg, E. (1928). Hormone mechanism for gallbladder contraction and evacuation. *Am. J. Physiol.*, **86**, 599–613.

Jeftinija, S., Miletic, V. and Randic, M. (1981). Cholecystokinin octapeptide excites dorsal horn neurons both in vivo and in vitro. *Brain Res.*, **213**, 231–236.

Kahn, R. S. and Wetzler, S. (1991). m-Chlorophenylpiperazine as a probe of serotonin function. *Biol. Psychiatry*, **30**, 1139–1166.

Keck, P. E., Taylor, V. E., Tugrul, K. C. *et al.* (1993). Valproate treatment of panic disorder and lactate-induced panic attacks. *Biol. Psychiatry*, **33**, 542–546.

Klein, E., Zohar, J., Geraci, M. F. *et al.* (1991). Anxiogenic effects of m-CCP in patients with panic disorder: comparison to caffeine's anxiogenic effects. *Biol. Psychiatry*, **30**, 973–984.

Kosaka, T., Katsumaru, H., Hama, K. *et al.* (1987). GABAergic neurons containing the Ca^{2+}-binding protein parvalbumin in the rat hippocampus and dentate gyrus. *Brain Res.*, **419**, 119–130.

Kramer, M. S., Cutler, N. R., Ballenger, J. C. *et al.* (1995). A placebo controlled trial of L-365,260, a CCK$_B$ antagonist, in panic disorder. *Biol. Psychiatry*, **37**, 462–466.

Kubota, K., Sugaya, K., Koizumi, Y. and Toda, M. (1989). Cholecystokinin antagonism by anthramycin, a benzodiazepine antibiotic, in the central nervous system in mice. *Brain Res.*, **485**, 62–66.

Liebowitz, M. R. (1985). Imipramine in the treatment of panic disorder and its complications. *Psychiatr. Clin. North Am.* **8**, 37–47.

Liebowitz, M. R., Fyer, A.J. and Gorman, J. M. (1984). Lactate provocation of panic attacks. I. Clinical and behavioral findings. *Arch. Gen. Psychiatry*, **41**, 764–770.

Liebowitz, M. R., Gorman, J. M., Fyer, A. *et al.* (1986). Possible mechanisms for lactate induction of panic. *Am. J. Psychiatry*, **143**, 495–502.

Lindefors, N., Lindén, A., Brené, S. *et al.* (1993). CCK peptides and mRNA in the human brain. *Progr. Neurobiol.*, **40**, 671–690.

Lines, C., Challenor, J. and Traub, M. (1995). Cholecystokinin and anxiety in normal volunteers: an investigation of the anxiogenic properties of pentagastrin and reversal by cholecystokinin receptor subtype B antagonist L-365,260. *Br. J. Pharmacol.*, **39**, 235–242.

Lotti, V. J., Pendleton, R. G., Gould, R. J. *et al.* (1987). *In vivo* pharmacology of L-364,718, a new potent nonpeptide peripheral cholecystokinin antagonist. *J. Pharmacol. Exp. Ther.*, **241**, 103–109.

Lydiard, R. B., Ballenger, J. C., Laraie, M. T. *et al.* (1992). CSF cholecystokinin concentrations in patients with panic disorder and in normal comparison subjects. *Am. J. Psychiatry*, **149**, 691–693.

Mantyh, P. W. and Hunt, S. P. (1984). Evidence for cholecystokinin-like immunoreactive neurons in the rat medulla oblongata which project to the spinal cord. *Brain Res.*, **291**, 49–54.

Morin-Surun, M. P., Demarchi, P., Champagnat, J. *et al.* (1983). Inhibitory effect of cholecystokinin octopeptide on neurons in the nucleus tractus solitarius. *Brain Res.*, **265**, 333–338.

Morley, J. E. (1990). Appetite regulation by gut peptides. *Annu. Rev. Nutr.*, **10**, 383–395.

Mutt, V. and Jorpes, J. E. (1971). Hormonal polypeptides of the upper intestine. *Biochem. J.*, **125**, 57–58.

Nair, N. P. V., Lal, S. and Bloom, D. M. (1985). Cholecystokinin peptides, dopamine and schizophrenia: a review. *Prog. Neuropsychopharmacol. Biol. Psychiatry*, **9**, 515–524.

Novak, M. A. and Suomi, S. J. (1988). Psychological well-being of primates in captivity. *Am. Psychol.*, **43**, 765–773.

Ortiz, A., Rainy, J. M. and Frohman, R. (1985). Effects of imipramine on lactate induced panic anxiety. World Congress of Biological Psychiatry, Philadelphia.

Palmour, R. M., Bradwejn, J. and Ervin, F. R. (1992). The anxiogenic effects of CCK-4 in monkeys are reduced by CCK-B antagonists, benzodiazepines and adenoside A2 agonists. *Eur. Neuropsychopharmacol.*, **2**, 193–195.

Paudice, P. and Raiteri, M. (1991). Cholecystokinin release mediated by 5-HT$_3$ receptors in rat cerebral cortex and nucleus accumbens. *Br. J. Pharmacol.*, **103**, 1790–1794.

Pearse, A. G. E. (1966). 5-Hydroxy-tryptophan uptake by dog thyroid C cells and its possible significance in polypeptide hormone production. *Nature*, **211**, 598–600.

Pinnock, R. D., Woodruff, G. N. and Boden, P. R. (1990). Cholecystokinin excites dorsal raphe neurones via a CCK$_A$ receptor. *Br. J. Pharmacol.*, **100**, 349P.

Pittaway, K. M. and Hill, R. G. (1987). Cholecystokinin and pain. *Pain Headache*, **9**, 213–246.

Powell, K. R. and Barrett, J. E. (1991). Evaluation of the effect of PD 134308 (CI-988), a CCK-B antagonist, on the punished responding of squirrel monkeys. *Neuropeptides*, **19**, 75–78.

Raiteri, M., Paudice, P. and Vallebuona, F. (1993a). Inhibition by 5-HT$_3$ receptor antagonists of release of cholecystokinin-like immunoreactivity from the frontal cortex of freely moving rats. *Naunyn Schmiedebergs Arch. Pharmacol.*, **347**, 111–114.

Raiteri, M., Paudice, P. and Vallebuona, F. (1993b). Release of cholecystokinin in the central nervous system: invited review. *Neurochem. Int.*, **22**, 519–527.

Rasmussen, K., Helton, D. R., Berger, J. E. and Scearce, E. (1993). The CCK-B antagonist LY288513 blocks effects of the diazepam withdrawal on auditory startle. *Neuroreport*, **5**, 154–156.

Rattray, M., Singhvi, S., Wu, P. Y. *et al.* (1993). Benzodiazepines increase preprocholecystokinin messenger RNA levels in rat brain. *Eur. J. Pharmacol.* (Mol. Pharmacol. Section), **245**, 193–196.

Rehfeld, J. F. (1978). Immunohistochemical studies on cholecystokinin. II. Distribution and molecular heterogenity in central nervous system and small intestine of man and dog. *J. Biol. Chem.*, **253**, 4022–4030.

Rehfeld, J. F. and Hansen, H. F. (1986). Characterization of preprocholecystokinin products in the porcine cerebral cortex. *J. Biol. Chem.*, **261**, 5832–5840.

Rex, A., Fink, H., Marsden, C. A. (1994a). Effects of BOC-CCK-4 and L-365,260 on cortical 5-HT release in guinea pigs on exposure to the elevated plus maze. *Neuropharmacology*, **33**, 559–565.

Rex, A., Barth, T., Voight, J.-P. *et al.* (1994b). Effects of cholecystokinin tetrapeptide and sulfated cholecystokinin octapeptide in rat models of anxiety. *Neurosci. Lett.*, **172**, 139–142.

Rifkin, A., Klein, D. F. and Dillon, D. (1981). Blockade by imipramine or desipramine of panic induced by sodium lactate. *Am. J. Psychiatry*, **138**, 676–677.

Rose, C., Camus, A. and Schartz, J. C. (1989). Protection by serine peptidase inhibitors of endogenous cholecystokinin released from brain slices. *Neuroscience*, **29**, 583–594.

Rupniak, N. M. J., Schaffer, L. and Iversen, S. D. (1993). Failure of intravenous pentagastrin challenge to induce panic-like effects in rhesus monkeys. *Neuropeptides*, **25**, 115–119.

Rybarczyk, M. C., Orosco, M., Rouch, C. *et al.* (1990). Interaction of cholecystokinin and diazepam: effects on brain monoamines. *Fundam. Clin. Pharmacol.*, **4**, 245–253.

Schalling, M., Friberg, K., Seroogy, K. *et al.* (1990). Analysis of expression of cholecystokinin in dopamine cells in the ventral mesenchephalon of serval species and in humans with schizophrenia. *Proc. Natl. Acad. Sci. USA*, **87**, 8427–8431.

Singh, L., Field, M. J., Hughes, J. *et al.* (1991). The behavioural properties of CI-988, a selective cholecystokinin$_B$ receptor antagonist. *Br. J. Pharmacol.*, **104**, 239–245.

Somogyi, P., Hodgson, A. J., Smith, A. D. *et al.* (1984). Different populations of GABAergic neurons in the visual cortex and hippocampus of cat contain somatostatin- or cholecystokinin-immunoreactive material. *J. Neurosci.*, **4**, 2590–2603.

Stengaard-Pedersen, K. and Larsson, L. I. (1984). Localization and opiate receptors binding of enkephalin, cholecystokinin, ACTH an β-endorphin in the rat central nervous system. *Peptides*, **23**, 715–718.

Tamminga, C. A., Lewitt, P. A. and Chase, T. N. (1985). Cholecystokinin and neurotensin gradients in human CSF. *Arch. Neurol.*, **42**, 354–355.

Turkelson, C. M., Solomon, T. E. and Hamilton, J. (1990). A cholecystokinin-metabolizing enzyme in the rat intestine. *Peptides*, **11**, 213–219

Van den Hout, M. A., and Griez, E. (1984). Panic symptoms after inhalation of carbondioxide. *Br. J. Psychiatry*, **144**, 503–507.

Vanderhaeghen, J. J., Signeau, J. C. and Gepts, W. (1975). New peptide in the vertebrate CNS reacting with antigastrin antibodies. *Nature*, **257**, 604–605.

Van der Kooy, D., Hunt, S. P., Steinbusch, H. W. M. and Verhofstad, A. A. J. (1981). Separate populations of cholecystokinin and 5-hydroxytryptamine-containing neuronal cells in the rat dorsal raphe, and their contribution to the ascending raphe projections. *Neurosci. Lett.*, **26**, 25.

Van Megen, H. J. G. M., Den Boer, J. A. and Westenberg, H. G. M. (1992). Single blind dose response study with cholecystokinin (CCK-4) in panic disorder patients. *Clin. Neuropharmacol.*, **15** (Suppl. 1), 532B.

Van Megen, H. J. G. M., Den Boer, J. A. and Westenberg, H. G. M. (1994a). Pentagastrin induced panic attacks: enhanced sensitivity in panic disorder patients. *Psychopharmacology*, **114**, 449–455.

Van Megen, H. J. G. M., Westenberg, H. G. M. and Den Boer, J. A. (1994b). Effect of the colecystokinin-B (CCK-B) receptor antagonist L-365, 260 on lactate induced panic attacks (PA). CINP 1994. *Psychopharmacology*, **10**, 3s (part 2).

Van Megen, H. J. G. M., Westenberg, H. G. M. and Den Boer, J. A. (1994c). Effect of the selective serotonin reuptake inhibitor (SRRI) fluvoxamine on CCK-4 induced panic attacks. CINP 1994. *Psychopharmacology*, **10**, 270.

Van Megen, H. J. G. M., Den Boer, J. A., Westenberg, H. G. M. and Bradwejn, J. (1994d). On the significance of cholecystokinin receptors in panic disorder. *Prog. Neuropsychopharmacol.*, **18**, 1235–1246.

Vasar, E., Peuranen, E., Oöpik, T. *et al.* (1993). Ondansetron, an antagonist of 5-HT$_3$ receptors, antagonizes the anti-exploratory effect of caerulein, an agonist of CCK receptors, in the elevated plus-maze. *Psychopharmacology*, **110**, 213–218.

Vasar, E., Lang, A., Harro, J. *et al.* (1994). Evidence for potentiation by CCK antagonists of the effect of cholecystokinin octapeptide in the elevated plus-maze. *Neuropharmacology*, **33**, 729–735.

Verhage, M., Ghijsen, W. E. J. M., Nicholls, D. G. and Wiegant, V. M. (1991).

Characterization of the release of cholecystokinin-8 from isolated nerve terminals and comparison with exocytosis of classical transmitters. *J. Neurochem.*, **56**, 1394–1400.

Wang, X. J., Wang, X. H. and Han, S. (1990). Cholecystokinin octapeptide antagonized opioid analgesia mediated by μg- and τ- but not δ-receptors in the spinal cord of the rat. *Brain Res.*, **523**, 5–10.

Westenberg, H. G. M. and Den Boer, J. A. (1994). The neuropharmacology of anxiety: a review on the role of serotonin. In *Handbook of Depression and Anxiety* (eds J. A. Den Boer and J. M. A. Sitsen), pp. 405–446. Marcel Dekker, New York.

Woodruff, G. N., Hill, D. R., Boden, P. *et al.* (1991). Functional role of brain CCK receptors. *Neuropeptides*, **19** (Suppl.), 45–46.

Yaksh, T. L., Furui, T., Kanawati, I. S. and Go, V. L. W. (1987). Release of cholecystokinin from rat cerebral cortex in vivo: role of GABA and glutamate receptor systems. *Brain Res.*, **406**, 207–214.

Zandbergen, J., Pols, H., Fernandez, I. and Griez, E. (1991). An analysis of panic symptoms during hypercarbia compared to hypocarbia in patients with panic attacks. *J. Affect. Disord.*, **23**, 131–136.

10 An Update on the Pharmacological Treatment of Panic Disorder

JAMES C. BALLENGER

Department of Psychiatry and Behavioral Science, Charleston, South Carolina, USA

INTRODUCTION

Recognition of the prevalence, chronicity, and morbidity associated with panic disorder (PD) has stimulated extensive research and the subsequent development of a number of effective treatments for this condition. The first psychopharmacological agents to be used for the treatment of PD included the tricyclic antidepressants (TCAs) and the monoamine oxidase inhibitors (MAOIs), followed by the benzodiazepines (BZDs), and more recently the selective serotonergic reuptake inhibitors (SSRIs). This chapter will provide the reader with a brief review of the traditional classes of medications used to treat this disorder. However, because there already exist extensive reviews describing the TCAs, MAOIs, and BZDs, more attention will be focused on the newer treatments, including the new reversible MAOIs and the SSRIs, as well as less frequently discussed treatment issues, including length of treatment, discontinuation, and relapse. Comparisons of the various agents with information on the advantages and disadvantages for each of the classes will be provided, as well as side effect profiles. Finally, information regarding research on the cholecystokinin (CCK) antagonists, one of the promising leads in the development of new antianxiety agents, will be provided as well.

TRADITIONAL TREATMENTS

TRICYCLIC ANTIDEPRESSANTS

The TCAs were one of the earliest and most extensively studied classes of medications found to be effective for the treatment of (PD). Imipramine, the most frequently used TCA, has been proven effective in the treatment of PD in over a dozen controlled (Ballenger *et al.*, 1977; Sheehan *et al.*, 1980; Zitrin *et al.*, 1983) and numerous uncontrolled trials (Ballenger *et al.*, 1984; Lydiard and Ballenger, 1988; Mavissakalian and Michelson, 1982; Mavissakalian *et al.*,

Advances in the Neurobiology of Anxiety Disorders. Edited by H. G. M. Westenberg, J. A. Den Boer and D. L. Murphy
©1996 John Wiley & Sons Ltd

1983; McNair & Kahn, 1981). However, its use is somewhat limited by the length of time required to achieve clinically significant improvement (i.e., generally 4–12 weeks) and associated side effects. For this reason, BZDs are sometimes used in conjunction with the TCAs early in treatment, in order to provide more rapid relief from anxiety symptomatology during this initial treatment phase (Ballenger, 1993).

In prescribing the TCAs, as well as any other antianxiety medication, the clinician should take into consideration the broad range of effective dosages required to achieve clinical improvement. Although most require doses greater than 150 mg per day, some patients can obtain therapeutic improvement at doses even as low as 25 mg per day (Zitrin et al., 1983). Particularly bothersome, some patients experience a "hyperstimulatory" effect, i.e., more intense and increased panic symptoms, rapid heart beat, insomnia, and general agitation, when beginning treatment with the TCAs. This hyperstimulation can be minimized in the majority of patients (Ballenger, 1991) if the medication is initiated at a low dose, with gradual increases. In addition, adequate patient education regarding the transient nature of this side effect, i.e., generally remits within a couple of weeks, is often helpful in maintaining medication compliance (Noyes et al., 1989). The clinician's encouragement and availability, as well as the patient's participation in activities that he or she finds relaxing, such as warm baths or long walks, are also useful until the hyperstimulation abates. Weight gain with the TCAs can also be troublesome to such a degree that the patient is unwilling to continue treatment with these agents (Noyes et al., 1989).

TCAs other than imipramine have demonstrated efficacy for the treatment of panic disorder, and include doxepin, nortriptyline, maprotiline, amitriptyline, and trimipramine (Lydiard and Ballenger, 1987). It has been shown that the TCAs are not as effective as the MAOIs, however, in the patient who suffers from PD and comorbid depression (Liebowitz, 1993; Quitkin et al., 1990).

MONOAMINE OXIDASE INHIBITOR ANTIDEPRESSANTS

The MAOIs, like the TCAs, have been extensively studied, with demonstrated efficacy for this condition. Again, similar to the TCAs, the MAOIs share the disadvantage of delayed onset of action, and require several weeks before clinically significant relief is obtained from anxiety symptoms. The MAOI most frequently used and studied is phenelzine, again with a large number of controlled (Ballenger et al., 1977; Mountjoy et al., 1977; Sheehan et al., 1980; Solyom et al., 1973, 1981; Tyrer et al., 1973) as well as several open studies (Ballenger et al., 1987; Buiges and Vallejo, 1987; Howell et al., 1987) that have demonstrated its effectiveness. The reader should be cautioned, however, that the studies with the MAOIs cannot be considered as conclusive as those with the TCAs because of the small sample sizes, mixed diagnoses, and low medication doses (Ballenger, 1992b). In addition, use of the MAOIs requires considerable dietary and medication restriction, often referred to as the "cheese reaction", because of the acute hypertensive reaction that can develop if the patient ingests aged cheeses, red wine, and/or a number of other foods and medicines. These restrictions, unfortunately, limit the utility of the MAOIs because of the almost "phobic" fear that most PD patients have about taking medication (Ballenger, 1993). For an in-depth review of these agents, the reader is referred to Johnson *et al.* (in press).

BENZODIAZEPINES

The BZDs, more recently studied, have also been proven to be extremely effective, with the advantage of rapid onset of action and the demonstrated ability to begin reducing the symptoms associated with anxiety within the first week of treatment (Ballenger *et al.*, 1988; Cross National Collaborative Panic Study, Second Phase Investigators, 1992). In addition, the BZDs, and more specifically alprazolam, have been found to have a more favorable side effect profile than the TCAs or MAOIs. These results have been confirmed in the large Cross National Trial and later replicated in the Cross National Phase II Trial (Ballenger *et al.*, 1988; Cross National Collaborative Panic Study, Second Phase Investigators, 1992). Both of these trials were carefully controlled, utilized a very large patient sample with sites in multiple countries, and in both studies the efficacy of alprazolam was confirmed. In addition to significantly reducing the primary symptoms of PD, alprazolam was also effective in improving the secondary disability associated with this condition. Open studies have also demonstrated and confirmed alprazolam's efficacy (Liebowitz *et al.*, 1986; Rizley *et al.*, 1986).

BZDs other than alprazolam have also been successfully used for this condition. Clonazepam has been shown to be effective in the treatment of PD in several studies (Pollack *et al.*, 1986; Tesar and Rosenbaum, 1985). Diazepam has also demonstrated efficacy in the treatment of PD, at doses approximately 10 times that required for alprazolam (Dunner *et al.*, 1986). Lorazepam, when compared to alprazolam, was shown to be approximately equally effective (Charney and Woods, 1989), although the patients on alprazolam rated themselves more improved than those on lorazepam. Other BZDs studied and shown to be effective include bromazepam (Beaudry *et al.*, 1984) and oxazepam (Fogelson, 1988).

Despite the effectiveness of the BZDs, considerable controversy exists regarding potential difficulty with discontinuation of this class of medication. This has been studied in depth (Fontaine *et al.*, 1984; Pecknold, 1990; Rickels *et al.*, 1990, 1993; Schweizer *et al.*, 1990; Sellers *et al.*, 1993) and reviewed by Ballenger *et al.* (1993) with clinical evidence that demonstrates that the majority of patients taking BZDs actually can be discontinued with minimal difficulty if the discontinuation is conducted gradually and slowly (over two to four months) and the patient is educated about what to expect during this process.

NEWER TREATMENT OPTIONS

REVERSIBLE MONOAMINE OXIDASE INHIBITORS

Although evidence strongly indicates the effectiveness of the MAOIs in the treatment of PD, their utility has been severely limited as described earlier, i.e., dietary and medication restrictions, hyperstimulatory effects, and weight gain. However, recent studies of reversible monoamine oxidase-A (MAO-A) inhibitors have demonstrated their clinical utility, particularly in the treatment of depression, without the hypertensive risk associated with the tyramine-potentiating effects generally associated with the earlier MAOIs.

Recently brofaromine, an MAO-A, has been studied, to determine its efficacy in the treatment of PD. Garcia-Borreguero et al. studied 14 inpatients with PD and agoraphobia, five of whom also suffered from depression. Patients were treated for four weeks at 150 mg brofaromine per day. Side effects were minimal, resulting in no drop-outs. In addition, patients' diets were not restricted, and there was no evidence of hypertensive reactions. Treatment with brofaromine was associated with improvement in both panic and depressive symptomatology, with no difference in treatment outcome between the groups (Garcia-Borreguero et al., 1992).

Bakish et al. (1993) have extended these preliminary findings in a double-blind, eight-week comparison of brofaromine and clomipramine. Ninety-three patients who were diagnosed with PD, with or without agoraphobia, were included. Of the 93 patients, 47 were assigned to brofaromine at initial doses of 50 mg per day and 46 to clomipramine, 25 mg per day. Medications were increased each week in 25 mg increments for clomipramine and 50 mg for brofaromine, to maximum tolerated doses. Although the medications were initiated at low doses, there was a high drop-out rate. Five of the initial patients did not begin treatment, leaving 45 patients assigned to brofaromine and 45 to clomipramine. Of the brofaromine group, 27 or 63% dropped out, compared to 22 or 49% of the clomipramine group. More than half of the drop-outs took place during the first two weeks of the study and were attributed to medication intolerance, at even the lowest doses. Therefore, only 16 brofaromine (37%) and 23 clomipramine (51%) patients completed the study, with both medications demonstrating comparable efficacy by significantly reducing panic attacks by week eight of the study. There were differences in the side effect profiles for the two drugs, with the brofaromine group experiencing more headache, nausea and insomnia and the clomipramine group constipation, urinary difficulty, excessive perspiration, and sexual difficulties. Because of the high drop-out rate, the authors suggest that even lower doses may be needed for initiating treatment with PD patients who often exhibit hypersensitivity to the effects of different medications (Bakish et al., 1993).

SELECTIVE SEROTONIN REUPTAKE INHIBITORS

Originally used successfully for the treatment of major depression (Boyer and

Feighner, 1991), this class of medication has also been shown in recent studies to be effective in a number of anxiety disorders including obsessive-compulsive disorder and PD (Boyer, 1992), with fewer side effects than the TCAs (Asberg and Martensson, 1993). The hypothesis that an abnormality in brain serotonin (5-HT) function is correlated with anxiety disorders has been supported by studies that demonstrated the ability of various agents that act on the monoamine neurotransmitter systems to induce panic attacks in PD patients but not control subjects. Yohimbine, sodium lactate and isoproterenol have been used successfully in laboratory settings to induce panic (Murphy and Pigott, 1990; Gorman et al., 1985, 1989). It has also been demonstrated, however, that if patients are given imipramine prior to lactate administration, panic symptoms do not occur (Klerman et al., 1993).

Animal studies suggested 5-HT overactivity in anxiety (Humble and Wistedt, 1992). However, there has been limited support for this hypothesis. Other studies have implicated a 5-HT deficit in anxiety, based on the ability of zimelidine to decrease anxiety in clinical populations (Evans and Moore, 1981; Hoes et al., 1980; Koczkas et al., 1981). Other indications of a 5-HT deficiency include the respiratory difficulties associated with PD, i.e., hyperventilation, uncontrolled breathing rate, and choking frequently experienced by PD patients (Gorman and Papp, 1990). In addition, the high incidence of suicide attempts associated with untreated PD (Weissman et al., 1989) further supports this theory since suicide has been linked to decreased 5-HT (Asberg et al., 1987).

More importantly, provocation studies with m-chlorophenylpiperazine (mCPP), a 5-HT agonist, induced panic attacks in PD patients but not controls or depressed patients (Kahn et al., 1988). Another study which utilized higher doses of mCPP induced panic attacks not only in PD subjects, but in normal controls as well (Charney et al., 1987). Challenge studies utilizing fenfluramine produced comparable results (Targum and Marshall, 1989).

Included in the SSRIs are fluoxetine, citalopram, fluvoxamine, sertraline, and paroxetine (Boyer, 1992). Also included in this section is clomipramine, a tricyclic antidepressant, whose primary mode of action is on the 5-HT system. Clinical evidence has demonstrated the superiority of clomipramine over other more traditionally used medications for the treatment of PD. In a 12-week study comparing clomipramine, imipramine, and placebo in PD patients, clomipramine was shown to be superior to imipramine in reduction of panic attacks and scores on the HAM-A (Modigh et al., 1992). In the group treated with clomipramine, panic attacks were reduced from 6 to 0, and at one to two years follow-up patients who were maintained on lower doses of the drug remained panic-free. In addition, none of the 22 clomipramine compared to four of the 29 imipramine and seven of the 17 placebo patients terminated participation in the study. A study comparing clomipramine and fluvoxamine demonstrated comparable efficacy with both drugs, with significant improvement in panic symptomatology including reduction in panic attacks and depressive/anxiety symptoms, as well as a 50% decrease on HAM-A scores. Although both drugs were shown to be effective, the effects of clomipramine were demonstrated earlier and were shown to be somewhat greater than those seen with fluvoxamine (Den Boer et al., 1987).

Gorman et al. (1987) conducted an open trial of fluoxetine, 20 mg per day, in 16 PD patients. Of the 16, seven responded; however, seven of the nine non-responders were unable to tolerate the hyperstimulatory effects of fluoxetine. Specifically, patients complained of increased agitation, gastrointestinal side effects that included diarrhea, insomnia, restlessness, and jitteriness. It is therefore recommended that fluoxetine be initiated at low dosages in the range of 2.5–5.0 mg per day, and that development of hyperstimulation be monitored closely. It should be noted that it has been demonstrated that the group of patients who experience the extreme hyperstimulatory reaction are also responsive to doses in the lower range (Coplan et al., 1992). For those patients for whom this hyperstimulation syndrome appears to be problematic, the dose should be titrated upward slowly and gradually.

Another open study (Schneier et al., 1990) conducted in 25 PD patients with and without agoraphobia utilized initial doses of fluoxetine at 5 mg per day, with gradual increases every five days. In 19 of the 25 patients (76%), a moderate to marked improvement was demonstrated; four (16%) could not tolerate the side effects, and two were not even moderately improved.

In a placebo-controlled study, 62% of the patients treated with fluvoxamine enjoyed complete cessation of panic attacks, compared to 18% of the patients who received placebo. In addition, 28% of the fluvoxamine group were completely free of associated disability, versus 13% of the placebo group (Woods et al., 1994). Another placebo-controlled study confirmed fluvoxamine's superiority over placebo in the treatment of PD (Hoehn-Saric et al., 1993). In this eight-week trial, 50 patients were studied, with clinically significant relief from panic attacks experienced by the fluvoxamine group in the third week of the study. At study conclusion, the fluvoxamine group achieved a much higher percentage of patients who were panic-free.

Den Boer and Westenberg (1988) compared maprotiline, a specific norepinephrine (NE) reuptake blocker with fluvoxamine, a specific 5-HT reuptake blocker, in a double-blind, six-week treatment study, at doses averaging 150 mg per day. This trial further supported the 5-HT abnormality hypothesis in panic. Fluvoxamine was effective in significantly decreasing panic attacks. Maprotiline, on the other hand, was able to decrease the depressive symptomatology to a minor degree, but had almost no effect on the panic symptoms experienced by this group (Den Boer and Westenberg, 1988). However, non-responders to maprotiline did respond when switched to fluvoxamine.

This same group conducted a comparison study of fluvoxamine and ritanserin (Westenberg and Den Boer, 1989). These investigators reasoned that because ritanserin blocks the postsynaptic 5-HT$_2$ receptors, it would work more quickly than fluvoxamine. However, in this eight-week trial, the efficacy of fluvoxamine was again demonstrated, with further evidence that phobic avoidance improved in the final two weeks of the trial. Ritanserin, on the other hand, had no effect on these patients. These findings would suggest that 5-HT receptor subtypes other than postsynaptic 5-HT$_2$ are involved in the pathophysiology of panic (Westenberg and Den Boer, 1989).

A study of 75 PD subjects compared fluvoxamine, placebo, and cognitive therapy in an eight-week trial. The fluvoxamine group was clinically superior to the cognitive therapy group on several measures, but the cognitive therapy group did not demonstrate superiority to fluvoxamine on any measure. In addition, the effects of fluvoxamine were experienced earlier than those of cognitive therapy (Black *et al.*, 1993).

Three studies have been conducted with zimelidine, a serotonergic reuptake blocker with excellent antidepressant effects and no anticholinergic side effects (Heel *et al.*, 1982). Evans and Moore (1981) treated seven agoraphobics with zimelidine, at doses up to 300 mg per day. Five of the seven showed marked improvement. Kockzas *et al.* (1981) replicated this finding in an open study of 13 patients at similar doses. These results demonstrated efficacy of zimelidine in seven of the 13 patients studied. Evans *et al.* (1986) conducted a double-blind trial of 44 agoraphobics with panic attacks, utilizing either zimelidine, imipramine, or placebo. Zimelidine was significantly superior to placebo on only one of the four scales used, whereas imipramine was not superior to placebo on any measure. Patients initiated medication at 50 mg per day and doses were increased to 150 mg per day. Of the total, only 13 zimelidine, 16 imipramine, and seven placebo patients were analyzed. Although zimelidine has shown some efficacy in reducing panic attacks as demonstrated in these three studies, it has been withdrawn because of the frequent occurrence of Gillain–Barré syndrome (Coplan *et al.*, 1992; Nilsson, 1983).

Citalopram was also shown to have good results and few side effects (Humble *et al.*, 1989), in an eight-week open trial. Thirteen of the 17 patients studied had greater than 50% improvement on global measures. At the conclusion of the study, four of the 17 were panic-free and six had only minor situational panic attacks. Of particular significance is the relatively rapid onset of action, with improvement seen in two weeks of drug therapy (Humble *et al.*, 1989). Following acute treatment, 16 patients were enrolled in a long-term maintenance study. Eleven patients completed this phase of treatment with maintenance of initial improvement as well as further treatment gains during this extended treatment period (Humble and Wistedt, 1992).

There is evidence that stimulation of the 5-HT$_{1A}$ receptor appears to be useful in some anxiety conditions, particularly generalized anxiety disorder (Asberg and Martensen, 1993). Included in this class of drugs are buspirone, gepirone, ipsapirone, and tandospirone (Asberg and Martensen, 1993). In addition, there is evidence that the 5-HT$_3$ antagonists may also have promise in the treatment of anxiety (Lader, 1991).

CHOLECYSTOKININ ANTAGONISTS

Recent evidence supports development of another treatment alternative for this condition. Animal studies have shown antagonism between BZDs and the cholecystokinin octapeptide (CCK_8) in the hippocampus (Bradwejn and de Montigny 1984), and "anxious" rats have demonstrated evidence of decreased CCK_8 receptors in the hippocampus (Harro et al., 1990).

Supporting these findings, studies in humans have shown CCK in the tetrapeptide form (CCK_4) to be anxiogenic (de Montigny, 1989; Bradwejn et al., 1990). However, when BZDs were administered to rats who had received CCK_4, the anxiety effects were alleviated (Bradwejn and de Montigny, 1984). A number of investigators have replicated these findings. De Montigny induced panic attacks in healthy volunteers by injecting CCK_4; the anxiogenic effects were antagonized by BZDs but not by the administration of meprobamate or naloxone (de Montigny, 1989). Bradwejn and colleagues were able to induce panic attacks in 11 patients through injection of CCK_4; however, none of the patients who received placebo panicked (Bradwejn et al., 1990). A recent study found a much higher percentage of PD patients compared to normal controls who panicked when administered CCK_4 (Bradwejn et al., 1991). Of 11 PD patients studied, 10 or 91% panicked when administered 25 µg of CCK_4 compared to only two of 12 normal controls (17%).

Lydiard et al. (1992) studied the cerebrospinal fluid (CSF) of 25 PD patients and 16 controls. Of the PD patients, eight also met diagnostic criteria for major depression. All subjects were instructed to remain medicine free for two weeks prior to the lumbar puncture procedure. Their findings demonstrated significantly lower concentrations of CCK in the CSF of the PD patients compared to the control subjects. There were no significant differences in CSF between the subset of PD patients who also suffered from depression and those who suffered from PD alone (Lydiard et al., 1992a).

These studies suggest that CCK antagonists may be effective as antipanic agents and are under active investigation. However, early trials have as yet been inconclusive (Kramer et al., 1995).

DOSAGE AND LENGTH OF TREATMENT

As mentioned earlier, the effective dosage range for psychopharmacological treatment of PD patients varies widely among individual patients and within each of the medication classes described. Other factors that should be considered when prescribing medications is the PD patient's frequent hypersensitivity to the effects of many substances, including caffeine and various medications. Although there is little formal documentation regarding this phenomenon, clinical reports and experience clearly describe in a large number of PD patients not only a hypersensitivity to certain substances but an extreme, almost phobic, reluctance to take any medication. The latter is often exaggerated to such a degree that the patient can only be convinced to initiate medication treatment while in the clinician's office, under his or her close supervision. The clinician should therefore consider the patient's previous medication history as well as the specific somatic symptoms described by the patient when choosing a medication. These same considerations should also be used in determining the dosage for initiating a medication, as well as the schedule for increasing dosage to a level that will allow the patient to attain maximum therapeutic efficacy.

Tricyclic antidepressants

Treatment with imipramine, the most frequently prescribed TCA, is usually initiated at 10 mg per day, with 10 mg increases every three to four days, until an optimal level has been attained. For most patients, this appears to be at least 150 mg per day (Klein, 1984; Mavissakalian et al., 1984). However, it has been demonstrated that some patients require significantly higher doses to attain clinically significant improvement. If the patient remains unimproved at 150 mg per day, the medication should be increased to 300 mg per day over a four- to eight-week period (Ballenger, et al. 1991). Evidence suggests that a threshold of serum imipramine and desipramine of 100–125 ng/ml is associated with clinical response (Ballenger et al. 1984; Lydiard, 1987; Mavissakalian and Jones, 1990). The TCAs generally require four to eight weeks before significant improvement is seen in anxiety symptomatology.

Monoamine oxidase inhibitors

Treatment with phenelzine, the most commonly used MAOI, is prescribed at initial doses of 15 mg per day, taken in the morning, with 15 mg increases every four to seven days, up to 90 mg per day (Hollander et al., 1990). It has been demonstrated that doses of at least 60 mg are generally necessary in order to achieve a good treatment response (Klerman et al., 1993). If the side effects associated with phenelzine, i.e., weight gain and sedation, are particularly troublesome, tranylcypromine can be substituted. In addition to being better tolerated by some patients, tranylcypromine is generally effective at lower doses than phenelzine and can be initiated at 10 mg per day with 10 mg increases every three to four days, up to a maximum daily dose of 80 mg (Hollander et al., 1990). As with the TCAs, slow onset of action is associated with the MAOIs, and 4–12 weeks is usually required to achieve clinically significant relief.

Because of the risk of a hypertensive episode with the MAOIs, some clinicians recommend that patients on these medications carry with them nifediprine, 20 mg, which works to rapidly lower blood pressure (Hollander et al., 1990). Although infrequent, the patient should be instructed about the symptoms preceding a hypertensive episode, generally identified by a pulsing, severe headache. If evidence exists that a hypertensive episode is imminent, the patient should present to an emergency room for assessment of blood pressure and treatment if indicated. The clinician should be reminded that the restrictions associated with the use of the MAOIs should be maintained for two weeks after these drugs are discontinued.

Benzodiazepines

Again, using alprazolam as the most frequently prescribed BZD, medication treatment should be initiated at low levels, generally 0.25–0.5 mg, to be taken three times a day. Increases of 0.25–0.5 mg per day can be made every four to six days, as tolerated and as indicated. Similar to the other medications, the dosage range for alprazolam is also widely variable, with many patients experiencing significant improvement at doses as low as 1–3 mg per day (Ballenger, 1986; Lydiard et al., 1992). On the other hand, clinical experience has demonstrated that it is not uncommon for many patients to require higher doses, in the range of 4–6 and 6–10 mg per day in order to achieve significant relief from anxiety symptomatology (Ballenger et al., 1988).

Selective serotonin reuptake inhibitors

Fluvoxamine has been compared at doses of 50, 100, and 150 mg per day, with approximately equal efficacy achieved at all three doses (J. A. Den Boer, unpublished communication, 1992). However, as might be expected, side effects were significantly more problematic at the higher doses of the drug. As described earlier, patients on the SSRIs can expect to have an exacerbation of anxiety symptoms during the first week or two of treatment.

LENGTH OF TREATMENT

Recent attention has focused on the chronic nature of PD, and the shift in emphasis from short- to longer-term, generally defined as more than six months, treatment for many patients (Klerman et al., 1993; Schatzberg and Ballinger, 1991). It was discovered that many patients relapsed after short-term pharmacotherapy (Fyer et al., 1987; Versianni et al., 1985), but recovered to prediscontinuation levels once medication was reinstituted. Although long-term treatment does have some drawbacks, such as the weight gain frequently experienced with long-term use of the TCAs and MAOIs, the benefits of continued treatment are generally considered far greater than their associated risks. With long-term treatment, the patient is able to maintain and extend initial treatment gains. Avoidant behaviors that have developed in conjunction with the PD can be addressed and the patient can resume a more normal, prepanic existence (Schatzberg and Ballenger, 1991).

The long-term treatment model proposed by Ballenger (1991) is comparable to that described by Kupfer (1991) during treatment of affective disorders. Essentially, there are three phases of treatment proposed. The first is referred to as the acute phase, lasting approximately one to three months, during which the clinician attempts to significantly reduce symptomatology associated with the disorder. The second stage, described as the maintenance phase, or treatment months 3–12, follows the patient's initial positive response to the medication. During this phase, initial treatment gains can be extended, and the patient can hopefully return to a more normal, prepanic lifestyle, enjoying activities that before treatment the patient had avoided or engaged in only with anxiety (Ballenger, 1991). The final stage of treatment generally begins 12–18 months after medication initiation. Described as the taper phase, attempts are made to discontinue medication treatment. The taper should be conducted slowly and gradually to cause the least disruption to the stability that the patient has attained over the preceding months.

DISCONTINUATION

The primary question to be addressed before discontinuation is initiated is whether the medication is still needed. Unfortunately, the only way to determine definitively the need for continued medication treatment is to discontinue the medication. It is imperative, however, that medications be tapered gradually and slowly.

The decision to discontinue medication treatment should be a collaborative one between patient and clinician, with adequate information and education regarding what the patient should expect once this process has been initiated. Timing of medication discontinuation is also of the utmost importance. For example, attempting to taper or discontinue medication from a student directly before exams or from a business person directly before a critical business meeting is strongly discouraged. However, once the patient has recovered fully, has resumed activities associated with the predisease state, and is at a stable point in his or her life, discontinuation can be conducted. The patient can expect to experience one of four outcomes during this process, i.e., continue to remain symptom-free, relapse, suffer from a withdrawal syndrome, or experience rebound (Ballenger, 1992). Relapse does not appear to be related to the type of medication that the patient has been taking. However, the time course for relapse is related to the class of medicine the patient has been taking, and the amount of time required to achieve the initial clinical response.

BENZODIAZEPINES

As a general statement, relapse seems to occur within the same timeframe as that required for initial response to the medication. For example, significant improvement is generally seen within the first week of treatment with the BZDs. If relapse occurs when the BZDs are discontinued, it usually occurs within the first week that the patient begins taper or becomes medication-free (Ballenger, 1992a).

Data show that withdrawal occurs in 35–90% of BZD patients when medication is discontinued (Rickels et al., 1993; Pecknold et al., 1988). Withdrawal symptoms generally improve or abate by the end of the first week following discontinuation. Symptoms associated with BZD withdrawal are considered mild, and again are transient (Ballenger, 1992).

Rebound is defined as a recurrence of pretreatment anxiety symptomatology, but at levels greater than those experienced pre treatment. During the Phase I trial, 35% of patients who were discontinued from alprazolam rapidly experienced rebound (Pecknold et al., 1988). Again, the short-term nature of these symptoms should provide some degree of reassurance to the patient who can expect symptoms to improve greatly by the seventh day of discontinuation and abate totally by day 14 (Ballenger, 1992).

The best strategy for avoiding or reducing the withdrawal syndrome is a slow, gradual taper, in a patient who is educated about the discontinuation process. As discovered by Pecknold during the Cross-National Phase I trial, a large percentage of patients who were tapered from alprazolam by 1 mg every three to four days suffered from rebound (35%) or withdrawal symptoms (35%) (Pecknold et al., 1988). Pecknold and his group subsequently studied patients who had received alprazolam for six weeks, but who were tapered slowly and gradually over a two- to four-month period (Pecknold et al., 1993). With this taper schedule, only 7% of patients suffered from any withdrawal syndrome and no patients experienced rebound. Similar results with this slower discontinuation schedule have been replicated in studies by Rickels et al. (Rickels, 1990; Schweizer et al., 1990). It is therefore recommended that the BZDs be tapered slowly and gradually over a two- to four-month period, with particular emphasis on the taper that occurs when the patient reaches a dosage of 1.5 mg or less (Rickels, 1990).

TRICYCLIC AND MONOAMINE OXIDASE INHIBITOR ANTIDEPRESSANTS

Similar to the timeframe described with the BZDs, withdrawal with the TCAs and/or the MAOIs is comparable to the period of time within which clinical improvement is seen, i.e., four to eight weeks. A gradual reduction in dosage of 25 mg per month is recommended when discontinuing the TCAs (Klerman et al., 1993). The clinician should be advised to monitor the discontinuation process closely, and to work with the patient regarding the return of panic symptomatology that is intolerable. The patient and clinician may decide that reinstitution of medication is indicated, a strategy that is almost always successful in regaining control of anxiety symptoms. However, the patient, if properly educated about the discontinuation process, may be better able to tolerate the transient withdrawal syndrome that frequently occurs when medication discontinuation is attempted.

TCAs, if discontinued suddenly, can result in nausea, tremor, and headaches. These side effects can be minimized if the taper or discontinuation process is conducted gradually over several weeks.

OUTCOME

Unfortunately, little is known about the long-term outcome for PD patients. As described in the preceding section, data regarding relapse is highly variable, but sufficient evidence exists to document the likelihood of relapse in a large number of PD patients.

Nagy and colleagues (1989) followed-up 60 PD patients 1.7–4 years, after they had been treated with alprazolam and behavioral therapy for four months. Most patients were maintained on lower doses of alprazolam than that used during the acute treatment phase, although 30% discontinued medication entirely. Initial treatment gains were maintained and an additional 9% of the patients became panic-free during the follow-up period (Nagy *et al.*, 1989).

In the largest follow-up study to date, 423 PD patients were followed three to six years post treatment with either imipramine or alprazolam. This study showed that 18.2% of patients had remained well throughout the follow-up period, 12.7% got well during follow-up and remained well, 23.6% experienced mild intermittent panic, 26.8% had mild panic symptoms continuously, and 18.6% suffered from full-blown PD during the entire follow-up period (Katschnig *et al.*, 1991).

One of the few prospective long-term follow-up studies conducted confirmed earlier studies that indicated that panic patients who also suffered from depression had a more chronic and severe illness as well as poorer prognosis (Cross-National Collaborative Panic Study, Second Phase Investigators, 1992; Noyes *et al.*, 1990; Wittchen *et al.*, 1991). This study involved 32 PD and 20 PD plus depression patients initially treated with either imipramine or doxepin. After patients had remained well for a three-month period, the drug was tapered, with increases as necessary to deal with the recurrence of panic symptoms. In addition to medication treatment, patients were provided psychotherapy for 1 h per week for six to eight months. At the end of the two-year follow-up period, 75% of the PD group were panic-free compared to only 35% of the comorbid (panic plus depression) group (Albus and Scheibe, 1993).

In conclusion, further studies are needed in order to adequately determine the long-term prognosis for these patients. Studies involving those newer agents described in this chapter are also warranted, as are comparisons with other more traditional pharmacotherapies and behavioral interventions.

REFERENCES

Albus, M. and Scheibe, G. (1993). Outcome of panic disorder with or without concomitant depression: a 2-year prospective follow-up study. *Am. J. Psychiatry*, **150**(12), 1878–1880.

Asberg, M. and Martensson, B. (1993). Serotonin selective antidepressant drugs: past, present, future. *Clinical Neuropharmacology*, Vol. S3, pp. S32–S44. Raven Press, New York.

Asberg, M., Schalling D., Traskman-Bendz, L. and Wagner, A. (1987). Psychobiology of suicide, impulsivity, and related phenomena. In *Psychopharmacology: The Third Generation of Progress* (ed. H. Y. Meltzer), pp. 655–668. Raven Press, New York.

Bakish, D., Saxena, B. M., Bowen, R. and D'Souza, J. D. (1993). Reversible monoamine oxidase-A inhibitors in panic disorder. *Clin. Neuropharmacol.*, **16**(2), S77–S82.

Ballenger, J. C. (1986). Acute fixed-dose alprazolam study in panic disorder patients. Presented at the Panic Disorder and Biological Research Workshop, Washington, DC, April 15–16, 1986.

Ballenger, J. C. (1991). Long-term pharmacologic treatment of panic disorder. *J. Clin. Psychiatry*, **52** (2S), 18–23.

Ballenger, J. C. (1992a). Medication discontinuation in panic disorder. *J. Clin. Psychiatry*, **53** (3S), 26–31.

Ballenger, J. C. (1992b). Overview of panic disorder. *Asean J. Psychiatry*, **2**(1), 13–27.

Ballenger, J. C. (1993). Panic disorder: efficacy of current treatments. *Psychopharmacol. Bull.*, **29**, 477–486.

Ballenger, J. C., Sheehan, D. V. and Jacobsen, G. (1977). Antidepressant treatment of severe phobic anxiety. In *Abstracts of the Scientific Proceedings of the 130th Annual Meeting of the American Psychiatric Association*, Toronto, May, 1977.

Ballenger, J. C., Peterson, G. A., Laraia, M. T. *et al.* (1984). A study of plasma catecholamines in agoraphobia and the relationship of serum tricyclic levels to treatment response. In *Biology of Agoraphobia* (ed. J. C. Ballenger), pp. 27–64. American Psychiatric Association Press, Washington, DC.

Ballenger, J. C., Howell, E. F., Laraia, M. and Lydiard, R. B. (1987). Comparison of four medicines in panic disorder. Presented at the 140th Annual Meeting of the American Psychiatric Association, Chicago, May 14, 1987.

Ballenger, J. C., Burrow, G. D., DuPont, R. L., Jr *et al.* (1988). Alprazolam in panic disorder and agoraphobia: results from a multicenter trial. I: Efficacy in short-term treatment. *Arch. Gen. Psychiatry*, **46**, 413–422.

Ballenger, J. C., Pecknold, J., Rickels, K. and Sellars, E. M. (1993), Medication discontinuation in panic disorder. *J. Clin. Psychiatry*, **54**, 15–21.

Beaudry, P., Fontaine, R. and Chouinard, G. (1984). Bromazepam, another high-potency benzodiazepine for panic attacks (letter). *Am. J. Psychiatry*, **141**, 464–465.

Black, D. W., Wesner, R., Bowers, W. *et al.* (1993). A comparison of fluvoxamine, cognitive therapy, and placebo in the treatment of panic disorder. *Arch. Gen. Psychiatry*, **50**, 44–50.

Boyer, W. F. (1992). Potential indications for the selective serotonin reuptake inhibitors. *Int. Clin. Psychopharmacol.*, **6**(S5), 5–12.

Boyer, W. F. and Feighner, J. P. (1991). The efficacy of selective serotonin reuptake inhibitors in depression. In *Selective Serotonin Reuptake Inhibitors*, (eds J. P. Feighner and W. F. Boyer), pp. 89–108. Wiley, Chichester.

Bradwejn, J. and de Montigny, C. (1984). Benzodiazepines antagonize cholecystokinin-induced activation of rat hippocampal neurones. *Nature*, **312** 363–365.

Bradwejn, J., Koszycki, D., and Meterissian, G. (1990). Cholecystokinin-tetrapeptide induces panic attacks in patients with panic disorder. *Can. J. Psychiatry*, **35**, 83–85.

Bradwejn, J., Koszycki, D. and Shriqui, C. (1991). Enhanced sensitivity to cholecystokinin tetrapeptide in panic disorder: clinical and behavioral findings. *Arch. Gen. Psychiatry*, **48**, 603–610.

Buiges, J. and Vallejo, J. (1987). Therapeutic response to phenelzine in patients with panic disorder and agoraphobia with panic attacks. *J. Clin. Psychiatry*, **48**, 55.

Charney, D. S. and Woods, S. W. (1989). Benzodiazepine treatment of panic disorder: a comparison of alprazolam and lorazepam. *J. Clin. Psychiatry*, **50**, 418–423.

Charney, D. S., Woods, S. W., Goodman, W. K. and Heninger, G. R. (1987). Serotonin function in anxiety. II. Effects of the serotonin agonist MCPP in panic disorder patients and healthy subjects. *Psychopharmacology*, **92**, 14–24.

Coplan, J. D., Gorman, J. M., and Klein, D. F. (1992). Serotonin related functions in panic–anxiety: a critical overview. *Neuropsychopharmacology*, **6**(3), 189–200.

Cross National Collaborative Panic Study, Second Phase Investigators (1992). Drug treatment of panic disorder: comparative efficacy of alprazolam, imipramine, and placebo. *Br. J. Psychiatry*, **160**, 191–202.

de Montigny, C. (1989). Cholecystokinin tetrapeptide induces panic-like attacks in healthy volunteers: preliminary findings. *Arch. Gen. Psychiatry*, **46**, 511–517.

Den Boer, J. A., and Westenberg, H. G. (1988). Effect of a serotonin and noradrenaline uptake inhibitor in panic disorder: a double-blind comparative study with fluvoxamine and maprotiline. *Int. Clin. Psychopharmacol.*, **3**, 59–74.

Den Boer, J. A. Westenberg, H. G. M., Kamerbeck, W. O. J. *et al* (1987). Effect of serotonin uptake inhibitors in anxiety disorders: a double-blind comparison of clomipramine and fluvoxamine, *Int. Clin. Psychopharmacol.* **2**, 21–32.

Dunner, D. L., Ishiki, D., Avery, D. H. *et al.* (1986). Effect of alprazolam and diazepam on anxiety and panic attacks in panic disorder: a controlled study. *J. Clin. Psychiatry*, **47**, 458–460.

Evans, L. and Moore, G. (1981). The treatment of phobic anxiety by zimelidine. *Acta Psychiatr. Scand.,* **63**, 342–345.

Evans, L., Kenardy, J., Schneider, P. and Hoey, H. (1986). Effect of a selective serotonin uptake inhibitor in agoraphobia with panic attacks: a double blind comparison of zimelidine, imipramine and placebo. *Acta Psychiatr. Scand.*, **73**, 49–53.

Fogelson, D. L., (1988). Lorazepam and oxazepam in the treatment of panic disorder (letter). *J. Clin. Psychopharmacol.*, **8**, 160.

Fontaine, R., Chouinard, G. and Annable, L. (1984). Rebound anxiety in anxious patients after abrupt withdrawal of benzodiazepine treatment. *Am. J. Psychiatry*, **141**, 848–852.

Fyer, A. J., Liebowitz, M. R., Gorman, J. M. *et al.* (1987). Discontinuation of alprazolam treatment in panic patients. *Am. J. Psychiatry,* **144**, 303–308.

Garcia–Borreguero, D., Lauer, C. J., Ozdaglar, A. *et al.* (1992). Brofaromine in panic disorder: a pilot study with a new reversible inhibitor of monoamine oxidase-A. *Pharmacopsychiatry*, **25**, 261–264.

Gorman, J. M. and Papp, L. A. (1990). Respiratory physiology of panic. In *Neurobiology of Panic Disorder* (ed. J. C. Ballenger), pp. 127–203. Liss, New York.

Gorman, J. M., Liebowitz, M. R., Fyer, A. J. *et al.* (1985). Lactate infusions in obsessive compulsive disorder. *Am. J. Psychiatry*, **142**, 864–866.

Gorman, J. M., Liebowitz, M. R., Fyer, A. J. *et al.* (1987). An open trial of fluoxetine in the treatment of panic attacks. *J. Clin. Psychopharmacol*, **7**, 329–332.

Gorman, J. M., Liebowitz, M. R., Fyer, A. J. *et al.* (1989). A neuroanatomical hypothesis for panic disorder. *Am. J. Psychiatry*, **146**, 148–161.

Harro, J., Kiivet, R.-A., Lang, A. and Vasar, E. (1990). Rats with anxious or nonanxious type of exploratory behavior differ in their brain CCK-8 and benzodiazepine receptor characteristics. *Behav. Brain Res.*, **39**, 63–71.

Heel, R. C., Morley, P. A., Brogden, R. N. *et al.* (1982). Zimelidine: a review of its pharmacological properties and therapeutic efficacy in depressive illness. *Drugs*, **28**, 169–206.

Hoehn-Saric, R., McLeod, D. R. and Hipsley, P. A. (1993). Effect of fluvoxamine on panic disorder. *J. Clin. Psychopharmacol.,* **13**(5), 321–326.

Hoes, M. J. A. J. M., Colla, P. and Folgering, H. (1980). Clomipramine treatment of hyperventilation syndrome. *Pharmacopsychiatry Neuropsychopharmacol.*, **13**, 25–28.

Hollander, E., Hatterer, J. and Klein, D. F. (1990). Antidepressants for the treatment of panic and agoraphobia. In *Handbook of Anxiety*, Vol. 4 (eds. R. Noyes Jr, M. Roth and G. D. Burrows), pp. 207–231. Elsevier, New York.

Howell, E. F., Laraia, M. T., Ballenger, J. C. and Lydiard, R. B. (1987). Lorazepam treatment of panic disorder. Presented at the 140th Annual Meeting of the American Psychiatric Association Meeting, Chicago, IL, 5/9–16, 1987.

Humble, M. and Wistedt, B. (1992) Serotonin, panic disorder and agoraphobia: short-term and long-term efficacy of citalopram in panic disorders. *Int. Clin. Psychopharmacol.*, **6**(5S), 21–39.

Humble, M., Koczkas, C. and Wistedt, B. Serotonin and anxiety: an open study of citalopram in panic disorder. In *Psychiatry Today: VIII World Congress of Psychiatry Abstracts* (eds C. N. Stefanis, C. R. Soldatos and A. D. Rabavilas), p. 151. Elsevier, New York.

Johnson, M. R., Lydiard, R. B., and Ballenger, J. C. (1994). Monoamine oxidase inhibitors in panic disorder and agoraphobia. In *Clinical Advances in MAOI Therapies:* Progress in Psychiatry series (ed. S. H. Kennedy). American Psychiatric Press, Washington, D. C.

Kahn, R. S., Asnis, G. M., Wetzler, S., and van Praag, H. M. (1988) Neuroendocrine evidence for serotonin receptor hypersensitivity in panic disorder. *Psychopharmacology*, **96**, 360–364.

Katschnig, H., Stolk, J., Klerman, G. *et al.* (1991). Discontinuation experiences and long-term treatment follow-up of participants in a clinical drug trial for panic disorder. In *Biological Psychiatry International Congress Series 968*, Vol.1 (eds G. Racagni, N. Brunello and T. Takuda), pp. 657–660. Elsevier, New York.

Klein, D. F. (1984) Psychopharmacologic treatment of panic disorder. *Psychosomatics*, **25**(10S), 32–35.

Klerman, G. L., Hirschfeld, R. M. A., Weissman, M. M. *et al.* (eds) (1993). *Panic Anxiety and its Treatments: A Task Force Report of the World Psychiatric Association*, p. 47. American Psychiatric Press, Washington, DC.

Koczkas, S., Holmberg, G. and Wedin, L. (1981). A pilot study of the effect of 5-HT uptake inhibitor, zimelidine, on phobic anxiety. *Acta Psychiatr. Scand.*, **64**, 1–11.

Kramer, M. S., Cutler, N. R., Ballenger, J. C. *et al.* (1995). A placebo controlled trial of L-365,260, a CCKB antagonist in panic disorder. *Biol. Psychiatry*, **37**, 462–466.

Kupfer, D. J. (1991). Lessons to be learned from long-term treatment of affective disorders: potential utility in panic disorder. *J. Clin. Psychiatry*, **52**(2S), 12–16.

Lader, M. (1991). Ondansetron in the treatment of anxiety. In *Biological Psychiatry: Proceedings of the 5th World Congress of Biological Psychiatry*, Florence, 9–14 June 1991, Vol. 2, pp. 885–887. Excerpta Medica, Amsterdam.

Liebowitz, M. R. (1993). Depression with anxiety and atypical depression. *J. Clin. Psychiatry*, **54**(2S), 10–14,

Liebowitz, M. R., Fyer, A. J., Gorman, J. M. *et al.* (1986). Alprazolam in the treatment of anxiety disorders. *J. Clin. Psychopharmacol.*, **6**, 13–20.

Lydiard, R. B. (1987). Desipramine in agoraphobia with panic attacks: an open, fixed-dose study. *J. Clin. Psychopharmacol.*, **7**, 258–260.

Lydiard, R. B. and Ballenger, J. C. (1987). Antidepressants in panic disorder and agoraphobia. *J. Affect. Disord.*, **13**, 153–168.

Lydiard, R. B. and Ballenger, J. C. (1988). Panic-related disorders: evidence for efficacy of the antidepressants. *J. Anxiety Dis.*, **2**, 77–94.

Lydiard, R. B., Ballenger, J. C., Laraia, M. T. *et al.* (1992a). CSF cholecystokinin concentrations in patients with panic disorder and in normal comparison subjects. *Am. J. Psychiatry*, **149**(5), 691–693.

Lydiard, R. B., Lesser, I. M., Ballenger, J. C. *et al.* (1992b). A fixed-dose study of alprazolam 2 mg, alprazolam 6 mg, and placebo in panic disorder. *J. Clin. Psychopharmacol.*, **12**(2), 96–103.

Mavissakalian, M. and Jones B. (1990). Comparative efficacy and interaction between drug and behavioral therapies for panic/agoraphobia. In *Handbook of Anxiety, Vol. 4: Treatment of Anxiety* (eds R. Noyes Jr, M. Roth and G. D. Burrow), pp. 73–86. Elsevier, Amsterdam.

Mavissakalian, M. and Michelson, L. (1982) Agoraphobia: behavioral and pharmacological treatment, preliminary outcome, and process findings. *Psychopharmacol. Bull.*, **18**, 91–103.

Mavissakalian, M., Michelson, L. and Dealy, R. S. (1983). Pharmacological treatment of agoraphobia: imipramine versus imipramine with programmed practice. *Br. J. Psychiatry*, **143**, 348–366.

Mavissakalian, M., Perel, J. and Michelson, L. (1984) The relationship of plasma imipramine and N-desmethylimipramine to improvement in agoraphobia. *J. Clin. Psychopharmacol.*, **4**, 36–40.

McNair, D. M. and Kahn, R. J. (1981). Imipramine compared with a benzodiazepine for agoraphobia. In *Anxiety: New Research and Changing Concepts* (eds D. F. Klein and J. G. Rabkin). Raven Press, New York.

Modigh, K., Westberg, P. and Eriksson, E. (1992). Superiority of clomipramine over imipramine in the treatment of panic disorder: a placebo-controlled trial. *J. Clin. Psychopharmacol.*, **12**, 251–261.

Mountjoy, C. Q., Roth, M., Garside, R. F. *et al.* (1977). A clinical trial of phenelzine in anxiety depressive and phobic neuroses. *Br. J. Psychiatry*, **131**, 486–492.

Murphy, D. L. and Pigott, T. A. (1990). A comparative examination of a role for serotonin in obsessive compulsive disorder, panic disorder, and anxiety. *J. Clin. Psychiatry*, **51**(4S), 53–58.

Nagy, L. M., Krystal, J. H., Woods, S. W. *et al.* (1989). Clinical and medication outcome after short-term alprazolam and behavioral group treatment in panic disorder: 2.5-year naturalistic follow-up study. *Arch. Gen. Psychiatry*, **41**, 993–999.

Nilsson, B. S. (1983). Adverse reactions in connection with zimelidine treatment: a review. *Acta Psychiatr. Scand. Suppl.*, **308**, 115–119.

Noyes, R., Jr, Garvey, M. G., Cook, B. L. *et al.* (1989). Problems with tricyclic antidepressant use in patients with panic disorder or agoraphobia: results of a naturalistic follow-up study. *J. Clin. Psychiatry*, **60**, 163–169.

Noyes, R., Jr, Reich, J., Christiansen, J. *et al.* (1990). Outcome of panic disorder: relationship to diagnostic subtypes and comorbidity. *Arch. Gen. Psychiatry*, **47**, 809–818,

Pecknold, J. C. (1990). Discontinuation studies: short-term and long-term treatment. Presented at the Panic Awareness for the Clinician Conference, Carlsbad, CA, November 29, 1990.

Pecknold, J. C., Swinson, R. P., Kuch, *et al.* (1988). Alprazolam in panic disorder and agoraphobia: results from a multicenter trial, III. Discontinuation effects. *Arch. Gen. Psychiatry*, **45**, 429–436.

Pecknold, J. Alexander, P. E. and Munjack, D. (1993). Alprazolam-XR in the management of anxiety: discontinuation. *Psychiatr. Ann.*, **23**, 38–44.

Pollack, M. H., Tesar, G. E., Rosenbaum, J. F. and Spier, S. A. (1986). Clonazepam in the treatment of panic disorder and agoraphobia: a one-year follow-up. *J. Clin. Psychopharmacol.*, **6**, 302–304.

Quitkin, F. M., McGrath, P. J., Stewart, J. W. *et al.* (1990) Atypical depression, panic attacks, and response to imipramine and phenelzine: a replication. *Arch. Gen. Psychiatry*, **47**, 935–941.

Rickels, K. (1990) Discontinuation studies with alprazolam (abstract). *J. Psychiatr. Res.*, **23**(1S), 57–58.

Rickels, K., Schweizer, B., Case, W. G. and Greenblatt, D. J. (1990). Long-term therapeutic use of benzodiazepines. I. Effects of abrupt discontinuation. *Arch. Gen. Psychiatry*, **47**, 899–907.

Rickels, K., Schweizer, E., Weiss, S. *et al.* (1993). Maintenance drug treatment for panic disorder. II. Short- and long-term outcome after drug taper. *Arch. Gen. Psychiatry*, **50**, 61–68.

Rizley, R., Kahn, R. J., McNair, D. M. and Frankenthaler, L. M. (1986). A comparison of alprazolam and imipramine in the treatment of agoraphobia and panic disorder. *Psychopharmacol. Bull.*, **22**, 167–172.

Schatzberg, A. F. and Ballenger, J. C. (1991). Decisions for the clinician in the treatment of panic disorder: when to treat, which treatment to use, and how long to treat. *J. Clin. Psychiatry*, **54**(S), 26–31.

Schneier, F. R., Liebowitz, M. R., Davies, S. O. *et al.* (1990). Fluoxetine in panic disorder. *J. Clin. Psychopharmacol.* **10**, 119–121.

Schweizer, E., Rickels, K., Case, W. G. and Greenblatt, D. J. (1990). Long-term therapeutic use of benzodiazepines. II. Effects of gradual taper. *Arch. Gen. Psychiatry*, **47**(10),

908–915.

Sellers, E. M., Ciraulo, D. A., DuPont, R. L. *et al.* (1993). Alprazolam and benzodiazepine dependence. *J. Clin. Psychiatry*, **54**, 64–75.

Sheehan, D. V., Ballenger, J. and Jacobsen, G. (1980). Treatment of endogenous anxiety with phobic, hysterical and hypochondriacal symptoms. *Arch. Gen. Psychiatry*, **37**, 61–69.

Solyom, L., Heseltine, G. F. D., McClure, D. J. *et al.* (1973) Behavior therapy versus drug therapy in the treatment of phobic neurosis. *Can. Psychiatr. Assoc. J.*, **18**, 26–32.

Solyom, C., Solyom, L., LaPierre, Y. *et al.* (1981). Phenelzine and exposure in the treatment of phobias. *Biol. Psychiatry,* **16**, 230–247.

Targum, S. D. and Marshall, L. E. (1989). Fenfluramine provocation of anxiety in patients with panic disorder. *Psychiatry Res.*, **28**, 295–306.

Tesar, G. E. and Rosenbaum, F. J. (1985). Successful use of clonazepam in patients with treatment-resistant panic disorder. *J. Nerv. Ment. Dis.*, **174**, 477–482.

Tyrer, P., Candy, J. and Kelly, D. (1973). A study of the clinical effects of phenelzine and placebo in the treatment of phobic anxiety. *Psychopharmacologia*, **32**, 237–264.

Versiani, M., Gentile, V., Paprocki, J. *et al.* (1985). Data about 508 cases of panic disorder and responses to treatment with alprazolam, clomipramine, imipramine, and tranyl-cypromine. In *Biological Psychiatry: Proceedings from the IVth World Congress of Biological Psychiatry* (eds C. Shagass, R. D. Josiassen, W. H. Bridger *et al.*). Elsevier, Amsterdam.

Weissman, M. M., Klerman, G. L., Markowitz, J. S. and Ouellette R. (1989). Suicidal ideation and suicide attempts in panic disorder and attacks. *N. Engl. J. Med.*, **321**, 1209–1214.

Westenberg, H. G. M. and Den Boer, J. A. (1989). Serotonin-influencing drugs in the treatment of panic disorder. *Psychopathology*, **22**(S1), 68–77.

Woods, S., Black, D., Brown, S. *et al.* (1994). Fluvoxamine in the treatment of panic disorder in outpatients: a double-blind, placebo-controlled study. Poster presented at the annual meeting of the College of International Neuropsychopharmacology, Washington, D. C.

Zitrin, C. M., Klein, D. F., Woerner, M. G. *et al.* (1983). Treatment of phobias. I. Comparison of imipramine hydrochloride and placebo. *Arch. Gen. Psychiatry*, **40**, 126–138.

Part III

OBSESSIVE-COMPULSIVE DISORDER

11 Animal Models of Obsessive-compulsive Disorder

MARGARET ALTEMUS AND DENNIS L. MURPHY
Laboratory of Clinical Science, National Institute of Mental Health, Bethesda, Maryland, USA

ANIMAL MODEL THEORY

Despite the recent surge of interest in obsessive-compulsive disorder (OCD) and a wide range of research studies, the specific pathophysiology of the illness is poorly understood. OCD is currently classified as an anxiety disorder in DSM-IV (American Psychiatric Association, 1994) and anxiety ratings in OCD patients equal those of patients with other anxiety disorders (Murphy *et al.*, 1990). Although there is a high degree of comorbidity of OCD with other anxiety disorders, OCD is distinguished by the presence of repetitive thoughts or obsessions and repetitive behaviors or compulsions. The most common obsessions in OCD patients concern contamination, unchecked dangers, symmetry, and incompleteness; patients also often describe intrusive violent and sexual thoughts. The most common compulsions are washing and cleaning, checking, hoarding, counting and other mental rituals, arranging, repeating movements and touching. These particular obsessions and compulsions seem to be similar across cultures (Akhtar *et al.*, 1975; Hinjo *et al.*, 1989; Khanna and Channabasavanna, 1987; Okasha *et al.*, 1994; Weissman *et al.*, 1994) Performance of compulsions is usually associated with a temporary reduction in anxiety, and attempts to resist performance of compulsions usually are associated with worsening of anxiety and obsessions. Twenty to thirty percent of OCD patients have no response to current standard pharmacological treatment with serotonin reuptake inhibitors, and those patients who do respond generally experience only partial relief of symptoms (McDougle *et al.*, 1993; Greist *et al.*, 1995).

Because techniques for examining central nervous system function in humans are limited, animal models of OCD may be useful in furthering our understanding of the pathophysiology of the illness and in developing new treatments. Specifically, animal models may allow investigation of neurochem-

Advances in the Neurobiology of Anxiety Disorders. Edited by H. G. M. Westenberg, J. A. Den Boer and D. L. Murphy
©1996 John Wiley & Sons Ltd

ical abnormalities, receptor adaptations, and other functional or structural changes in brain systems associated with repetitive behaviors. In addition because the illness responds selectively to serotonin reuptake inhibitors (Murphy *et al.*, this volume), identification of behaviors and neural processes which are differentially affected by serotonin-selective antidepressants may also shed light on the disorder.

It is very doubtful that an exact animal model can be found for any psychiatric syndrome. To be useful, however, an animal model need not reproduce all of the signs, symptoms, pathophysiology, and treatment response characteristics of a human disorder (Guttmacher *et al.*, 1983; Henn and McKinney, 1987). Different animal models of OCD may shed light on different aspects of the disorder. Moreover, it is doubtful that a single consistent pathology underlies all cases of OCD. Animal models actually may help to define clinical subgroups which are differentiated by phenomenology, comorbidity or treatment response. For example, OCD associated with motor tics is more common in males, more strongly familial, presents at a younger age and has a better response to neuroleptic augmentation of serotonin reuptake inhibitor treatment (Swedo *et al.*, 1992a; McDougle *et al.*, 1994; Pauls *et al.*, 1995).

Henn and McKinney have identified four categories of animal models of psychiatric illness: phenomenological, etiologic, physiological, and drug response models (Henn and McKinney, 1987). Some proposed animal models of OCD may be considered under more than one of these four categories.

Phenomenological models

Models which simulate behaviors or symptoms associated with OCD and other repetitive behavior syndromes may be used to examine potential associated physiological mechanisms and to test etiologic theories. If neurobiological abnormalities associated with the model are identified, they may be evaluated in clinical studies to determine their possible relevance to the human disorder.

There are multiple examples of species-typical animal behaviors such as grooming or nesting which are inappropriately expressed after environmental or pharmacological manipulation and appear analogous to the repetitive intentional motor acts (checking, washing, hoarding) characteristic of OCD. In addition, several pharmacologic agents and a few specific brain lesions seem to enhance expression of repetitive behaviors in animals. Inappropriately repetitive expression of species-typical behaviors in animals has been labeled by researchers in different disciplines as stereotypy, displacement behavior and adjunctive behavior. These terms will be used interchangeably in this review. Of course an animal model will never be able to reproduce human mental experiences such as intrusive thoughts or cognitively elaborated obsessions, but the experience of fear, preoccupation, or uncertainty in an animal may be indirectly observable through facial expressions and behaviors.

Models meeting the criteria of phenomenological similarity have face validity for OCD. Although these models are intuitively appealing, the methods used to produce repetitive behaviors in these animal models, i.e., environmental manipulations, drug administration, lesions, and use of susceptible strains, may not necessarily correspond to etiologic factors in the human disorder. Moreover, the neurobiological processes underlying these behaviors in animals may not correspond to the pathophysiology in humans and may not respond to the same treatment regimens. In other words, these models may have face validity but not necessarily construct or predictive validity.

Etiologic models

Animal models may also be designed specifically to test etiologic theories. If successful, such models would have construct validity. OCD probably does not have a single etiology, and different variables may be more or less important in different individuals. The advantage of using animal models to test etiologic theories is that potential etiologic variable can be manipulated while other developmental, social and biological variables are kept relatively constant. Proposed etiologic mechanisms which could be tested in this type of model include candidate genes, autoimmune pathology, neuropeptide, neurotransmitter and hormonal abnormalities, and the importance of stress and avoidance learning.

Physiological models

Animal models may also be designed to study biological or physiological mechanisms thought to play a role in expression or maintenance of the disorder. Such models, if correct, would have construct validity. Some of these models may not resemble phenomenologically the actual illness but could nevertheless help to sort out functional interactions of anatomic systems. For example, certain neurotransmitter pathways may be shown to stimulate particular patterns of basal ganglia activation, or feedback systems may be identified which normally act to restrain activated motor or limbic pathways.

Drug response models

Finally, animal models may be developed to mimic or predict clinical pharmacologic effectiveness. If such models are able to distinguish effective and ineffective agents for OCD treatment, they have predictive validity. Outcome measures in these tests may be quite different from the actual phenomenology of OCD. Thus these models may have predictive validity but not construct or face validity. Also despite the need for chronic treatment in OCD, predictive validity in some animal models may be found based on acute pharmacological treatment effects. Attempts to model repetitive behaviors, as well as other behaviors which respond preferentially to serotonin reuptake blockers, may have relevance for a broad range of disorders in addition to OCD. Recent studies suggest beneficial effects of serotonin reuptake blockers in the treatment of stereotypies in individuals with autism, mental retardation, and schizophrenia as well as in the treatment of stuttering, nail-biting, trichotillomania, self-mutilation syndromes, and anorexia nervosa (Swedo et al., 1989c; Gwirtsman et al., 1990; Markowitz 1990; Leonard et al., 1991; Kaye et al., 1992; Winchel et al., 1992; Gordon et al., 1993, 1995; Zohar et al., 1993).

A major limitation of animal models of OCD and repetitive behaviors is the possibility that findings may not generalize to the human disorder. Species differences in the metabolism and neurobiological effects of drugs and in the function of neuropeptides, neurotransmitters and anatomical systems are also significant stumbling blocks. As Willner stated in a review of animal models of psychiatric illness, "The major contribution of animal models may well be that they encourage clinicians to apply a similar rigor to the analysis of disordered behavior" (Willner, 1991).

ANIMAL MODELS OF OBSESSIVE-COMPULSIVE DISORDER/REPETITIVE BEHAVIORS

NATURALISTIC MODELS

Phenomenology–etiology

A number of ethological models in which repetitive behaviors occur in response to environmental stimuli have been described and may be used to test etiologic theories and identify neurophysiological mechanisms possibly associated with OCD in humans. Recent studies suggest that some of these ethological models also may be used to predict pharmacological efficacy.

Learning theory defines the compulsive rituals of OCD in humans as reinforced avoidance behaviors performed in response to anxiety-provoking stimuli. Performance of compulsions reduces anxiety and this in turn is thought to be experienced as reinforcement, thus strengthening the compulsive response and allowing it to generalize to other anxiety-provoking stimuli (Rachman and Hodgson, 1980). Traditional psychodynamic understanding of OCD also has emphasized the defensive nature of compulsions as an aid to manage frightening thoughts or impulses (Freud, 1959). These psychological processes in humans seem to be analogous to the tendency of animals to develop displacement behaviors or stereotypies in response to stressors such as novelty, environmental deprivation, conflict over territory, and frustration of appetitive drives (Skinner, 1948; Maier, 1949; Tinbergen, 1953; Hediger, 1955; Lorenz, 1981; Dantzer, 1986b; Swedo, 1989; Leuscher et al., 1991; Mason, 1991).

Displacement behaviors and environmentally induced stereotypies in animals are inappropriate expressions of adaptive, often innate, behaviors such as grooming, territorial displays, attack behavior, chewing, vocalization, pacing, freezing, foraging, and nest-building. Normal, functional expressions of these behaviors are provoked by environmental stimuli and internal developmental and hormonal events. Displacement or stereotypy refers to expression of these behaviors in an excessive, repetitive fashion which serves no apparent purpose. Related phenomena, "adjunctive behaviors", can be induced by administering reward on a regular schedule while the animal is in a state of partial deprivation for food or water (Falk, 1971; Staddon, 1977). Adjunctive behaviors include excessive water-drinking (Falk, 1961), attack behaviors (Flory, 1969), wheel-running (Epling et al., 1983; Rieg et al., 1993), grooming (Lawler and Cohen, 1988) and licking at an air stream (Mendelson and Chillag, 1970). Available stimuli are the major determinant of the type of stereotypy which develops in many adjunctive and displacement paradigms (Wayner, 1974). In addition, particular types of displacement behaviors are more likely to occur in certain species and breeds of animals. Doberman pinschers are more prone to flank-sucking, tail-chewing is more commonly seen in German shepherds, and wool-chewing is seen only in Siamese cats (Leuscher et al., 1991). Only small foraging animals seem to develop excessive wheel-running. As in humans with OCD, displacement behavior in animals can be reduced by removal of the conflict or frustration, by distracting the animal with a more urgent task or stimulus and by providing for expression of more alternative behaviors (Leuscher et al., 1991).

Displacement behaviors or stereotypies can be simple movements such as licking or may involve relatively complex motor sequences. Many of these behaviors closely resemble the compulsive behaviors demonstrated by humans with OCD (Holland, 1974; Pitman, 1989; Swedo, 1989). For example, grooming stereotypies mimic washing rituals, nesting behavior is similar to hoarding compulsions, and territorial displays resemble arranging and ordering compulsions. Another similarity to human OCD symptoms is that, once initiated, displacement behaviors continue to completion. However, because displacement behavior and stereotypies are so species-specific it may be unreasonable to expect a close homology between animal behaviors and human behaviors. Even stereotypies like tail-chasing which do not resemble human symptoms, still may provide useful models of pathophysiology.

In humans with OCD there is a wide variation in symptoms among individuals. However, the most common OCD symptoms in humans can be grouped under a relatively small number of themes which are consistent across cultures (Akhtar et al., 1975; Khanna and Channabasavanna, 1987; Hinjo et al., 1989; Okasha et al., 1994; Weissman et al., 1994). These concerns—contamination, protection against aggression, territoriality, and hoarding—seem to be basic to survival and to be phylogenetically adaptive. Studies have found that in humans with phobias or OCD, the content of phobias and obsessions most commonly involves objects that posed a threat for early primates and humans, i.e. spiders, snakes and enclosed spaces, and less commonly involves objects which are dangerous in current society such as cars, high-tension wires or knives and guns

(Seligman, 1971; DeSilva *et al.*, 1977). Further support for the notion of biologically or evolutionarily based predispositions to acquire certain fears comes from studies showing that laboratory-reared rhesus monkeys can be taught to fear toy snakes but they cannot be taught to fear flowers by observing edited video tapes of monkeys meeting fearfully to flowers by observing video tapes of wild-reared monkeys reacting fearfully to snakes (Mineka and Cook, 1993).

Several studies demonstrate aspects of the development of displacement behaviors which may be relevant to the generalization of OCD symptoms in humans. Displacement behaviors or stereotypies that are initially expressed in response to a specific situation may become generalized to any stressful or arousal-producing situation or even be expressed without any clear stimulus (Davenport and Menzel, 1963; Stolba *et al.*, 1983). Similarly, rats which learn an avoidance response to reduce fear or frustration may express that same response when experiencing frustration or fear in a different situation (Ross, 1964; Rescorla and LoLordo, 1965; Amsel and Rashotte, 1969). Restricted opportunities for expression of more complex alternative behaviors would increase the likelihood of generalization of displacement behaviors (Dantzer, 1986). The avoidance-learning literature also indicates that the frequency of occurrence of avoidance responses is enhanced in paradigms where the aversive stimulus appears without warning (Sidman, 1955; Teasdale, 1974). Although beyond the scope of this review, Mineka (1985) extends this work by discussing the use of displacement models to study the mechanism of action of behavioral treatment for OCD.

Consistent with the familial nature of OCD in humans (Pauls *et al.*, 1995), some kindreds within a species or strain are more prone to develop stereotypies. Inherited temperament traits such as avoidance, sensitivity to novelty and excitability (MacKenzie *et al.*, 1986) may contribute to the expression of displacement behaviors within a species (Vecchiotti and Galant, 1986; Dallaire, 1993). Examining neurobiological differences between strains or between animals within a strain that are prone to stereotypies and those that are more resistant may be a fruitful avenue of research.

Finally, as in humans with OCD, increases in generalized arousal in animals seem to increase performance of displacement behaviors. A variety of arousing environmental stimuli can set off stereotypies in domestic animals, zoo animals and laboratory animals (Dantzer, 1986; Odberg, 1987; Mason, 1991). Consistent with the importance of a sense of danger or threat, autogrooming stereotypies are performed more frequently by socially subordinate rats and primates (Goosen, 1974; Raab *et al.*, 1986).

A number of ethologists have suggested that ritualized display may reduce the tension associated with arousal, conflict or frustration and thereby have a rewarding reinforcement effect (Tinbergen, 1953; Dantzer, 1983; Delius, 1988). Behaviors like grooming may be associated with soothing memories of early maternal care or, alternatively, performance of stereotypies may isolate the animal from disturbing internal or external stimuli. A few observations in animals support this hypothesis. Rats exposed to inescapable shock had less pituitary–adrenal axis activation if given the opportunity to fight with another animal (Conner *et al.*, 1971). In another study, calves which displayed tongue-rolling had less severe stomach ulcers than calves which did not perform this stereotypy (Wiepkema, 1987).

Physiological mechanisms

There has been some investigation of the neurobiological substrates of these naturalistic inductions of displacement behaviors and stereotypies. Lesion studies have implicated mesolimbic dopamine reward systems in the generation of a variety of adjunctive and displacement behaviors. The mesolimbic dopaminergic systems originate in the ventral tegmental area and innervate forebrain limbic areas including the nucleus accumbens, striatum and frontal cortex. In one study, mesolimbic 6-hydroxydopamine (6-OHDA) lesions prevented development of adjunctive drinking without affecting drinking in response to water deprivation (Robbins and Koob, 1980). Hoarding of food pellets by rats also has been prevented by 6-OHDA lesions of the mesolimbic, but not other dopaminergic subsystems, and restored by administration of the dopamine precursor *l*-dopa (Blundell *et al.*, 1977; Kelley and Stinus, 1985). Furthermore, some stereotypies in animals have responded to treatment with dopamine antagonists (Cools and Van Rossum, 1970; Wise, 1982; Odberg *et al.*, 1987) and dopamine depletion (Odberg *et al.*, 1987).

It is unclear from these studies, however, whether mesolimbic dopamine systems play a role in determining the repetitive nature of displacement behaviors and stereotypies. Mesolimbic dopamine systems may be necessary only to generate the motivational force or arousal needed to develop and maintain stereotypies. One proposed explanation of adjunctive behaviors is that during conditions of food restriction the motivational excitement induced by food presentation is not relieved by satiety or feedback from adequate food consumption so the motivational excitement is directed toward other stimuli (Lawrence and Terlouw, 1993). In support of this model, brief encounters with reinforcers such as food have been shown to increase activity (Killeen *et al.*, 1978). Moreover, stereotypic behavior occurs much more commonly in large farm animals and fowl if food intake is restricted (Appleby and Lawrence, 1987; Savoy *et al.*, 1992), and it occurs predominantly in the postprandial period (Rushen, 1984).

A role for serotonergic processes in displacement behavior is suggested by the work of Jacobs and coworkers using electrophysiologic recording which documented that a subgroup of neurons in the dorsal raphe nucleus in cats is activated when the animal repetitively licks, chews, bites or grooms with its mouth. Firing of these neurons is not affected by environmental or metabolic challenges which activate noradrenergic systems. These findings raise the possibility that repetitive behaviors may function to correct deficits in serotonergic firing or to increase serotonergic firing to correct other dysfunctional systems

(Jacobs *et al.*, 1990; Jacobs, 1993). Changes in serotonergic function also have been noted in an environmentally induced adjunctive behavior model of OCD. In this model, known as 'schedule-induced polydipsia', hungry rats exposed to the periodic presentation of small pellets of food, with regular temporal delay, develop persistent, excessive drinking (Falk, 1961). In the brains of animals who developed this syndrome, binding of a ligand for the serotonin transporter was substantially reduced (Roehr *et al.*, 1995).

There is also evidence that gonadal hormones may play a role in induction of displacement behaviors in animals and in OCD symptoms in humans. Onset of symptoms during puberty is common in both humans with OCD, dogs with acral lick dermatitis (Rapoport *et al.*, 1992) and wool-sucking Siamese cats (Leuscher *et al.*, 1991). In humans, pregnancy seems to be another time of increased risk for onset of OCD (Nezeroglu *et al.*, 1992). Sows also have been noted to have increased amounts of stereotypies during pregnancy (Cronin and Wiepkema, 1984). OCD behaviors during pregnancy in humans may be an exaggeration of adaptive nesting behaviors which occur during pregnancy in humans and other species. Further support for the role of gonadal steroids comes from several case reports of decreases in OCD symptoms following blockade of gonadal hormone activity (Casas *et al.*, 1986; Leonard, 1989).

Drug treatment response

Several recent studies have found preferential improvement in displacement behavior after chronic treatment with serotonin reuptake blockers compared to treatment with non-serotonin selective antidepressants, further strengthening the similarity of these phenomena to OCD in humans. Canine acral lick in dogs may be the best-studied displacement behavior as a model for drug treatment response in OCD. Also known as lick granuloma, the condition occurs mainly in Labrador retrievers, setters, Great Danes and German shepherds, and within these breeds vulnerability seems to run in families. Dogs with this disorder lick the lower anterior portion of the leg excessively, which leads to localized alopecia and granulomatous lesions (Rapoport *et al.*, 1992). There is a sense that the condition is exacerbated by stress, but this has not been studied systematically. The disorder responds to chronic treatment with clomipramine, fluoxetine, and sertraline, but not fenfluramine or desipramine, paralleling the treatment results in humans with OCD (Rapoport *et al.*, 1992).

Two other forms of adjunctive behavior have also been shown to be selectively responsive to treatment with serotonin reuptake blockers. Schedule-induced polydypsia was reversed by chronic treatment with serotonin reuptake blocking agents, but not by non-serotonin selective antidepressants, benzodiazepines (Woods *et al.*, 1993) or naloxone (Cooper and Holtzman, 1983). Furthermore, neuroleptic treatment suppressed the behavior (Sanger and Blackman, 1978; Woods *et al.*, 1993), consistent with reports of relief of human OCD symptoms after addition of neuroleptic agents to serotonin reuptake blockers and with relief of repetitive behaviors by neuroleptic treatment in Tourette's syndrome (McDougle *et al.*, 1994).

In another adjunctive behavior paradigm, rats which are food-restricted and given access to a running wheel develop severe weight loss, excessive wheel-running and a paradoxical decrease in food intake often leading to death (Epling *et al.*, 1983). This syndrome also appears to be differentially responsive to chronic treatment with a serotonin reuptake blocker compared to a less selective tricyclic antidepressant. In addition, development of the syndrome was exacerbated by treatment for 10 days with PCPA, a serotonin-depleting agent (Altemus *et al.*, 1996).

Anxiolytic drugs seem to reduce novelty-induced grooming (Moody *et al.*, 1988) but are ineffective at reducing more inappropriately expressed and more maladaptive stereotypies such as canine acral lick or adjunctive running or drinking. These findings are consistent with the lack of response of OCD patients to benzodiazepine treatment. There also have been reports of opiate blockade leading to attenuation of development of stereotypies, but not reduced expression of stereotypies once they are established (Feldman, 1962; Cronin *et al.*, 1985; Dodman *et al.*, 1987; Kennes *et al.*, 1988).

DRUG-INDUCED MODELS

Administration of a number of pharmacologic agents is associated with the expression of stereotypies and displacement behaviors. All of these agents enhance arousal, and it is unclear whether any of these agents act specifically to induce repetitive behaviors or whether enhanced expression of repetitive behaviors after drug treatment is due simply to increased general arousal. Another problem with drug-induced models of OCD is that the induced stereotypies are typically of short duration and not problematic for functioning of the animal. It may be informative to examine differences between strains of rodents which are more or less prone to developing stereotypies when aroused.

Dopaminergic agents

Chronic amphetamine use in humans can lead to complex repetitive behaviors resembling compulsive rituals including checking and skin picking (Lowe *et al.*, 1982; Koizumi, 1985; Fishman, 1987), but these are not clearly related to concerns about contamination or danger. Dopaminergic exacerbation of symptoms is more clear in Tourette's syndrome and tic disorders (Valenstein, 1980) and dopamine antagonists are a primary method of treatment of these disorders. While neuroleptics alone are not effective treatments for OCD, treatment response to serotonin reuptake inhibitors in the subgroup of OCD patients with comorbid tic disorders seems to be augmented by dopamine blocking agents (McDougle *et al.*, 1994).

In animals, stimulation of ascending dopaminergic tracts or administration of dopamine agonists or amphetamine reliably produces stereotyped behaviors

(Wilner *et al.*, 1970; Creese and Iverson, 1974; Kelley *et al.*, 1988). Like environmentally induced displacement behaviors, stereotypies provoked by amphetamine vary according to species (Randrup and Munkvad, 1967; Ellinwood and Kilbey, 1975).

Disruption of the normal spontaneous alternation of choice of arms in a T-maze by adult rats has also been used as a model of the indecision characteristic of OCD (Yadin *et al.*, 1991). A selective dopamine D_1 receptor agonist has been reported to inhibit spontaneous alternation and to produce a vacillatory behavior at the choice point in neonatal rats (Molino *et al.*, 1989), following which appropriate decision-making can be restored by simultaneous acute administration of clomipramine and 5-HT_{1A} agonists but not benzodiazepines (Whitaker-Azmitia *et al.*, 1990). One explanation of the age dependency of this model is that modulatory systems which protect the animal from the effects of D_1 receptor stimulation are not yet in place. There also has been a report of induction of perseverative patterns of exploration by the D_2 agonist quinpirole (Eilam *et al.*, 1989).

Serotonergic agents

OCD patients seem to experience exacerbation of OCD symptoms with acute administration of *m*-chlorophenylpiperazine (mCPP) (Zohar *et al.*, 1987; Pigott *et al.*, 1993), a 5-HT_{2C} agonist, which does not occur after administration of other anxiogenic agents or stimulants (Gorman *et al.*, 1985; Rasmussen *et al.*, 1987; Griez *et al.*, 1990). This selective action of mCPP in OCD suggests a specific role for the 5-HT_{2C} subsystem in exacerbation of OCD (Murphy *et al.*, this volume). However, *de novo* production of obsessive or compulsive symptoms does not occur after mCPP administration in normals or in patients with other psychiatric illnesses. Normals given mCPP experience generalized anxiety or activation/euphoria and patients with panic disorder experience increases in panic symptoms (Kahn *et al.*, 1988; Murphy *et al.*, 1991). Patients with other psychiatric disorders which are characterized by hypoarousal, such as seasonal affective disorder and premenstrual syndrome, may actually experience a reduction in symptoms with mCPP (Joseph-Vanderpool *et al.*, 1993; Jacobsen *et al.*, 1994; Su *et al.*, 1994). Together these mCPP data suggest that the 5-HT_{2C} subsystem modulates emotional arousal and anxiety but may not necessarily play a specific role in generation of obsessions or compulsions. It may be a general "anxiogenic" effect of mCPP in OCD that stimulates worsening of OCD symptoms, and mCPP may be more effective than other challenge agents because it generates more anxiety than other agents in OCD patients. Currently, however, there is no available data to support this speculation.

Administration of 5-HT_{2C} agonists to rats and mice produces effects which resemble the challenge responses seen in OCD patients. The 5-HT_{2C} agonists mCPP and trifluoromethylphenylpiperazine (TFMPP) appear to be anxiogenic in rodents (Kennett *et al.*, 1989; Curzon *et al.*, 1991) and can induce stereotypic chewing behaviors in adult rats while 5-HT_{1A} agonists do not (Stewart *et al.*,

1989). mCPP and TFMPP are also the only serotonin agonists which increase grooming and produce stereotyped oral movements in rat pups (Jackson and Kitchen, 1989). There is some evidence from microdialysis studies that 5-HT_{2C} agonists also facilitate dopamine release in the striatum (Benloucif and Galloway, 1991), which possibly could mediate production of stereotypies after 5-HT_{2C} agonist administration.

In the spontaneous alternation model of OCD, acute administration of a nonselective serotonin agonist, 5-methoxy-N,N-dimethyltryptamine, and a more selective 5-HT_{1A} agonist, 8-hydroxy-2-(di-n-propylamino)tetralin (8-OH-DPAT), both disrupted spontaneous alternation, producing more perseverative choices of arms of the T-maze (Yadin et al., 1991). Chronic administration of the serotonin reuptake inhibitor fluoxetine reduced the amount of disruption of spontaneous alternation produced by 5-HT_{1A} agonists, an effect suggested to be due to downregulation of 5-HT_{1A} receptors (Yadin et al., 1991). This model of OCD is limited by observations that a number of other pharmacological agents have been shown to disrupt spontaneous alternation, and it is unclear whether protection from disruption of spontaneous alternation is specific to treatment with serotonin reuptake blockers or whether it would occur after chronic administration of non-serotonin-selective antidepressants. Other serotonergic manipulations, including parachloroamphetamine and parachlorophenylalanine, and serotonin depletion with administration of the serotonin antagonist methysergide, did not disrupt or enhance spontaneous alternation (Yadin et al., 1991).

Neuropeptides

Recent reports suggest that some stress-responsive, arousal-producing neuropeptides, i.e. corticotropin-releasing hormone, vasopressin and somatostatin, are secreted in larger amounts into the cerebrospinal fluid of patients with OCD (Kruesi et al., 1990; Altemus et al., 1992b, 1993) and are reduced by pharmacologic treatment (DeBellis et al., 1993; Altemus et al., 1994). Vasopressin and somatostatin activity may be differentially inhibited by this class of antidepressants (Kakigi et al., 1990; Altemus et al., 1992a), suggesting that hypersecretion of these peptides may be associated with the selective response of OCD to serotonin reuptake inhibitors.

A number of displacement behaviors can be elicited in animals by central administration of these peptides. Neuropeptide-induced grooming has been studied most extensively. Grooming similar to that seen in novel environments can be elicited or exacerbated by central administration of several arousal-producing neuropeptides, including adrenocorticotropic hormone, somatostatin, corticotropin-releasing hormone and vasopressin (Dunn et al., 1979; Winslow and Insel, 1991; Spruijt et al., 1992). Central administration of these peptides also enhances the expression of other behaviors associated with stress and activates the sympathetic nervous system (Koob, 1991). Thus, in addition to activating the animal behaviorally to cope with stress these peptides may also initiate the process of dearousal through grooming and other displacement behaviors and thus model a possible sustaining physiological mechanism observed in OCD.

The responses of peptide-induced grooming to pharmacologic manipulation resembles the responses of novelty-induced grooming to pharmacologic manipulations. In both conditions, grooming is decreased by opiate antagonists and enhanced by morphine. γ-Aminobutyric acid (GABA) agonists and 5-HT$_{1A}$ agonists both also reduce novelty and adrenocorticotropic hormone-induced grooming (Spruijt et al., 1992), highlighting the non-specific arousal aspects of the behavior. Adrenocorticotropic hormone-induced grooming has also been blocked by administration of dopamine antagonists systemically and into the striatum and exacerbated by apomorphine (Traber et al., 1988). A specific D$_1$ receptor antagonist also blocked vasopressin-induced grooming in rats (Guild and Dunn, 1982; Van Wimersma-Greidanus et al., 1989). Finally, destruction of serotonergic neurons seems to increase corticotropin grooming (Lucki and Kucharick, 1988).

Flank-marking in hamsters, which can be induced by central vasopressin administration, is another potential behavioral model of OCD. The behavior is stereotyped, lasting 5–6 min and consists of grooming of the flank glands and rubbing the glands against objects in the environment in a characteristic posture. The behavior functions as a communication of dominance and territoriality (Ferris et al., 1986, 1990).

Modulation of cocaine-induced stereotypies by neuropeptides has also been examined. Central administration of oxytocin, a peptide which often has behavioral effects which oppose those of vasopressin, produced a dose-dependent attenuation of cocaine-induced stereotypies, while vasopressin tended to augment cocaine-induced stereotyped behaviors (Sarnyai et al., 1991).

BRAIN LESION MODELS

Two lines of evidence—functional brain imaging studies and associations of OCD with specific neurological disorders—suggest possible localization of OCD-related changes to specific brain regions.

Neuroimaging studies using positron emission tomography (PET) scanning to measure cerebral metabolic rate, while not completely consistent, generally demonstrate hyperactivity of the caudate nucleus as well as orbital prefrontal and cingulate cortices in OCD patients (Baxter and Brodie, this volume; Baxter et al., 1986; Nordahl et al., 1989; Swedo et al., 1989b; Benkelfat et al., 1990). These abnormalities in OCD patients do not seem to be associated with morphological changes since magnetic resonance imaging studies have failed to detect any consistent abnormalities seem to (Garber et al., 1989; Kellner et al., 1991). In addition, the PET scan abnormalities seem to resolve after pharmacologic or behavioral treatment of OCD (Benkelfat et al., 1990; Baxter et al., 1992; Swedo et al., 1992b) and increase during symptom provocation (Rauch et al., 1994). At this point, it is unclear if these changes are specific to OCD or whether other anxiety states may be associated with similar changes.

Associations between obsessive-compulsive symptoms and motor tic and choreiform disorders linked to basal ganglia pathology have been described for more than 100 years (de la Tourette, 1885; Schilder, 1938; Devinsky, 1983; Rapoport and Wise, 1988; Insel, 1992) and more recently linked in controlled comorbidity (Swedo et al., 1989a; Leonard et al., 1993) and family studies (Pauls et al., 1995; Lenane et al., 1990).

Researchers in this area have proposed an anatomically based "dysfunctional circuit" model to integrate the observed abnormalities from imaging studies in OCD patients with the known functions, anatomical interconnections and neuro-pharmacology of the implicated brain areas (Rapoport and Wise, 1988; Stahl, 1988; Modell et al., 1989; Pitman, 1989; Insel, 1992). Uncertainty regarding the functional role of some of the identified neurotransmitters and structures has led to some differences in the proposed models.

The basal ganglia are subcortical nuclei (caudate, putamen and globus pallidus) closely associated with cortical and limbic structures. The basal ganglia are hypothesized to be sites for integration of information from sensory, association and limbic cortex areas and subsequent control and sequencing of specific directed behavioral responses as well as inhibition of unwanted or inappropriate responses. Alexander et al. (1986) reviews evidence that the basal ganglia consist of at least five parallel, segregated anatomical circuits or loops connecting specific areas of the basal ganglia, thalamic nuclei and cortical areas. The most well known, more lateral, loops have been demonstrated to play an important role in the modulation of motor activity. Two more medial circuits have been identified in anatomic and physiologic studies which may be particularly relevant to OCD. In the first of the two circuits, the lateral orbitofrontal cortex projects to the ventromedial caudate, then to the dorsomedial pallidum, then to medial parts of the thalamus and back to the lateral orbitofrontal cortex. An additional anatomical loop has been proposed linking the anterior cingulate, amygdala, hippocampus and some areas of temporal cortex and posterior medial orbitofrontal cortex to the ventromedial striatum and nucleus accumbens with projections from there to the ventral pallidum and in turn to the thalamus and then back to prefrontal and cingulate cortex.

There is relatively little experimental evidence regarding the functional activities of these loops, but they include several of the areas shown to be hypermetabolic on PET scans of OCD patients. Perhaps analogous to the disinhibition of motor controls seen in Huntington's disease, tardive dyskinesia and Tourette's syndrome—diseases linked to basal ganglia motor dysfunction (Modell et al., 1989)—impairment of more ventromedial basal ganglia activity may be associated with inappropriate expression of stereotyped rituals or intrusive doubts in patients with OCD. Evidence that frontal and orbitofrontal lesions produce emotional lability, indifference and impaired ability to plan (Goldman-Rakic, 1987) suggests that increased frontal activity noted on PET scans of OCD patients may reflect a converse behavioral syndrome, the excessive worry and emotional constriction characteristic of OCD.

Derangements of modulatory inputs which could contribute to impairment of frontal–basal ganglia–thalamic loop function in OCD include increased inhibitory dopaminergic input from the midbrain to the palladum or reductions in inhibitory serotonergic input to the medial caudate and nucleus accumbens or from the brainstem raphe nuclei to the striatum or orbital frontal cortex. Serotonergic fibers from the raphe project predominantly to the medial caudate and accumbens nuclei in the basal ganglia (Molliver, 1987; Parent, 1990), which may contribute to the differential responses to pharmacologic treatment in OCD and Tourette's syndrome. Because motor loops travel through more lateral aspects of the striatum, the motor compulsions of Tourette's syndrome may be less responsive than the cognitive obsessions of OCD to treatment with serotonin reuptake inhibitors.

A number of lesion studies in humans support the importance of frontal–basal ganglia–thalamic circuits in generation of OCD symptoms. There is evidence for attenuation of OCD symptoms in humans when surgery interrupts these circuits. Examples include lesions of the orbital frontal cortex (Corsellis and Jack, 1977; Scovill and Bettis, 1977; Hay et al., 1993), cingulotomy (Mitchell-Heggs et al., 1976; Tippin and Henn, 1982; Jenike et al., 1991), medial thalamotomy (Hassler and Kieckmann, 1977) and anterior internal capsulotomy (Fodstad et al., 1982; Mindus et al., 1987; Chiocca and Martuza, 1990; Baer et al., 1995). In addition there have been reports of several patients with selective basal ganglia lesions and associated OCD symptoms (Pulst et al., 1983; Laplane et al., 1989; Levin and Duchowny, 1991; Penisson-Besnier et al., 1992). Finally, electrical stimulation of the cingulum in humans seems to produce stereotypy (Talairach et al., 1973) and perseveration (Meyer et al., 1973).

Phenomenology: etiology

There have been a few descriptions of brain lesions in animals that seem to produce stereotypic behaviors. Acaudate cats have been noted to exhibit stereotypy, perseveration, hyperactivity and compulsive approach behavior (Villablanca and Olmstead, 1982). In primates, lesions of orbitofrontal cortex or ventromedial caudate produce perseveration and interference with the ability to make appropriate switches in behavioral set (Divac et al., 1967; Mishkin and Manning, 1978). Lesions of the medial prefrontal cortex in rats seem to delay extinction of conditioned freezing behavior (Morgan et al., 1993), a phenomenon which may be analogous to inappropriate expression of avoidance behavior in humans with OCD.

Hippocampal lesions also seem to potentiate development of stereotypies. Eight weeks after lesions of hippocampal pyramidal cells by intraventricular administration of kainic acid, rats developed stereotypies when exposed to a conditioned reward paradigm; these could be blocked by dopamine antagonists (Devenport et al., 1981). Rats with bilateral hippocampal lesions also demonstrate other behaviors which resemble OCD symptoms in humans, including enhanced acquisition of shuttlebox avoidance (Pitman, 1982; Port *et al.*, 1991), delayed extinction of conditioned behavior (Schmaltz and Isaacson, 1967), reductions in spontaneous alternation (Roberts *et al.*, 1962) and enhanced adjunctive drinking (Devenport, 1978). The hippocampus also may play an important role in suppression of arousal and stereotyped behaviors by inhibiting responses of the amygdala to fear-associated stimuli (Gray, 1982). Anatomic studies point to the amygdala as playing a central role in generation of conditioned fear and arousal (LeDoux, 1986; Davis, 1992).

In addition, two studies describe disruption of stereotyped or displacement behaviors by lesions of the basal ganglia frontal cortex circuit. In rats, hoarding behavior can be disrupted by lesions of the caudate, dorsomedial thalamus and prefrontal cortex (Kolb, 1974, 1977; Borker and Gogate, 1980). In the squirrel monkey, a common stereotypic display (vocalization, thigh spread, and penile erection) produced in response to threat or as a greeting is decreased by medial globus pallidus lesions while other motor behaviors remain intact (MacLean, 1978).

Modulation of stereotypies by lesions of basal ganglia circuits seems less likely than pharmacologically induced models to be a non-specific response to arousal and more likely to reflect a specific link to repetitive behaviors. Behavioral effects of hippocampal lesions, on the other hand, which are more global in scope, may be due to a more non-specific enhancement of arousal.

Treatment response

There have been no studies of the response of these lesion models to chronic treatment with serotonin reuptake blockers, but such studies could help to validate these lesion effects as models of OCD.

TREATMENT RESPONSE MODELS

Chronic treatment with serotonin reuptake inhibitors

As mentioned above, several displacement behavior models have been shown to respond differentially to chronic treatment with serotonin reuptake inhibitors, including acral lick dermatitis in dogs, and food restriction-induced hyperactivity and schedule-induced polydipsia in rodents.

At this time, the mechanism of action of the serotonin reuptake inhibitors to reduce expression of repetitive behaviors is unclear. The long-term neurochemical effects of serotonin reuptake inhibitors which are not shared by the noradrenergic uptake inhibitors are the effects most likely to be relevant to antiobsessional efficacy. Although acute administration of serotonin reuptake blockers decreases raphe firing through stimulation of autoreceptors, electrophysiologic and other studies of the effects of chronic treatment with these agents indicate that some other measures of serotonergic neurotransmission appear to be enhanced (Blier *et al.*, 1990; Fuller, 1994). This is consistent with studies of the effects of serotonin manipulations on the acquisition and retention of conditioned behaviors. Manipulations which generally decrease serotonin activity tend to improve retention and those that increase serotonergic activity tend to impair acquisition and retention of conditioned behaviors (Tenen, 1967; Beninger and Phillips, 1979; Altman and Normile, 1988; Soubrie, 1988).

The effect of chronic treatment with serotonin reuptake inhibitors on specific serotonergic receptors and second messenger systems and on neuronal transmission in different serotonergic pathways is only beginning to be examined (Maj and Moryl, 1992; Watanabe *et al.*, 1993). At least 14 serotonin receptor subtypes have been molecularly identified in recent years, some of which may have separate and opposing actions in mediating anxiety and anxiety-related behaviors (Sandou and Hen, 1994; Humphrey *et al.*, 1993; Hoyer *et al.*, 1994). Anatomic subsystems of serotonergic projections and serotonin receptors also may have opposing roles. Development of drugs which are more selective for specific serotonin receptor subsystems and use of anatomically specific modes of administration may provide means to sort out the roles of these different subsystems.

Drug discrimination based on acute treatment

Two stress-induced behaviors in rats have been shown to respond differentially to acute administration of serotonin reuptake inhibitors. In the first, serotonergic and catecholaminergic reuptake inhibitors have been distinguished by having opposite effects on the ultrasonic isolation calls of rat pups (Winslow and Insel, 1990). These vocalizations are emitted during separation and have been used as probes for a variety of environmental and pharmacological stimuli. In a comparison of effects of acute administration of antidepressant agents, desipramine, a norepinephrine reuptake blocker, increased calling, while several different serotonin reuptake inhibitors reduced calling. This model is weakened by observations that pup ultrasonic vocalizations are also reduced by low doses of benzodiazepines and by opiates, two agents which are relatively ineffective for treatment of OCD.

In another model, the resident–intruder paradigm, grooming by the intruder on exposure to the empty cage of the resident mouse was enhanced by desipramine, a selective norepinephrine reuptake blocker, and was blocked by clomipramine, a serotonin reuptake blocker. On exposure to the resident mouse, grooming by the intruder mouse was decreased by clomipramine and not affected by desipramine (Winslow and Insel, 1989).

ANIMAL MODELS OF RELATED BEHAVIORS

ANIMAL MODELS OF ANXIETY AND DEPRESSION

Hyperarousal and depression seem to be important contributory factors to the initiation and exacerbation of OCD as well as most other anxiety disorders and psychiatric illnesses. This is consistent with the high degree of comorbidity among OCD and depression and other anxiety disorders, including panic disorder, social phobia, generalized anxiety disorder and post-traumatic stress disorder. Although hyperarousal and depression are non-specific processes and cannot account for the unique behavioral manifestations and treatment responsiveness of OCD, models which produce hyperarousal or "anxiety" and signs of behavioral "depression" may shed light on the role of these contributory factors in the generation of OCD symptoms in humans. Well-studied animal models of anxiety and depression include punishment paired with a reinforced response, separation, novel environments, fear potentiated startle and learned helplessness.

Unfortunately, stereotypic responses, if they occur at all, are rarely measured in most investigations of animal models of anxiety and stress. Increased incidence of stereotyped behavior has been noted in infant macaques separated from their mothers (Suomi *et al.*, 1971) and repeated separation from peers also generated high levels of stereotypic behavior in young adult rhesus monkeys (Mineka *et al.*, 1981). Domesticated dogs also may exhibit stereotypic behaviors when left alone at home (McCrave, 1991).

ANIMAL MODELS OF AGGRESSION

Some of the more common OCD symptoms in adults are intrusive violent and sexual thoughts and a sense of having hurt someone else. These thoughts are ego dystonic and virtually never acted out, but may reflect increased aggressive and sexual drives in some OCD patients. The role of aggressive impulses in OCD deserves special attention since aggression has been linked to reduced serotonergic activity and enhanced androgenic activity, and manipulation of each of these systems also has been reported to modulate OCD symptoms. A recent autoradiographic study indicated that similar brain areas including the striatum and dorsal thalamus are activated during ritualized displays of aggression in the lizard as during episodes of OCD in humans (Baxter *et al.*, 1993).

There have been two case reports of reduction in OCD symptoms after pharmacologic reduction of androgen activity (Casas *et al.*, 1986; Leonard *et al.*, 1989). The mechanism of action of this effect remains to be determined but may involve reduction in intrusive aggressive and sexual thoughts. There have been multiple reports of distinct increases in aggressive behavior when animals and humans are chronically treated with testosterone (Pope, 1988; Hannan *et al.*, 1991; Bonson and Winter, 1992; Yates *et al.*, 1992; Su *et al.*, 1993) and decreases in aggressive behavior in animals after castration (de Jong *et al.*, 1986; Albert *et al.*, 1992; Bonson and Winter, 1992).

Two OCD-related neurotransmitter systems affected by androgens, the serotonergic and vasopressinergic systems, may be particularly important in modulation of aggression. There is preliminary evidence that reductions in androgenic steroids are associated with enhancement of central serotonergic activity (Van de Kar *et al.*, 1978; Vacas and Carinali, 1979; Fischette *et al.*,

1983, 1984; Matsuda et al., 1991; Bonson et al., 1994). Conversely, administration of testosterone has been associated with reductions in central serotonergic activity (Martinez-Conde et al., 1985; Mendelson and McEwen, 1990). Pharmacological manipulations which decrease central serotonergic neurotransmission have been associated with increases in aggressive and sexual behaviors in several species (Sheard, 1969; Ferguson et al., 1970; Shillito, 1970; Katz and Thomas, 1976; Raleigh et al., 1986; Chamberlain et al., 1987; Vergnes et al., 1988) while increases in central serotonergic activity have been associated with lessening of aggression and enhancement of affiliative behaviors (DiChiara et al., 1971; Pucilowski and Kostowski, 1983; Raliegh et al., 1986; Chamberlain et al., 1987; Chojnacka-Wojcik and Przegalalinski, 1991; Bonson and Winter, 1992). Studies of aggressive or dominant non-human primates and of violent criminals have reported lower levels of the serotonin metabolite, 5-hydroxyindoleacetic acid (5-HIAA), in brain and cerebrospinal fluid (Raleigh et al., 1984; Yodyinggual et al., 1985; Linnoila et al., 1989; Higley et al., 1992). In addition, lower central levels of 5-HIAA have been associatede with impaired social affiliation in primates and humans (Kruesi, et al., 1992; Mehlman et al., 1995). Studies also have reported increased cerebrospinal fluid testosterone in impulsive violent offenders (Virkkunen et al., 1994) and increased plasma testosterone in dominant primates (Sapolosky, 1986). Soubrie (1988) in a review of preclinical data on serotonin and behavior proposed that reduced serotonergic transmission is associated with impulsivity or an inability to delay expressions of a wide range of drive behaviors which are normally suppressed, including aggression, sexuality and punished responding.

If both OCD patients and violent criminals show evidence of decreased serotonergic activity, the reason for the differing behavioral manifestations may be the degree of anxiety associated with aggressive and sexual impulses in the two populations. Two studies suggest that neurotransmitter systems which seem to increase OCD or anxiety symptoms can also act to decrease aggressive behavior. In one report, the 5-HT$_2$ agonist TFMPP but not the 5-HT$_{1A}$ agonist 8-OH-DPAT decreased stereotyped aggressive attack behaviors in rats elicited by electrical stimulation (Kruk et al., 1987). In another study, comparison of Roman High Avoidance and Roman Low Avoidance rat strains indicated that the strain with high central levels of vasopressin, Roman Low Avoidance, was more likely to freeze than to perform a directed escape or attack behavior when threatened (Roozendaal et al., 1992).

Reductions in gonadal steroids are also associated with decreases in central vasopressin activity (DeVries et al., 1985; Miller et al., 1992). Centrally, vasopressin is an anxiogenic substance which, like serotonin, also seems to modulate aggressive behavior. Flank-marking in hamsters, a ritualized response to threat, is expressed more by dominant animals and this can be blocked by vasopressin antagonists (Ferris et al., 1986). Non-ritualized aggression toward a juvenile intruder can also be blocked by central administration of a vasopressin antagonist (Ferris and Potegal, 1988).

CONCLUSIONS

Most likely, OCD is a disorder of several different etiologies with a final common pathway of expression through phylogenetically old patterns of behavior. These behaviors may emerge through displacement mechanisms or possibly via activation of localized anatomic systems. Clearly, expression of the illness can be modulated by hormones, neurotransmitters and stress. Animal models can be used to investigate each of these aspects of OCD, with the caveat that phenomenological models are limited to observable repetitive behaviors since repetitive thoughts or doubts in animals cannot be assessed.

The neural substrate of the core distinctive feature of OCD, repetitive thoughts and behaviors, remains elusive. Conflicts can be managed and anxiety expressed in non-repetitive ways in both animals and humans. More clinical studies comparing different anxiety disorders and more studies of anxiety generation in anxiety disorder patients, normal controls and animals are needed to sort out the non-specific effects of arousal from manipulations that specifically modulate repetitive behaviors.

One of our most compelling clues to the pathophysiology of repetitive behaviors is the differential treatment efficacy of serotonin reuptake inhibitors. Although the behavioral effects of particular serotonergic receptor agonists and antagonists may be due to non-specific modulation of arousal, chronic administration of serotonin reuptake blockers seems to have selective effects on performance of repetitive behaviors. More work is needed to identify specific biochemical effects of chronic administration of serotonin reuptake blockers, distinct from the effects of non-serotonergic antidepressants. Finally, preliminary evidence that neuropeptides and gonadal hormones may modulate expression of repetitive behaviors deserves further attention and study.

REFERENCES

Akhtar, S., Wig, N., Varma, V. *et al.* (1975). A phenomenological analysis of symptoms in obsessive-compulsive disorder. *Br. J. Psychiatry*, **127**, 342–348.

Albert, D. J., Jonik, R. H. and Walsh, M. L. (1992). Hormone-dependent aggression in male and female rats: experiential, hormonal and neural foundations. *Neurosci. Biobehav. Rev.*, **16**, 177–192.

Alexander, G. E., DeLong, M. R. and Strick, P. L. (1986). Parallel organization of functionally segregated circuits linking basal ganglia and cortex. *Annu. Rev. Neurosci.*, **9**, 357–381.

Altemus, M., Cizza, G. and Gold, P. W. (1992a). Chronic fluoxetine treatment reduces hypothalamic vasopressin secretion *in vitro*. *Brain Res.*, **593**, 311–313.

Altemus, M., Pigott, T. A., Kalogeras, K. T. *et al.* (1992b). Abnormalities in the regulation of vasopressin and corticotropin releasing factor secretion in obsessive-compulsive disorder. *Arch. Gen. Psychiatry*, **49**, 9–20.

Altemus, M., Pigott, T., L'Heureux, F. *et al.* (1993b). CSF somatostatin in obsessive-compulsive disorder. *Am. J. Psychiatry*, **150**, 460–464.

Altemus, M., Swedo, S. E., Leonard, H. L. *et al.* (1994). Changes in CSF neurochemistry during treatment of OCD with clomipramine. *Arch. Gen. Psychiatry*, **51**, 794–803.

Altemus, M., Glowa, J., Galliven, E. *et al.* (1996). Effects of serotonergic agents on food restriction-induced hyperactivity. *Pharmacol. Biochem. Behav.,* **53**, 123–131.

Altman, H. J. and Normile, H. J. (1988). What is the nature of the role of the serotonergic nervous system in learning and memory: prospects for development of an effective treatment strategy for senile dementia. *Neurobiol. Aging,* **9**, 627–638.

American Psychiatric Association (1994). *Diagnostic and Statistical Manual of Mental Disorders, DSM-IV.* American Psychiatric Press, Washington, DC.

Amsel, A. and Rashotte, M. G. (1969). Transfer of experimenter-imposed slow response patterns to the extinction of a continuously rewarded response. *J. Comp. Physiol. Psychol.,* **69**, 185–189.

Appleby, M. C. and Lawrence, A. B. (1987). Food restriction as a cause of stereotypic behavior in tethered gilts. *Anim. Prod.,* **45**, 103–110.

Baer, L., Rausch, S. L., Ballantine, H. T. *et al.* (1995). Cingulotomy for intractable obsessive-compulsive disorder. Prospective long-term follow-up of 18 patients. *Arch. Gen. Psychiatry.,* **52**, 384–392.

Baxter, L., Phelps, M. and Mazziotti, J. (1986). Local cerebral glucose metabolic rates of obsessive compulsive disorder compared to unipolar depression and normal controls. *Arch. Gen. Psychiatry,* **44**, 211–218.

Baxter, L. R., Schwartz, J. M., and Bergman, K. S. (1992). Caudate glucose metabolic rate changes with drug and behavior therapy for obsessive-compulsive disorder. *Arch. Gen. Psychiatry,* **49**, 681–689.

Baxter, L. R., Colgan, M., Baxter, J. E. G. *et al.* (1993). Brain activation patterns during ritual territorial aggression and its extinction in *anolis carolinesis. Proceedings of the American College of Neuropsychopharmacology,* 32nd Annual Meeting (abstract), p. 198.

Beninger, R. J. and Phillips, A. G. (1979). Possible involvement of serotonin in extinction. *Pharmacol. Biochem. Behav.,* **10**, 37–41.

Benkelfat, C., Nordahl, T. E. and Semple, W. E. (1990). Local cerebral glucose metabolic rates in obsessive-compulsive disorder: patients treated with clomipramine. *Arch. Gen. Psychiatry,* **47**, 840–848.

Benloucif, S. and Galloway, M. P. (1991). Facilitation of dopamine release *in vivo* by serotonergic agonists: studies with microdialysis. *Eur. J. Pharmacol.,* **200**, 1–8.

Blier, P. B., deMontigny, C. and Chaput, Y. (1990). A role for the serotonin system in the mechanism of action of antidepressant treatments: preclinical evidence. *J. Clin. Psychiatry,* **51**, 14–20.

Blundell, J. E., Strupp, B. J. and Latham, C. J. (1977). Pharmacological manipulation of hoarding: further analysis of amphetamine isomers and pimozide. *Physiol. Psychol.,* **5**, 462–468.

Bonson, K. R. and Winter, J. C. (1992). Reversal of testosterone-induced dominance by the serotonergic agonist quipazine. *Pharmacol. Biochem. Behav.,* **42**, 809–813.

Bonson, K. R., Johnson, R. G., Fiorella, D. *et al.* (1994). Serotonergic control of androgen-induced dominance. *Pharmacol. Biochem. Behav.,* **49**, 313–322.

Borker, A. S. and Gogate, M. G. (1980). Hoarding in caudate lesioned rats. *Indian J. Exp. Biol.,* **18**, 690–692.

Casas, M., Alvarez, E., Duro, P. *et al.* (1986). Antiandrogenic treatment of obsessive-compulsive neurosis. *Acta Psychiatr. Scand.,* **73**, 221–222.

Chamberlain, B., Ervin, F., Pihl, R. O. and Young, S. N. (1987). The effect of raising or lowering tryptophan levels on aggression in vervet monkeys. *Pharmacol. Biochem. Behav.,* **28**, 503–510.

Chiocca, E. A. and Martuza, R. L. (1990). Neurosurgical therapy of the obsessive-compulsive disorder. In *Obsessive-compulsive Disorders: Theory and Management* (eds M. A. Jenike, L. Baer and W. E. Minichiello), 2nd edn, pp. 283–284. Mosby–Yearbook Medical, Chicago.

Chojnacka-Wojcik, E. and Przegalalinski, E. (1991). Evidence for the involvement of 5-HT1A receptors in the anti-conflict effect of ipsapirone in rats. *Neuropharmacology*, **30**, 703–709.

Conner, R. L., Vernicos-Danellis, J. and Levine, S. (1971). Stress, fighting and neuroendocrine function. *Nature*, **234**, 564–566.

Cools, A. R. and Van Rossum, J. M. (1970). Caudal dopamine and stereotypy behavior of cats. *Arch. Int. Pharmacodyn. Ther.*, **187**, 163–173.

Cooper, S. J. and Holtzman, S. G. (1983). Patterns of drinking in the rat following the administration of opiate antagonists. *Pharmacol. Biochem. Behav.*, **19**, 505–511.

Corsellis, J. and Jack, A. B. (1977). Neuropathological observations on tritium implants and on undercutting in the orbito-frontal areas of the brain. In *Surgical Approaches in Psychiatry: Proceedings of the Third International Congress of Psychosurgery* (eds L. V. Laitinen and K. V. Livingston), pp. 189–197. University Park Press, Baltimore.

Creese, I. and Iverson, S. D. (1974). The role of forebrain dopamine systems in amphetamine induced stereotyped behavior in the rat. *Psychopharmacologia*, **39**, 345–357.

Cronin, G. M. and Wiepkema, P. R. (1984). An analysis of stereotyped behavior in tethered sows. *Ann. Rech. Vet.*, **15**, 263–270.

Cronin, G. M., Wiepkema, P. R. and VanRee, J. M. (1985). Endogenous opioids are involved in abnormal stereotyped behaviors of tethered sows. *Neuropeptides*, **6**, 527–530.

Curzon, G., Gibson, E. L., Kennedy, A. J. *et al.* (1991). Anxiogenic and other effects of m-CPP, a 5-HT$_{1C}$ agonist. In *New Concepts in Anxiety* (eds M. Briley and S. E. File), pp. 154–167. Macmillan, London.

Dallaire, A. (1993). Stress and behavior in domestic animals: temperament as a predisposing factor to stereotypies. *Ann. NY Acad. Sci.*, **697**, 269–274.

Dantzer, R. (1983). De-arousal properties of stereotyped behavior: evidence from pituitary adrenal correlation in pigs. *Appl. Anim. Ethol.*, **10**, 244.

Dantzer, R. (1986). Behavioral, physiological and functional aspects of stereotypic behavior: a review and re-interpretation. *J. Anim. Sci.*, **62**, 1776.

Davenport, R. K. and Menzel, E. W. (1963). Stereotyped behaviors of the infant chimpanzee. *Arch. Gen. Psychiatry*, **8**, 99–104.

Davis, M. (1992). The role of the amygdala in fear and anxiety. *Annu. Rev. Neurosci.*, **15**, 353–375.

de Jong, F. H., Eerland, E. M. J. and van de Poll, N. E. (1986). Sex-specific interactions between aggressive and sexual behavior in the rat: effects of testosterone and progesterone. *Horm. Behav.*, **20**, 432–444.

DeBellis, M. D., Gold, P. W., Geracioti, T. D. *et al.* (1993). Association of fluoxetine treatment with reductions in CSF concentrations of corticotropin-releasing hormone and arginine vasopressin in patients with major depression. *Am. J. Psychiatry*, **150**, 656–657.

de la Tourette, G. (1885). Etude sur une affection nerveuse caraterisee par de l'incoordination motrice accompagnee d'echolalie et de coprolie. *Arch. Neurol.*, **9**, 19–42.

Delius, J. D. (1988). Preening and associated comfort behavior in birds. *Ann. NY Acad. Sci.*, **525**, 40–55.

DeSilva, P., Rachman, S. and Seligman, M. (1977). Prepared phobias and obsessions: therapeutic outcomes. *Behav. Res. Ther.*, **15**, 65–78.

Devenport, L. D. (1978). Schedule-induced polydipsia in rats: adrenocortical and hippocampal modulation. *J. Comp. Physiol. Psychol.*, **92**(4), 651–660.

Devenport, L. D., Davenport, J. A. and Holloway, F. A. (1981). Reward-induced stereotypy: modulation by the hippocampus. *Science*, **212**, 1288–1289.

Devinsky, D. (1983). Neuroanatomy of Gilles de la Tourette's syndrome: possible midbrain involvement. *Arch. Neurol.*, **40**, 508–514.

DeVries, G. J., Bujis, R. M., Van Leeuwen, F. W. *et al.* (1985). The vasopressinergic innervation of the brain in normal and castrated rats. *J. Comp. Neurol.*, **233**, 236–254.

DiChiara, G., Camba, R. and Spano, P. F. (1971). Evidence for inhibition by brain serotonin of mouse killing behavior in rats. *Nature*, **233**, 272–273.

Divac, I., Rosvold, H. E. and Szwarcbart, M. K. (1967). Behavioral effects of selective ablation of the caudate nucleus. *J. Comp. Physiol. Psychol.*, **63**, 184–190.

Dodman, N. H., Shuster, L. and White, S. D. (1987). Use of narcotic antagonists to modify stereotypic self-licking, self-chewing and scratching behavior in dogs. *J. Am. Vet. Med. Assoc.*, **193**, 815–819.

Dunn, A. J., Green, E. J. and Isaacson, R. L. (1979). Intracerebral adrenocorticotropic hormone mediates novelty-induced grooming in the rat. *Science*, **203**, 281–283.

Eilam, D., Golani, I. and Szechtmna, H. (1989). D2-agonist quinpirole induces perseveration of routes and hyperactivity but no perserveration of movements. *Brain Res.*, **490**, 255–267.

Ellinwood, E. H. and Kilbey, M. M. (1975). Species differences in response to amphetamine. In *Psychopharmacolgenetics* (ed. B. E. Eleftheriou) pp. 324–375. Plenum Press, New York.

Epling, W. F., Pierce, W. D. and Stefan, L. (1983). A theory of activity-based anorexia. *Int. J. Eat. Disord.*, **3**, 27–46.

Falk, J. L. (1961). Production of polydipsia in normal rats by an intermittent food schedule. *Science*, **133**, 195–196.

Falk, J. L. (1971). The nature and determinants of adjunctive behaviour. *Physiol. Behav.*, **6**, 577–588.

Feldman, R. S. (1962). The prevention of fixations with chlordiazepoxide. *J. Neuropsychiatry*, **3**, 154–259.

Ferguson, J., Henrickson, S., Cohen, J. *et al.* (1970). Hypersexuality and behavioral changes in cats caused by administration of p-chlorophenylalanine. *Science*, **168**, 499–501.

Ferris, C. F. and Potegal, M. (1988). Vasopressin receptor blockade in the anterior hypothalamus suppresses aggression in hamsters. *Physiol. Behav.*, **44**, 235–239.

Ferris, C. F., Meenan, D. M., Axelson, J. F. and Albers, H. E. (1986). A vasopressin antagonist can reverse dominant/subordinate behavior in hamsters. *Physiol. Behav.*, **38**, 135–138.

Ferris, C. F., Albers, H. E., Weselowski, S. M. *et al.* (1990). Vasopressin injected into the hypothalamus triggers a stereotypic behavior in Golden hamsters. *Science*, **224**, 521–523.

Fischette, C. T., Biegon, A. and McEwen, B. S. (1983). Sex differences in serotonin₁ receptor binding in rat brain. *Science*, **22**, 333–335.

Fischette, C. T., Biegon, A. and McEwen, B. S. (1984). Sex steroid modulation of the serotonin behavioral syndrome. *Life Sci.*, **35**, 1197–1206.

Fishman, M. W. (1987). Cocaine and amphetamines. In *Psychopharmacology: The Third Generation of Progress* (ed. H. Y. Meltzer), pp. 1543–1553. Raven Press, New York.

Flory, R. K. (1969). Attack behavior as a function of minimum inter-food interval. *J. Exp. Anal. Behav.*, **12**, 825–828.

Fodstad, H., Strandman, E. and Karlsson, B. (1982). Treatment of chronic obsessive compulsive states with stereotactic anterior capsulotomy or cingulotomy. *Acta Neurochir.*, **62**, 1–23.

Freud, S. (1959). Obsessive actions and religious practices. In *Collected Psychological Works*, Vol. 9, pp. 177–127. Hogarth Press, London.

Fuller, R. W. (1994). Uptake inhibitors increase extracellular serotonin concentration measured by brain microdialysis. *Life Sci.*, **55**, 163–7.

Garber, H., Ananth, J., Chiu, L. *et al.* (1989). Nuclear magnetic resonance study of obsessive-compulsive disorder. *Am. J. Psychiatry*, **146**, 1001–1005.

Goldman-Rakic, P. S. (1987). Circuitry of primate prefrontal cortex and regulation of behaviour by representational memory. In *Secondary Circuitry of Primate Prefrontal Cortex and Regulation of Behaviour by Representational Memory* (eds V. B. Moncastle, F. Plum and S. R. Geiger), pp. 373–417. American Physiological Society, Bethesda, MD.

Goosen, C (1974). Some casual factors in autogrooming behaviour of adult stumptailed macaques (Macaca arctoides). *Behaviour*, **49**, 111–129.

Gordon, C. T., Cotelingam, G. M., Stager, S. *et al.* (1995). A double-blind comparison of clomipramine and desipramine in the treatment of developmental stuttering. *J. Clin. Psychiatry*, **56**, 238–242.

Gordon, C. T., State, R. C., Nelson, J. E. *et al.* (1993). A double-blind comparison of clomipramine desipramine and placebo in the treatment of autistic disorder. *Arch. Gen. Psychiatry*, **50**, 441–447.

Gray, J. A. (1982). *The Neuropsychology of Anxiety: An Enquiry into the Functioning of the Septohippocampal System.* Oxford University Press, New York.

Greist, J. H., Jefferson, J. W., Kobak, K. A. *et al.* (1995). Efficacy and tolerability of serotonin transport inhibitors in obsessive-compulsive disorder. *Arch. Gen. Psychiatry*, **52**, 53–60.

Griez, E., deLoff, C., Pols, H. *et al.* (1990). Specific sensitivity of patients with panic attacks to carbon dioxide inhalation. *Psychiatry Res.*, **31**, 193–199.

Guild, A. L. and Dunn, A. J. (1982). Dopamine involvement in ACTH-induced grooming behavior. *Pharmacol. Biochem. Behav.*, **17**, 31–36.

Guttmacher, L. B., Murphy, D. L. and Insel, T. R. (1983). Pharmacological models of anxiety. *Compr. Psychiatry*, **24**, 312–326.

Gwirtsman, H., Guze, B., Yager, J. *et al.* (1990). Fluvoxetine treatment of anorexia nervosa: an open clinical trial, *J. Clin. Psychiatry*, **51**, 378–382.

Hannan, C. J., Friedl, K. E., Zold, A. *et al.* (1991). Psychological and serum homovanillic acid changes in men administered androgenic steroids. *Psychoneuroendocrinology*, **16**, 335–343.

Hassler, R. and Kieckmann, G. (1977). Relief of obsessive-compulsive disorders, phobias and tics by stereotactic coagulation of the rostral intralaminar and medial-thalamic nuclei. In *Neurosurgical Treatment in Psychiatry, Pain and Epilepsy* (eds W. H. Sweet, S. Obrador and J. Marin-Rodriguez), pp. 206–212. University Park Press, Baltimore.

Hay, P., Sachdev, P., Cumming, S. *et al.* (1993). Treatment of obsessive-compulsive disorder by psychosurgery. *Acta Psychiatr. Scand.*, **87**, 197–207.

Hediger, H. (1955). *Studies in the Psychology and Behavior of Captive Animals in Zoos and Circuses.* Dover Press, London.

Henn, F. A. and McKinney, W. T. (1987). Animal models in psychiatry. In *Psychopharmacology: The Third Generation of Progress* (ed. H. Y. Meltzer), pp. 687–696. Raven, New York.

Higley, J. D., Mehlman, P., Taub, D. *et al.* (1992). Cerebrospinal fluid monoamine and adrenal correlates of aggression in free-ranging rhesus monkeys. *Arch. Gen. Psychiatry*, **49**, 436–441.

Hinjo, S., Hirano, C., Murase, S. *et al.* (1989). Obsessive-compulsive symptoms in childhood and adolescence. *Acta Psychiatr. Ann.*, **2**, 80–87.

Holland, H. C. (1974). Displacement activity as a form of abnormal behavior in animals. In *Obsessional States* (ed. H. R. Bech), pp. 189–198. Methuen, London.

Hoyer, D., Clarke, D. E., Fozard, J. R. *et al.* (1994). International Union of Pharmacology classification of receptors for 5-hydroxytryptamine (serotonin). *Pharmacological Reviews*, **46**, 157–203.

Humphrey, P. P. A., Hartig, P. and Hoyer, D. (1993). A proposed new nomenclature for 5-HT receptors. *Trends Pharmacol. Sci.*, **14**, 233–236.

Insel, T. R. (1992). Toward a neuroanatomy of obsessive-compulsive disorder. *Arch. Gen. Psychiatry*, **49**, 739–744.

Jackson, H. C. and Kitchen, I. (1989). Behavioral profiles of putative 5-hydroxytryptamine receptor agonists and antagonists in developing rats. *Neuropharmacology*, **28**, 635–642.

Jacobs, B. L. (1993). Obsessive compulsive disorder: a neurobiological hypothesis. In *Serotonin* (ed. P. M. Vanhoutte), pp. 231–237. Kluwer, Dordrecht.

Jacobs, B. L., Fornal, C. A. and Wilkenson, L. O. (1990). Neurophysiological and neurochemical studies of brain serotonergic neurons in behaving animals. In *The*

Neuropharmacology of Serotonin (eds P. M. Whitaker-Azmitia and S. J. Peroutka), pp. 260–271. New York Academy of Sciences, New York.

Jacobsen, F. M., Mueller, E. A., Rosenthal, N. E. *et al.* (1994). Behavioral responses to intravenous meta-chlorophenylpiperazine in patients with seasonal affective disorder and control subjects before and after phototherapy. *Psychiatry Res.*, **52**, 181–197.

Jenike, M. A., Baer, L. and Griest, J. H. (1990). Clomipramine versus fluoxetine in obsessive-compulsive disorder: a retrospective comparison of side effects and efficacy. *J. Clin. Psychopharmacol.*, **10**, 122–124.

Jenike, M. A., Baer, L. and Ballantine, H. T. (1991). Cingulomotomy for refractory obsessive-compulsive disorder: a long-term follow-up of 33 patients. *Arch. Gen. Psychiatry*, **48**, 548–555.

Joseph-Vanderpool, J. R., Jacobsen, F. M. *et al.* (1993). Seasonal variation in behavioral responses to m-CPP in patients with seasonal affective disorder and controls. *Biol. Psychiatry*, **33**, 496–504.

Kahn, R. S., Wetzler, S., vanPraag, H. M. *et al.* (1988). Behavioral indications for serotonin receptor hypersensitivity in panic disorder. *Psychiatry Res.*, **25**, 101–104.

Kakigi, T., Tanimoto, K. and Maeda, K. (1990). The effect of various antidepressants on the concentration of somatostatin in the rat brain. *Jpn. J. Psychiatry Neurol.*, **44**, 145.

Katz, R. J. and Thomas, E. (1976). Effects of para-chlorophenylalanine upon brain stimulated affective attack in the cat. *Pharmacol. Biochem. Behav.*, **5**, 391–394.

Kaye, W., Weltzin, T., Nsu, L. and Bulik, C. (1992). An open trial of fluoxetine in patients with anorexia nervosa. *J. Clin. Psychiatry,* **52**, 464–471.

Kelley, A. E. and Stinus, L. (1985). Disappearance of hoarding behavior after 5-hydroxy-dopamine lesions of the mesolimbic dopamine neurons and its reinstatement with L-dopa. *Behav. Neurosci.*, **99**, 531–545.

Kelley, A. E., Lang, C. G. and Gauthier, A. M. (1988). Induction of oral stereotypy following amphetamine microinjection into a discrete subregion of the striatum. *Psychopharmacology*, **95**, 556–559.

Kellner, C. H., Jolle, R. R. and Holgate, R. C. (1991). Brain MRI in obsessive-compulsive disorder. *Psychiatry Res.*, **36**, 45–49.

Kennes, D., Odberg, F. O., Bouquet, Y. and DeRycke, P. H. (1988). Changes in naloxone and haloperidol effects during the development of captivity-induced jumping stereotypy in bank voles. *Eur. J. Pharmacol.*, **153**, 19–24.

Kennett, G. A., Whitton, P., Shah, K. and Curzon, G. (1989). Anxiogenic-like effects of m-CPP and TFMPP in animal models are opposed by 5-HT_{1c} receptor antagonists. *Eur. J. Pharmacol.*, **164**, 445–454.

Khanna, S. and Channabasavanna, S. (1987). Toward a classification of compulsions in obsessive-compulsive neurosis. *Psychopathology*, **20**, 23–28.

Killeen, P. R., Hanson, S. J. and Osbourne, S. R. (1978). Arousal: its genesis and manifestation as response rate. *Psychol. Rev.*, **85**, 571–581.

Koizumi, H. M. (1985). Obsessive-compulsive symptoms following stimulants. *Biol. Psychiatry*, **20**, 1332–1337.

Kolb, B. (1974). Prefrontal lesions alter eating and hoarding behavior in rats. *Physiol. Behav.*, **12**, 507–511.

Kolb, B. (1977). Studies on the caudate, putamen and the dorsomedial thalamic nuclei of the rat: implications for mammalian frontal lobe functions. *Physiol. Behav.*, **18**, 237–244.

Koob, G. F. (1991). Behavioral responses to stress. In *Stress: Neurobiology and Neuroendocrinology* (eds M. R. Brown, G. R. Koob and C. Rivier), pp. 255–271. Marcel Dekker, New York.

Kruesi, M. J. P., Swedo, S., Leonard, H. *et al.* (1990). CSF somatostatin in childhood psychiatric disorders: a preliminary investigation. *Psychiatry Res.*, **33**, 277–284.

Kruesi, M., Hibbs, E. O., Zahn, T. P. *et al.* (1992). A 2-year prospective follow-up study of children and adolescents with disruptive behavior disorders: prediction by cerebrospinal fluid 5-hydroxy-indoleacetic acid, homovanillic acid and anatomic measures? *Arch. Gen. Psychiatry,* **49**, 429–435.

Kruk, M. R., Van er Poel, A. M., Lammers, J. H. C. M. *et al.* (1987). *Ethnopharmacology of Hypothalamic Aggression in the Rat.* Martinus Nijhoff, Dordrecht.

Laplane, D., Levasseur, M., Pillon, B. *et al.* (1989). Obsessive-compulsive and other behavioral changes with bilateral basal ganglia lesions. *Brain,* **112**, 699–725.

Lawler, C. P. and Cohen, P. S. (1988). Paw grooming induced by intermittent positive reinforcement in rats. *Ann. NY Acad. Sci.,* **525**, 417–419.

Lawrence, A. B. and Terlouw, E. M. C. (1993). A review of behavioral factors involved in the development and continued performance of stereotypic behavior in pigs. *J. Anim. Sci.,* **71**, 2815–2825.

LeDoux, J. E. (1986). The neurobiology of emotion. In *Mind and Brain, Dialogues in Cognitive Neuroscience* (eds J. E. LeDoux and W. Hirst), pp. 301–358. Cambridge University Press, New York.

Lenane, M. C., Swedo, S. E., Leonard, H. *et al.* (1990). Psychiatric disorders in first degree relatives of children and adolescents with obsessive compulsive disorder. *J. Am. Acad. Child Adolesc. Psychiatry,* **29**, 407–412.

Leonard, H. L. (1989). Drug treatment of obsessive-compulsive disorder. In *Obsessive-compulsive Disorder in Children and Adolescents* (ed. J. L. Rapoport), pp. 217–236. American Psychiatric Press, Washington, DC.

Leonard, H. L., Lenane, M. C., Swedo, S. E. *et al.* (1991). A double-blind comparison of clomipramine and desipramine treatment of severe onychophagia (nail biting). *Arch. Gen. Psychiatry,* **48**, 922–927.

Leonard, H. L., Swedo, S. E., Lenane, M. C. *et al.* (1993). A 2- to 7-year follow-up of 54 obsessive compulsive children and adolescents. *Arch. Gen. Psychiatry,* **50**, 429–439.

Leuscher, U. A., McKeown, D. B. and Halip, J. (1991). Stereotypic or obsessive-compulsive disorders in dogs and cats. *Vet. Clin. North Am. Small Anim. Pract.,* **21**, 401–413.

Levin, B. and Duchowny, M. (1991). Childhood obsessive-compulsive disorder and cingulate epilepsy. *Biol. Psychiatry,* **30**, 1049–1055.

Linnoila, M., de Jonge, J. and Virkkunen, M. (1989). Family history of alcoholism in violent offenders and impulsive fire setters. *Arch. Gen. Psychiatry,* **46**, 613–616.

Lorenz, K. (1981). *The Foundations of Ethology.* Springer-Verlag, New York.

Lowe, T. L., Cohen, D. J., Detlor, J. *et al.* (1982). Stimulant medications precipitate Tourette's syndrome. *JAMA,* **247**, 1729–1731.

Lucki, I. and Kucharick, R. F. (1988). Selective enhancement of grooming behavior by the D-1 agonist SKF 38393 in rats following the destruction of serotonin neurons. *Ann. NY Acad. Sci.,* **525**, 420–422.

MacKenzie, S. A., Oltenacu, E. A. B. and Howpt, K. A. (1986). Canine behavioral genetics: a review. *Appl. Anim. Behav. Sci.,* **15**, 365–393.

MacLean, P. D. (1978). Effects of lesions of globus pallidus on species-typical display behavior of squirrel monkeys. *Brain Res.,* **149**, 175–196.

Maier, N. (1949). *Frustration and Conflict.* McGraw Hill, New York.

Maj, J. and Moryl, E. (1992). Effects of sertraline and citalopram given repeatedly on the responsiveness of 5-HT receptor subpopulations. *J. Neural Transm.,* **88**, 143–156.

Markowitz, P. I. (1990). Fluoxetine treatment of self-injurious behavior in mentally retarded patients. *J. Clin. Psychopharmacol.,* **10**, 299–300.

Martinez-Conde, E., Leret, M. L. and Diaz, S. (1985). The influence of testosterone in the brain of the male rat on levels of serotonin (5-HT) and 5-hydroxyindoleacetic acid (5-HIAA). *Comp. Biochem. Physiol.,* **80**C, 411–414.

Mason, G. J. (1991). Stereotypies: a critical review. *Anim. Behav.,* **41**, 1015–1037.

Matsuda, T., Nakano, Y., Kanda, T. *et al.* (1991). Gonadal hormones affect the hypothermia induced by serotonin1A (5-HT1A) receptor activation. *Life Sci.,* **48**, 1627–1632.

McCrave, E. (1991). Diagnostic criteria for separation anxiety in the dog. *Vet. Clin. North Am. Small Anim. Proc.,* **21**, 247–256.

McDougle, C. J., Goodman, W. K., Leckman, J. F. and Price, L. H. (1993). The psychophar-macology of obsessive compulsive disorder: implications for treatment and pathogenesis. *Psychiatr. Clin. North Am.*, **16**(4), 749–766.

McDougle, C. J., Goodman, W. K., Leckman, J. F. *et al.* (1994). Haloperidol addition in flu-voxamine-refractory obsessive compulsive disorder: a double-blind, placebo-controlled study in patients with and without tics. *Arch. Gen. Psychiatry*, **51**, 302–308.

Mehlman, P. T., Higley, J. D., Faucher, I. *et al.* (1995). Correlation of CSF 5-HIAA concen-tration with sociality and the timing of emigration in free-ranging primates. *Am. J. Psychiatry*, **152**, 907–913.

Mendelson, J. and Chillag, D. (1970). Schedule-induced air licking in rats. *Physiol. Behav.*, **5**, 535–537.

Mendelson, S. D. and McEwen, B. A. (1990). Testosterone increases the concentration of (3H)8-hydroxy-2-(di-n-propylamino)tetralin binding at 5-HT1A receptors in the medial preoptic nucleus of the castrated male rat. *Eur. J. Pharmacol.*, **181**, 329–331.

Meyer, G., McElhaney, M., Martin, W. and McGraw, C. P. (1973). Stereotactic cingulotomy with results of acute stimulation and serial psychological testing. In *Surgical Approaches to Psychiatry* (eds I. V. Latinen and K. E. Livingstone), pp. 39–58. MTP, Lancaster.

Miller, M. A., DeVries, G. J., al-Shamma, H. A. and Dorsa, D. M. (1992). Decline of vaso-pressin immunoreactivity and mRNA levels in the bed nucleus of the stria terminalis fol-lowing castration. *J. Neurosci.*, **12**, 2881–2887.

Mindus, P., Bergstrom, K. and Levander, S. E. (1987). Magnetic resonance images related to clinical outcome after psychosurgical intervention in severe anxiety disorder. *J. Neurol. Neurosurg. Psychiatry*, **50**, 1288–1293.

Mineka, S. (1985). Animal models of anxiety-based disorders: their usefulness and limita-tions. In *Anxiety and the Anxiety Disorders* (ed J. Master and A. Turner), pp. 199–244. Erlbaum, Hillsdale, NJ.

Mineka, S. and Cook, M. (1993). Mechanisms involved in the observational conditioning of fear. *J. Exp. Psychol. (Gen.)*, **122**, 23–38.

Mineka, S., Suomi, S. J. and Delizio, R. (1981). Multiple peer separations in adolescent mon-keys: an opponent process interpretation. *J. Exp. Psychol. (Gen.)*, **110**, 56–85.

Mishkin, M. and Manning, F. J. (1978). Nonspatial memory after selective prefrontal lesions in monkeys. *Brain Res.*, **143**, 313–323.

Mitchell-Heggs, N., Kelly, D. and Richardson, A. (1976). Stereotactic limbic leucotomy: a follow-up at 16 months. *Br. J. Psychiatry*, **128**, 226–240.

Modell, J. G., Mountz, J. M., Curtis, G. C. and Greden, J. F. (1989). Neurophysiologic dys-function in basal ganglia/limbic striatal and thalamocortical circuits as a pathogenetic mechanism of obsessive-compulsive disorder. *J. Neuropsychiatry*, **1**, 27–36.

Molino, L. J., Shemer, A. V. and Whitaker-Azmitia, P. (1989). SKF 38393: vacillatory behavior in immature rats. *Eur. J. Pharmacol.*, **161**, 223–225.

Molliver, M. E. (1987). Serotonergic neuronal systems: what their anatomic organization tells us about function. *J. Clin. Psychopharmacol.*, **7**(6), 3S–23S.

Moody, T. W., Meralli, Z. and Crawley, J. N. (1988). The effects of anxiolytics and other agents on rat grooming behavior. *Ann. NY Acad. Sci.*, **525**, 281–289.

Morgan, M. A., Romanski, L. M. and LeDoux, J. E. (1993). Extinction of emotional learn-ing: contribution of medial prefrontal cortex. *Neurosci. Lett.*, **163**, 109–113.

Murphy, D. L., Lesch, K. P., Aulakh, C. S. and Pigott, T. A. (1991). Serotonin-selective arylpiperazines with neuroendocrine, behavioral, temperature, and cardiovascular effects in humans. *Pharmacol. Rev.*, **43**(4), 527–552.

Murphy, D. L., Pigott, T. A. and Insel, T. R. (1990). Obsessive-compulsive disorder and anx-iety. In *Handbook of Anxiety: The Neurobiology of Anxiety* (ed G. D. Burrows, R. Noyes and M. Roth), Vol. 3, pp. 269–287. Elsevier, Amsterdam.

Nezeroglu, F., Anemone, R. and Yaryura-Tobias, J. (1992). Onset of obsessive-compulsive disorder in pregnancy. *Am. J. Psychiatry*, **149**, 947–950.

Nordahl, T. E., Benkelfat, C. and Semple, W. E. (1989). Cerebral glucose metabolic rates in obsessive-compulsive disorder. *Neuropsychopharmacology*, **2**, 23–28.

Odberg, F. D. (1987). The influence of cage size and environmental enrichment on the development of stereotypies in bank voles. *Behav. Proc.*, **14**, 155–173.

Odberg, F. O., Kennes, D., DeRycke, P. H. and Bouquet, Y. (1987). The effect of interference in catecholamine biosynthesis on captivity-induced jumping stereotypy in bank voles. *Arch. Int. Pharmacodyn. Ther.*, **285**, 34–42.

Okasha, A., Saad, A., Khalil, A. H. *et al.* (1994). Phenomenology of obsessive-compulsive disorder: a transcultural study. *Comp. Psychiatry*, **35**, 141–147.

Parent, A. (1990). Serotonergic innervation of the basal ganglia. *Comp. Neurol.*, **209**, 1–16.

Pauls, D. L., Alsobrook, J. P., Goodman, W. *et al.* (1995). A family study of obsessive-compulsive disorder, *Am. J. Psychiatry,* **152**, 76–84.

Penisson-Besnier, I., LeGall, D. and Dubas, F. (1992). Obsessive-compulsive behavior (arithmomania): atrophy of the caudate nuclei. *Rev. Neurol. (Paris)*, **148**, 262–267.

Pigott, T. A., Hill, J. L., Grady, T. A. *et al.* (1993). A comparison of the behavioral effects of oral versus intravenous m-CPP administration in OCD patients and the effect of metergoline prior to IV m-CPP. *Biol. Psychiatry*, **33**, 3–14.

Pitman, R. K. (1982). Neurological etiology of obsessive-compulsive disorders? *Am. J. Psychiatry*, **139**, 139–140.

Pitman, R. K. (1989). Animal models of compulsive behavior. *Biol. Psychiatry*, **26**, 189–198.

Pope, H. G. (1988). Affective and psychotic symptoms associated with anabolic steroid use. *Am. J. Psychiatry*, **145**, 487–490.

Port, R. L., Sample, J. A. and Seybold, K. S. (1991). Partial hippocampal pyramidal cell loss alters behavior in rats: implications for an animal model of schizophrenia. *Brain Res. Bull.*, **26**, 993–996.

Pucilowski, O. and Kostowski, W. (1983). Aggressive behavior and the central serotonergic systems. *Behav. Brain Res.*, **9**, 33–48.

Pulst, S. M., Walshe, T. M. and Romero, J. A. (1983). Carbon monoxide poisoning with features of Gilles de la Tourette syndrome. *Arch. Neurol.*, **10**, 443–444.

Raab, A., Dantzer, R., Michaud, B. *et al.*(1986). Behavioral physiological and immunological consequences of social status and aggression in chronically coexisting resident and intruder dyads of male rats. *Physiol. Behav.*, **36**, 223–228.

Rachman, S. J. and Hodgson, R. J. (1980). *Obsessions and compulsions*. Prentice Hall, Englewood Cliffs, NJ.

Raleigh, M. J., McGuire, M. T., Brammer, G. L. and Yuwiler, A. (1984). Social and environmental influences on blood serotonin concentrations in monkeys. *Arch. Gen. Psychiatry*, **41**, 405–410.

Raleigh, M. J., Brammer, Ritvo, E. R. *et al.* (1986). Effects of chronic fenfluramine on blood serotonin, cerebrospinal fluid metabolites and behavior in monkeys. *Psychopharmacology,* **90**, 503–508.

Raleigh, M. J., Branme, G. L., Ritvo, E. R. *et al.* (1986). Effects of chronic fenfluramine on blood serotonin, cerebrospinal fluid metabolites and behavior in monkeys. *Psychopharmacology*, **90**, 503–508.

Randrup, A. and Munkvad, I. (1967). Stereotyped activities produced by amphetamines in several animal species and man. *Psychopharmacologia (Berl.)*, **11**, 300–310.

Rapoport, J. L. and Wise, S. P. (1988). Obsessive-compulsive disorder: evidence for basal ganglia dysfunction. *Psychopharmacol. Bull.*, **24**, 380–384.

Rapoport, J. L., Ryland, D. and Kriete, M. (1992). Drug treatment of canine acral lick: an animal model of obsessive-compulsive disorder. *Arch. Gen. Psychiatry*, **49**, 517–521.

Rasmussen, S. A., Goodman, W. K., Woods, S. W. *et al.* (1987). Effects of yohimbine in obsessive compulsive disorder. *Psychopharmacology*, **93**, 308–313.

Rauch, S. L., Jenike, M. A. and Alpert, N. M. (1994). Regional cerebral blood flow measured during symptom provocation in obsessive-compulsive disorder using oxygen 15-labeled carbon dioxide and positron emission tomography. *Arch. Gen. Psychiatry*, **51**, 62–70.

Rescorla, R. A. and LoLordo, V. M. (1965). Inhibitory avoidance behavior. *J. Comp. Physiol. Psychol.*, **59**, 406–412.

Rieg, T. S., Doerries, E., O'Shea, J. G. and Aravich, P. F. (1993). Water deprivation produces an exercise-induced weight loss phenomenon in the rat. *Physiol. Behav.*, **53**, 607–610.

Robbins, T. W. and Koob, G. F. (1980). Selective disruption of displacement behavior by lesions of the mesolimbic dopamine system. *Nature*, **285**, 409–412.

Roberts, W. W., Dember, W. N. and Brodwick, M. (1962). Alternation and exploration in rats with hippocampal lesions. *J. Comp. Physiol. Psychol.*, **55**, 695–698.

Roehr, J., Woods, A., Corbett, R. *et al.* (1995). Changes in paroxetine binding in the cerebral cortex of polydipsic rats. *Eur. J. Pharmacol.*, **278**, 75–78.

Roozendaal, B., Wiersma, A., Driscoll, P. *et al.* (1992). Vasopressinergic modulation of stress responses in the central amygdala of the roman high-avoidance and low-avoidance rat. *Brain Res.*, **596**, 35–40.

Ross, R. R. (1964). Positive and negative partial reinforcement extinction effects carried through continuous reinforcement changed motivation and changed response. *J. Exp. Psychol.*, **68**, 492–502.

Rushen, J. (1984). Stereotypic behavior, adjunctive drinking and the feeding period of tethered sows. *Anim. Behav. Sci.*, **14**, 137–145.

Sandou, F and Hen, R. (1994). 5-Hydroxytryptamine receptor subtypes: molecular and functional diversity. *Adv. Pharmacol.,* **30**, 327–380.

Sanger, D. J. and Blackman, D. E. (1978). Effects of drugs on adjunctive behavior. In *Contemporary Research in Behavioral Pharmacology* (eds D. E. Blackman and D. J. Sanger), pp. 213–261. Plenum, New York.

Sapolsky, R. M. (1986). Stress-induced elevation of testosterone concentrations in high ranking baboons: role of catecholamines. *Endocrinology*, **118**, 1630–1635.

Sarnyai, Z., Babarczy, E., Zkrivun, M. *et al.* (1991). Selective attenuation of cocaine-induced stereotyped behavior by oxytocin: putative role of basal forebrain target sites. *Neuropeptides*, **19**, 51–56.

Savoy, C. J. E., Seawright, E. and Watson, A. (1992). Stereotyped behaviors in broiler breeders in relation to husbandry and opiod receptor blockade. *Appl. Anim. Behav. Sci.*, **33**, 17–24.

Schilder, P. (1938). The organic background of obsessions and compulsions. *Am. J. Psychiatry*, **94**, 1397–1414.

Schmaltz, L. W. and Isaacson, R. L. (1967). Effect of bilateral hippocampal destruction on the acquisition and extinction of an operant response. *Physiol. Behav.*, **2**, 291–298.

Scovill, W. B. and Bettis, D. B. (1977). Results of orbial undercutting today: a personal series. In *Neurosurgical Treatment in Psychiatry, Pain and Epilepsy* (eds W. H. Sweet, S. Obrador and J. Marin-Rodriguez), pp. 189–197. University Park Press, Baltimore.

Seligman, M. E. P. (1971). Phobias and preparedness. *Behav. Ther.*, **2**, 307–320.

Sheard, M. (1969). The effect of p-chlorophenylalanine on behavior in rats: relation to brain serotonin and 5-hydroxyindoleacetic acid. *Brain Res.*, **15**, 524–528.

Shillito, E. E. (1970). The effect of parachlorophenylalanine on social interaction of male rats. *Br. J. Pharmacol.*, **38**, 305–315.

Sidman, M. (1955). Some properties of warning stimulus in avoidance behavior. *L. Comp. Physiol. Psychol.*, **48**, 444–450.

Skinner, B. F. (1948). Superstition in the pigeon. *J. Exp. Psychol.*, **38**, 168–172.

Soubrie, P. (1988). Serotonin and behavior, with special regard to animal models of anxiety, depression and waiting ability. In *Neuronal Serotonin* (eds N. N. Osborne and M. Hamon), pp. 255–270. Wiley, New York.

Spruijt, B. M., VanHooff, J. and Gispen, W. H. (1992). Ethology and neurobiology of grooming behavior. *Physiol. Rev.*, **72**, 825–852.

Staddon, J. E. R. (1977). Schedule-induced behavior. In *Handbook of Operant Behavior* (eds W. K. Honig and J. E. R. Staddon), pp. 125–152. Prentice Hall, Englewood Cliffs, NJ.

Stahl, S. M. (1988). Basal ganglia neuropharmacology and obsessive-compulsive disorder: the obsessive-compulsive disorder hypothesis of basal ganglia dysfunction. *Psychopharmacol. Bull.*, **24**, 370–374.

Stewart, B. R., Jenner, P. and Marden, C. D. (1989). Induction of purposeless chewing behavior in rats by 5-HT agonist drugs. *Eur. J. Pharmacol.*, **162**, 101–107.

Stolba, A., Baker, N. and Wood-Gush, D. G. M. (1983). The characterization of stereotyped behavior in stalled sows by informational redundancy. *Behavior*, **87**, 157–182.

Su, T. P., Pagliaro, M., Ollo, C. *et al.* (1993). Neuropsychiatric effects of anabolic steroids. *JAMA*, **269**, 2760–2764.

Su, T. P., Danaceau, M. A., Schmidt, P. J. *et al.* (1994). Effect of menstrual cycle phase on biochemical and behavioral response to m-CPP (abstract). *Biol. Psychiatry*, **35**, 661.

Suomi, S. J., Seaman, S. F., Lewis, J. K. *et al.* (1971). Effects of imipramine treatment of separation-induced social disorders in rhesus monkey. *Arch. Gen. Psychiatry*, **35**, 321–325.

Swedo, S. E. (1989). Rituals and releasers: an ethological model of obsessive-compulsive disorder. In *Obsessive-compulsive Disorder in Children and Adolescents* (ed. J. L. Rapoport), pp. 269–288. American Psychiatric Press, Washington, DC.

Swedo, S. E., Rapoport, J. L. and Cheslow, D. L. (1989a). High prevalence of obsessive-compulsive symptoms in patients with Sydenham's chorea. *Am. J. Psychiatry*, **146**, 246–249.

Swedo, S. E., Shapiro, M. B. and Grady, C. L. (1989b). Cerebral glucose metabolism in childhood-onset obsessive-compulsive disorder. *Arch. Gen. Psychiatry*, **46**, 518–523.

Swedo, S. E., Leonard, H. L., Rapoport, J. L. *et al.* (1989c). A double-blind comparison of clomipramine and desipramine in the treatment of trichotillomania (hair pulling). *N. Engl. J. Med.* **321**, 497–501.

Swedo, S. E., Leonard, H. L. and Rapoport, J. L. (1992a). Childhood-onset obsessive-compulsive disorder. *Psych. Clin. North Am.*, **15**, 767–775.

Swedo, S. E., Pietrini, P. and Leonard, H. L. (1992b). Cerebral glucose metabolism in childhood-onset obsessive-compulsive disorder: revisualization during pharmacotherapy. *Arch. Gen. Psychiatry*, **49**, 690–694.

Talairach, J., Bancaud, J. and Geier, S. (1973). The cingulate gyrus and human behavior. *Electroencephalogr. Clin. Neurophysiol.*, **34**, 45–52.

Teasdale, J. D. (1974). Learning models of obsessive-compulsive disorder. In *Obsessional States* (ed. H. R. Beech), pp. 197–229. Methuen, London.

Tenen, S. S. (1967). The effects of p-chlorophenylalanine a serotonin depletor on avoidance acquisition, pain sensitivity and related behaviors in the rat. *Psychopharmacologia (Berl.)*, **10**, 204–219.

Tinbergen, H. (1953). *Social Behavior in Animals*. Holt, Rinehart & Winston, London.

Tippin, J. and Henn, F. A. (1982). Stereotactic limbic leucotomy: a follow-up at 16 months. *Br. J. Psychiatry*, **128**, 226–240.

Traber, J., Spencer, D. G., Glaser, T. and Gispen, W. H. (1988). Actions of psychoactive drugs on ACTH- and novelty-induced behavior in the rat. *Ann. NY Acad. Sci.*, **525**, 270–280.

Vacas, M. I. and Carinali, D. P. (1979). Effects of castration and reproductive hormones on pineal serotonin metabolism in rats. *Neuroendocrinology*, **28**, 187–195.

Valenstein, E. S. (1980). Stereotypy and sensory-motor changes evoked by hypothalamic stimulation: possible relation to schizophrenic behavior patterns. In *Biology of Reinforcement: Facets of Brain-Stimulation Reward* (ed. A. Routtenberg), pp. 39–52. Academic Press, New York.

Van de Kar, L., Levine, J. and Ordern, L. S. (1978). Serotonin in hypothalamic nuclei:

increased content after castration of male rats. *Neuroendocrinology*, **27**, 186–192.

Van Wimersma-Greidanus, T. B., Tornm, M. C., Ronner, E. *et al.* (1989). Dopamine D-1 and D-2 receptor agonists and antagonists and neuropeptide-induced excessive grooming. *Eur. J. Pharmacol.*, **173**, 227–231.

Vecchiotti, G. G. and Galant, R. (1986). Evidence of heredity of cribbing, weaving and stall-walking in thoroughbred horses. *Livest. Prod. Sci.*, **14**, 91–95.

Vergnes, M., Depaulis, A., Boehrer, A. and Kempf, E. (1988). Selective increase of offensive behavior in the rat following intrahypothalamic 5,7-DHT-induced serotonin depletion. *Behav. Brain Res.*, **29**, 85–91.

Villablanca, S. R. and Olmstead, C. E. (1982). The striatum: a fine tuner of the brain. *Acta Neurobiol. Exp. (Warsz.)*, **42**, 227–299.

Virkkunen, M., Rawlings, R., Tokola, R. *et al.* (1994). CSF biochemistries, glucose metabolism, and diurnal activity rhythms in alcoholic, violent fire setters and healthy volunteers. *Arch. Gen. Psychiatry*, **51**, 20–27.

Watanabe, Y., Sakai, R. R., McEwan, B. S. and Mendelson, S. (1993). Stress and antidepressant effects on hippocampal and cortical and 5-HT$_2$ receptors and transport sites for serotonin. *Brain Res.*, **615**, 87–94.

Wayner, M. J. (1974). Specificity of behavioral regulation. *Physiol. Behav.*, **12**, 851–869.

Weissman, M. M., Bland, R. C., Canino, G. J. *et al.* (1994). The cross national epidemiology of obsessive compulsive disorder. *J. Clin. Psychiatry*, **55** (Suppl.), 5–10.

Whitaker-Azmitia, P., Molino, L. J., Caruso, J. and Shemer, A. V. (1990). Serotonergic agents restore appropriate decision-making in neonatal rats displaying dopamine D1 receptor-mediated vacillatory behavior. *Eur. J. Pharmacology*, **180**, 305–309.

Wiepkema, P. R. (1987). Developmental aspects of motivated behavior in domestic animals. *J. Anim. Sci.*, **65**, 1220–1227.

Willner, P. (1991). Behavior models in psychopharmacology. In *Behavioral Models in Psychopharmacology: Theoretical, Industrial and Clinical Perspectives* (ed. P. Willner), pp. 3–18. Cambridge University Press, Cambridge.

Wilner, J. H., Samach, M. and Angrist, B. M. (1970). Drug-induced stereotyped behavior and its antagonism in dogs. *Commun. Behav. Biol.*, **5**, 135–142.

Winchel, R. R., Jones, J. S., Stanley, B. *et al.* (1992). Clinical characteristics of trichotillomania and its response to fluoxetine. *J. Clin. Psychiatry*, **53**, 304–308.

Winslow, J. T. and Insel, T. R. (1989). Neuroethological models of obsessive-compulsive disorder. In *Psychobiological Approaches to Obsessive-Compulsive Disorder* (eds. J. Zohar, S. Rasmussen and T. R. Insel), pp. 208–226. Springer, New York.

Winslow, J. T. and Insel, T. R. (1990). Serotonergic and catecholaminergic reuptake inhibitors have opposite effects on the ultrasonic isolation calls of rat pups. *Neuropsychopharmacology*, **3**, 51–59.

Winslow, J. and Insel, T. R. (1991). Vasopressin modulates male squirrel monkey's behavior during social separation. *Eur. J. Pharmacol.*, **200**, 95.

Woods, A., Smith, C., Szewczak, M. *et al.* (1993). Selective serotonin reuptake inhibition decreases schedule-induced polydipsia in rats: a potential model for obsessive-compulsive disorder. *Psychopharmacology*, **112**, 195–198.

Yadin, E., Friedman, E. and Bridger, W. H. (1991). Spontaneous alternation behavior: an animal model for obsessive-compulsive disorder. *Pharmacol. Biochem. Behav.*, **40**, 311–315.

Yates, W. R., Perry, P. and Murray, S. (1992). Aggression and hostility in anabolic steroid users. *Biol. Psychiatry*, **31**, 1232–1234.

Yodyingyuad, U., de la Riva, C., Abbott, D. M. *et al.* (1985). Relationship between dominance hierarchy, CSF level of 5-HIAA and cortisol in monkeys. *Neuroscience*, **16**, 851–858.

Zohar, J., Mueller, E. A., Insel, T. R. *et al.* (1987). Serotonergic responsivity in obsessive-compulsive disorder: comparison of patients and healthy controls. *Arch. Gen. Psychiatry*, **44**, 946–951.

Zohar, J., Kaplan, Z and Benjamin, J. (1993). Clomipramine treatment of obsessive-compulsive symptomatology in schizophrenic patients. *J. Clin. Psychiatry,* **54**, 385–388.

12 The Neuropharmacology and Neurobiology of Obsessive-compulsive Disorder: An Update on the Serotonin Hypothesis

DENNIS L. MURPHY,[1] BENJAMIN GREENBERG,[1] MARGARET ALTEMUS,[1] JONATHAN BENJAMIN,[1] TANA GRADY[2] AND THERESA PIGOTT[3]

[1]Laboratory of Clinical Science, National Institute of Mental Health, Bethesda, Maryland, [2]Department of Psychiatry, Duke University Medical Center, Durham, North Carolina, and [3]Department of Psychiatry, Georgetown University Medical Center, Washington, DC, USA

INTRODUCTION

Many neuropsychiatric disorders are thought to be importantly related to brain serotonin (5-HT) subsystems, and 5-HT alterations have been hypothesized to be either contributory factors to these disorders or to the mechanisms involved in effective psychopharmacologic treatment. This is not surprising, as changes in brain 5-HT function resulting from experimental lesions or from drugs that selectively alter brain 5-HT synthesis, metabolism, or the 13-plus molecularly identified 5-HT receptors modulate almost every major physiological function, including food intake, temperature, sleep and other circadian rhythms, sexual activity, pain, memory, neuroendocrine systems, motor activity, and other behaviors and affects (Humphrey et al., 1993; Lesch et al., 1993a). Thus, hypotheses implicating 5-HT abound, and extensive clinical and animal model studies suggest a role for 5-HT in the anxiety disorders, affective disorders, eating disorders, schizophrenia, migraine, alcoholism, Parkinson's disease, Alzheimer's disease and other incompletely understood neuropsychiatric disorders (Coccaro and Murphy, 1990; Sandler et al., 1991).

What makes the 5-HT hypothesis for obsessive-compulsive disorder (OCD) different from that for these other disorders is the neuropharmacological data suggesting a tight linkage between changes in OCD symptoms and 5-HT- selective drug effects, both therapeutic and adverse. While other disorders have a complex pharmacology, with drugs of at least several different classes and modes of

Advances in the Neurobiology of Anxiety Disorders. Edited by H. G. M. Westenberg, J. A. Den Boer and D. L. Murphy
©1996 John Wiley & Sons Ltd

action influencing symptoms, there is only very sparse data suggesting that non-5HT-selective agents alter OCD-related behaviors. As we concluded several years ago, "at present, OCD remains the neuropsychiatric disorder for which there is the strongest evidence of a possible selective involvement of a brain serotonin subsystem" (Murphy *et al.*, 1992). This chapter provides an update and re-evaluation of the data supportive of—or discordant with—this viewpoint.

Two initial caveats need to be addressed at the outset. First, most of the evidence linking OCD symptoms is indirect, based on evidence that agents with primary, initial actions on serotonergic transmission alter OCD symptoms (Insel *et al.*, 1985a; Murphy *et al.*, 1989b). It cannot be assumed that secondary consequences of these agents, either via direct interactions with other neurotransmitter systems or via longer-term, adaptive changes at sites distant from the initial drug actions, are not a more likely basis for the clinical changes observed; in fact, in this review we consider some substantive evidence for the latter possibility.

Secondly, direct studies aimed at identifying a primary 5-HT neurochemical abnormally or, for that matter, any physiological abnormality in any system that is etiologically linked to OCD, have not been successful. Attempts during the last decade to investigate possible serotonergic abnormalities using peripheral measures such as 5-HT binding sites, 5-HT uptake or 5-HT receptors in platelets led to no clear-cut differences. These direct approaches have been previously reviewed (Bastani *et al.*, 1991), and will not be summarized here. Brain studies using postmortem tissue from OCD patients are essentially non-existent, and neuroimaging studies using ligands which can quantitatively assess serotonin neurons, their terminals and their receptors which have not yet been accomplished in patients with OCD. While a few earlier studies hinted at abnormalities in the 5-HT metabolite, 5-hydroxyindoleacetic acid (5-HIAA), measured in cerebrospinal fluid, two recent studies with larger samples reported normal 5-HIAA levels (Altemus *et al.*, 1992; Swedo *et al.*, 1992). Current strategies using molecular biological approaches are searching for polymorphisms and possible abnormalities in the structure or regulation of genes for 5-HT receptors, transporters, and enzymes but only preliminary data are available (Lesch *et al.*, 1993a; Altemus *et al.*, in press; Brett *et al.*, 1995).

TREATMENT STUDIES USING SELECTIVE SEROTONIN REUPTAKE-INHIBITING DRUGS AND OTHER SEROTONIN ALTERING DRUGS IN PATIENTS WITH OBSESSIVE-COMPULSIVE DISORDER

Involvement of the brain 5-HT neurotransmitter system in OCD was originally suggested on the basis of therapeutic effects found with the semi-selective 5-HT uptake inhibitor, clomipramine. A series of case reports and open studies dating back to the 1960s (Fernandez and Lopez-Ibor, 1967) was eventually supplemented by six small controlled studies in the early 1980s, all of which reported that clomipramine was superior to placebo in OCD patients, both adults and children, and both with or without concomitant depression (reviews: McTavish and Benfield, 1990; Murphy and Pigott, 1990).

Two large multicenter treatment trials of clomipramine, involving more patients than all prior studies combined, conclusively demonstrated that clomipramine led to improvement as measured on the Yale–Brown Obsessive-Compulsive Scale (YBOCS) averaging an approximately 40% reduction in symptoms versus a negligible (~5%) change with placebo (Clomipramine Collaborative Study Group, 1991; DeVeaugh-Geiss et al., 1992). Overall, about 60% of patients were considered "much improved" or "very much improved." Patients who were not depressed responded as well as those who had depression symptoms. Sustained improvement was observed over a one-year double-blind extension of clomipramine treatment (Katz and DeVeaugh-Geiss, 1990).

While clomipramine's 5-HT uptake-inhibiting potency is more than 10-fold greater than that of its inhibitory actions on norepinephrine (NE) or dopamine uptake, its metabolite, desmethylclomipramine, has less selective effects; clomipramine, like other tricyclics, also has substantial affinity for cholinergic, histaminergic, and α-adrenergic receptors, as well as somewhat greater affinity for dopamine D_2 receptors than do other tricyclics (Hyttel and Larsen, 1985). Studies of changes in monoamine metabolites in cerebrospinal fluid from patients treated with clomipramine revealed greater reductions in the 5-HT metabolite, 5-HIAA, than the NE metabolite, 3-methoxy-4-hydroxyphenethy-lineglycol (MHPG), while the reverse was found for other antidepressants (review: Murphy, 1990b). There were also hints that responders to clomipramine had greater reductions in 5-HIAA than non-responders, and that the magnitude of therapeutic response correlated more highly with plasma levels of clomipramine than of desmethylclomipramine (Thoren et al., 1980). While these data suggested a primary serotonergic mode of action for clomipramine's efficacy in OCD, other interpretations, including a possible combination of several pharmacological effects, remained plausible.

The emergence of several selective serotonin reuptake inhibitors (SSRIs) with greater relative selectivity for 5-HT versus NE uptake inhibition and with, for the most part, negligible affinity for most neurotransmitter system receptors has provided strong support for the hypothesis that 5-HT uptake inhibition is the primary, initiating mechanism of action of clomipramine and the newer SSRIs. These newer SSRIs that have been studied in OCD patients include fluvoxamine, fluoxetine and sertraline. Fluvoxamine was the first of these shown to be effective in OCD in several placebo-controlled smaller studies (Perse et al., 1987; Cottraux et al., 1990; Goodman et al., 1990); two multicenter trials, not yet completely published, have confirmed fluvoxamine's efficacy in OCD (Greist, 1992; Montgomery and Manceaux, 1992).

A multicenter center study of sertraline yielded significantly greater improvement in OCD patients given this drug versus placebo; however, YBOCS differences were modest (sertraline, –16%, placebo, –7%) and patients rated as "much improved" or "very much improved" constituted 25% of the sertraline-treated group versus 11% of the placebo-treated group (Chouinard et al., 1990; Murdoch and McTavish, 1992). Fluoxetine also has been shown to be significantly better than placebo in OCD patients in multicenter studies conducted in Europe (Montgomery et al., 1993) and the USA (Wood et al., 1993); the latter has not yet been reported in full detail. In the European study which included 214 patients, YBOCS scale reductions in the 60 mg per day fluoxetine group averaged –28.5% versus –17.5% with placebo; the proportions of patients rated "much improved" or "very much improved" were 48% after fluoxetine and 26% after placebo (Montgomery et al., 1993).

Table 1. Double-blind comparisons of 5-HT-selective antidepressants versus other antidepressants and antianxiety agents in patients with OCD

Result	Design, N	Reference
Clomipramine (CMI)		
CMI ≥ nortriptyline	Parallel, 35	Thoren et al. (1980)
CMI ≥ amitriptyline	Parallel, 20	Ananth et al. (1981)
CMI > clorgyline	Cross-over, 13	Insel et al. (1983)
CMI > imipramine	Parallel, 16	Volavka et al. (1985)
CMI > desipramine	Cross-over, 10	Zohar and Insel (1987)
CMI > desipramine	Cross-over, 48	Leonard et al. (1989)
CMI = buspirone	Parallel, 20	Pato et al. (1991)
CMI = phenelzine	Parallel, 30	Vallejo et al. (1992)
CMI = clonazepam > diphenhydramine, clonidine	Cross-over, 28	Hewlett et al. (1992)
CMI > alprazolam = placebo	Parallel, 46	Stein et al. (1992)
Other 5-HT-selective antidepressants		
Fluvoxamine > desipramine	Parallel, 35	Goodman et al. (1990)
Fluvoxetine = clomipramine	Parallel, 32	Pigott et al. (1990)

The comparative efficacy of the SSRIs over that of other antidepressants (Table 1) quite sharply differentiates OCD patients from depressed patients and several other neuropsychiatric patient populations (e.g. panic disorder patients) who manifest similar treatment responses to different classes and types of antidepressant agents (Murphy and Pigott, 1990).

The contrasting efficacy of the 5-HT-selective drugs versus desipramine in several studies of OCD patients (Table 1) and also in some additional studies of patients with syndromes characterized by OCD-like features including trichotillomania (Swedo *et al.*, 1989) and onychophagia (nail-biting) (Leonard *et al.*, 1991a) is particularly noteworthy. In one double-blind cross-over study, patients who had improved with clomipramine treatment developed an acute recurrence of OCD symptoms when they were switched to desipramine (Leonard *et al.*, 1991b). This rapid return of symptoms had earlier been observed during double-blind switches of OCD patients from clomipramine to placebo during a discontinuation study (Pato *et al.*, 1988) and also in apparent response to placebo substitution during a cross-over study (Pigott *et al.*, 1990), raising the question of whether continuing effects of treatment with 5-HT uptake inhibitor agents are required for symptom suppression (Pigott *et al.*, 1990).

A study investigating this question used a four-day cross-over treatment period of metergoline (4 mg) or placebo in OCD patients receiving clomipramine on a long-term basis. Relative to the placebo phase, the patients receiving the 5-HT antagonist became progressively more anxious and obsessional (Benkelfat *et al.*, 1989). In an ongoing replication study using a larger (8 mg), single dose of metergoline in fluoxetine-treated patients, a similar delayed worsening of OCD symptoms was observed (Greenberg *et al.*, 1994). While these exact metergoline treatment paradigms have not been investigated in untreated OCD patients, single 4 mg doses of metergoline had no similar effects in these patients (Zohar *et al.*, 1987; Pigott *et al.*, 1991). A likely hypothesis, therefore, is that metergoline is reversing some ongoing serotonergic changes produced by clomipramine or fluoxetine.

Despite the recent success of 5-HT uptake inhibitors in the pharmacological treatment of OCD, most patients respond to these agents with only a partial reduction in OCD symptoms, and a distinct subgroup of patients are non-responders. Consequently, studies have been conducted with adjuvant agents in combination with 5-HT uptake inhibitors in an attempt to maximize antiobsessive response. Due to the preferential benefit from 5-HT-selective drugs in OCD, most of the adjuvant agents that have been utilized also possess 5-HT-enhancing properties, including lithium carbonate, tryptophan, fenfluramine, and buspirone. An exception was the adjuvant use of haloperidol in OCD patients with or without concurrent tic disorders who were refractory to treatment with fluvoxamine; haloperidol was found to be an effective adjunct in OCD patients with tic disorders (8 of 8 were responders), but less so in OCD patients without tic disorders (3 of 9 were responders) (McDougle *et al.*, 1994). There have been several case reports and uncontrolled studies of the successful use of adjuvant lithium (Rasmussen, 1984; Feder, 1988; Golden *et al.*, 1988), fenfluramine (Hollander *et al.*, 1990), L-tryptophan (Yaryura-Tobias and Bhagavan, 1977; Rasmussen, 1984) and buspirone (Markovitz *et al.*, 1990; Jenike *et al.*, 1991) in patients with OCD; however, controlled studies of adjuvant agents have been much less promising.

Our group has recently completed four controlled studies of adjuvant agents in patients with OCD who had been previously stabilized on either clomipramine or fluoxetine monotherapy. In the first study, adjuvant lithium carbonate or thyroid hormone was not associated with significant further reduction in OCD symptoms attained during continued clomipramine treatment (Pigott et al., 1991). McDougle and colleagues (1991) also completed a controlled adjuvant lithium study in patients with OCD and reported that adjuvant lithium therapy was not significantly different from fluvoxamine alone. More recently, our group also completed two separate studies of adjuvant buspirone in clomipramine- or fluoxetine-treated patients with OCD (Pigott et al., 1992b; Grady et al., 1993). Neither study demonstrated significant further reductions in OCD or anxiety symptoms. In a fourth study—a controlled trial of adjuvant clonazepam in clomipramine- or fluoxetine-treated patients with OCD—clonazepam treatment was associated with significant further reductions in anxiety symptoms, and also significant reductions on one of the three OCD rating scales (Pigott et al., 1992a). There is considerable evidence from human and animal studies indicating that clonazepam has indirect serotonergic properties that are distinct from those of the other benzodiazepines (Chadwick et al., 1977; Pranzatelli, 1989; Lima, 1991; Lima et al., 1993).

There are a number of possible reasons for the discrepancy between the open reports and the controlled trials in addition to the potential observer and patient bias inherent in uncontrolled studies. Many of the open reports included patients who had received an inadequate duration of treatment with 5-HT uptake inhibitors prior to the addition of adjuvant medication, so that any further improvement noted and attributed to the adjuvant medication may have been in fact attributable to the longer treatment duration of the 5-HT uptake inhibitor alone. The previously described controlled trials only included patients that had been stabilized on their primary medication for at least 10 weeks prior to the addition of adjuvant medication. Of course, adjuvant medications like lithium and buspirone may be unable to promote further symptom reductions because their mechanisms or sites of action have already been saturated by the primary medication—something that would also pertain to the controlled as well as open studies.

SEROTONIN AGONISTS IN PATIENTS WITH OBSESSIVE-COMPULSIVE DISORDER AND CONTROLS

Drugs with 5-HT-selective effects have been administered to patients with OCD and other neuropsychiatric disorders in order to assess the functional status of brain serotonergic pathways in these disorders (reviews: Murphy, 1990a; Kahn and Wetzler, 1991; Murphy et al., 1991). Many 5-HT agonists produce increases in plasma prolactin, cortisol and adrenocorticotropic hormone (ACTH) concentrations, some agonists increase temperature, and some also alter behavior (Murphy et al., 1991). In a small number of studies, the neuroendocrine responses to 5-HT agonists have been found to be diminished in OCD patients relative to healthy controls (Table 2), but a fully consistent pattern of neuroen-

Table 2. Comparison of the neuroendocrine responses to serotonergic agents in OCD patients compared to healthy controls

Agent	Hormone response relative to controls				Reference
	Prolactin	Cortisol	ACTH	Growth hormone	
mCPP	Same	Blunted	ND	ND	Zohar *et al.* (1987)
mCPP (oral)	Blunted	Same	ND	ND	Hollander *et al.* (1992)
mCPP (i.v.)	Blunted (F)	Same	ND	Same	Charney *et al.* (1988)
mCPP (i.v.)	Same	Same	Blunted	ND	Pigott *et al.* (1992c)
L-Tryptophan	Increased	ND	ND	Same	Charney *et al.* (1988)
MK-212	Same	Blunted	ND	ND	Bastani *et al.* (1990)
Ipsapirone	ND	Same	Same	ND	Lesch *et al.* (1991)
Fenfluramine	Same	Same	ND	ND	Hollander *et al.* (1992)
Fenfluramine	Same	ND	ND	ND	McBride *et al.* (1992)
Fenfluramine	Blunted	Blunted	ND	ND	Lucey *et al.* (1993)
Buspirone	Same	Same	Same	ND	Pigott *et al.* (1992c)

ND, not determined, F, female OCD patients only.

docrine response differences has not emerged.

The provocation of brief exacerbations of OCD symptoms by one serotonergic agent, *m*-chlorophenylpiperazine (mCPP), has aroused greatest interest among these pharmacologic challenge paradigms, and mCPP has become the most-studied pharmacologic challenge agent in OCD patients (Tables 3 and 4). Our research group's initial studies with mCPP demonstrated that it led to highly reproducible, dose-dependent effects on prolactin, cortisol, and temperature in normal volunteers (Mueller *et al.*, 1985a, 1985b; Murphy *et al.*, 1989a) and rhesus monkeys (Aloi *et al.*, 1984). These neuroendocrine and temperature effects of mCPP were blocked by the $5\text{-}HT_1/5\text{-}HT_2$ antagonist, metergoline, in human volunteers (Mueller *et al.*, 1986). Small, statistically significant increases on two of the six subscales of the NIMH Self-Rating Scale—"activation/euphoria" and "anxiety"—were found after oral mCPP doses (0.5 mg/kg) were given to healthy volunteers (Mueller *et al.*, 1985a; Murphy *et al.*, 1989a). Larger increases followed intravenous administration of mCPP (0.1 mg/kg) (Murphy *et al.*, 1989a).

In the first study of mCPP in OCD patients, responses to single doses (0.5 mg/kg orally) of mCPP in patients with OCD and in normal controls compared with responses to placebo under double-blind, random-assignment conditions (Zohar *et al.*, 1987). Relative to healthy controls, the patients with OCD became more anxious and depressed. Of greatest interest, a transient but objectively verifiable exacerbation of the patients' OCD symptoms occurred. Approximately

Table 3. Effects of serotonergic agents on OCD symptoms and other psychological symptoms in OCD patients: I. Orally administered mCPP

Agent	OCD symptoms	Anxiety	Depression	Reference
mCPP	↑	↑	↑	Zohar *et al.* (1987, 1988)
mCPP	↑	0	0	Hollander *et al.* (1988, 1992)
mCPP	0	0	0	Pigott *et al.*, (1993)

Table 4. Effects of serotonergic agents on OCD symptoms and other psychological symptoms in OCD patients: II. Intravenously administered mCPP

Agent	OCD symptoms	Anxiety	Depression	Reference
mCPP	0	↑	↑	Charney *et al.* (1988)
mCPP	↑	↑	↑	Broocks *et al.* (1992)
mCPP	↑	↑	↑	Pigott *et al.* (1993)

half of the patients spontaneously described emergence of new obsessions or reoccurrence of obsessions that had not been present for sometime. The response to placebo as well as the side effects in both groups were minimal and did not differ significantly between the patients and the controls (Zohar and Insel, 1987; Zohar *et al.*, 1988).

A second independent study also reported transient exacerbations in OCD symptoms after orally administered mCPP (0.5 mg/kg), which were statistically significant for the group as a whole and represented meaningful clinical changes in 11 of 20 (55%) of the OCD patients (Hollander *et al.*, 1988, 1992). Visual analog scales did not indicate any differential non-OCD-related mood or anxiety changes in the patients compared to the controls. A third study using orally administered mCPP did not find a significant increase in OCD symptoms, nor any differential anxiety or other changes in self-ratings between OCD patients and healthy controls (Table 3) (Pigott *et al.*, 1993).

There have also been three studies of mCPP given intravenously to OCD patients (Table 4). In all three studies, considerably greater increases in anxiety and other self-ratings were found than had been reported with orally administered mCPP. Nonetheless, the first of these studies reported no increase in OCD symptoms following mCPP versus placebo (Charney et al., 1988). The other two studies, one using the same mCPP dose (0.1 mg/kg) (Pigott et al., 1993) and the other, a smaller mCPP dose (0.08 mg/kg) (Broocks et al., 1992) reported statistically significant increases in ratings of OCD symptoms after mCPP but not after placebo. There were some differences between the first study and the other two in terms of duration of intravenous administration of mCPP (20 min vs 90s) and the mode and timing of OCD symptom assessment, but evaluations of these differences remain incomplete. Likewise, while we have speculated in detail about possible reasons for the different results found among these studies of mCPP in OCD patients (Pigott et al., 1993), no simple explanations are available at this time.

Table 5. Effects of serotonergic agents on OCD symptoms and other psychological symptoms in OCD patients and controls: III. 5-HT precursors, releasing agents and other receptor agonists besides mCPP

Agent	OCD symptoms	Anxiety	Depression	Reference
L-Tryptophan	0	↑	0	Charney et al. (1988)
Fenfluramine	0	0	0	Hollander et al. (1988, 1992)
Fenfluramine	0	ND	ND	McBride et al. (1992)
MK-212	0	↑	↑	Bastani et al. (1990)
Ipsapirone	0	0	0	Lesch et al. (1991)
Buspirone	0	0	0	Pigott et al. (1992b)

ND, not determined.

As summarized in Table 5, a 5-HT metabolic precursor (L-tryptophan), a 5-HT releasing agent (fenfluramine), and several 5-HT receptor agonists, including the $5-HT_{1A}$ selective partial agonists, ipsapirone and buspirone, as well as MK-212, which has some chemical and pharmacological similarities to mCPP, have been administered to OCD patients. Unlike mCPP, none of these agents have been reported to produce OCD symptom exacerbations. In addition, most of these agents, with the exception of MK-212, produced only minimal behavioral effects of any kind. Lowering plasma tryptophan using a tryptophan-free amino acid challenge did not affect OCD symptoms in patients being treated with SSRIs; in this study, however, significant increases in depressive symptoms occurred, resembling those previously observed in depressed patients receiving this challenge during SSRI treatment (Barr et al., 1994).

ATTENUATION OR BLOCKADE OF mCPP'S EFFECTS IN OBSESSIVE-COMPULSIVE DISORDER PATIENTS AND HEALTHY CONTROLS BY SEROTONIN ANTAGONISTS AND BY CHRONIC TREATMENT WITH SEROTONIN-SELECTIVE UPTAKE INHIBITORS

To evaluate whether mCPP's behavioral effects in patients with OCD might be attributable to actions at 5-HT receptors, two studies investigated pretreatment with a single dose (4 mg) of the 5-HT antagonist, metergoline, prior to mCPP. In an earlier, preliminary study, metergoline given alone produced a small but significant increase on one of three OCD rating scales (Zohar and Insel, 1987); however, when this same study was extended to include a larger number of OCD patients, metergoline was not found to significantly change OCD symptoms or anxiety ratings (Zohar et al., 1988). Metergoline did block or significantly attenuate the plasma prolactin, cortisol, ACTH, and temperature responses to orally administered mCPP in healthy controls (Mueller et al., 1986; Kahn et al., 1990). Metergoline provided a less complete blockade of intravenously administered mCPP's effects, significantly reducing the plasma prolactin, temperature, and blood pressure increases found after mCPP, but not the plasma cortisol, growth hormone, or NE changes (Pigott et al., 1993). Less complete studies with two other 5-HT antagonists, methysergide and ritanserin, also provided evidence that these agents reduced mCPP's neuroendocrine effects in humans (Kahn et al., 1990).

Table 6. Effects of pretreatment with clomipramine, fluoxetine, metergoline, or ondansetron on behavioral responses to mCPP in OCD patients

Agent	Behavioral responses to mCPP			Reference
	OCD symptoms	Anxiety	Depression	
Orally administered mCPP				
Clomipramine (4 months)	Significantly attenuated	Significantly attenuated	Blocked	Zohar et al. (1988)
Fluoxetine (3 months)	Blocked	ND	ND	Hollander et al. (1991)
Metergoline	Blocked	Blocked	Blocked	Pigott et al. (1991)
Intravenously administered mCPP				
Metergoline	Blocked	Blocked	Blocked	Pigott et al. (1993)
Ondansetron	Unchanged	Unchanged	Unchanged	Broocks et al. (1992)

ND, not determined.

As summarized in Table 6, metergoline pretreatment was associated with essentially complete blockade of the increase in OCD symptoms and the other behavioral effects of mCPP given either orally or intravenously (Pigott et al., 1991, 1993). mCPP-induced plasma prolactin increases were also blocked by metergoline pretreatment in these patients. In contrast, the highly selective antagonist of 5-HT$_3$ receptors, ondansetron, was without effects on OCD symptoms elicited by intravenous mCPP (Broocks et al., 1992). In none of these studies with mCPP and metergoline in patients with OCD were mCPP plasma levels altered by metergoline pretreatment.

As metergoline has high, equivalent potency at all 5-HT$_1$ and 5-HT$_2$ receptor sites, and mCPP's order of binding affinity, is 5-HT$_{2C}$>5-HT$_3$>5-HT$_{2A}$>5-HT$_{1A}$ and other 5-HT$_1$ sites; these results are most compatible with the hypothesis that mCPP's behavioral effects in OCD patients are primarily mediated by its 5-HT$_{2C}$ agonist properties (Hoyer, 1988; Hoyer and Schoeffter, 1991; Murphy, 1991b). Studies of mCPP's behavioral effects in animal models have previously attributed mCPP's apparent anxiogenic actions to 5-HT$_{2C}$-mediated effects (Kennett and Curzon, 1988; Lucki et al., 1989; Murphy, 1991b), with some qualifications (Review: Murphy, 1991b).

Several attempts have been made to determine whether the behavioral and other responses of patients with OCD to mCPP might be modified by therapeutic agents that improve OCD symptoms. Patients with OCD treated for an average of four months with the partially selective 5-HT uptake inhibitor, clomipramine, were found to have attenuated behavioral responses to mCPP, with no significant exacerbation of OCD symptoms after mCPP treatment (Zohar et al., 1988). Temperature responses to mCPP were also attenuated, but prolactin and cortisol increases were no different from non-clomipramine-treated patients with OCD given mCPP. Plasma mCPP concentrations were approximately two-fold higher in patients studied during clomipramine treatment compared to their pretreatment values. As the patients receiving clomipramine treatment had improved approximately 40% at the end of the mCPP study, the question of whether the altered behavioral response to mCPP might be related to the altered clinical state rather than a primary pharmacological effect or biochemical adaptational change produced by clomipramine remains open.

Treatment with the more highly selective 5-HT uptake inhibitor, fluoxetine, also led to an attenuation of the exacerbation of obsessive-compulsive symptoms produced by orally administered mCPP in patients with OCD (Hollander et al., 1991b). Four-fold higher plasma concentrations of mCPP were found in the fluoxetine-treated patients. Plasma prolactin and cortisol responses to mCPP were enhanced during fluoxetine treatment, perhaps reflecting mCPP's altered pharmacokinetics.

CONCLUSIONS

OCD is classified in the USA as one of the anxiety disorders, and OCD patients' self-ratings of anxiety on standard scales are as high as those of patients with panic disorder and generalized anxiety disorder (review: Murphy *et al.*, 1990). OCD patients are also intermittently depressed, sometimes quite severely. In fact, the prominent depressive symptoms originally found in OCD patients seeking psychiatric treatment, combined with OCD patients' therapeutic responses to clomipramine, and their lack of response to anxiolytic drugs like the benzodiazepines, originally led clinicians to consider the possibility that OCD might be an affective disorder variant (Insel *et al.*, 1985b). More recently, treatment response data have indicated that depression and anxiety in OCD patients often do not improve unless OCD symptoms improve, confirming the primary nature of OCD symptoms in patients with OCD (Montgomery *et al.*, 1991, 1993).

The hallmarks of the disorder, compulsive rituals and intrusive, obsessional thoughts, associated with functional impairment, comprise the core of this syndrome which recent community survey data suggests may afflict approximately 2.5% of the US population (Karno *et al.*, 1988). While comorbidity with some of the anxiety disorders, including phobias and panic disorder, as well as with depression and alcohol and other substance abuse exists, epidemiologic data support OCD as a distinct entity (Flament *et al.*, 1988; Karno *et al.*, 1988; Rasmussen and Eisen, 1992). In fact, among all the "official" DSM-III-R anxiety disorders, OCD has recently been reported to share the least anxiety disorder comorbidity (Angst, 1993). As reviewed above, OCD neuropharmacology is also distinctly different from that of both the affective disorders and the other anxiety disorders.

This review has narrowly focused on pharmacologic studies using 5-HT-selective agents in patients with OCD. Other important aspects of the psychobiology of OCD have been reviewed elsewhere (Rapoport, 1989, 1991; Insel and Winslow, 1992). The possible contributions of brain 5-HT function changes to the disorder and to its treatment reviewed in this chapter represent hypotheses that need to be integrated into the "whole picture" of this syndrome as additional information becomes available.

In the areas of acute pharmacologic challenges and treatment involving OCD symptoms, there are recent examples of symptom improvement reported after non-serotonergic interventions, including single doses of the α_2-adrenergic agonist, clonidine (Hollander *et al.*, 1991a), and longer-term adjunctive treatment with the dopamine receptor antagonist, pimozide (McDougle *et al.*, 1990). However, a small controlled study of the dopamine receptor antagonist, haloperidol, and a six-week study of clonidine provided no evidence of efficacy in OCD treatment (O'Regan, 1970; Hewlett *et al.*, 1992). As the catecholamine and 5-HT neurotransmitter subsystems in brain also exhibit many interactions, it is not possible at the present time to fully dissect and define the relative contributions of these major neurotransmitter systems to therapeutic drug actions in OCD.

As to the other side of the coin, OCD is obviously not the only neuropsychiatric disorder in which brain 5-HT function is thought to be important. In the last decade, evidence suggesting serotonergic dysregulation in many different neuropsychiatric disorders has accumulated, and a recent review, which focused only on investigations of specific 5-HT receptor subtype-mediated responses, listed studies of depression, schizophrenia, alcoholism, migraine, sexual dysfunction, and Alzheimer's disease, as well as, of course, the anxiety disorders, including OCD and panic disorder (Coccaro and Murphy, 1990). Panic disorder is an especially interesting case among these disorders, as, reminiscent of the findings in OCD, there is good evidence of the precipitation of panic attacks by mCPP (Kahn *et al.*, 1988; Klein *et al.*, 1991), and some evidence that panic disorder patients respond well to treatment with 5-HT-selective uptake inhibitors (Den Boer and Westenberg, 1991). However, in contrast to OCD, panic attacks are also precipitated by other agents such as lactate, yohimbine, and carbon dioxide, which do not affect anxiety or OCD ratings in OCD patients; likewise, patients with panic disorder respond well to treatment with other types of tricyclic and monoamine oxidase-inhibiting antidepressants which are ineffective in treating OCD patients (reviews: Murphy *et al.*, 1990; Den Boer and Westenberg, this volume). Thus, at present, OCD continues as the neuropsychiatric disorder for which there is the strongest evidence of a possible selective involvement of a brain 5-HT subsystem.

It remains premature to speculate about which 5-HT subsystem is most likely involved. Microanatomical features indicate that two different types of axons project to some discrete and also some overlapping terminal fields: one type from the dorsal raphe nucleus and the other from the medial raphe nucleus (Molliver, 1987). Electrophysiological, pharmacological and lesion studies also support important differences in functional aspects of the two raphe nuclei and perhaps for the other B1–B9 nerve cell groups containing 5-HT (Murphy, 1991a; Jacobs and Azmitia, 1992). In addition to these cell body and projection subsystems, there exist at least 13 molecularly identified 5-HT receptors in synaptic terminals; these receptors use three main signal transduction pathways: adenylyl cyclase, phosphotidylinositol hydrolysis and ion channel changes, alone or in combination (Humphrey *et al.*, 1993). As some brain cells have been identified that contain two or more of these receptors, some with opposing actions on cell function, and as there is evidence from pharmacologic studies of other opposing or potentiating actions of 5-HT-selective agents or physiologic events, it is clear that much further work is needed to clarify the identity and functional nature of these multiple subsystems, and ultimately, to perhaps relate their functions to complex neuropsychiatric disorders like OCD.

ACKNOWLEDGMENT

We thank Mrs Wilma Davis for valuable assistance in the editing of this chapter.

REFERENCES

Aloi, J. A., Insel, T. R., Mueller, E. A. and Murphy, D. L. (1984). Neuroendocrine and behavioral effects of m-chlorophenylpiperazine administration in rhesus monkeys. *Life Sci.*, **34**, 1325–1331.

Altemus, M., Pigott, T. A., Kalogeras, K. T. *et al.* (1992). Abnormalities in the regulation of vasopressin and corticotropin releasing factor secretion in obsessive-compulsive disorder. *Arch. Gen. Psychiatry*, **49**, 9–20.

Altemus, M., Murphy, D. L., Greenberg, B and Lesch, K. P. (in press). Intact coding region of the serotonin transporter gene in obsessive-compulsive disorder. *Am. J. Med. Genet. (Neuropsychiatr. Genet.).*

Ananth, J., Pecknold, J. C., vandenSteen, N. and Engelsmann, F. (1981). Double-blind comparative study of clomipramine and amitriptyline in obsessive neurosis. *Prog. Neuropsychopharmacol. Biol. Psychiatry,* **5**, 257–262.

Angst, J. (1993). Comorbidity of anxiety, phobia, compulsion and depression. *Int. Clin. Psychopharmacol.*, **8** (Suppl. 1), 21–25.

Barr, L. C., Goodman, W. K., McDougle, C. J. *et al.* (1994). Tryptophan depletion in patients with obsessive-compulsive disorder who respond to serotonin reuptake inhibitors. *Arch. Gen. Psychiatry*, **51**, 309–317.

Bastani, B., Arora, R. C. and Meltzer, H. Y. (1991). Serotonin uptake and imipramine binding in the blood platelets of obsessive-compulsive disorder patients. *Biol. Psychiatry*, **30**(2), 131–139.

Bastani, B., Nash, J. F. and Meltzer, H. Y. (1990).

Benkelfat, C., Murphy, D. L., Zohar, J. *et al.* (1989). Clomipramine in obsessive-compulsive disorder: further evidence for a serotonergic mechanism of action. *Arch. Gen. Psychiatry*, **46**, 23–28.

Brett, P. M., Curtis, D., Robertson, M. M. and Gurling, H. M. D. (1995). Exclusion of the 5-HT$_{1A}$ serotonin neuroreceptor and tryptophan oxygenase genes in a large British kindred multiply affected with Tourette's syndrome, chronic motor tics, and obsessive-compulsive behavior. *Am. J. Psychiatry,* **152**, 437–440.

Broocks, A., Pigott, T. A., Canter, S. *et al.* (1992). Acute administration of ondansetron and m-CPP in patients with obsessive-compulsive disorder (OCD) and controls: behavioral and biological results. *Biol. Psychiatry*, **31**, 174A.

Chadwick, D., Hallett, M., Harris, R. *et al.* (1977). Clinical, biochemical, and physiological features distinguishing myoclonus responsive to 5-hydroxytryptophan, tryptophan with a monoamine oxidase inhibitor, and clonazepam. *Brain*, **100**, 455–487.

Charney, D. S., Goodman, W. K., Price, L. H. *et al.* (1988). Serotonin function in obsessive-compulsive disorder: a comparison of the effects of tryptophan and m-chlorophenylpiperazine in patients and healthy subjects. *Arch. Gen. Psychiatry*, **45**, 177–185.

Chouinard, G., Goodman, W., Greist, J. *et al.* (1990). Results of a double-blind placebo controlled trial of a new serotonin uptake inhibitor, sertraline, in the treatment of obsessive-compulsive disorder. *Psychopharm. Bull.*, **26**, 279–284.

Clomipramine Collaborative Study Group (1991). Clomipramine in the treatment of patients with obsessive compulsive disorder. *Arch. Gen. Psychiatry*, **46**, 730–738.

Coccaro, E. F. and Murphy, D. L. (1990). *Serotonin in Major Psychiatric Disorders.* American Psychiatric Press, Washington, DC.

Cottraux, J., Mollard, E., Bouvard, M. *et al.* (1990). A controlled study of fluvoxamine and exposure in obsessive-compulsive disorder. *Int. Clin. Psychopharmacol.*, **5**, 17–30.

Den Boer, J. A. and Westenberg, H. G. M. (1991). Do panic attacks reflect an abnormality in serotonin receptor subtypes? *Hum. Psychopharmacol.*, **6**, S25–30.

DeVeaugh-Geiss, J., Moroz, G., Biederman, J. *et al.* (1992). Clomipramine hydrochloride in childhood and adolescent obsessive compulsive disorder: a multicenter trial. *J. Am. Acad. Child Adolesc. Psychiatry*, **31**, 45–49.

Feder, R. (1988). Lithium augmentation of clomipramine. *J. Clin. Psychiatry*, **49**, 458.

Fernandez, E. and Lopez-Ibor, J. (1967). Clomipramine in resistant psychiatric disorders and other treatments. *Actas Luso Esp. Neurol. Psiquiatr. Cienc. Afines*, **26**, 119.

Flament, M. F., Whitaker, A. and Rapoport, J. L. (1988). Obsessive compulsive disorder in adolescence: an epidemiologic study. *J. Am. Acad. Child Adolesc. Psychiatry*, **27**,

764–771.

Golden, R. N., Morris, J. E. and Sack, D. A. (1988). Combined lithium–tricyclic treatment of obsessive-compulsive disorder. *Biol. Psychiatry*, **23**, 181–185.

Goodman, W. K., McDougle, C. J., Price, L. H. *et al.* (1990). Beyond the serotonin hypothesis: a role for dopamine in some forms of obsessive compulsive disorder? *J. Clin. Psychiatry*, **51**(8, Suppl.), 36–43.

Grady, T., Pigott, T. A., L'Heureux, F. *et al.* (1993). Double-blind study of adjuvant buspirone for fluoxetine-treated patients with obsessive-compulsive disorder. *Am. J. Psychiatry*, **150**, 819–821.

Greenberg, B. D., Benjamin, J. and Murphy, D. L. (1994). Biphasic effects of metergoline in fluoxetine-treated OCD patients. *Biol Psychiatry*, **35**, 615.

Greist, J. H. (1992). A multicentre parallel design double-blind placebo-controlled trial. XVIIIth CINP Congress, Nice, France.

Hewlett, W. A., Vinogradov, S. and Agras, W. S. (1992). Clomipramine, clonazepam, and clonidine treatment of obsessive-compulsive disorder. *J. Clin. Psychopharmacol.* **12**, 420–430.

Hollander, E., Fay, M., Cohen, B. *et al.* (1988). Serotonergic and noradrenergic sensitivity in obsessive-compulsive disorder: behavioral findings. *Am. J. Psychiatry*, **145**, 1015–1017.

Hollander, E., DeCaria, K. M., Schneier, F. R. *et al.* (1990). Fenfluramine augmentation of serotonin reuptake blockade antiobsessional treatment. *J. Clin. Psychiatry*, **51**, 119–122.

Hollander, E., DeCaria, C., Gully, R. *et al.* (1991a). Effects of chronic fluoxetine treatment on behavioral and neuroendocrine responses to meta-chloro-phenylpiperazine in obsessive-compulsive disorder. *Psychiatry Res.*, **36**, 1–17.

Hollander, E., DeCaria, C., Nitescu, A. *et al.* (1991b). Noradrenergic function in obsessive-compulsive disorder: behavioral and neuroendocrine responses to clonidine and comparison to healthy controls. *Psychiatry Res.*, **37**, 161–177.

Hollander, E., DeCaria, C. M., Nitescu, A. *et al.* (1992). Serotonergic function in obsessive-compulsive disorder: behavioral and neuroendocrine responses to oral m-chlorophenylpiperazine and fenfluramine in patients and healthy volunteers. *Arch. Gen. Psychiatry*, **49**(1), 21–28.

Hoyer, D. (1988). Functional correlates of serotonin 5-HT$_1$ recognition sites. *J. Recept. Res.*, **8**, 59–81.

Hoyer, D. and Schoeffter, P. (1991). 5-HT receptors: subtypes and second messengers. *J. Recept. Res.*, **11**, 197–214.

Humphrey, P. P. A., Hartig, P. and Hoyer, D. (1993). A proposed new nomenclature for 5-HT receptors. *Trends Pharmacol. Sci.*, **14**, 233–236.

Hyttel, J. and Larsen, J.-J. (1985). Serotonin-selective antidepressants. *Acta Pharmacol. Toxicol. (Copenh.)*, **56**(1), 146–153.

Insel, T. R. and Winslow, J. T. (1992). Neurobiology of obsessive compulsive disorder. *Psychiatr. Clin. North Am.*, **15**, 813–824.

Insel, T. R., Murphy, D. L., Cohen, R. M. *et al.* (1983). Obsessive-compulsive disorder: a double-blind trial of clomipramine and clorgyline. *Arch. Gen. Psychiatry*, **40**, 605–612.

Insel, T. R., Mueller, E. A., Alterman, I., Linnoila, M. and Murphy, D. L. (1985a). Obsessive-compulsive disorder and serotonin: is there a connection? *Biol. Psychiatry*, **20**, 1174–1188.

Insel, T. R., Mueller, E. A., Gillin, J. C. *et al.* (1985b). Tricyclic response in obsessive compulsive disorder. *Prog. Neuropsychopharmacol. Biol. Psychiatry*, **9**, 25–31.

Jacobs, B. L. and Azmitia, E. C. (1992). Structure and function of the brain serotonin system. *Physiol. Rev.*, **72**, 165–229.

Jenike, M. A., Baer, L. and Buttolph, L. (1991). Buspirone augmentation of fluoxetine in patients with obsessive-compulsive disorder. *J. Clin. Psychiatry*, **52**, 13–14.

Kahn, R. S. and Wetzler, S. (1991). m-Chlorophenylpiperazine as a probe of serotonin function. *Biol. Psychiatry*, **30**, 1139–1166.

Kahn, R. S., Wetzler, S., vanPraag, H. M. *et al.* (1988). Behavioral indications for serotonin receptor hypersensitivity in panic disorder. *Psychiatry Res.*, **25**, 101–104.

Kahn, R. S., Wetzler, S., Asnis, G. M. *et al.* (1990). Effects of serotonin antagonists on m-chlorophenylpiperazine-mediated responses in normal subjects. *Psychiatry Res.*, **33**, 189–198.

Karno, M., Golding, J. M., Sorenson, S. B. and Burnam, M. A. (1988). The epidemiology of obsessive-compulsive disorder in five US communities. *Arch. Gen. Psychiatry*, **45**, 1094–1099.

Katz, R. J. and DeVeaugh-Geiss, J. (1990). The antiobsessional effects of clomipramine do not require concomitant affective disorder. *Psychiatry Res.*, **31**, 121–129.

Kennett, G. A. and Curzon, G. (1988). Evidence that m-CPP may have behavioral effects mediated by central 5-HT$_{1C}$ receptors. *Br. J. Pharmacol.*, **94**, 137–147.

Klein, E., Zohar, J., Geraci, M. F. *et al.*, (1991). Anxiogenic effects of m-CPP in patients with panic disorder: comparison to caffeine's anxiogenic effects. *Biol. Psychiatry*, **30**, 973–984.

Leonard, H. L., Swedo, S. E., Rapoport, J. L. *et al.* (1989). Treatment of obsessive-compulsive disorder with clomipramine and desipramine in children and adolescents: a double-blind crossover comparison. *Arch. Gen. Psychiatry*, **46**, 1088–1092.

Leonard, H., Lenane, M. C., Swedo, S. E., *et al.* (1991a). A double-blind comparison of clomipramine and desipramine treatment of severe onychophagia (nail biting). *Arch. Gen. Psychiatry*, **48**, 821–827.

Leonard, H. L., Swedo, S. E., Lenane, M. C., *et al.* (1991b). A double-blind desipramine substitution during long-term clomipramine treatment in children and adolescents with obsessive-compulsive disorder. *Arch. Gen. Psychiatry*, **48**, 922–927.

Lesch, K. P., Hoh, A., Disselkamp, T. J. *et al.* (1991). 5-Hydroxytryptamine$_{1A}$ (5-HT$_{1A}$) receptor responsivity in obsessive-compulsive disorder: comparison of patients and controls: *Arch. Gen. Psychiatry*, **48**, 540–547.

Lesch, K. P., Aulakh, C. S. and Murphy, D. L. (1993b). Brain serotonin subsystem complexity and receptor heterogeneity: therapeutic potential of selective serotonin agonists and antagonists: in *Clinical Pharmacology in Psychiatry: Strategies in Psychotropic Drug Development* (ed. L. F. Graft *et al.*), pp. 52–69. Springer-Verlag, Berlin.

Lesch, K. P., Wolozin, B. L., Murphy, D. L. and Reiderer, P. (1993b). Primary structure of the human platelet serotonin uptake site: identity with the brain serotonin transporter. *J. Neurochem.*, **60**, 2319–2322.

Lima, L. (1991). Region-selective reduction of brain serotonin turnover rate and serotonin agonist-induced behavior in mice treated with clonazepam. *Pharmacol. Biochem. Behav.*, **39**, 671–676.

Lima, L., Salazar, M. and Trejo, E. (1993). Modulation of 5-HT$_{1A}$ receptors in the hippocampus and the raphe area of rats treated with clonazepam. *Prog. Neuropsychopharmacol. Biol. Psychiatry*, **17**, 663–677.

Lucey, J. V., Butcher, G., Clare, A. W. and Dinan, T. G. (1993). The anterior pituitary responds normally to protirelin in obsessive-compulsive disorder: evidence to support a neuroendocrine serotonergic deficit. *Acta Psychiatr. Scand.*, **87**, 384–388.

Lucki, I., Ward, H. R. and Fraxer, A. (1989). Effect of 1-(m-chlorophenyl)piperazine and 1-(m-trifluoromethylphenyl)piperazine on locomotor activity. *J. Pharmacol. Exp. Ther.*, **249**, 155–164.

Markovitz, P. J., Stagno, S. J. and Calabrese, J. R. (1990). Buspirone augmentation of fluoxetine in obsessive-compulsive disorder. *Am. J. Psychiatry*, **147**, 798–800.

McBride, P. A., DeMeo, M. D., Sweeney, J. A. *et al.* (1992). Neuroendocrine and behavioral responses to challenge with the indirect serotonin agonist dl-fenfluramine in adults with obsessive-compulsive disorder. *Biol. Psychiatry*, **31**, 19–34.

McDougle, C. J., Goodman, W. K., Price, L. H. *et al.* (1990). Neuroleptic addition in fluvoxamine-refractory obsessive-compulsive disorder. *Am. J. Psychiatry*, **147**, 652–654.

McDougle, C. J., Price, L. H., Goodman, W. K. *et al.* (1991). A controlled trial of lithium augmentation in fluvoxamine-refractory obsessive-compulsive disorder: lack of efficacy. *J. Clin. Psychopharmacol*, **11**, 175–184.

McTavish, D. and Benfield, P. (1990). Clomipramine: an overview of its pharmacological properties and a review of its therapeutic use in obsessive compulsive disorder and panic disorder. *Drugs*, **39**(1), 136–153.

Molliver, M. E. (1987). Serotonergic neuronal systems: what their anatomic organization tells us about function. *J. Clin. Psychopharmacol.*, **7**(6), 3S–23S.

Montgomery, S. A. and Manceaux, A. (1992). Fluvoxamine in the treatment of obsessive compulsive disorder. *Int. Clin. Psychopharmacol.*, **7**(Suppl. 1), 5–9.

Montgomery, S. A., Bullock, T. and Fineberg, N. (1991). Serotonin selectivity for obsessive compulsive and panic disorders. *J. Psychiatry Neurosci.*, **16**, 30–35.

Montgomery, S. A., McIntyre, A., Osterheider, M. *et al.* (1993) A double-blind, placebo-controlled study of fluoxetine in patients with DSM-III-R obsessive-compulsive disorder. *Eur. Neuropsychopharmacol.*, **3**, 143–152.

Mueller, E. A., Murphy, D. L. and Sunderland, T. (1985a). Neuroendocrine effects of m-chlorophenylpiperazine, a serotonin agonist, in humans. *J. Clin. Endocrinol.*, **61**, 1179–1184.

Mueller, E. A., Murphy, D. L., Sunderland, T. and Jones, J. (1985b). A new postsynaptic serotonin receptor agonist suitable for studies in humans. *Psychopharmacol. Bull.*, **21**, 701–704.

Mueller, E. A., Murphy, D. L. and Sunderland, T. (1986). Further studies of the putative serotonin agonist m-chlorophenylpiperazine: evidence for a serotonin receptor mediated mechanism of action in humans. *Psychopharmacology*, **89**, 388–391.

Murdoch, D. and McTavish, D. (1992). Sertraline: a review of its pharmacodynamic and pharmacokinetic properties, and therapeutic potential in depression and obsessive-compulsive disorder. *Drugs*, **44**(4), 604–624.

Murphy, D. L. (1990a). Neuropsychiatric disorders and the multiple human brain serotonin receptor subtypes and subsystems. *Neuropsychopharmacology*, **3**, 457–471.

Murphy, D. L. (1990b). Peripheral indices of central serotonin function in humans. *Ann. NY Acad. Sci.*, **600**, 282–296.

Murphy, D. L. (1991a). An overview of serotonin neurochemistry and neuroanatomy. In *5-Hydroxytryptamine in Psychiatry: A Spectrum of Ideas* (eds M. Sandler, A. Coppen and S. Harnett), pp. 23–36. Oxford University Press, London.

Murphy, D. L. (1991b). The serotonin connection in OCD: comments on "Recent advances in obsessive-compulsive disorder." *Neuropsychopharmacology*, **84**, 29–32.

Murphy, D. L. and Pigott, T. A. (1990). A comparative examination of a role for serotonin in obsessive compulsive disorder, panic disorder, and anxiety. *J. Clin. Psychiatry*, **51**(4), 53–58.

Murphy, D. L., Mueller, E. A., Hill, J. L. *et al.* (1989a). Comparative anxiogenic, neuroendocrine, and other physiologic effects of m-chlorophenylpiperazine given intravenously or orally to healthy volunteers. *Psychopharmacology*, **98**, 275–282.

Murphy, D. L., Zohar, J., Benkelfat, C. *et al.* (1989b). Obsessive-compulsive disorder as a 5-HT subsystem-related behavioural disorder. *Br. J. Psychiatry*, **155**(8), 15–24.

Murphy, D. L., Pato, M. T. and Pigott, T. A. (1990). Obsessive-compulsive disorder: treatment with serotonin-selective uptake inhibitors, azapirones, and other agents. *J. Clin. Psychopharmacol.*, **10**(3), 91S–100S.

Murphy, D. L., Lesch, K. P., Aulakh, C. S. and Pigott, T. A. (1991). Serotonin-selective arylpiperazines with neuroendocrine, behavioral, temperature, and cardiovascular effects in humans. *Pharmacol. Rev.*, **43**(4), 527–552.

Murphy, D. L., Pigott, T. A., Grady, T. A. *et al.* (1992). Neuropharmacological investigations of brain serotonin subsystem functions in obsessive-compulsive disorder. In *Serotonin, CNS Receptors and Brain Function* (ed. P. B. Bradley *et al.*), pp. 271–285. Pergamon Press, Oxford.

Nielsen, D. A., Goldman, D., Virkkunen, M. *et al.* (1994). Suicidality and 5-hydroxyindoleacetic acid concentration associated with a tryptophan hydroxylase polymorphism. *Arch. Gen. Psychiatry*, **51**, 34–38.

O'Regan, B. (1970). Treatment of obsessive-compulsive neurosis with haloperidol. *Can. Med. Assoc. J.*, **103**, 167–168.

Pato, M. T., Zohar-Kadouch, R., Zohar, J. and Murphy, D. L. (1988). Return of symptoms after discontinuation of clomipramine in patients with obsessive-compulsive disorder. *Am. J. Psychiatry*, **145**, 1521–1525.

Pato, M. T., Pigott, T. A., Hill, J. L. *et al.* (1991). Controlled comparison of buspirone and clomipramine in obsessive-compulsive disorder. *Am. J. Psychiatry*, **148**, 127–129.

Perse, T. L., Greist, J. H., Jefferson, J. W. *et al.* (1987). Fluvoxamine treatment of obsessive-compulsive disorder. *Am. J. Psychiatry*, **144**, 1543–1548.

Pigott, T. A., Pato, M. T., Bernstein, S. E. *et al.* (1990). Controlled comparisons of clomipramine and fluoxetine in the treatment of obsessive-compulsive disorder. *Arch. Gen. Psychiatry*, **47**, 926–932.

Pigott, T. A., Pato, M. T., L'Heureux, F. *et al.* (1991). A controlled comparison of adjuvant lithium carbonate or thyroid hormone in clomipramine-treated OCD patients. *J. Clin. Psychopharmacol.*, **11**, 242–248.

Pigott, T. A., L'Heureux, F., Bernstein, S. E. *et al.* (1992a). A controlled comparative therapeutic trial of clomipramine and m-chlorophenylpiperazine (m-CPP) in patients with obsessive-compulsive disorder. *NCDEU Annual Meeting*, Marco Island, FL.

Pigott, T. A., L'Heureux, F., Hill, J. L. *et al.* (1992b). A double blind study of adjuvant buspirone hydrochbride in clomipramine-treated patients with obsessive-compulsive disorder. *J. Clin. Psychopharmacol.*, **12**(1), 11–18.

Pigott, T. A., Grady, T. A., Bernstein, S. E. *et al.* (1992c). A comparison of oral and IV m-CPP in patients with OCD. *Biol. Psychiatry*, **31**, 173A.

Pigott, T. A., Hill, J. L., Grady, T. A. *et al.* (1993). A comparison of the behavioral effects of oral versus intravenous m-CPP administration in OCD patients the effect of metergoline prior to IV m-CPP. *Biol. Psychiatry*, **33**, 3–14.

Pranzatelli, M. R. (1989). Benzodiazepine-induced shaking behavior in the rat: structure–activity and relation to serotonin and benzodiazepine receptors. *Exp. Neurol.*, **104**, 241–250.

Rapoport, J. L. (1989). The neurobiology of obsessive-compulsive disorder. *JAMA*, **260**(19), 2888–2890.

Rapoport, J. L. (1991). Recent advances in obsessive-compulsive disorder. *Neuropsychopharmacology*, **5**(1), 1–10.

Rasmussen, S. A. (1984). Lithium and tryptophan augmentation in clomipramine-resistant obsessive-compulsive disorder. *Am. J. Psychiatry*, **141**, 1283–1285.

Rasmussen, S. A. and Eisen, J. L. (1992). The epidemiology and differential diagnosis of obsessive compulsive disorder. *J. Clin. Psychiatry*, **53**(4), 4–10.

Sandler, M., Coppen, A. and Harnett, S. (1991). *5-Hydroxytryptamine in Psychiatry: A Spectrum of Ideas*. Oxford University Press, London.

Stein, D. J., Hollander, E., Mullen, L. S. *et al.* (1992). Comparison of clomipramine, alprazolam and placebo in the treatment of obsessive-compulsive disorder. *Hum. Psychopharmacol.*, **7**, 389–395.

Swedo, S. E., Leonard, H. L., Rapoport, J. L. *et al.* (1989). A double-blind comparison of clomipramine and desipramine in the treatment of trichotillomania (hair pulling). *N. Engl. J. Med.*, **321**, 497–501.

Swedo, S. E., Leonard, H. L., Kruesi, M. J. P. *et al.* (1992). Cerebrospinal fluid neurochemistry in children and adolescents with obsessive-compulsive disorder. *Arch. Gen. Psychiatry*, **49**, 29–36.

Thoren, P., Asberg, M., Cronholm, B. *et al.* (1980). Clomipramine treatment of obsessive-compulsive disorder I: A controlled clinical trial. *Arch. Gen. Psychiatry*, **37**, 1281–1285.

Vallejo, J., Olivares, J., Marcos, T. *et al.* (1992). Clomipramine versus phenelzine in obsessive-compulsive disorder: a controlled clinical trial. *Br. J. Psychiatry*, **161**, 665–670.

Volavka, J., Neziroglu, F. and Yaryura-Tobias, J. A. (1985). Clomipramine and imipramine in obsessive-compulsive disorder. *Psychiatry Res.*, **14**, 83–91.

Wood, A., Tollefson, G. D. and Birkett, M. (1993). Pharmacotherapy of obsessive compulsive disorder: experience with fluoxetine. *Int. Clin. Psychopharmacol.*, **8**, 301–306.

Yaryura-Tobias, J. A. and Bhagavan, H. N. (1977). L-Tryptophan in obsessive-compulsive disorders. *Am. J. Psychiatry*, **134**, 1298–1299.

Zohar, J., and Insel, T. R. (1987). Obsessive-compulsive disorder: psychobiological approaches to diagnosis, treatment, and pathophysiology. *Biol. Psychiatry*, **22**, 667–687.

Zohar, J., Mueller, E. A., Insel, T. R. *et al.* (1987). Serotonergic responsivity in obsessive-compulsive disorder: comparison of patients and healthy controls. *Arch. Gen. Psychiatry*, **44**, 946–951.

Zohar, J., Insel, T. R., Zohar-Kadouch, R. C. *et al.* (1988). Serotonergic responsivity in obsessive-compulsive disorder: effects of chronic clomipramine treatment. *Arch. Gen. Psychiatry*, **45**, 167–172.

13 New Compounds for the Treatment of Obsessive-compulsive Disorder

ORNAH T. DOLBERG, YEHUDA SASSON, DONATELLA
MARAZZITI, MOSHE KOTLER, SETH KINDLER
AND JOSEPH ZOHAR
Department of Psychiatry, Chaim Sheba Medical Center, Ramat Gan, Israel

INTRODUCTION

Traditionally, obsessive-compulsive disorder (OCD) was considered to be a rare, chronic disorder refractory to treatment. The realization that OCD is much more prevalent than previously assumed has stimulated research regarding the therapy of OCD, pharmacological was well as behavioral and surgical. Previously, little hope was offered in the way of treatment but current approaches allow considerable improvement for those afflicted.

In this chapter we will review the progress made in the therapy of OCD, as well as interventions for the treatment-resistant patient and augmentation strategies.

TREATMENT WITH SEROTONERGIC DRUGS

OCD stands apart from all anxiety and effective disorders, in that it demonstrates a high selectivity for drug response. Only compounds with a serotonergic profile have been documented to be consistently effective in this disorder (Zohar *et al.*, 1992).

The specific response of OCD to antidepressants possessing serotonergic properties has been investigated in several comparative drug studies between serotonergic and non-serotonergic drugs. These studies have demonstrated a preferential response to serotonergic drugs such as clomipramine (CMI), versus a lack of response to non-serotonergic drugs, such as placebo, desipramine (DMI), nortriptyline, amitriptyline, and clorgyline (Zohar *et al.*, 1992). CMI and amitriptyline were compared in a four-week, randomized, double-blind study of 20 OCD patients, by Ananth *et al.* (1981). They reported that statistically significant improvement was demonstrated with CMI but not with amitriptyline. In a study by Insel *et al.* (1983), 12 patients were given CMI

Advances in the Neurobiology of Anxiety Disorders. Edited by H. G. M. Westenberg, J. A. Den Boer and D. L. Murphy
©1996 John Wiley & Sons Ltd

versus clorgyline in a placebo-controlled, randomized, cross-over design. Significant improvement was noted for OCD patients while on CMI but not on clorgyline. A 12-week, double-blind study was conducted using CMI compared to imipramine in 23 OCD patients (Volavka *et al.*, 1985). Of the 16 patients who completed the study, partial improvement was noted on both medications, although CMI was found to be slightly superior to imipramine. More recently, CMI was examined against desmethylimipramine (DMI), by Zohar and Insel (1987). In a double-blind, randomized, cross-over study of 10 OCD patients, CMI was found to have significantly more antiobsessional effects in these patients than DMI. In 48 children and adolescents with OCD, CMI was compared to DMI, and was shown to be significantly superior (Leonard *et al.*, 1989).

CLOMIPRAMINE

Among the wide variety of medications used in the treatment of OCD patients, an effective drug is the serotonergic tricyclic, CMI, which has been the most extensively studied.

Combining data from several studies, the tricyclic CMI was found to be effective in several placebo-controlled studies, which included more than 700 patients with OCD (Zohar *et al.*, 1992). The results of a multicenter trial with CMI was published in 1991 (Clomipramine Collaborative Study Group, 1991). Twenty-one centers participated in two studies with a total of 520 patients. They examined the efficacy, safety and tolerability of up to 300 mg per day of CMI. On the two main scales assessing OCD, the Yale–Brown Obsessive-Compulsive Scale (YBOCS), and the National Institute of Mental Health Global Obsessive-Compulsive Scale (NIMH GOCS), CMI was significantly more effective than placebo. The mean reduction in the YBOCS score at the end of 10 weeks of treatment was 38% in one study, and 44% in the second study.

One of the first controversies regarding treatment of OCD patients with CMI was whether the patients benefited from CMI's antidepressant effects or whether the improvement was actually due to an antiobsessive effect. The early studies reported on the efficacy of CMI in depressed OCD patients, such as the study done by Marks *et al.* (1980). However, further reports demonstrated that the antiobsessive effectiveness of CMI is independent from its antidepressive effects (Ananth *et al.*, 1981; Flament *et al.*, 1985; Mavissakalian *et al.*, 1985; Montgomery, 1980; Thoren *et al.*, 1980; Volavka *et al.*, 1985; Zohar and Insel, 1987). A double-blind study presented by Insel *et al.* (1982), which compared the response of depressed versus non-depressed OCD patients to CMI treatment, found that both groups of patients responded similarly regarding their OC symptoms.

It has been shown that a relatively long period is needed for CMI to be significantly effective. Thoren *et al.* (1980) reported that only at week 5 do the differences between CMI and other treatments become evident. Volavka *et al.* (1985) are more extreme, and have found that at least 12 weeks are required for CMI to exceed imipramine's effects.

The question of how long to treat OCD patients with CMI is still an open one. It has been demonstrated that length of treatment should be considerable, and that most patients will relapse with premature discontinuation. Few studies have addressed this question. In one such study by Pato *et al.* (1988), 16 of 18 patients with OCD relapsed within seven weeks after stopping CMI, although some had been treated for nearly a year. Leonard *et al.* (1991) examined the effect of DMI substitution during long-term CMI treatment in 26 children and adolescents with OCD. Mean duration of CMI treatment was 17 months. Half were blindly assigned to two months of DMI treatment, and then CMI was reinstituted. Almost 90% relapsed during the two-month substitution period. Further studies are required in order to determine length of maintenance CMI treatment.

FLUOXETINE

CMI differs from other tricyclics in its potency as a serotonin reuptake blocker. Other, non-tricyclic, serotonin (5-HT) reuptake blockers are gaining acceptance as effective alternatives to CMI treatment of OCD.

In the Lilly European OCD study group, 214 patients with OCD were treated with fluoxetine or placebo, in a double-blind manner, for eight weeks. Patients received either 40 mg or 60 mg of fluoxetine. Fluoxetine was demonstrated to be significantly superior to placebo. One hundred and sixty-one patients continued to a 16-week extension evaluation.

The rate of discontinuation due to adverse effects was low, and not significantly different between placebo and fluoxetine (Montgomery *et al.*, 1993). Fluoxetine was compared to CMI in a study presented by Pigott *et al.* (1990), where 11 patients with OCD were treated with fluoxetine for 10 weeks and then were crossed-over to treatment with CMI. No significant differences were noted regarding clinical efficacy, but significant differences were present when comparing side effects. Patients reported significantly fewer side effects while treated with fluoxetine. A second group of 21 OCD patients were treated initially with CMI and then with fluoxetine. After 10 weeks of fluoxetine administration, results were similar to those achieved while on CMI treatment. Higher doses of antidepressants have been used in the treatment of OCD than for the treatment of depression, though empirical data supporting this practice is scant. Fixed-dose studies using selective serotonin reuptake inhibitors (SSRIs) such as fluoxetine and sertraline have found no advantage for the use of higher doses, with the lower dose being as effective. Dominguez (1992) reported a double-blind trial of three doses of fluoxctine (20 mg, 40 mg, 60 mg) versus placebo in 51 patients with OCD. Fluoxetine was superior to placebo, but no significant differences were noted between the three fixed doses, with 20 mg being as

effective as the 40 mg or 60 mg dose. It appears that fluoxetine produces therapeutic effects equivalent to those of CMI in OCD patients. The difference in
side-effect profile is perhaps the guideline for preferring one over the other.

FLUVOXAMINE

Another, recently included, non-tricyclic SSRI is fluvoxamine. Fluvoxamine
has been compared to placebo in three studies, including in all 96 patients, and
has been found superior to it (Goodman *et al.*, 1989; Jenike *et al.*, 1990a; Perse
et al., 1988). Lately, Westenberg *et al.* (1992) confirmed these previous studies,
in 20 patients with OCD, treated with fluvoxamine in a double-blind placebo-
controlled design, in an incremental dosing fashion, beginning at 50 mg up to
300 mg depending on response and emergence of adverse effects. The study
was conducted for eight-weeks. Fluvoxamine was found to be significantly
superior to placebo. Goodman *et al.* (1990) compared fluvoxamine and DMI in
35 patients with OCD in an eight-week-long study, and found fluvoxamine to
be superior to DMI.

   Both fluoxetine and fluvoxamine are important alternatives to CMI treatment, since they lack the anticholinergic side effects of CMI, which seem to be
troublesome to many patients: dry mouth, blurred vision, urinary retention, constipation, sedation, weight gain. On the other hand, it is important to keep in
mind that these drugs do have several side effects, including headaches, nausea
and sleep disturbance.

SERTRALINE

With the growing evidence for the effectiveness of SSRIs in the treatment of
OCD, several new agents have been investigated, among them sertraline, which
has been approved for the treatment of depression in several countries.
Chouinard *et al.* (1990) reported on 87 OCD patients who were randomized to
receive either placebo or sertraline titrated upwards, at doses ranging from 50
mg to 200 mg maximally, during the first two weeks of the study, which lasted
for eight weeks. Sertraline was found to be significantly more effective than
placebo, and was well tolerated. Only 2% of the patients discontinued treatment
with sertraline due to adverse reactions. The most common side effects with
sertraline treatment were: nausea 30%, insomnia 26%, dyspepsia 21% and ejac-
ulatory failure 19%. Sertraline was also compared to placebo in a fixed-dose
study which included 325 non-depressed OCD patients who were randomized
to 12 weeks of double-blind treatment with either placebo or 50 mg, 100 mg or
200 mg of sertraline. On all efficacy measures, sertraline-treated patients fared
significantly better than those on placebo. No significant differences were noted
between the three sertraline dosage groups (Chouinard, 1992; Greist *et al.*,
1993a). The usefulness of sertraline was also examined in long-term treatment
(Greist *et al.*, 1993b). Of the 118 patients that had improved moderately or
markedly, in the previously reported 12-week study conducted by this group, 96

had been receiving sertraline. These 96 patients entered a long-term treatment phase. The patients continued to improve and were able to tolerate treatment.

Common side effects were headaches, insomnia, nausea, diarrohea, decreased libido and anorexia, in decreasing order of frequency. With the exception of headaches, the other adverse reactions seem to decrease significantly with time. In contrast to these reports, Jenike *et al.* (1990b) compared the effect of sertraline in 10 patients with OCD versus nine patients on placebo, and found sertraline to be ineffective on four measures of obsessive-compulsive symptoms. This trial included only 19 patients, while the above studies explored the effects of sertraline in 400 patients, which may explain the difference in the results.

PAROXETINE

Paroxetine, one of the SSRIs, has mainly been studied in depression. Data regarding its efficacy in OCD is practically non-existent. The role of paroxetine in OCD is currently being investigated in multicenter trials, and until more evidence is available no definite conclusions can be drawn.

TRAZODONE

Trazodone is an antidepressant unrelated to any known group of antidepressants, and is a 5-HT reuptake inhibitor. Trazodone has mostly been described in case reports that included few patients, and in open trials. Pigott *et al.* (1992a) conducted a double-blind, placebo-controlled study of trazodone in 21 patients with OCD. At the end of the 10-week study, there were no significant differences regarding depressive or OC symptoms in the 17 patients who completed the study, between trazodone versus placebo. They conclude that despite being a 5-HT reuptake inhibitor, trazodone shows little promise as an antiobsessive drug. In contrast, Hermesh *et al.* (1990) reported on nine patients who failed to respond to CMI or CMI plus lithium. As a group, the patients showed mild but significant improvement. Currently the data regarding the efficacy of trazodone in OCD remains inconclusive.

BUSPIRONE

Buspirone, while not being of the SSRI class, appears to exert its effects through the serotonergic system. It is an anxiolytic drug that acts as an agonist on $5-HT_{1A}$ type receptors. Its effectiveness has been examined in a double-blind study versus CMI, in 18 OCD patients by Pato *et al.* (1991). They report that both drugs led to statistically significant and similar improvements on various scales for OCD and depression. Jenike *et al.* (1988) reported on 14 patients with OCD that entered an eight-week open trial of buspirone. At the end of the study period, none of the patients had improved. With such conflicting results, it is evident that further studies are required in order to verify the therapeutic role of buspirone in OCD.

Table 1. Double-blind drug treatment studies in OCD patients

Study	Treatment	Design/(N)	Duration weeks	Result
Drug versus placebo				
DeVeaugh *et al.* (1989)	CMI 100–250 mg	PL (384)	10	CMI>P
Flament *et al.* (1985)	CMI 141 mg	CO (19)	5	CMI>P (childhood OCD)
Foa *et al.* (1987)	IMI 233 mg	PL (37)	6	IMI=P
Goodman *et al.* (1989)	FLUV 255 mg	PL (42)	6–8	FLUV>P
Jenike *et al.* (1990)	FLUV 294 mg	PL (38)	10	FLUV>P
Marks *et al.* (1980)	CMI 183 mg	PL (40)	4	CMI>P
Mavissakalian *et al.* (1985)	CMI 228 mg	PL (15)	6	CMI>P
Montgomery (1980)	CMI 75 mg	CO (14)	4	CMI>P
Perse *et al.* (1988)	FLUV 300 mg	CO (16)	8	FLUV>P
Thoren *et al.* (1980)	CMI 150 mg NOR 150 mg	PL (35)	5	CMI>P NOR not>P
Bick and Hackett (1989)	SER 50, 200 mg	PL (87)	8	SER>P
Greist *et al.* (1993)	SER 50, 100, 200 mg	PL (325)	12	SER>P
Drug versus drug				
Ananth *et al.* (1981)	CMI 133 mg vs AMI 197 mg	PL (20)	6	MI>BASE-LINE AMI=BASE-LINE
Goodman *et al.* (1990)	FLUV 213 mg vs DMI 188 mg	PL (35)	8	FLUV>DMI
Insel *et al.* (1983)	CMI 236 mg vs CLG 28 mg	CO (13)	4+6	CMI>CLG
Leonard *et al.* (1988)	CMI vs DMI 3 mg/kg	CO (21)	6	CMI>DMI (childhood OCD)
Pigott *et al.* (1990)	CMI 200 mg vs FLU 80 mg	CO (32)	10	CMI+FLU
Volavka *et al.* (1985)	CMI 275 mg vs IMI 265 mg	PL (16)	6	CMI>IMI
Zohar and Insel (1987)	CMI 235 mg vs DMI 290 mg	CO (10)	6	CMI>DMI

CMI, clomipramine; NOR, nortriptyline; AMI, amitriptyline; CLG, clorgiline; IMI, imipramine; DMI, desipramine; FLU, fluoxetine; FLUV, fluvoxamine; P, placebo; SER, sertraline; PL, parallel; CO, cross-over; ">" signifies greater therapeutic effects than; "=" signifies equivalent therapeutic effects.

TREATMENT WITH ANXIOLYTICS

OCD is considered an anxiety disorder according to the *Diagnostic and Statistical Manual of Mental Disorders*, third edition, revised (DSM-III-R). It is therefore not surprising that anxiolytics have been used in the treatment of OCD patients. However, present data stems mostly from case reports, as extensive double-blind placebo-controlled studies have not been undertaken. Alprazolam was reported to cause moderate to marked improvement in four patients (Tollefson, 1985). Clonazepam has been reported to be effective in three patients (Hewlett *et al.*, 1990). More recently, Hewlett *et al.* (1992) reported in a double-blind, randomized, multiple cross-over study of 28 OCD patients that clonazepam was as effective as CMI and more effective than diphenhydramine, a control medication. It is apparent that with such a small number of studies no substantive conclusions can be drawn, and further investigation is required. Moreover, since OCD is a chronic disease, the use of anxiolytics raises concern regarding the dependency brought about by long-term use of compounds from the benzodiazepine class.

TREATMENT WITH ANTIPSYCHOTICS

Most of the information regarding the role of antipsychotics in OCD stems from few case reports. A study by McDougle *et al.* (1990) found that nine of 17 patients with OCD, who were considered non-responders, after an adequate trial with fluvoxamine responded upon the addition of an antipsychotic to ongoing fluvoxamine treatment. The efficacy of antipsychotics in OCD requires further verification, especially when considering the long-term adverse effects associated with antipsychotic treatment. Currently the role of antipsychotics in OCD seems to be reserved to a specific subgroup of OCD patients with a comorbid tic disorder, such as Tourette's syndrome (McDougle *et al.*, 1993).

TREATMENT WITH ELECTROCONVULSIVE THERAPY

OCD is not considered to be responsive to electroconvulsive therapy (ECT), although few past case reports have demonstrated its efficacy in the individual patient (Mellman *et al.*, 1992). However, in a recent review of eight OCD patients who received ECT, only one had a good antiobsessional response that was sustained (Guttmacher, personal communication). The apparent lack of response of OCD to such a powerful antidepressant treatment modality as ECT may lend further support to the hypothesis that the antiobsessive response to treatment is distinct from the antidepressant response.

OTHER TREATMENTS

Few uncontrolled trials reported on the beneficial effects of monoamine oxidase inhibitors (MAOIs) in OCD. However, Insel *et al.* (1983) compared CMI to clorgyline, a selective MAOI, and found no support for the antiobsessive effects of MAOIs. Vallejo *et al.* (1992) compared CMI to phenelzine in a double-blind manner in 30 OCD patients. They found that obsessive-compulsive symptoms improved significantly in both drug groups, and noted no differences between the groups.

Den Boer and Westenberg (1992) treated 12 OCD patients with intranasal administration of oxytocin spray (18 IU per day) in a double-blind placebo-controlled design. The results revealed no support for the role of oxytocin in OCD.

NEUROSURGICAL TREATMENT

With the increasing effectiveness of drug therapy in OCD, the use of psychosurgery has decreased in the last 20 years. In the past a cingulectomy or cingulotomy was recognized as effective. A second procedure, an anterior capsulotomy, is a variant of the original frontal lobotomy, which has been reported to decrease the symptoms of OCD. In a retrospective study by Jenike *et al.* (1991a), the records of 18 patients who underwent a cingulotomy for treatment of OCD several years previously were examined, and their current status was evaluated with a battery of questionnaires. The authors conclude that between 25% and 30% of these patients benefited substantially from this procedure. They also report on four patients who were followed for several months after a cingulotomy. One patient showed a 100% decrease in YBOCS score; the other three showed slight to no improvement and they underwent a second procedure.

Current neurosurgical techniques, involving stereotactic surgery, permitting a high degree of accuracy, with a minority of side effects, are rapidly gaining acceptance. Understandably, studies done in this field contain several methodological issues, such as the lack of control patients, and therefore it is difficult to assess the efficacy of these interventions. In order to address this issue, double-blind studies are required. The availability of the gamma-knife technique makes it possible to start double-blind studies, employing sham procedures. Currently, this controversial mode of therapy is reserved for OCD patients with a severe and intractable illness of several years duration, who have failed to respond to both pharmacological and psychological interventions.

AUGMENTATION STRATEGIES

Although the last decade has produced a myriad of pharmacological interventions, still only approximately 50% of OCD patients ultimately improve in any given pharmacologic treatment trial (Insel, 1992). In order to enhance response, research has been concentrating on augmentation regimens, but so far results seem far from encouraging. Lithium carbonate has been reported to be effective as an adjuvant agent in several open reports, which combined lithium with a serotonergic drug. However, two double-blind studies have failed to demonstrate evidence of significant further improvement in OCD symptoms in comparison to CMI treatment alone or fluvoxamine treatment alone (Pigott et al., 1991, 1992b; McDougle et al., 1991).

The combination of two serotonergic compounds has been another approach for the treatment-refractory patient. Buspirone has been added to ongoing fluoxetine treatment in 10 patients, and improved clinical response, compared to those treated with fluoxetine alone (Jenike et al., 1991b). Thirteen OCD patients were given adjuvant buspirone while being treated with fluoxetine, or placebo, for four weeks. No differences were noted between the two groups (Grady et al., 1993). Eleven OCD patients participated in an open-label trial of fluoxetine followed by buspirone augmentation. The combination therapy was found to be superior to monotherapy with fluoxetine (Markovitz et al., 1990). Buspirone was also added to CMI treatment in a double-blind 10-week study of 14 patients (Pigott et al., 1992c). Before the addition of buspirone, the patients as a group had shown a partial but incomplete reduction of OCD symptoms (average 28%). Although adjuvant treatment was well tolerated regarding adverse reactions, mean obsessive-compulsive and depressive symptoms did not significantly differ from baseline scores.

However, individual patients (four out of 14) did have an additional 25% reduction in OCD symptoms after adjuvant buspirone treatment. The results of this study indicate that there may be a subgroup of OCD patients responsive to this intervention.

Fenfluramine was added to either fluvoxamine or CMI in seven patients, who were unable to tolerate therapeutic doses of either medication owing to side effects. Dose of fenfluramine ranged from 20 mg to 60 mg. Therapy was well tolerated and caused further decrease in obsessive-compulsive symptoms in six of these patients (Hollander et al., 1990).

Browne et al. (1993) reported on the use of CMI–fluoxetine combination in four patients with severe OCD. In two patients, the combination was effective, when either drug used alone was not. In the other two cases, fluoxetine augmentation enhanced benefits, without the emergence of additional side effects.

CLINICAL STRATEGIES FOR THE TREATMENT-REFRACTORY PATIENT

The approach to the treatment-refractory OCD patient is similar to that employed in other disorders in psychiatry. The first steps include examination of the pharmacological agent employed. Failure to provide an adequate dose of medication for adequate periods of time may be the most common cause of "treatment resistance" (Coplan *et al.*, 1993). Secondly, the clinician must determine whether further diagnoses have emerged since the original evaluation. Depression and substance abuse are especially implicated in treatment failures. Several studies have shown that concomitant personality disorders predict poorer outcomes of treatment. These additional diagnoses must be addressed in order to enhance response (Baer *et al.*, 1992). The clinician must also evaluate compliance whether by pill counts or plasma drug levels, which may also be useful for identifying patients who are rapid metabolizers.

The most commonly employed first-line pharmacological approach to nonresponders include changing to a different SRI or combining SRIs. Despite the lack of controlled studies, there are several case-report examples of therapeutic achievements with one SRI following failure with a different SRI. Goodman *et al.* (1993) recommend switching to a different SRI if there has been no improvement at all following an adequate trial with one SRI. If there have been partial gains, they suggest a combination approach. The principles of combination therapy include combining SRIs with behavioral therapy, adding agents that enhance serotonergic function, adding another SRI, or adding an antipsychotic drug. Combination treatments that have shown the most promise include adding buspirone or an antipsychotic to ongoing SRI therapy.

It is clearly evident that clinical trials are needed for patients with treatment-resistant OCD. Identification of the various subtypes of OCD and clinical or biological markers of those subtypes is the future path to be explored, since subtype markers may serve as predictors of response and may help select the appropriate treatment (Goodman *et al.*, 1993).

CONCLUSIONS

5-HT reuptake inhibitors, such as clomipramine, fluvoxamine, fluoxetine, and sertraline, have been shown to be effective in the treatment of OCD patients, both with and without depression. Other non-serotonergic antidepressants and antianxiety agents do not appear to be consistently effective.

Despite the numerous gains made in the treatment of OCD, several issues await further investigation, such as length of maintenance therapy, the approach to the treatment refractory patient, and the role of behavioral therapy and neurosurgical therapy alone and in combination with pharmacological treatment.

Further research is required in order to differentiate the non-responsive patients into various subgroups and application of specific approaches for each such group.

REFERENCES

Ananth, J., Pecknold, J. C., Van Den Steen, N. and Engelsmann, F. (1981). Double blind comparative study of clomipramine and amitriptyline in obsessive neurosis. *Prog. Neuropsychopharmacol.*, **5**, 257–262.

Baer, L., Jenike, M. A., Black, T. W. *et al.* (1992). Effect of axis II diagnoses on treatment outcome with clomipramine in 55 patients with obsessive-compulsive disorder. *Arch. Gen. Psychiatry*, **49**, 862–866.

Bick, P. A. and Hackett, E. (1989). Sertraline is effective in obsessive-compulsive disorder. In *Psychiatry Today: VIII World Congress of Psychiatry Abstracts* (eds C. N. Stefanis, C. R. Soldatos and A. D. Rabavilas), p. 152, Elsevier, New York.

Browne, M., Horn, E. and Jones, T. T. (1993). The benefits of clomipramine–fluoxetine combination in obsessive compulsive disorder. *Can. J. Psychiatry*, **38**, 242–243.

Chouinard, G. (1992). Sertraline in the treatment of obsessive compulsive disorder: two double-blind, placebo-controlled studies. *Int. Clin. Psychopharmacol.*, **7s**, 37–41.

Chouinard, G., Goodman, W., Greist, J. *et al.* (1990). Results of a double-blind placebo controlled trial of a new serotonin uptake inhibitor, sertraline, in the treatment of obsessive compulsive disorder. *Psychopharmacol. Bull.*, **26**, 279–284.

Clomipramine Collaborative Study Group (1991). *Arch. Gen. Psychiatry*, **48**, 730–738.

Coplan, J. D., Tiffon, L. and Gorman, J. M. (1993). Therapeutic strategies for the patient with treatment-resistant anxiety. *J. Clin. Psychiatry*, **54s**, 69–74.

Den Boer, J. A. and Westenberg, H. G. (1992). Oxytocin in obsessive compulsive disorder. *Peptides*, **13**, 1083–1085.

DeVeaugh Geiss, J., Landau, P. and Katz, R. (1989). Treatment of obsessive-compulsive disorder with clomipramine. *Psychiatr. Ann.*, **19**, 97.

Dominguez, R. A. (1992). Serotonergic antidepressants and their efficacy in obsessive compulsive disorder. *J. Clin. Psychopharmacol.*, **53s**, 56–59.

Flament, M. F., Rapoport, J. L., Berg, C. J. *et al.* (1985). Clomipramine treatment of childhood obsessive compulsive disorder: a double-blind controlled study. *Arch. Gen. Psychiatry*, **42**, 977.

Foa, E. B., Steketee, G., Kozak, M. J. and Dugger, D. (1987). Effects of imipramine on depression and obsessive-compulsive symptoms. *Psychiatry Res.*, **21**, 123.

Goodman, W. K., Price, L. H. and Rasmussen, S. A. (1989). Efficacy of fluvoxamine in obsessive-compulsive disorder: a double-blind comparison of fluvoxamine and placebo. *Arch. Gen. Psychiatry*, **46**, 36–40.

Goodman, W. K., Price, L. H., Delgado, P. L. *et al.* (1990). Specificity of serotonin reuptake inhibitors in the treatment of obsessive-compulsive disorder: comparison of fluvoxamine and desipramine. *Arch. Gen. Psychiatry*, **47**, 577–585.

Goodman, W. K., McDougle, C. J., Barr, L. C. *et al.* (1993). Biological approaches to treatment-resistant obsessive-compulsive disorder. *J. Clin. Psychiatry*, **54s**, 16–26.

Grady, T. A., Pigott, T. A., L'Heureux, F. *et al.* (1993). Double-blind study of adjuvant buspirone for fluoxetine-treated patients with obsessive-compulsive disorder. *Am. J. Psychiatry*, **150**, 819–821.

Greist, J., Chouinard, G., DuBoff, E. *et al.* (1993a). Double-blind comparison of three doses of sertraline and placebo in the treatment of outpatients with obsessive compulsive disorder. 9th World Congress of Psychiatry, Rio de Janeiro, Brazil, June 1993, pp. 18–19.

Greist, J., Chouinard, G., DuBoff, E. *et al.* (1993b). Long-term sertraline treatment of obsessive compulsive disorder: a 52-week double blind comparative study versus placebo. 9th World Congress of Psychiatry, Rio de Janeiro, Brazil, June 1993, pp. 20–21.

Guttmacher, L. B. (personal communication). Electroconvulsive therapy for patients with obsessive-compulsive disorder.

Hermesh, H., Aizenberg, D. and Munitz, H. (1990). Trazodone treatment of clomipramine-resistant obsessive-compulsive disorder. *Clin. Neuropharmacol.*, **13**, 322–328.

Hewlett, W. A., Vinogradov, S. and Argas, W. S. (1990). Clonazepam treatment of obsessions and compulsions. *J. Clin. Psychiatry*, **51**, 158–161.

Hewlett, W. A., Vinogradov, S. and Agras, W. S. (1992). Clomipramine, clomazepam and clonidine treatment of obsessive-compulsive disorder. *J. Clin. Psychopharmacol.*, **12**, 420–430.

Hollander, E., DeCaria, C. M., Schneier, F. R. *et al.* (1990). Fenfluramine augmentation of serotonin reuptake blockade antiobsessional treatment. *J. Clin. Psychiatry*, **51**, 119–123.

Insel, T. R. (1992). Toward a neuroanatomy of obsessive-compulsive disorder. *Arch. Gen. Psychiatry*, **49**, 739–744.

Insel, T. R., Alterman, I. and Murphy, D. L. (1982). Antiobsessional and anti-depressant effects of clomipramine in the treatment of obsessive-compulsive disorder. *Psychopharmacol. Bull.*, **18**, 115–117.

Insel, T. R., Murphy, D. L., Cohen, R. M. *et al.* (1983). Obsessive-compulsive disorder: a double-blind trial of clomipramine and clorgyline. *Arch. Gen. Psychiatry*, **40**, 605–612.

Jenike, M. A. and Baer, L. (1988). An open trial of buspirone in obsessive-compulsive disorder. *Am. J. Psychiatry*, **145**, 1285–1286.

Jenike, M. A., Hyman, S., Baer, L. *et al.* (1990a). A controlled trial of fluvoxamine in obsessive-compulsive disorder. *Am. J. Psychiatry*, **147**, 1209–1215.

Jenike, M. A., Baer, L., Summergrad, P. *et al.* (1990b). Sertraline in obsessive compulsive disorder: a double blind comparison with placebo. *Am. J. Psychiatry*, **147**, 923–928.

Jenike, M. A., Baer, L., Ballantine, T. *et al.* (1991a). Cingulotomy for refractory obsessive-compulsive disorder. *Arch. Gen. Psychiatry*, **48**, 548–555.

Jenike, M. A., Baer, L. and Buttolph, L. (1991b). Buspirone augmentation of fluoxetine in patients with obsessive compulsive disorder. *J. Clin. Psychiatry*, **52**, 13–14.

Leonard, H. L., Swedo, S. E., Rapoport, J. L. *et al.* (1988). Treatment of childhood obsessive compulsive disorder with clomipramine and desipramine: a double blind crossover comparison. *Psychopharmacol. Bull.*, **24**, 93.

Leonard, H., Swedo, S., Koby, E. *et al.* (1989). Treatment of obsessive-compulsive disorder with clomipramine and desmethylimipramine in children and adolescents: a double-blind crossover comparison. *Arch. Gen. Psychiatry*, **46**, 1088–1092.

Leonard, H., Swedo, S. E., Lenane, M. C. *et al.* (1991). A double-blind desipramine substitution during long-term clomipramine treatment in children and adolescents with obsessive-compulsive disorder. *Arch. Gen. Psychiatry*, **48**, 922–927.

Markovitz, P. J., Stagno, S. J. and Calabrese, J. R. (1990). Buspirone augmentation of fluoxetine in obsessive-compulsive disorder. *Am. J. Psychiatry*, **147**, 798–800.

Marks, I. M., Stern, R. S., Mawson, D. *et al.* (1980). Clomipramine and exposure for obsessive-compulsive rituals: I. *Br. J. Psychiatry*, **136**, 1–25.

Mavissakalian, M., Turner, S. M., Michelson, L. and Jacob, R. (1985). Tricyclic antidepressants in obsessive-compulsive disorder: antiobsessional or antidepressant agents? *Am. J. Psychiatry*, **142**, 572.

McDougle, C. J., Goodman, W. K. and Price, L. H. (1990). Neuroleptic addition in fluvoxamine-refractory obsessive-compulsive disorder. *Am. J. Psychiatry*, **147**, 652–654.

McDougle, C. J., Price, L. H., Goodman, W. K. *et al.* (1991). A controlled trial of lithium augmentation in fluvoxamine-refractory obsessive-compulsive disorder. *J. Clin. Psychopharmacol.*, **11**, 175–184.

McDougle, C. J., Goodman, W. K. and Price, L. H. (1993). The pharmacotherapy of obsessive-compulsive disorder. *Pharmacopsychiatry*, **26s**, 24–29.

Mellman, L. A. and Gorman, J. M. (1992). Successful treatment of obsessive-compulsive disorder with ECT. *Am. J. Psychiatry*, **141**, 596.

Mindus, P. and Jenike, M. A. (1992). Neurosurgical treatment of malignant obsessive compulsive disorder. In *Obsessional Disorders. Psychiatr. Clin. North Am.*, **15**, 921–938.

Montgomery, S. A. (1980). Clomipramine in obsessional neurosis: a placebo controlled trial. *Pharm. Med.*, **1**, 89.

Montgomery, S. A., McIntyre, A., Osterheider, M. *et al.* (1993). A double-blind, placebo-controlled study of fluoxetine in patients with DSM-III-R obsessive-compulsive disorder. The Lilly European OCD Study Group. *Eur. Neuropsychopharmacol.*, **3**, 143–152.

Pato, P. T., Zohar-Kadouch, R. C., Zohar, J. and Murphy, D. L. (1988). Return of symptoms after discontinuation of clorimipramine in patients with obsessive compulsive disorder. *Am. J. Psychiatry*, **145**, 1521–1525.

Pato, P. T., Pigott, T. A., Hill, J. L. *et al.* (1991). Controlled comparison of buspirone and clomipramine in obsessive-compulsive disorder. *Am. J. Psychiatry*, **148**, 127–129.

Perse, T. L., Greist, J. H., Jefferson, R. H. *et al.* (1988). Fluvoxamine treatment of obsessive-compulsive disorder. *Am. J. Psychiatry*, **144**, 1543–1548.

Pigott, T. A., Pato, M. T., Bernstein, S. E. *et al.* (1990). Controlled comparisons of clomipramine and fluoxetine in the treatment of obsessive compulsive disorder: behavioral and biological results. *Arch. Gen. Psychiatry*, **47**, 926–932.

Pigott, T. A., Pato, M. T., L'Heureux, F. *et al.* (1991). A controlled comparison of adjuvant lithium carbonate or thyroid hormone in clomipramine-treated OCD patients. *J. Clin. Psychopharmacol.*, **11**, 242–248.

Pigott, T. A., L'Heureux, F., Rubinstein, C. S. *et al.* (1992a). Double-blind, placebo-controlled study of trazodone in patient with obsessive-compulsive disorder. *J. Clin. Psychopharmacol.*, **12**, 156–162.

Pigott, T. A., L'Heureux, F. and Murphy, D. L. (1992b). Pharmacological approaches to treatment-resistant OCD patients. *Proceedings of the 18th CINP Congress*, Nice, pp. 123–125.

Pigott, T. A., L'Heureux, F., Hill, J. L. *et al.* (1992c). A double-blind study of adjuvant buspirone hydrochloride in clomipramine-treated patients with obsessive-compulsive disorder. *J. Clin. Psychopharmacol.*, **12**, 11–18.

Robins, L. N., Helzer, J. E., Weissman, M. M. *et al.* (1984). Lifetime prevalence of specific psychiatric disorders in three sites. *Arch. Gen. Psychiatry*, **41**, 949–959.

Thoren, P., Asberg, M., Gronholm, B. *et al.* (1980). Clomipramine treatment of obsessive-compulsive disorder. I. A controlled clinical trial. *Arch. Gen. Psychiatry*, **37**, 1281–1285.

Tollefson, G. (1985). Alprazolam in the treatment of obsessive symptoms. *J. Clin. Psychopharmacol.*, **5**, 39–42.

Vallejo, J., Olivares, J., Marcos, T. *et al.* (1992). Clomipramine versus phenelzine in obsessive compulsive disorder: a controlled clinical trial. *Br. J. Psychiatry*, **161**, 665–670.

Volavka, J., Neziroglu, F. and Yaryura-Tobias, J. A. (1985). Clomipramine and imipramine in obsessive-compulsive disorder. *Psychiatry Res.*, **14**, 85–93.

Westenberg, H. G. M., De Leeuw, A. S. and Den Boer, J. A. (1992). Serotonin reuptake blockers in obsessive compulsive disorder: a controlled trial with fluvoxamine. *Proceedings of the 18th CINP Congress*, Nice, p. 116.

Zohar, J. and Insel, T. (1987). Obsessive-compulsive disorder: psychobiological approaches to diagnosis, treatment, and pathophysiology. *Biol. Psychiatry*, **22**, 667–687.

Zohar, J., Zohar-Kadouch, R. C. and Kindler, S. (1992). Current concepts in the pharmacological treatment of obsessive-compulsive disorder. *Drugs*, **2**, 210–218.

14 Neuroimaging in Obsessive-compulsive Disorder: Advances in Understanding the Mediating Neuroanatomy

ARTHUR L. BRODY AND LEWIS R. BAXTER JR
UCLA Neuropsychiatric Institute and Hospital Center for the Health Sciences, Los Angeles, California, USA

INTRODUCTION

This chapter reviews brain imaging studies of obsessive-compulsive disorder (OCD) and related conditions. We start with studies of brain structure using computed tomography (CT) and magnetic resonance imaging (MRI). Then we move to an overview of functional brain imaging techniques, before describing studies of brain function using single-photon emission computed tomography (SPECT) and positron emission tomography (PET). We and our collaborators have published several previous reviews of brain imaging studies in OCD (Baxter, 1991; Baxter and Guze, 1992; Baxter *et al.*, 1990a, 1990b, 1991) and, by necessity, much of the material here is a repetition of these previous reviews. The purpose of this chapter is to update work in the field. In this regard, recent work with functional brain imaging allows firmer conclusions to be drawn about the brain mediation of OCD symptoms.

STUDIES OF BRAIN STRUCTURE IN OCD PATIENTS

CT STUDIES

The first CT study had negative findings. Insel and associates (1983) studied 10 OCD patients: two with abnormalities on electroencephalography (EEG), four with abnormalities on neuropsychological testing and four other OCD patients chosen at random from other study groups. Controls were age- and gender-matched patients without evidence of psychiatric illness or central nervous system (CNS) illness, although seven had other known "peripheral illnesses".

Advances in the Neurobiology of Anxiety Disorders. Edited by H. G. M. Westenberg, J. A. Den Boer and D. L. Murphy
©1996 John Wiley & Sons Ltd

There were no significant differences between OCD subjects and controls when examining an index ratio of ventricle to brain matter (VBR).

A CT study of childhood-onset OCD (Behar *et al.*, 1984), however, did find VBRs that were significantly larger in the OCD subjects than in controls. Several of the 17 OCD subjects had "secondary" depression. The 16 control subjects had CT scans that were not "questionable clinically" and were not from individuals with altered consciousness, psychiatric symptoms, or "hard" neurologic signs. All controls were suspected of having CNS pathology at time of scanning, however. While VBRs were larger in the OCD group, they did not show a significant correlation with demographic, disease severity, or prior treatment variables. VBRs were higher in patients with compulsions alone than in those with both obsessions and compulsions.

This same laboratory also did a second CT study of late adolescents with childhood-onset OCD (Luxenberg *et al.*, 1988). They studied 10 male subjects with OCD and 10 male controls, and found that volumes of the caudate nuclei were significantly smaller in OCD subjects than in controls.

MAGNETIC RESONANCE IMAGING STUDIES

To date there have been three published series of OCD patients studied with magnetic resonance imaging (MRI). In the first, Garber and colleagues (1989) studied 32 patients with OCD who were taking either clomipramine ($n = 19$) or placebo ($n = 13$) during a double-blind treatment study. These patients were compared with normal controls. There were no distinct structural abnormalities noted in the MRI scans by gross visual inspection, but neuroanatomic structure, volume and other morphologic measurements were not done. In both patients and controls, a variety of non-specific T_2 hyperintensity loci were seen in white matter, but the authors also used the controversial approach of T_1 intensity mapping to compare OCD subjects to controls. OCD subjects with a positive family history had more T_1 abnormalities in the anterior cingulate gyrus than did other patients or normals. Right minus left T_1 differences for the orbital cortex were also calculated. There was a significant positive correlation between these differences and symptom severity in unmedicated patients and patients with a family history positive for OCD.

Kellner *et al.* (1991) studied 12 OCD subjects and 12 age- and sex-matched healthy controls and found no differences between the groups with MRI. Scanning was for T_1- and T_2-weighted images and measures were made of the area of the head of the caudate, cingulate gyrus thickness, intracaudate/frontal horn ratio, and the area of the corpus callosum.

Scarone *et al.* (1992) looked specifically at the volume of the head of the caudate nucleus using T_1-weighted MRI in 20 OCD patients (treated with clomipramine or fluvoxamine) and 16 normal controls. They found a significant increase in the volume of the right side of the head of the caudate nucleus in OCD subjects when compared with controls. Nevertheless, they found no significant correlations between MRI caudate volumes and age, age at onset, or Yale–Brown Obsessive-Compulsive Scale (YBOCS) parameters.

Thus, the first study implicated the right orbital cortex and the anterior cingulate gyrus in the expression of OCD. The second showed no significant differences on certain measures between OCD patients and controls. And the third showed a significant increase in the volume of the right side of the head of the caudate nucleus in OCD subjects (see Table 1).

Table 1. Structural neuroimaging studies in OCD

Reference	Technique	Subjects	Results
Insel *et al.* (1983)	CT	10 OCD patients 10 normal controls	OCD = controls
Behar *et al.* (1984)	CT	17 OCD (several with secondary dependency) 16 controls	VBRs larger in OCD subjects
Luxenberg *et al.* (1988)	CT	10 male OCD adolescents 10 male adolescents	Decreased caudate in OCD
Garber *et al.* (1989)	MRI	32 treated OCD patients 14 normal controls	T_1 abnormals in anterior cingulate gyrus and orbital cortex
Kellner *et al.* (1991)	MRI	12 OCD subjects 12 matched controls	OCD = controls
Scarone *et al.* (1992)	MRI	20 treated OCD patients 16 normal controls	Increased head of caudate in OCD

STUDIES OF BRAIN PHYSIOLOGY AND BIOCHEMISTRY WITH FUNCTIONAL BRAIN IMAGING IN OCD

FUNCTIONAL BRAIN IMAGING TECHNIQUES

Functional brain imaging uses CT techniques to obtain information about brain function *in vivo*. All functional brain imaging studies of OCD published to date have used PET or SPECT (though magnetic resonance spectroscopy (MRS) also has the potential to measure cerebral biochemistry). PET and SPECT are high-resolution imaging techniques in which tracer amounts of biochemicals of interest are labeled with radiation emitters and injected, and whose local concentrations are subsequently measured in the brain by the scanner.

Unstable atoms that emit positrons—positively charged antimatter particles that correspond to the negatively charged electrons—are used to label compounds of interest for PET. Positrons annihilate with electrons to give two γ photons, emitted simultaneously and at an angle of 180° from each other. SPECT employs radiation emitters, such as ^{133}Xe, ^{123}I, and [99]mTc which give off only a single photon to provide the signal for tomographic localization. The double signal of PET, which allows precise computer-assisted localization of the tracer, is what presently allows it to have higher resolution than SPECT. Image resolution refers to the distance two structures need to be apart to be detected as distinct by the instrument, while axial resolution equals slice thickness.

Many important physiologic substances have been studied with PET and SPECT, but only a handful have been used to study OCD. To date, PET work in OCD has employed radiolabeled deoxyglucose, glucose, or oxygen to look at brain glucose metabolism or blood flow. For cerebral glucose metabolism, the tracers [^{18}F]fluorodeoxyglucose (FDG) and [^{11}C]glucose have been used, while for blood flow, inhaled carbon dioxide or injected water has been used. Under non-starvation conditions, glucose and oxygen are by far the predominant energy substrates in the human brain and have been shown to be a highly sensitive indicator of cerebral function (Phelps and Mazziotta, 1985; Phelps et al., 1986). Under most circumstances, cerebral blood flow is highly correlated with glucose metabolic rates.

SPECT studies have used either the gas ^{133}Xe or [99]mTc-labeled d,l-hexamethyl propyleneamine oxime (HMPAO) to estimate regional blood flow. [133]Xe SPECT uses measures of the flux of this inert gas in the brain to estimate cerebral blood flow. Thus, ^{133}Xe is inhaled by the subject. Because of technical limitations, ^{133}Xe can only measure blood flow on the cortical surface of dorsal aspects of the brain.

HMPAO, on the other hand, is injected. This tracer is a highly lipophilic compound that crosses the lipophilic blood–brain barrier quickly, but once in cells is converted to a hydrophilic form that, in the presence of a fully functional blood–brain barrier, is trapped in the brain at concentrations roughly proportional to the blood flow through the region. Thus, although HMPAO uptake usually is interpreted as a valid method of estimating the blood flow of one brain structure relative to that of another, there may be circumstances when local rates of the metabolic conversion from the lipophilic to the hydrophilic form and local functional properties of the blood–brain barrier are more of a factor than is usually reported in the SPECT literature.

Although FDG and [^{11}C]glucose PET both measure a form of cerebral glucose metabolic rate, evidence indicates that they are not always equivalent. Unfortunately, this is not always recognized, even by investigators in the field, leading to confusion. For this reason, the basics of each technique will be briefly described. Readers interested in more detail are referred elsewhere (Blomqvist et al., 1985; Lear and Ackermann, 1991; Phelps et al., 1986).

FDG is phosphorylated and transported into cells proportional to glucose transport, but once in the cell it undergoes no further metabolism and is trapped.

Thus, not only is FDG PET scanning done after uptake is complete, but it also reflects total glucose uptake, whether that glucose is being used for aerobic or anaerobic processes.

[^{11}C]glucose, on the other hand, undergoes metabolism rapidly and the ^{11}C label is lost, eventually as [^{11}C]CO$_2$. Glucose metabolism in non-stimulated ("baseline condition") mammalian brain regions is thought to be mainly aerobic. Rat studies in the baseline state have shown that where glucose labeled with ^{11}C in the 1- or 6-position gives metabolic rates comparable to deoxyglucose, labeling in the other four possible positions of the glucose molecule gives severe underestimations of glucose metabolic rates as measured with deoxyglucose. Glucose metabolic rate underestimation, even with glucose labeled in the 6-position, is worse in brain regions undergoing physiologic stimulation, where the underestimation of glucose metabolic rates can be as high as 10% in rats even just 6 min after administration of the tracer. And with ^{11}C labeled at other positions, the error is even higher. Although the exact reason for this markedly increased underestimation of brain glucose metabolic rates in stimulated regions is still somewhat controversial, it is probably accounted for by the fact that under physiologic stimulation a significant amount of cerebral glucose is metabolized anaerobically due to near-saturation of the pyruvate dehydrogenase complex. Here, the tracer is quickly converted into lactate, which is carried off and not available for counting in PET.

^{15}O can be used to label various simple compounds (oxygen, carbon monoxide, carbon dioxide, nitrous oxide and water) to study blood flow with PET. ^{15}O has a half-life of about 2 min and therefore can be used to study the same subject under varying conditions. It is usually either inhaled in the carbon dioxide form, or given in bolus intravenous injections in the water form and is assumed to be in equilibrium at the time of scanning. Thus, its flux through the brain tracks regional blood flow.

STUDIES OF BRAIN PHYSIOLOGY AND BIOCHEMISTRY IN OCD

^{133}Xe SPECT FOR CEREBRAL BLOOD FLOW

Zohar et al. (1989) and Rubin et al. (1992) have reported ^{133}Xe SPECT studies of blood flow in OCD. However, because the Rubin study used both ^{133}Xe and HMPAO SPECT, with the former the more minor part of the report, the results of that study are reviewed in the next section.

In the Zohar et al. (1989) study, 10 subjects, all with washing compulsions and reports of focal stimuli for their obsessions concerning contamination, were studied. The design was complicated. Subjects underwent two single-blind "placebo Xe" test runs in an attempt to diminish test-situation anxiety. All studies were done with eyes closed for 16 min, with 30 min intervals in between. The subjects underwent, in sequence, Xe flow studies (1) in a relaxation state,

(2) during imaginal flooding, and (3) during *in vivo* exposure to stimuli that, in the past, had tended to induce contamination obsessions and washing rituals. All three stimulus state studies were done during a 4 h period on the same day. The relaxation stimulus was done with an audio tape of a "relaxation scene" (same for all subjects), whereas the flooding was done with an audio tape of a situation specific to the subject's individual contamination fears. Exposure *in vivo* was done with the flooding tape, accompanied by placing the contaminating object in contact with the dorsum of the right hand. In an attempt to gain information as to whether results were biased by the fixed sequence of presentation, three subjects returned, 5–10 days later, for testing in which exposure was given before flooding.

As predicted by the authors, both symptom rating scale scores and peripheral physiologic measures gave highest values during *in vivo* exposure and were lowest during relaxation. However, in contrast to what the authors expected, cerebral blood flow was increased non-significantly overall in the imaginal flooding, but *decreased* significantly in virtually all surface superior cortical regions during *in vivo* exposure. The temporal cortex was the only area that showed a significant increase in cerebral blood flow during *in vivo* exposure.

A number of different speculative explanations were offered to account for these results. Differences in the sensory modalities of the stimuli (i.e., auditory versus touch) could have been important. Imaginal flooding might require more active cortical involvement than the passive touch situation, but this explanation was not favored because of patient reports of the degree of conscious activity in the various situations. Another possible explanation was that, in the highly anxiety-provoking *in vivo* exposure situation, blood was being shunted away from the surface cortical areas of the brain to other areas, such as the caudate nucleus or orbital gyri (see section on PET studies), which cannot be visualized with the Xe flow method.

HMPAO SPECT FOR CEREBRAL BLOOD FLOW

HMPAO studies of OCD have looked at both untreated and treated states. A first group of researchers looked at pretreatment OCD and at brain response to fluoxetine in OCD. Another looked at pretreatment OCD. And a more recent group looked at "markedly symptomatic" patients who were being treated with either clomipramine or fluoxetine.

In the first study (Machlin *et al.*, 1991), 10 non-depressed, medication-free OCD subjects were compared to a comparison group of eight Johns Hopkins' employees or students, matched by age, race, and sex. Studies were done on the Toshiba GCA-90B single rotating Anger camera (Toshiba, Japan), resolution 16 mm and slice thickness 11 mm. Patients had a significantly higher ratio of medial–frontal cortex to whole cortex HMPAO concentration than controls (109.7% ± 3.7% of cortical mean vs 102.9% ± 3.6%). This gave a significant correlation with anxiety ($r = -0.84$, $p = 0.002$), *not* OCD severity ($p > 0.50$).

Orbital metabolic rates were not significantly different between the two groups.

Three factors complicate the interpretation of these findings. First, the significant correlation was only with anxiety and not OCD symptoms; there was no other patient group to control for anxiety. Second, the SPECT camera used is of low resolution. It is doubtful that the orbital region, which is not trivial to localize with higher-resolution PET, could always be identified reliably. Third, "partial volume effects," described elsewhere, could lead to serious overestimations of activity in midline structures, like the one reported.

This same research group also examined six of these OCD subjects after three to four months of treatment with 80–100 mg fluoxetine per day (Hoehn-Saric *et al.*, 1991). Ratios of medial–frontal cortex to mean cortex showed significant decreases with treatment, as did OCD and anxiety symptoms. The orbital region of the brain was not found to change pre to post treatment.

Another group (Rubin *et al.*, 1992) used the much higher-resolution Shimadzu Headtome (Shimadzu, Japan), Model SET/031 SPECT system (8–9.6 mm resolution) to study 10 untreated males with OCD and 10 matched controls using both ^{133}Xe- and HMPAO-measured blood flow. With ^{133}Xe, they found no significant differences in regional cerebral blood flow (rCBF) between groups, though they did find a significant positive correlation in patients between OCD severity and rCBF. This correlation was not found with HMPAO.

Instead, HMPAO scanning revealed that patients had significantly increased ^{99m}Tc-labeled HMPAO uptake (normalized to cerebellar and whole cerebral cortex uptake) in the high dorsal parietal cortex bilaterally, the left posterofrontal cortex, and the orbital frontal cortex bilaterally. They also found decreased uptake in the head of the caudate bilaterally in OCD patients. Although the most likely reason for detecting differences with HMPAO and not with ^{133}Xe is the resolution difference between the two methods, the authors also thought an HMPAO-sensitive difference between patients and controls in blood–brain barrier permeability or a difference in the rate of HMPAO trapping through hydrophilic conversion might be responsible.

A more recent study (Adams *et al.*, 1993) looked at 11 symptomatic patients (treated with either clomipramine or fluoxetine), using a General Electric 400 AC/T rotating gamma camera (Milwaukee, Wisconsin), resolution 12 mm. The control group used was from a separate study of normal ranges for cerebral perfusion in a healthy population. They found asymmetric perfusion of the basal ganglia in eight of the 11 scans, with left hypoperfusion in six scans and right hypoperfusion in two. The authors felt that their findings were consistent with PET studies showing alterations in basal ganglia glucose metabolism in OCD (see Table 2).

FDG PET FOR CEREBRAL GLUCOSE METABOLIC RATES

Our group at the University of California at Los Angeles (UCLA) examined 14 OCD patients (nine with concurrent major depression), 14 patients with unipo-

Table 2. SPECT Studies of OCD subjects versus controls

Reference	*N*	Technique	Results
Zohar *et al.* (1989)	10 OCD	Xe—symptoms provoked	Increased overall flow in imaginal flooding, decrease with *in vivo* experiment
Machlin *et al.* (1991)	10 OCD 8 controls	HMPAO	Increased median frontal cortex in OCD
Rubin *et al.* (1992)	10 OCD 10 controls	Xe and HMPAO	Xe—OCD = controls HMPAO—increased parietal and frontal cortex, decreased caudate
Adams *et al.* (1993)	11 OCD controls—from another study	HMPAO	Decreased left basal ganglia

lar depression only, and 14 normal controls (Baxter *et al.*, 1987). All subjects were matched for age, and OCD and depressed subjects had similar Hamilton Depression Rating Scale and Brief Psychiatric Rating Scale tension and anxiety item scores. Although nine of the OCD subjects were drug-free for at least two weeks, the other five were taking a variety of antidepressants, benzodiazepines, and neuroleptics. The normal and depressed subjects were drug-free.

FDG PET scanning was done with the Neuro ECAT (Seimens-CTI, Knoxville, Tennessee, in-plane resolution 11 mm, axial 12.5 mm) in the eyes and ears open state, without specific stimuli. Absolute glucose metabolic rates were determined for the whole cerebral hemispheres, hippocampal–parahippocampal complexes, anterior cingulate gyri, heads of the caudate nuclei, putamen nuclei, and thalamic nuclei, as well as various gyri in the prefrontal and temporal cortices. A one-way analysis of variance (ANOVA) was run among the subject groups for each structure, using the first seven subjects only. For those structures yielding significant results, a second prospective analysis was run using the second group of seven. A separate analysis also was done, excluding treated OCD subjects. Neuroanatomic regions of interest had to pass all tests to be considered significant.

Absolute glucose metabolic rates for the whole cerebral hemispheres, caudate nuclei, and orbital gyri were found to be significantly elevated in OCD patients in comparison with control groups. Furthermore, metabolic rates in the left orbital gyrus, normalized to the ipsilateral hemisphere, were significantly higher than those found in normals on the left. There was a trend for this to be the case on the right. Normalized caudate metabolic rates in OCD were not different from those in normal controls.

The subject groups in this first FDG PET study had several problems: (1) unequal numbers of male and female across experimental groups; (2) most of the OCD subjects also had concomitant major depression; (3) some of the OCD subjects were taking medication; and (4) handedness was not equal across groups. Therefore, a second study (Baxter *et al.*, 1988) was undertaken to compare a new group of drug-free, non-depressed, right-handed OCD patients to normal control subjects of similar age scanned under the same conditions as before.

Glucose metabolic rates in the cerebral hemispheres, heads of the caudate nuclei, and orbital gyri were examined, and the results of this study were similar to those of the previous study. The OCD subjects had significantly higher glucose metabolic rates for the whole cerebral hemispheres, heads of the caudate nuclei, and orbital gyri than those found in normal control subjects. Normalized orbital rates also were elevated in OCD patients when compared with normals, but in this second study this finding was significant bilaterally.

At the same time that researchers at UCLA were conducting their second study, two separate groups at the National Institute of Mental Health (NIMH) were performing similar studies independently.

Nordahl *et al.* (1989) compared eight non-depressed OCD subjects with 30 normal volunteers with no personal or family history of psychiatric problems using FDG PET. During uptake of FDG, subjects had their eyes closed and performed an auditory continuous performance task which involved identifying the lowest tone in a series. This task was used for almost all FDG PET scans at NIMH. Scans were performed with a Scanditronix scanner (in-plane resolution 5–6 mm). Sixty regions of interest were compared using two-tailed Student *t*-tests, except for areas found significant in earlier UCLA work, where a one-tailed *t*-test was used.

The authors found significant hypermetabolism in both orbital frontal regions in OCD patients. However, they did not observe differences in global metabolic rates or normalized metabolism of basal ganglia structures as observed at UCLA. Of the many other regions examined, they found hypometabolic differences in normalized values in the right parietal and left occipital–parietal regions. The authors noted that because of the small number of subjects scanned and the large number of structures investigated, the findings require further investigation and are subject to both type I and type II errors.

The other NIMH group (Horwitz *et al.*, 1991; Swedo *et al.*, 1989) examined nine men and nine women with severe, childhood-onset OCD but no concurrent psychiatric or physical disorders. All subjects were drug-free for at least two weeks and were compared with 18 healthy volunteers. FDG PET scanning was done using a Scanditronix PC-1024-7B (in-plane resolution 6 mm) in the eyes and ears closed condition, and both absolute and normalized values (using the mean of cortical gray matter) were used to compare regions of interest. The authors also measured OCD severity and anxiety in patients while being scanned. They chose to be overinclusive in their data analyses and recognized the potential for type I error, given the large number of comparisons and the small differences in metabolism measured.

In OCD subjects, 11 of 46 regions showed altered metabolism. As hypothesized by the authors, increased metabolic activity was found in left and right prefrontal, left orbital frontal, left premotor, right sensorimotor, and bilateral anterior cingulate areas. They also found increased metabolism in the right thalamus, right inferior temporal, left paracentral, and right cerebellar regions. There were no significant between-group differences in whole brain or caudate nuclei metabolism.

The authors also found a significant positive correlation between OCD severity and absolute and normalized right orbitofrontal metabolism. In addition, patients with increased anxiety during scanning had increased prefrontal or orbital frontal activity. Further, all patients were treated with clomipramine after scanning and the six patients who did not respond had higher right anterior cingulate and right orbital metabolism than did those who did respond.

Another recent FDG PET study (Martinot et al., 1990a) found results at odds with those of the above PET studies. Sixteen OCD patients were compared with eight normal controls in the resting state. Both absolute glucose metabolic rates and rates normalized to whole brain were analyzed. All brain regions examined were reported to show lower absolute rates in the OCD subjects than in the controls. In addition, for normalized values, the lateral prefrontal cortex had significantly *lower* rates in the OCD subjects than in normal controls. They could not confirm orbital abnormalities.

Given the similarity between these results and the UCLA group's data on depressed OCD subjects, it is particularly important to note that the authors of this report assure us that no subjects were depressed at the time of PET scanning, and results of drug-free subjects were similar to those scanned on medication. It is possible, however, that a different threshold of depression severity for a diagnosis of major depression was applied in this study than was applied in those studies done in the USA. In a PET study of depression by this same group, "recovered" patients had a mean score of 32 on the 26-item Hamilton Depression Rating Scale (Martinot et al., 1990b).

Thus, in summary, four separate FDG PET studies have found evidence for inferior prefrontal (orbital) cortex abnormalities in OCD, whereas one has not.

^{15}O-LABELED CARBON DIOXIDE, OXYGEN AND CARBON MONOXIDE PET STUDY OF OBSESSIONAL SLOWNESS

A British group (Sawle et al., 1991) studied six patients with obsessional slowness compared to six normal controls using PET. These male patients all had a diagnosis of DSM-III-R OCD, and all experienced difficulty in performing routine activities related to repetitive, time-consuming rituals. Three patients were being treated with antidepressants and other medications and three were untreated. PET scans were performed using the CTI 931/12/8 (CTI, Knoxville, Tennessee). Regional cerebral metabolic oxygen metabolism data were normalized to global metabolic rate.

Using an unpaired two-tailed *t*-test, patients with obsessional slowness showed bilateral hypermetabolism in the orbital frontal, premotor, and mid-frontal cortices. Caudate metabolism values did not differ significantly between groups. In noting the new findings of increased premotor and midfrontal metabolism, the authors hypothesized that these results could have been due to differences in scanner resolution, scanning technique (oxygen vs FDG), or patient differences.

These authors also performed ^{18}F-labeled dopa PET scans on five of these six patients to evaluate the integrity of the presynaptic nigrostriatal system. No significant differences were found between the two groups (see Table 3).

Table 3. PET studies of OCD subjects versus controls

Reference	N	Ligand	Results
Baxter *et al.* (1987)	14 OCD(9 with depression) 14 Depressed 14 Control	FDG	Increased orbital gyri and caudate
Baxter *et al.* (1988)	10 OCD 10 Controls	FDG	Increased orbital gyri and caudate
Nordahl *et al.* (1989)	8 OCD 30 Controls	FDG	Increased orbital frontal, decreased parietal regions
Swedo *et al.* (1989)	18 OCD-childhood onset 18 Controls	FDG	Increased orbital frontal, prefrontal, anterior cingulate and others
Martinot *et al.* (1990b)	16 OCD 8 Controls	FDG	Decreased lateral prefrontal
Sawle *et al.* (1991)	6 OCD with obsessional slowness 6 Controls	[15]O	Increased orbital frontal, premotor and midfrontal

[11C]GLUCOSE PET STUDY OF OCD

One group has used [11C]glucose to measure cerebral glucose metabolism in five patients with treatment-refractory OCD 10 days before and one year after surgical capsulotomy (Mindus *et al.*, 1991). Two were females; drug status was not specified. These scans were compared with 10 healthy males.

The orbital and caudate metabolic rates in patients were significantly higher before surgery than they were after surgery, but it is not clear whether these are absolute or normalized metabolic rates. In addition, although the orbital region was not determined in normals, the Brodmann area 11 was higher in the five normal controls in whom it could be located than was the orbital cortex in the OCD patients before treatment.

This study is problematic. Besides multiple questions about patient status and results, there are basic problems with the [^{11}C]glucose method itself, as discussed previously. If the orbital region of the brain is overstimulated in OCD, as supported by most FDG studies and theories advanced about brain function in OCD, then the [^{11}C]glucose method would systematically underestimate the glucose metabolic rate in OCD patients versus normals.

FDG PET STUDIES OF OCD TREATMENT EFFECTS

Benkelfat *et al.* (1990) restudied eight subjects from their earlier NIMH cohort after an average of 16 weeks treatment with clomipramine. With treatment, the group as a whole showed a significant decrease in normalized regional glucose metabolism in the left caudate and three of five orbital frontal areas (medial frontal cortex, right posterior, and right anterior orbital frontal cortex). They also found a significant increase in right anterior putamen metabolism. When good responders ($n=4$, $\geq 50\%$ decrease in Comprehensive Psychiatric Rating Scale OC subscore) were compared with partial or poor responders, they showed a significantly greater decrease in normalized left caudate values (change from baseline: $-10.9 \pm 5\%$ (mean $\pm$ SD) vs $-2.1\% \pm 3.6\%$). There was a similar, but not statistically significant, directional change difference between these groups for the right caudate ($-7.4\% \pm 18.6\%$ vs $0.07\% \pm 8.7\%$).

Swedo *et al.* (1992) restudied 13 of their OCD patients after a mean of 20 months. Eight were taking clomipramine, two were taking fluoxetine, and three were off medication. At the time of rescanning, mean scores on all measures of symptomatology were significantly improved. Seven of the patients taking medication had treatment response, while the others had no significant improvement. The group as a whole showed significant decreases in normalized right and left orbital frontal metabolic rates. Further, medication responders had a significantly greater decrease in left orbitofrontal metabolism (normalized) than did non-responders ($9.0\% \pm 9.7\%$ vs $0.4\% \pm 6.1\%$). Unexpectedly, there was a strong *positive* correlation between post-treatment clomipramine plus desmethylclomipramine (a clomipramine metabolite) levels and normalized right orbitofrontal metabolism. The authors cautioned that their number of subjects was small, but speculated that the orbitofrontal region may be the site of action for clomipramine.

Baxter *et al.* (1992) studied OCD patients pre and post treatment with either fluoxetine ($n=9$) or behavior therapy ($n=9$). The two treatment groups were matched for OCD severity, anxiety, age, and sex. All were drug-free on initial scan and none had major depression. They were rescanned after 10 weeks of treatment. The high-resolution (6 × 6 mm in-plane, 6.75 mm axial) Seimens/CTI 831 tomograph (Seimens-CTI, Knoxville, Tennessee) was used.

In both groups, normalized right caudate metabolic rates decreased significantly in treatment responders ($-5.2\% \pm 2.3\%$ for drug treatment and $-8.0\% \pm 4.8\%$ for behavior treatment) but not in non-responders ($0.3\% \pm 1.0\%$ and $2.6\% \pm 3.2\%$, respectively), and the differences between responders and non-responders were significant within each treatment group. Results in OCD treatment responders were also significant compared with right caudate changes in a small group of normals ($0.4\% \pm 2.0\%$) rescanned after a similar interval. Further, percentage change in normalized right caudate glucose metabolic rates gave a significant correlation with percentage change on the YBOCS for drug treatment, and there was a trend for this in subjects treated with behavior therapy (see Table 4). In addition, the normalized left caudate glucose metabolic rate decreased in responders to each treatment, but not significantly. Right anterior cingulate gyrus and left thalamus metabolism decreased with fluoxetine, but not with behavior modification.

Table 4. FDG PET studies of OCD subjects pre and post treatment

Authors	N/treatment	Results
Benkelfat *et al.* (1990)	8 treated with clomipramine for mean 16 weeks	Decreased left caudate and three orbital frontal areas
Swedo *et al.* (1992)	13 subjects—8 on clomipramine, 2 on fluoxetine and 3 off medications at mean 20 months	Decreased bilateral orbital frontal
Baxter *et al.* (1992)	9 with fluoxetine, 9 with behavior therapy at 10 weeks	Decreased right caudate— both groups

Table 5. Correlations (Kendall's tau) found in treatment-responsive OCD patients before and after treatment

Brain region	Pre treatment	Post treatment
L caudate to L orbit	0.49*	0.00
R caudate to R orbit	0.44*	−0.03
L orbit to L thalamus	0.33	−0.21
R orbit to R thalamus	0.41*	−0.21
L caudate to L cingulate	−0.10	0.41*
R caudate to R cingulate	−0.04	−0.03

L, left; R, right.
*$p<.05$.

Table 6. Correlations (Kendall's tau) found in normal control subjects and unipolar depression patients

Brain region	Normal	Depressed
L caudate to L orbit	−0.09	−0.20
R caudate to R orbit	0.05	−0.20
L orbit to L thalamus	0.09	−0.24
R orbit to R thalamus	0.13	−0.11
L caudate to L cingulate	0.00	−0.29
R caudate to R cingulate	−0.18	−0.11

*L, left; R, right.

When all responders to treatment (n=13) were lumped together, significant correlations (Kendall's tau) between metabolism in different brain regions were found before and after treatment (see Table 5). All the correlations, except the right caudate to right cingulate, showed significant pre- to post-treatment differences, indicating that treatment disrupts the association of glucose metabolism that exists pre treatment.

Although obtained with the lower resolution NeuroECAT PET tomograph (11 mm in-plane and 12.5 mm axial), data from patients with unipolar depression (n=10) and normal control subjects (n=12) that were otherwise obtained in an identical manner as part of another project are presented in Table 6 for comparison with those of the OCD patients. None of these correlations for normal controls and patients with unipolar depression were significant.

These results in normals and depressives are informative in that they resemble those in OCD treatment responders after effective treatment, except the relationship of the head of the caudate nucleus to the cingulate gyrus. Thus, treatment-responsive OCD may be characterized by abnormal, disease-specific functional relationships between these brain regions in the symptomatic state. There also may be an unusual relationship between the caudate and cingulate after symptomatic improvement of OCD.

CRITIQUE OF FDG PET OCD TREATMENT STUDIES

Our group noted the conflicts in the three PET reports of treatment effects on the brains of OCD patients (Baxter *et al.*, 1992). These could relate to specific differences in the drugs chosen for each study (clomipramine vs fluoxetine), different stimulus conditions at time of scanning, or other factors. It was pointed out, however, that both the report of Benkelfat *et al.* (1990) and that of Baxter *et al.* (1992) found decreases in normalized caudate metabolic rates bilaterally; they differed only on which side made statistical significance. More importantly, time interval differences between pretreatment and posttreatment scans among these three studies may have been a critical factor. Our group has argued previously (Baxter *et al.*, 1990a) that orbital cortex changes should come some time after those in the caudate. In addition, other PET work done at UCLA (Mazziotta *et al.*, 1991) has shown that as a person learns to execute a task more efficiently, the brain region that mediates the behavior shows a decrease in both the extent and degree of activation on PET scanning as compared with the scan when the task was new. With time, the caudate might become more efficient in limiting OCD symptoms, and its change in a critical function might no longer be detectable with present FDG PET methods (Baxter *et al.*, 1992). It is interesting that the study with the shortest interval between scans (Baxter *et al.*, 1992) found only caudate changes and the study with the longest interval (Swedo *et al.*, 1992) found only orbital changes, but the study of intermediate length (Benkelfat *et al.*, 1990) found both.

rCBF STUDY WITH ^{15}O PET DURING SYMPTOM PROVOCATION

Recently, Rauch *et al.* (1994) studied eight OCD subjects (five men and three women) during a resting and a provoked (symptomatic) state using [^{15}O]CO$_2$ PET to measure rCBF changes. All subjects were free from psychoactive drugs for at least two weeks before the study.

The subjects underwent PET scanning (Scanditronix PC4096, General Electric, Milwaukee, Wisconsin; axial resolution 6.0 mm) twice in a resting state, while responding to an innocuous control stimulus and twice again in a provoked state, while responding to a provocative stimulus that was tailored to induce each patient's symptoms. The subjects participated in the process of identifying stimuli that would produce sufficient but not overwhelming stimuli.

The authors found statistically significant increases in relative rCBF during the symptomatic state versus the resting state in the right caudate nucleus ($p<0.006$), the left anterior cingulate cortex ($p<0.045$), and the bilateral orbitofrontal cortices ($p<0.008$). There was also a trend toward increase blood flow in the left thalamus ($p=0.07$).

A THEORY OF THE FUNCTIONAL NEUROANATOMY MEDIATING THE SYMPTOMS OF OCD

Many of the brain imaging studies reviewed here provide evidence for symptom-related abnormalities in the orbital prefrontal cortex in OCD. The caudate nucleus, although less consistently implicated, has been found in several pretreatment studies to show abnormalities. In addition, two studies have demonstrated decreases in caudate glucose metabolism after treatment with clomipramine, fluoxetine, and behavior modification, while another study demonstrated increases in rCBF to the caudate with symptom provocation.

Particularly in light of the pretreatment to posttreatment correlation data

A   Symptomatic Treatment – Responsive OCD

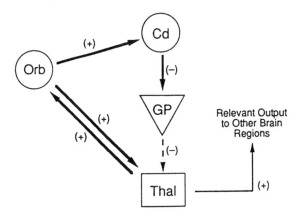

B   Successfully Treated OCD

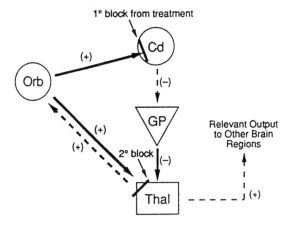

Figure 1 Although known connections among brain systems proposed to be involved in OCD symptom mediation are complex, a subsystem (A) may be the locus of pathologic dysfunction. Pretreatment correlations suggest that "worry" outputs from the orbital region of the brain may be driving OCD-relevant circuits in the caudate, and thus increase inhibitory output to relevant regions of the globus pallidus. This would reduce inhibition of the thalamus, making it vulnerable to being driven by the orbit as well. The excitatory connections between thalamus and orbit make this a potentially self-sustaining circuit, and thus difficult to break. With effective treatment (B), increases in "filtering" functions in the caudate may reduce its inhibitory output to the globus pallidus, which in turn would increase inhibitory output to the thalamus. This would result in an uncoupling of this fixed "worry circuit", and allow the patient to more easily terminate OCD behaviours. With time, orbital "worry activity" may also decrease. Arrows indicate effect of stimulating one brain region at the rate of neuronal firing in the other. (+), excitatory; (–), inhibitory. Broken lines represent reduced effect. Cd, head of caudate nucleus; GP, globus pallidus; Orb, orbital prefrontal cortex; Thal, thalamus (From Baxter, L. R., Schwartz, J. M., Bergman, K. S. *et al.*, Caudate glucose metabolic rate changes with both drug and behavior therapy for obsessive-compulsive disorder. *Arch. Gen. Psychiatry*, **49**, 681–689, 1992; copyright 1992 by the American Medical Association; with permission)

between these regions presented in Tables 5 and 6, our group at UCLA pointed out how brain imaging data can be used to support theories of how the brain mediates OCD symptoms that were first put forward by Rapoport and Wise (1988) and Insel (1988; Insel and Winslow, 1990), but in most detail by Modell *et al.* (1989). Figure 1 summarizes our group's present working model of OCD symptom mediation. It is distilled from those earlier theories, but now includes a proposed mechanism for symptom reduction after treatment.

What is not clear in this model is what neurotransmitter or second messenger system(s) might mediate the proposed critical change(s) in caudate function that may facilitate OCD treatment response. PET and SPECT studies with more specific tracers—especially ones for the serotonin system—are clearly needed.

REFERENCES

Adams, B. L., Warneke, L. B., McEwan, A. J. B. *et al.* (1993) Single photon emission computerized tomography in obsessive-compulsive disorder: a preliminary study. *J. Psychiatr. Neurosci.*, **18**, 109–112.

Baxter, L. R. (1991). PET studies of cerebral function in major depression and obsessive-compulsive disorder: the emerging prefrontal consensus. *Ann. Clin. Psychiatry*, **3**, 103–109.

Baxter, L. R. and Guze, B. H. (1992). Neuroimaging in Tourette's and related disorders. In *Handbook of Tourette's and Related Tic and Behavioral Disorders* (ed. R. Kurland). Marcel Dekker, Paris.

Baxter, L. R., Phelps, M. E., Mazziotta, J. C. *et al.* (1987). Local cerebral glucose metabolic rates in obsessive-compulsive disorder: a comparison with rates in unipolar depression and in normal controls. *Arch. Gen. Psychiatry*, **44**, 211–218.

Baxter, L. R., Schwartz, J. M., Mazziotta, J. C. *et al.* (1988). Cerebral glucose metabolic rates in non-depressed obsessive-compulsives. *Am. J. Psychiatry*, **145**, 1560–1563.

Baxter, L. R., Schwartz, J. M., Guze, B. H. *et al.* (1990a). Neuroimaging in obsessive-compulsive disorder: seeking the mediating neuroanatomy. In *Obsessive-Compulsive Disorders: Theory and Management*, 2nd edn (eds M. A. Jenicke, L. Baer and W. E. Minichiello), pp. 167–188. Year Book Medical Publishers, Chicago.

Baxter, L. R., Schwartz, J. M., Guze, B. H. *et al.* (1990b). PET imaging in obsessive-compulsive disorder with and without depression. *J. Clin. Psychiatry*, **51**(s), 61–69.

Baxter, L. R., Schwartz, J. M. and Guze, B. H. (1991). Brain imaging: toward a neuroanatomy of OCD. In *The Psychobiology of Obsessive-Compulsive Disorder* (eds Y. Zohar, T. R. Insel and S. Rasmussen), pp. 101–125. Springer-Verlag, New York.

Baxter, L. R., Schwartz, J. M., Bergman, K. S. *et al.* (1992). Caudate glucose metabolic rate changes with both drug and behavior therapy for obsessive-compulsive disorder. *Arch. Gen. Psychiatry*, **49**, 681–689.

Behar, D., Rapoport, J. L., Berg, C. J. *et al.* (1984). Computerized tomography and neuropsychological test measures in adolescents with obsessive-compulsive disorder. *Am. J. Psychiatry*, **141**, 363–369.

Benkelfat, C., Nordahl, T. E., Semple, W. E. *et al.* (1990). Local cerebral glucose metabolic rates in obsessive-compulsive disorder: patients treated with clomipramine. *Arch. Gen. Psychiatry*, **47**, 840–848.

Blomqvist, G., Bergstrom. K., Bergstrom, M. *et al.* (1985). Models for ^{11}C-glucose. In *The Metabolism of the Human Brain Studied with Positron Emission Tomography* (eds T. Greitz, D. H. Ingvar and L. Widen), pp. 185–194, Raven Press, New York.

Garber, H. J., Ananth, J. V., Chiu, L. C., *et al.* (1989). Nuclear magnetic resonance study of obsessive-compulsive disorder. *Am. J. Psychiatry*, **146**, 1001–1005.

Hoehn-Saric, R., Pearlson, G. D., Harris, G. J. *et al.* (1991). Effects of fluoxetine on regional cerebral blood flow in obsessive-compulsive patients. *Am. J. Psychiatry*, 1243–1245.

Horwitz, B., Swedo, S. E., Grady, C. L. *et al.* (1991). Cerebral metabolic pattern in obsessive-compulsive disorder: altered intercorrelations between regional rates of glucose utilization. *Psychiatry Res.*, **40**, 221–237.

Insel, T. R. (1988). Obsessive-compulsive disorder: a neuroethological perspective. *Psychopharmacol. Bull.*, **24**, 365–369.

Insel, T. R. and Winslow, J. T. (1990). Neurobiology of obsessive-compulsive disorder. In *Obsessive-Compulsive Disorders: Theory and Management*, 2nd edn (eds M. A. Jenicke, L. Baer and W. E. Minichiello), pp. 116–131. Year Book Medical Publishers, Chicago.

Insel, T. R., Donnelly, E. F., Lalakea, M. L. *et al.* (1983). Neurological and neuropsychological studies of patients with obsessive-compulsive disorder. *Biol. Psychiatry*, **18**, 741–751.

Kellner, C. H., Jolley, R. R., Holgate, R. C. *et al.* (1991). Brain MRI in obsessive-compulsive disorder. *Psychiatry Res.*, **36**, 45–49.

Lear, J. L. and Ackermann, R. F. (1991). Autoradiographic comparison of FDG-based and GLU-based measurements of cerebral glucose transport and metabolism: normal and activated conditions. In *Brain Work and Mental Activity: Quantitative Studies with Radioactive Tracers* (eds N. A, Lassen, D. H. Ingvar, M. E. Raichle and L. Friberg), pp. 142–157. 31st Alfred Benson Symposium. Munksgaard, Copenhagen.

Luxenberg, J. S., Swedo, S. E., Flamant, M. F. *et al.* (1988). Neuroanatomical abnormalities in obsessive-compulsive disorder determined with quantitative x-ray computed tomography. *Am. J. Psychiatry*, **145**, 1089–1093.

Machlin, S. R., Harris, G. J., Pearlson, G. D. *et al.* (1991). Elevated medial–frontal cerebral blood flow in obsessive-compulsive patients: a SPECT study. *Am. J. Psychiatry*, **148**, 1240–1242.

Martinot, J. L., Allilaire, J. F., Mazoyer, B. M. *et al.* (1990a). Obsessive-compulsive disorder: a clinical, neuropsychological and positron emission tomography study. *Acta Psychiatr. Scand.*, **82**, 233–242.

Martinot, J. L., Hardy, P., Feline, A. *et al.* (1990b). Left prefrontal glucose hypometabolism in the depressed state: a confirmation. *Am. J. Psychiatry*, **147**, 1313–1317.

Mazziotta, J. C., Grafton, S. T. and Woods, R. C. (1991). The human motor system studied with PET measurements of cerebral blood flow: topography and motor learning. In *Brain Work and Mental Activity: Quantitative Studies with Radioactive Tracers* (eds N. A., Lassen, D. H. Ingvar, M. E. Raichle and L. Friberg), pp. 280–293. 31st Alfred Benson Symposium. Munksgaard, Copenhagen.

Mindus, P., Nyman, H., Mogard, J. *et al.* (1991). Orbital and caudate glucose metabolism studied by positron emission tomography (PET) in patients undergoing capsulotomy for obsessive-compulsive disorder. In *Understanding Obsessive-Compulsive Disorder (OCD)* (eds M. A. Jenicke and M. Asberg), pp. 52–57. Hogrefe & Huber, Toronto.

Modell, J. G., Mountz, J. M., Curtis, G. C. *et al.* (1989). Neurophysiologic dysfunction in basal ganglia/limbic striatal and thalamocortical circuits as a pathogenetic mechanism of obsessive-compulsive disorder. *J. Neuropsychiatry*, **1**, 27–36.

Nordahl, T. E., Benkelfat, C., Semple, W. E. *et al.* (1989). Cerebral glucose metabolic rates in obsessive-compulsive disorder. *Neuropsychopharmacology*, **2**, 23–28.

Phelps, M. E. and Mazziotta, J. C. (1985). Positron emission tomography: human brain function and biochemistry. *Science*, **228**, 799–809.

Phelps, M. E. and Mazziotta, J. C. and Shelbert, H. R. (eds) (1986). *Positron Emission Tomography and Autoradiography*. Raven Press, New York.

Rapoport, J. L. and Wise, S. P. (1988). Obsessive-compulsive disorder: is it a basal ganglia dysfunction? *Psychopharmacol. Bull.*, **24**, 380–384.

Rauch, S. L., Jenike, M. A., Alpert, N. M. *et al.* (1994). Regional cerebral blood flow measured during symptom provocation in obsessive-compulsive disorder using oxygen 15-labeled carbon dioxide and positron emission tomography. *Arch. Gen. Psychiatry*, **51**, 62–70.

Rubin, R. T., Villanueva-Meyer, J., Ananth, J. *et al.* (1992). Regional ^{133}Xe cerebral blood flow and cerebral ^{99m}HMPAO uptake in unmedicated obsessive-compulsive disorder patients and matched normal control subjects: determination by high-resolution single-photon emission computed tomography. *Arch. Gen. Psychiatry*, **49**, 695–702.

Sawle, G. V., Hymas, N. F., Lees, A. J. *et al.* (1991). Obsessional slowness: functional studies with positron emission tomography. *Brain*, **114**, 2191–2202.

Scarone, S., Colombo, C., Livian, S. *et al.* (1992). Increased right caudate nucleus size in obsessive-compulsive disorder: detection with magnetic resonance imaging. *Psychiatry Res.*, **45**, 115–121.

Swedo, S. E., Schapiro, M. G., Grady, C. L. *et al.* (1989). Cerebral glucose metabolism in childhood onset obsessive-compulsive disorder. *Arch. Gen. Psychiatry*, **46**, 518–523.

Swedo, S. E., Pietrini, P., Leonard, H. L. *et al.* (1992). Cerebral glucose metabolism in childhood-onset obsessive-compulsive disorder: revisualization during pharmacotherapy. *Arch. Gen. Psychiatry*, **49**, 690–694.

Zohar, J., Insel, T. R., Berman, K. F. *et al.* (1989). Anxiety and cerebral blood flow during behavioral challenge: dissociation of central from peripheral and subjective measures. *Arch. Gen. Psychiatry*, **46**, 505–510.

Part IV

GENERALIZED ANXIETY DISORDER

15 Serotonin-selective Drugs in Generalized Anxiety Disorder: Achievements and Prospects

DEBRA A. GLITZ AND RICHARD BALON
Wayne State University, Detroit, Michigan, USA

INTRODUCTION

Throughout the era of modern psychopharmacology there has been an ongoing search for an "ideal" anxiolytic drug. Benzodiazepines (BZDs), the most widely used anxiolytics, are highly effective, generally well tolerated and much safer than their predecessors, the barbiturates. However, their potential side effects (primarily sedation and cognitive/motor impairment) and unwanted pharmacological properties (potential for interactions with other central nervous system (CNS) depressants, withdrawal reactions and development of tolerance) make them less than an ideal group of medications. Consequently, some clinicians use BZDs somewhat hesitantly and may fail to adequately treat patients with generalized anxiety disorder (GAD). Although the magnitude of their abuse potential remains debatable, BZDs are generally not the medications of first choice for anxious patients with concurrent substance abuse problems.

In the early 1960s, Donald Klein suggested that two syndromes with differential drug responsiveness (i.e., panic anxiety and generalized anxiety) could be delineated among patients with anxiety (Klein, 1964). This led to a subsequent split in the pharmacotherapy of these disorders. Panic anxiety was believed to be amenable to tricyclic antidepressants (TCAs) and monoamine oxidase inhibitors (MAOIs), while GAD was primarily treated with BZDs. Over the past decade we have witnessed a blurring of this pharmacotherapeutic division. New (e.g., alprazolam) (Chouinard *et al.*, 1982) and old (e.g., diazepam) (Dunner *et al.*, 1986) BZDs have been found to be effective for panic attacks and various antidepressants have been shown to be beneficial for GAD (Kahn *et al.*, 1987; Rickels and Schweizer, 1993). Although the older antidepressants (i.e., the TCAs and MAOIs) have proven effective for some patients with GAD, these medications also have significant drawbacks including various side effects and a delayed therapeutic response.

Advances in the Neurobiology of Anxiety Disorders. Edited by H. G. M. Westenberg, J. A. Den Boer and D. L. Murphy
©1996 John Wiley & Sons Ltd

During this same time period, a new class of anxiolytics, the azaspirode-canediones or azaspirones, emerged; buspirone being the first one widely studied (Ortiz *et al.*, 1987). Buspirone was first synthesized in 1972 as a potential antipsychotic agent. However, it proved to be ineffective in clinical trials for the treatment of schizophrenia. However, the discovery of its inhibition of aggressive behavior in rhesus monkeys (Tompkins *et al.*, 1980) led to clinical trials in the treatment of anxiety. Buspirone was approved by the FDA (Food and Drug Administration, USA) for use in the treatment of anxiety in the USA in October 1986. The search for the mechanism of action of this novel anxiolytic and the discovery of its primary involvement with the serotonergic neurotransmitter system led to further investigations into the role of serotonin (5-hydroxytryptamine, 5-HT) in the modulation of anxiety. Interest in 5-HT-selective drugs as potential therapeutic agents for GAD has been further enhanced by the success of such medications in the treatment of other anxiety disorders, including obsessive-compulsive disorder and panic disorder (Den Boer *et al.*, 1987; Murphy *et al.*, 1990). A variety of different types of 5-HT-selective drugs have been developed and are currently in testing as potential anxiolytics.

Rigorous investigation into the possible involvement of 5-HT in the underlying pathophysiology of GAD and the potential role for 5-HT-selective drugs (with the possible exception of the azaspirones) in the treatment of this disorder has been less systematic and rather limited in comparison with similar studies of the more dramatic forms of anxiety disorders (e.g., panic and obsessive-compulsive disorders). This chapter will initially focus on some possible reasons for the relative lack of such investigations involving the disorder known as GAD, including diagnostic uncertainties and discrepant hypotheses concerning the role of 5-HT in anxiety. We will then provide an overview of studies to date investigating the therapeutic potential for 5-HT-selective drugs in GAD and their possible advantages over other anxiolytics.

DIAGNOSTIC CRITERIA FOR GAD

In order to accurately interpret and compare the results of different treatment studies, it is necessary to consider whether the studies utilized the same patient population. This consideration is especially important for studies of GAD since this diagnostic category is relatively new and has been continuously modified with each successive revision of the various diagnostic classification systems (e.g., DSM-III-R) (American Psychiatric Association, 1987). Although the core symptoms have remained relatively stable over the last 13 years, certain specific features have been modified. This reflects the continuing debate over the essential features of this loosely defined and probably heterogeneous disorder. Since many investigators have questioned the validity of past and present diagnostic criteria for GAD, this may have contributed to the relative lack of intensive study into this disorder. The following is a brief review of the development and evolution of the diagnostic criteria for GAD.

The diagnostic term, GAD, first came into existence in 1980 with the publication of DSM-III (American Psychiatric Association, 1980). Prior to then all patients with prominent anxiety symptoms were lumped into one general diagnostic category termed anxiety neurosis. Other descriptive terms, such as vasomotor neurosis, neurasthenia, and neurocirculatory asthenia also appeared in the pre-DSM-III literature. Early neurobiological studies usually focused on state or trait anxiety rather than on psychiatric diagnosis. The decision to subdivide the category of anxiety neurosis into separate and distinct anxiety disorders stemmed in part from Klein's work and conceptualizations (Klein, 1980). Klein split anxiety neurosis into panic disorder with or without agoraphobia (responsive to imipramine), and into a residual diagnostic category (unresponsive to imipramine). The latter category became the basis for the new DSM-III category called GAD.

In DSM-III, GAD was defined as generalized and persistent anxiety of at least one month duration manifested by symptoms from three of the following four categories: (1) motor tension; (2) autonomic hyperactivity; (3) apprehensive expectation; and (4) vigilance and scanning. The anxiety could not be due to another mental disorder and only included patients over the age of 18. This definition was considerably more specific than the corresponding diagnosis in the contemporary ICD-9 diagnostic classification system. ICD-9 defined a GAD of at least six months duration in which the predominant feature was limited to diffuse and persistent anxiety without the specific symptoms that characterize phobic disorders, panic disorder, or obsessive disorder. In essence it was a residual or "wastebasket" category for anxious patients who failed to meet criteria for any other specific anxiety disorder.

These early definitions of GAD troubled various authors who suggested revising this diagnostic classification with additional more specific criteria. One major problem was the considerable overlap between the defining symptoms of GAD and the symptoms of other anxiety and affective disorders. Cameron et al. suggested that it was inappropriate to attempt to differentiate such disorders as GAD, panic disorder, and agoraphobia with or without panic attacks from one other on the basis of such overlapping symptoms (Cameron et al., 1986). They suggested that alternative criteria were needed to better define and differentiate these disorders. Another related problem with the early definitions of GAD was the absence of any essential and characteristic feature which differentiated it from the many other psychiatric disorders where anxiety may be a prominent symptom. Barlow et al. studied the phenomenology of 108 patients with anxiety (Barlow et al., 1986). Almost all of the patients studied across the various anxiety disorder diagnostic categories had the four basic features which defined GAD in DSM-III. Hence, although these early symptomatic criteria were likely to be present in this yet to be adequately defined disorder, the DSM-III criteria failed to effectively delineate GAD as a distinct disorder. In essence, the DSM-

III diagnosis, like the ICD-9 definition, appeared to be a diagnosis of exclusion. Their findings suggested, however, a possible differentiating feature within the DSM-III cluster of symptoms for GAD. They proposed utilizing the symptom of "apprehensive expectation" as a cardinal and essential feature to attempt to further delineate a more distinct and potentially homogeneous disorder characterized as a group of "chronic worriers."

DSM-III-R (American Psychiatric Association, 1987) utilized this proposed criterion and combined it with a more elaborate version of the symptomatic criteria from DSM-III. The result was a more stringent and detailed definition. The first DSM-III-R diagnostic criterion incorporated Barlow's suggested cardinal feature and was the presence of "unrealistic or excessive anxiety and worry about two or more life circumstances for a period of six months or longer." The second DSM-III-R criterion (i.e., the focus of the anxiety and worry could not be exclusively related to another axis I disorder) attempted to further separate GAD from other anxiety and affective disorders. The remaining additional DSM-III-R criteria changed only the detail and not the basic concepts of the other DSM-III criteria. Although the DSM-III-R criteria were much more detailed and elaborate, critics have continued to complain that the resulting diagnostic category remains imprecise and heterogeneous.

The Task Force on DSM-IV of the American Psychiatric Association (Task Force on DSM-IV, 1991) focused on two main problems with the DSM-III-R criteria for GAD: (1) unclear boundaries with other disorders (especially obsessive-compulsive disorder and hypochondriasis) and with normality; and (2) the "cumbersome and user unfriendly" nature of the first and fourth criteria (the description of anxiety and worry, and the presence of at least six out of 18 specific symptoms, respectively). Thus the DSM-IV criteria (American Psychiatric Association, 1994) for GAD (which now also includes overanxious disorder of childhood) attempt to rectify these problems. The first criterion has been modified to require the presence of excessive anxiety and worry about a number of events and activities on more days than not for at least six months. The symptomatic criterion (the third criterion in DSM-IV) has also been simplified and requires the presence of only three symptoms (instead of six as in DSM-III-R) from six groups of symptoms (restlessness or feeling keyed up or on the edge; easily fatigued; difficulty concentrating; irritability; muscle tension; and sleep disturbance). The non-specific symptoms of autonomic hyperactivity which commonly occur in other anxiety disorders as well have been eliminated. New additional criteria include requirements that the person finds it difficult to control the worry and that the anxiety causes significant distress or impairment in various areas (e.g., social or occupational functioning). This apparently is an attempt to better delineate this disorder from normal anxiety associated with realistic stressors in everyday life. Other criteria remain essentially unchanged. It remains to be seen whether these new criteria will improve the validity of this diagnostic category and possibly stimulate further neurobiological study of this disorder.

In addition, although the GAD symptoms discussed above are rather common, they frequently occur in association with other psychiatric disorders and some contend that they rarely occur in isolation. Careful scrutiny frequently uncovers the presence of other diagnoses. Indeed studies have demonstrated high comorbidity rates for GAD with alcohol dependence (Cloninger et al., 1990), other anxiety disorders (phobias) (Brawman-Mintzer et al., 1993) and depression (Merikangas, 1990; Weissman, 1990). One study found 42% of the patients with GAD had experienced at least one major depressive episode during their lifetime (Brawman-Mintzer et al., 1993). Hence some debate continues over the very existence of GAD as a distinct diagnostic entity.

Since the co-occurrence of symptoms of GAD and depression is so common, it is important to recall that DSM-III utilized hierarchical conventions which considered anxiety symptoms as secondary if a major depressive illness was also present. This precluded the DSM-III-R practice of giving multiple concurrent diagnoses whenever sufficient criteria are met for each individual disorder. Hence early GAD studies utilizing DSM-III criteria may have employed potentially purer samples of GAD patients. Although such pure diagnostic samples do not always accurately reflect clinical reality, they may be necessary to gain a better understanding of the underlying pathophysiology. Such high comorbidity rates also suggest the need to carefully consider which exclusion criteria for other major psychiatric disorders were utilized for any particular study in interpreting and comparing the results. Such factors as concurrent diagnoses (if not excluded) or other symptoms (e.g., depression) may function as confounding variables and further complicate the interpretation of GAD studies. All of these factors may have contributed to the apparent decreased interest in neurobiological studies of this particular anxiety disorder.

5-HT AND ANXIETY

Although there is considerable evidence to suggest that 5-HT is involved in the pathophysiology of anxiety (Charney et al., 1990), the specific nature and direction of that involvement remain unclear. Undoubtedly, other neurotransmitter (e.g., γ-aminobutyric acid (GABA) and norepinephrine) systems also play a role and may interact with 5-HT in the modulation of anxiety (Cloez-Tayarani et al., 1992; Gillespie et al., 1988: López-Rubalcava et al., 1992). 5-HT neurons (the majority of cell bodies are located in the brain stem raphe and tegmental nuclei) project to all levels of the neuroaxis, including several neuroanatomical structures considered likely to be involved in the regulation of anxiety (e.g., locus coeruleus, frontal cortex, septum, hippocampus and amygdala).

Some authors have suggested that anxiety is a 5-HT excess disease (Eison, 1990). This hypothesis is partially based on the fact that m-chlorophenylpiperazine (mCPP), a non-selective 5-HT agonist, induces marked anxiety in human subjects (Charney et al., 1987; Kahn et al., 1988a). In addition, BZDs decrease

5-HT turnover, release (in the cortex) and neuronal firing even though they have no direct effect on 5-HT receptors (Chase et al., 1970; Collinge and Pycock, 1982; Dominic et al., 1975; Laurent et al., 1983; Pratt et al., 1979, 1985; Trulson et al., 1982; Wise et al., 1972). However, BZDs increase 5-HT release in the raphe nuclei (Collinge and Pycock, 1982). Furthermore, the anxiolytic actions of BZDs are probably mediated via BZD–GABA receptors and may be unrelated to effects on 5-HT activity. The non-BZD anxiolytics, the azaspirones (e.g., buspirone), also acutely decrease 5-HT function (Sharp et al., 1989). However, chronic administration of gepirone, another azaspirone anxiolytic, increases 5-HT function (Blier and de Montigny, 1987). Chronic effects are more likely than acute effects to be related to the therapeutic mechanisms of such compounds since the azaspirones appear to have a delayed onset of therapeutic action similar to antidepressants (Enkelmann, 1991).

Other evidence supporting an anxiogenic role for 5-HT comes from some of the studies utilizing animal behavioral models of anxiety. A variety of animal models predictive for "anxiolytic" activity have been developed based on the effect of BZDs on these models. The relationship between these animal models and human anxiety is debatable. p-Chlorophenylalanine (PCPA), an inhibitor of 5-HT synthesis, as well as 5-HT neurotoxins, mimics the effects of BZDs when studied using animal conflict models of anxiety (Geller and Blum, 1970; Johnston and File, 1986; Tye et al., 1977). Furthermore, in some studies 5-HT antagonists also mimic the effects of BZDs (Geller et al., 1974), while 5-HT agonists suppress BZD-like effects (Aprison and Hingtgen, 1972) in animal conflict models. These observations have been interpreted as further evidence supporting the hypothesis that anxiety is a 5-HT excess disease.

In contrast, direct observation of animals given PCPA reveals behavior associated with anxious states (e.g., hyperexcitability and increased reactivity) (Brody, 1970). Furthermore, PCPA has been reported to precipitate anxiety when given to human subjects (Mendels and Frazer, 1974). 5-HT antagonists do not consistently display anticonflict activity (Commissaris and Rech, 1982; Kilts et al., 1982). 5-Hydroxytryptophan (5-HTP), a 5-HT precursor, has been reported to have both "anxiolytic" and "anxiogenic" properties in animal models (Geller and Blum, 1970; Kilts et al., 1982). Furthermore, one small clinical study reported a significant reduction in anxiety after treatment with 5-HTP and carbidopa (a peripheral decarboxylase inhibitor) in mixed group of 10 patients with DSM-III anxiety disorders (Kahn and Westenberg, 1985). In addition, serotonergic pathways to the hippocampus and amygdala (structures felt to be associated with the generation of anxiety) are inhibitory (Eriksson and Humble, 1990). These findings suggest that a 5-HT-deficient state might promote anxiety.

One possible explanation for the discrepancy between the observed behavioral effects of agents like PCPA and the suggested effects of these agents based on animal models of anxiety is that these animal paradigms may be testing for something other than anxiety reduction. Soubrie has suggested that animal conflict paradigms may actually be investigating impulsivity rather than anxiety (Soubrie, 1986). Furthermore, 5-HT appears to be involved in mediating some, but not all, of the behavioral responses interpreted as being related to anxiety or fear in the different models (Charney et al., 1990). It is apparent that no simple theory about 5-HT and anxiety can account for the diversity of findings reviewed above. Such contradictory hypotheses for the role of 5-HT in the regulation of anxiety relate in part to complexities in the regulation of serotonergic neurotransmission.

Four main classes of 5-HT receptor subtypes have been identified: $5-HT_1$, $5-HT_2$, $5-HT_3$ and $5-HT_4$ receptors. Within the $5-HT_1$ class of receptors, at least four different receptor subtypes have been identified: $5-HT_{1A}$, $5-HT_{1B}$, $5-HT_{1C}$ and $5-HT_{1D}$ (Bradley et al., 1986; Eriksson and Humble, 1990; Monferini et al., 1993; Peroutka and Snyder, 1979). There is evidence to suggest that $5-HT_{1A}$ agonists, $5-HT_2$ and $5-HT_3$ antagonists, as well as 5-HT reuptake inhibitors, may all have anxiolytic properties and prove to be useful for GAD.

5-HT-SELECTIVE DRUGS

$5-HT_{1A}$ RECEPTOR AGONISTS

The discovery that buspirone is a $5-HT_{1A}$ receptor partial agonist triggered considerable interest in this receptor subtype and investigations into its possible role in the modulation of anxiety. Several buspirone analogs which are also $5-HT_{1A}$ agonists have been developed, including gepirone, ipsapirone (TVXQ 7821) and tandospirone (SM-3997/metanopirone). $5-HT_{1A}$ receptor agonists have been shown to directly inhibit neurons that send excitatory projections to the spinal sympathetic outflow tracts (Wang and Lovick, 1992). $5-HT_{1A}$ receptors are also found in the cortex, raphe nuclei, amygdala and hippocampus (Pazos et al., 1987). The $5-HT_{1A}$ receptor subtype includes both postsynaptic receptors as well as somatodendritic, but not terminal, autoreceptors which provide feedback inhibition on neuronal firing (Hjorth and Magnusson, 1988; Sprouse and Aghajanian, 1988; Verge et al., 1985). Possible inhibition of 5-HT function is suggested by reports of $5-HT_{1A}$ agents decreasing levels of 5-hydroxyindoleacetic acid (5-HIAA, a 5-HT metabolite) (Gleeson et al., 1989). The overall balance between inhibition of serotonergic neurotransmission via stimulation of autoreceptors in the raphe nuclei and direct stimulation of 5-HT postsynaptic receptors may vary in different areas of the brain. Hence one could theoretically see some physiological or psychological effects associated with overall inhibition of serotonergic activity in one area of the brain and other effects related to enhancement of serotonergic neurotransmission in other brain areas with the same compound.

Compounds with affinity for $5-HT_{1A}$ receptors include both partial and full agonists. Mixed facilatory and inhibitory actions may also be related to the partial agonist (partial antagonist) nature of some of these compounds and be dose or concentration dependent (Söderpalm et al., 1989). Partial agonists have less intrinsic activity than full agonists. 5-HT_{1A} partial agonists act as net agonists or net antagonists depending on the amount of endogenous ligand present. Thus partial agonists may boost deficient 5-HT activity or decrease excessive 5-HT activity. Hence the net effect of 5-HT_{1A} partial agonists on 5-HT neurotransmission may not only be variable in different brain regions, but also be dependent on the underlying state of the 5-HT system. 5-HT_{1A} partial agonists appear to function as full agonists in the raphe nuclei and partial agonists (antagonists) in the hippocampus (Andrade and Nicoll, 1987; Dourish et al., 1986; Martin and Mason, 1987; Rowan and Anwyl, 1986; Sprouse and Aghajanian, 1988). The underlying mechanism and site of the anxiolytic actions for these compounds have not yet been definitively established. 5-HT_{1A} partial agonists could reduce anxiety by facilitating serotonergic inhibitory effects in the hippocampus via stimulation of postsynaptic receptors (in a 5-HT-deficient state) or by activating 5-HT autoreceptors and consequently decreasing 5-HT neurotransmission in the raphe nucleus (in a 5-HT-excess disease state).

To further complicate matters, since the anxiolytic effects of 5-HT_{1A} receptor agonists generally develop over a period of one to three weeks, chronic modulation of 5-HT receptors is probably necessary for their therapeutic activity. This suggests that acute receptor events may be only indirectly related to the therapeutic actions of these compounds. Indeed, acute administration of buspirone causes an increase in locus coeruleus activity (Sanghera et al., 1983), which is the opposite effect predicted by the locus coeruleus hypothesis of anxiety. Chronic administration of 5-HT_{1A} agonists causes desensitization of 5-HT_{1A} somatodendritic autoreceptors in the dorsal raphe nuclei (Blier and de Montigny, 1987) without affecting 5-HT_{1A} postsynaptic or terminal autoreceptor sensitivity (Godbout et al., 1991). This suggests that possible enhanced tonic activation of normosensitive 5-HT_{1A} postsynaptic receptors may occur with chronic treatment. There also appears to be possible downregulation of 5-HT_2 receptors associated with chronic 5-HT_{1A} agonist administration. Eison et al. reported a decreased sensitivity in cortical 5-HT_2 receptor sensitivity after continuous gepirone treatment (Eison and Yocca, 1985). Similarly, 5-HT_2 receptor density has been reported to be reduced after chronic treatment with tandospirone (Wieland et al., 1993). Another study failed to show any effect on 5-HT_2 mediated responses with subchronic treatment ($\times 21$ days) with ipsapirone (Baudrie et al., 1993). However, another study reported that gepirone treatment caused an initial enhancement of 5-HT_2 receptor-mediated behavior (at 3, 7 and 14 days) despite downregulation of 5-HT_2 receptor numbers. This was subsequently followed by a significant decrease in the same 5-HT_2-mediated behavioral response after 28 days of treatment (Yocca et al., 1991). Hence the duration of administration appears to be a significant factor. These studies suggest that secondary effects on other 5-HT receptor subtypes may also be involved in the therapeutic actions of 5-HT_{1A} agonists.

Numerous studies have demonstrated that 5-HT_{1A} partial agonists have activity in putative animal models predictive of anxiolytic activity. The highly selective 5-HT$_{1A}$ receptor agonist 8-hydroxy-2-(di-n-propylamino)tetralin (8-OH-DPAT) has demonstrated anticonflict activity in animal models (Engel et al., 1984; Shimizu et al., 1992a). Buspirone has also shown BZD-like activity in multiple animal models of anxiety (Amano et al., 1993; Higgins et al., 1988). Likewise, several other 5-HT$_{1A}$ agonists under investigation, including gepirone (Eison and Yocca, 1985), tandospirone (Shimizu et al., 1992a, 1992b), ipsapirone (Kaltwasser, 1991), BMY 7378 (Gleeson et al., 1989), E 4424 (Costall et al., 1992) and NDO 008 (Kostowski et al., 1992), have all shown possible anxiolytic potential based on studies utilizing animal models. Wy-47846 and Wy-48723, also 5-HT$_{1A}$ agonists, antagonized isolation-induced aggression suggesting possible non-sedating anxiolytic potential for these compounds as well (White et al., 1991). Eltoprazine, a mixed 5-HT$_{1A/B}$ agonist, has also been reported to reduce aggressive behavior in animal studies (Miczek et al., 1989; Olivier et al., 1989). However, these antiaggressive properties may be mediated via 5-HT$_{1B}$ receptors (Mos et al., 1992).

The 5-HT$_{1A}$ agonists vary both in their affinity for the 5-HT$_{1A}$ receptor and their agonist properties. Buspirone has high affinity, but only relative selectivity, for the 5-HT$_{1A}$ receptor (Peroutka, 1985). It also has both dopaminergic antagonistic and agonistic properties (Taylor et al., 1982; Temple et al., 1982). Although gepirone has less binding affinity than buspirone, it has greater agonist properties (Yocca, 1990). Gepirone and ipsapirone lack the direct dopaminergic properties of buspirone. In addition, the "anxiolytic" activity of buspirone, gepirone and ipsapirone in these animal models has been shown to be associated with their serotonergic properties (Carli et al., 1989; Eison et al., 1986; Fernández-Guasti and López-Rubalcava, 1990). E 4424, (2-(4-[4-(4-chloro-1-pyrazolyl)butyl]-1-piperazinyl)pyrimidine), has a greater antagonist/agonist ratio than either buspirone or ipsapirone (Costall et al., 1992). There is evidence to suggest that the "anxiolytic" response seen with the Vogel conflict model (punished responding) is mediated via stimulation of 5-HT$_{1A}$ postsynaptic receptors (Shimizu et al., 1992b).

However, while the 5-HT$_{1A}$ partial agonists produce "anxiolytic" effects in some animal conflict paradigms, they are inactive or "anxiogenic" in others. Sanger failed to find any anticonflict activity of buspirone in the Vogel conflict procedure (Sanger et al., 1984). Buspirone also failed to demonstrate BZD-like activity in conditioned defensive burying (Craft et al., 1988) and schedule-controlled behavior (Wettstein, 1988) tests. Ipsapirone failed to demonstrate any "anxiolytic" effects with either acute or chronic administration in the plus-maze model of anxiety (Wright et al., 1992). Hence animal model findings are inconsistent in predicting anxiolytic activity for these agents. One possible explanation for such inconsistencies, in addition to the reasons previously discussed, is that there is evidence to suggest that chronic treatment with 5-HT$_{1A}$ agonists may be necessary to achieve the full "anxiolytic" effect with some of the animal behavioral models utilized (Bodnoff et al., 1989; Schefke et al., 1989).

Buspirone, the only 5-HT_{1A} receptor partial agonist currently available in the USA, has undergone the most extensive clinical testing for the treatment of GAD. Several controlled clinical studies have found buspirone to be superior to placebo for GAD (Feighner and Cohn, 1989) and to have similar therapeutic efficacy compared to multiple BZDs, including diazepam (Cohn and Rickels, 1989; Pecknold et al., 1989), lorazepam (Petracca et al., 1990), oxazepam (Strand et al., 1990), clobazam (Böhm et al., 1990) and alprazolam (Enkelmann, 1991). Other 5-HT_{1A} agonists with evidence of clinical efficacy in GAD include gepirone (Csanalosi et al., 1987; Harto et al., 1988) and ipsapirone (Borison et al., 1990; Sramek et al., 1993). CGS-18102A, a mixed 5-HT_{1A} agonist and 5-HT_2 antagonist, is also currently undergoing clinical trials for the treatment of GAD. Enciprazine, a 5-HT_{1A} agonist and propanolamine derivative, which is chemically distinct from the azaspirones, has also undergone favorable preliminary clinical testing. In an open trial with a mixed group of anxious and anxious-depressed outpatients (Scheibe et al., 1990) and one double-blind placebo-controlled study for GAD (Schweizer et al., 1990), enciprazine was reported to be effective as an anxiolytic.

Multiple studies have shown that these 5-HT_{1A} receptor agonists are safe and well tolerated. The most common side effects appear to be gastrointestinal disturbances, headaches, dizziness, nervousness and lightheadedness (Borison et al., 1990; Enkelmann, 1991; Harto et al., 1988; Jann, 1988). Enciprazine was reported to have low levels of sedative and asthenic side effects (Schweizer et al., 1990). Long-term buspirone therapy also appears to be safe and effective (Feighner, 1987; Rakel, 1990). Furthermore, buspirone is well tolerated by elderly patients (Hart et al., 1991; Robinson et al., 1988). There is no evidence to suggest the potential for abuse or withdrawal reactions with these medications (Balster, 1990; Costall et al., 1992; Feighner and Boyer, 1989; Goldberg, 1984; Goudie and Leathley, 1991; Murphy et al., 1989; Rakel, 1990; Rickels et al., 1988; Sannerud et al., 1993; Schuckit, 1984). Interestingly, E 4424, but not buspirone, prevented the behavioral withdrawal syndrome associated with cocaine, alcohol, nicotine and diazepam discontinuation in one animal study (Costall et al., 1992). It is unknown whether this difference relates in any way to the previously mentioned differences in the antagonist/agonist ratio of these compounds.

5-HT_2 RECEPTOR ANTAGONISTS

5-HT_2 receptors may also be involved in the modulation of anxiety. These postsynaptic receptors are actually found in only low numbers in areas of dense 5-HT innervation (e.g., hippocampus). The highest numbers are found in the claustrum (where there are no 5-HT nerve terminals), olfactory tubercle and neocortex. This suggests that other endogenous substances unrelated to 5-HT may be active at this receptor or possibly that this receptor subtype is non-physiological and redundant. This does not imply that 5-HT_2 receptors can not be involved in the mediation of the anxiolytic effects of serotonergic medications. The high numbers of these receptors in the neocortex and its probable role in interpreting sensory stimuli from emotionally significant events such as those involving threat (Charney et al., 1990) suggest possible involvement of these receptors in the contribution of the neocortex to anxiety or fear. The indirect inhibitory effect of 5-HT on locus coeruleus firing also appears to be mediated by 5-HT$_2$ receptors (Gorea and Adrien, 1988; Rasmussen and Aghajanian, 1986). In addition, there is evidence to suggest that 5-HT$_2$ receptors may decrease the inhibitory and increase the excitatory effects produced by activation of 5-HT$_1$ receptors. In the prefrontal cortex, 5-HT$_2$ activation opposes the depressant effects of 5-HT on cell firing (Lakoski and Aghajanian, 1985). Therefore 5-HT$_2$ antagonists (or downregulation of these receptors via chronic administration of 5-HT$_{1A}$ agonists or TCAs) may potentiate the depressant effects of 5-HT on cell firing. However, some reports have failed to support any functional interaction between 5-HT$_{1A}$ and 5-HT$_2$ receptors (Li et al., 1992). Like the 5-HT$_{1A}$ agonists, chronic treatment with 5-HT$_2$ antagonists has also been reported to downregulate 5-HT$_2$ receptors (Leysen et al., 1986). 5-HT$_2$ receptor antagonists include ritanserin, ketanserin, serazepine and setoperone.

Some studies utilizing animal conflict models suggest possible "anxiolytic" activity for 5-HT$_2$ antagonists (Katz et al., 1993). Ketanserin and ritanserin, relatively selective 5-HT$_2$ receptor antagonists, have both been reported to increase the punished responding in rats (Gleeson et al., 1989; Stefanski et al., 1992). Ritanserin has also been reported to increase the entry ratio in the plus-maze model of anxiety (Critchley and Handley, 1987). However, as with other 5-HT-selective drugs, 5-HT$_2$ receptor antagonists do not show consistent "anxiolytic" effects in animal models of anxiety (Gardner, 1986). Similar to the 5-HT$_{1A}$ agonists, there may be a delayed onset of "anxiolytic" effects. In one study, chronic (×14 days), but not acute, administration of ritanserin resulted in a significant "anxiolytic" response in the plus-maze model (Wright et al., 1992).

5-HT$_2$ antagonists have undergone only limited clinical investigation as anxiolytics. One double-blind, placebo-controlled study of ritanserin found that 10 mg per day, but not 5 mg per day, was as effective as lorazepam (4 mg per day) in a study involving 83 patients with GAD (Ceulemans et al., 1985). Similarly, in another double-blind study with GAD patients, Bressa et al. reported ritanserin (20 mg per day) to be as effective as lorazepam (5 mg per day) (Bressa et al., 1987). Serazepine (CGS-15040A), a highly specific 5-HT$_2$ antagonist, also reportedly significantly reduced generalized anxiety in another double-blind, placebo-controlled clinical trial (Katz et al., 1993). Ritanserin has been reported to be safe and tolerable, with somnolence and fatigue being the most frequently reported side effects (Barone et al., 1986). Studies with ritanserin indicate little or no potential for tolerance development, withdrawal reactions or abuse (Idzikowski et al., 1987; Kamali et al., 1992). Further clinical investigation is needed to confirm and extend the preclinical and preliminary clinical studies suggesting possible anxiolytic actions for 5-HT$_2$ receptor antagonists.

5-HT$_3$ RECEPTOR ANTAGONISTS

5-HT$_3$ receptors are found in the brain (including the enthorinal cortex, amygdala, hippocampus and nucleus accumbens), as well as peripheral organs. This receptor subtype is a ligand-gated ion channel receptor, unlike other 5-HT receptor subtypes which are G protein-coupled. There is evidence to suggest that 5-HT$_3$ antagonists may block 5-HT-mediated inhibition of GABA release (Cloez-Tayarani *et al.*, 1992). 5-HT$_3$ antagonists may also prevent the 5-HT-mediated release of cholecystokinin (CCK), an "anxiogenic" neuropeptide (Raiteri *et al.*, 1993). Hence, 5-HT$_3$ antagonists could theoretically decrease anxiety by enhancing GABA-mediated anxiolytic effects or by blocking CCK-mediated "anxiogenic" influences in the CNS. A variety of 5-HT$_3$ antagonists have been developed, including ondansetron, granisetron, tropisetron, MDL 72222 and zacopride. Tropisetron has been shown to be a non-selective compound, exhibiting 5-HT$_4$ receptor antagonism at high concentrations. 5-HT$_3$ receptor antagonists have been used clinically as antiemetics for nausea associated with chemotherapy, for migraine and the carcinoid syndrome.

Some preclinical studies have suggested that drugs blocking 5-HT$_3$ receptors may have "anxiolytic" properties. 5-HT$_3$ receptor antagonists have been reported to stimulate a "return to normal behavior" in animals disturbed by exposure to aversive stimuli without reportedly modifying normal behavior (Costall and Naylor, 1992). The 5-HT$_3$ antagonists ondansetron (GR 38032F) and WAY 100289 reportedly demonstrated BZD-like responses in two animal models of anxiety: the mouse two-compartment light/dark box and the rat potentiated acoustic startle response paradigm (Bill *et al.*, 1992). In another study, ondansetron demonstrated BZD-like effects in all but one (the water lick conflict test in the rat) of several other animal behavioral models (Jones *et al.*, 1988). However, in other studies of 5-HT$_3$ antagonists, MDL 72222 failed to show "anxiolytic" properties in punished response tests, while results with ondansetron and tropisetron (ICS 205-930) were inconsistent (Gleeson *et al.*, 1989; Stefanski *et al.*, 1992). Mixed or negative results in other animal studies with 5-HT$_3$ antagonists have been reported for granisetron, zacopride, BRL 43964 and DAU 6215 (File and Johnston, 1989; Filip *et al.*, 1992). These mixed "BZD-like" results in animal models again suggest that 5-HT-selective drugs may act via different mechanisms than the BZDs and therefore not all BZD-based tests for "anxiolytic" activity are valid in predicting clinical efficacy for these drugs. As with other 5-HT-selective drugs, the duration of treatment may be the basis for some inconsistent results. Like ritanserin, only chronic administration of ondansetron resulted in "anxiolytic" effects in the plus-maze model of anxiety (Wright *et al.*, 1992). Furthermore, many of these compounds have exhibited U-shaped dose–response curves with reduce "anxiolytic" efficacy in animal models at very high doses. This is not found with the "second genera-tion" of 5-HT$_3$ antagonists such as GR 68755C and BRL 46470 (Costall and Naylor, 1992). Therefore the dosage utilized in each study may be an extremely important factor to consider in interpreting the results with some of these com-pounds.

Preliminary reports from clinical studies involving tropisetron, zacopride and ondansetron have all suggested anxiolytic efficacy accompanied by only a few side effects with no apparent rebound anxiety on discontinuation of treatment (Costall and Naylor, 1992). Clinical studies utilizing ondansetron as an antiemetic have also reported no significant adverse effects (Gandara et al., 1993; Green et al., 1989; Marty et al., 1989). The most common side effect appears to be headaches (Grunberg et al., 1993). There is no evidence to sug-gest the potential for tolerance development or withdrawal symptoms with ondansetron (Costall et al., 1989). Furthermore, some animal studies have sug-gested that ondansetron may help suppress the withdrawal symptoms associated with chronic BZD administration and therefore might be particularly useful for patients who have received prolonged BZD therapy (Costall et al., 1989; File and Andrews, 1993). However, conflicting evidence exists concerning ondansetron's potential efficacy in the treatment of BZD withdrawal (Prather et al., 1993). Further clinical studies using 5-HT$_3$ antagonists are needed to con-firm whether such compounds are effective for GAD and to determine their possible clinical efficacy in the suppression of BZD withdrawal symptoms.

5-HT-SELECTIVE REUPTAKE INHIBITORS

5-HT-selective reuptake inhibitors (SSRIs) (e.g., fluoxetine, paroxetine, sertra-line and fluvoxamine) are now widely used for the treatment of depression. Their possible clinical utility for the treatment of GAD has not yet been adequately studied. However, several factors suggest possible therapeutic roles for these agents in GAD. As mentioned previously, TCAs, with non-selective 5-HT reup-take inhibitory properties, have proven to be effective in treating GAD, but with a delayed onset of therapeutic activity. The anxiolytic properties of TCAs appear to be unrelated to their antidepressant actions (Kahn et al., 1987). Both TCAs and SSRIs may facilitate 5-HT neurotransmission acutely via reuptake blockade by increasing the concentration of 5-HT in the synaptic cleft and non-selectively stimulating 5-HT postsynaptic receptors. However, this effect may be lessened by the concurrent stimulation of 5-HT terminal autoreceptors and the associated decrease in 5-HT synthesis and release. Chronic administration of SSRIs has been shown to increase 5-HT neurotransmission and appears to occur secondary to desensitization of both the somatodendritic and terminal 5-HT autoreceptors (Chaput et al., 1986). Although chronic administration of TCAs may also increase 5-HT neurotransmission, it may be via a different mechanism. Chronic administration of TCAs downregulates 5-HT$_2$ receptors (Eison, 1990), while SSRIs have no effect on this receptor subtype. It is unknown whether such possible differences in the underlying mechanisms of action of these medications may result in selective efficacy for different illnesses or symptoms.

There has been only limited preclinical and clinical investigation of the anxiolytic potential of the SSRIs. Chronic, but not acute administration of fluoxetine has demonstrated "anxiolytic" properties similar to diazepam in an animal model utilizing novelty-suppressed feeding (Bodnoff et al., 1989). Acute administration of fluvoxamine and citalopram failed to demonstrate "anxiolytic" properties in the elevated plus-maze test (Durcan et al., 1988). One double-blind comparative clinical trial found fluvoxamine to be as effective as lorazepam in a group of patients with mixed anxiety and depression in a general practice setting (Laws et al., 1990). Another double-blind controlled study found paroxetine to be as effective as amitriptyline in the relief of symptoms of anxiety in a group of patients with depression and associated anxiety (Stahl and Aitken, 1993). While several studies have also demonstrated the efficacy of these drugs in obsessive-compulsive disorder (Goodman et al., 1992) and panic disorder (Den Boer and Westenberg, 1988; Gorman et al., 1987; Hoehn-Saric et al., 1993; Schneier et al., 1990; Westenberg and Den Boer, 1989), no known studies involving SSRIs for GAD have been published to date. Nefazodone, an analog of the antidepressant drug trazodone, recently recommended for approval by the FDA in the USA, blocks both presynaptic 5-HT reuptake and postsynaptic 5-HT$_2$ receptors. It is unknown whether this dual mechanism for possible enhancement of 5-HT neurotransmission might prove to be beneficial for patients with GAD.

The widespread usage of the relatively new SSRIs for depression stems in large part from their safety and side-effects profile. These medications lack most of the characteristic side effects of the non-selective TCAs. Potential side effects with these agents include decreased appetite, nausea, headache, dizziness, tremor, sweating, anxiety and sexual dysfunction. However, they are generally well tolerated. Controlled studies with SSRIs for GAD are definitely needed.

CONCLUSION

The findings reviewed above suggest that a variety of 5-HT selective drugs may have potential efficacy for patients with GAD. Much progress has recently been made in increasing our understanding of the complexities of the 5-HT neurotransmitter system. This has been facilitated by the associated development of increasingly selective and specific 5-HT receptor subtype agonists and antagonists. However, except for the azaspirones, controlled clinical studies with the 5-HT-selective drugs are insufficient at present to assess their true potential value as anxiolytics. Further refinement and improvement of the diagnostic criteria for GAD may serve to enhance such research. The side-effect profiles of the various 5-HT-selective drugs appear to make them useful alternatives to the

BZDs in the treatment of GAD. Although the majority of patients tolerate BZDs well and develop tolerance quickly to their sedative effects, significant cognitive and motor impairment sometimes goes unrecognized by clinicians. In addition, the low abuse potential and the absence of cross-tolerance with alcohol makes the 5-HT-selective drugs preferable to the BZDs as anxiolytics in the substance abuse patient population. The absence of withdrawal symptoms and any evidence suggesting the potential to develop tolerance to their therapeutic effects also gives these agents significant advantages over the BZDs for long-term maintenance. Although short-term therapy has often been advocated for anxiolytics, it appears that many GAD patients may require long-term therapy (Rickels, 1987). By the selective nature of their neurotransmitter interactions, the 5-HT-selective drugs generally have fewer side effects than the non-selective TCAs and MAOIs, which were the main alternatives to the BZDs for the treatment of anxiety prior to the arrival of buspirone.

5-HT$_{1A}$ partial agonists (e.g., buspirone) have proven efficacy for GAD and may have additional therapeutic benefits for patients with concurrent depressive features, alcohol abuse tendencies, suicidal ideation or impulse control problems (Glitz and Pohl, 1991). These drugs could also be useful in conditions complicated by serious physical illnesses such as AIDS (Batki, 1990). Given the high comorbidity of depression associated with GAD, 5-HT-selective drugs may be especially useful given the possible antidepressant properties of not only the SSRIs, but also the 5-HT$_{1A}$ agonists and 5-HT$_2$ antagonists (Amsterdam, 1992; Bressa et al., 1987; Heller et al., 1990; Hingtgen et al., 1985; Jenkins et al., 1990; Rausch et al., 1990; Robinson et al., 1989). For patients with mixed anxiety and depression, 5-HT-selective drugs may also be preferable because depression is a potential side effect associated with the BZDs (Sramek et al., 1993). Preclinical and preliminary clinical observations also suggest potential therapeutic application for 5-HT$_3$ receptor antagonists in an even wider range of emotional disturbances, including schizophrenia, age-related memory impairment and drug withdrawal syndromes (Costall and Naylor, 1992; Higgins et al., 1991).

Given all of the above and the ongoing widespread usage of the BZDs, it appears that buspirone may be currently underutilized in the treatment of GAD. One possible reason for this is its delayed therapeutic response, in comparison to the rapid relief achievable with the BZDs. However, this distinct disadvantage, which may be true of the other types of 5-HT-selective drugs with anxiolytic potential as well, is also the case with the SSRIs, which have rapidly gained popularity in the treatment of depression, obsessive-compulsive disorder and to a lesser extent panic disorder. This suggests that there may be ongoing clinical skepticism concerning the efficacy of buspirone. Past experience with the BZDs may make both patients and clinicians potentially biased and lead to early disappointment and premature abandonment of buspirone trials. This would suggest the need to further educate both patients and clinicians alike concerning the anticipated delay in achieving therapeutic effects, absence of the immediate calming effects typical of the BZDs and the importance of completing adequate medication trials in both duration and dosage. To achieve rapid relief of GAD symptoms, a combined pharmacotherapeutic strategy may prove beneficial for some patients. Patients could be started on both an azaspirone and a BZD initially, then tapered off the BZD once stabilized so that they are maintained on the azaspirone alone for long-term maintenance. Similar combined drug therapy is frequently utilized employing both BZDs and antidepressants initially in the treatment of panic attacks. Another explanation for the relatively limited usage of buspirone for GAD is the possibility that it may not be as effective in actual practice as previous research studies have suggested. Outcome studies in clinical practice settings evaluating both adequacy of medication trials and efficacy would help clarify these issues. In addition, the ongoing controversy concerning this diagnostic category and high comorbidity rates may also have impacted on the prescribing practices of clinicians.

Further preclinical studies are also needed to better identify which putative animal models are the most reliable predictors of anxiolytic activity for non-BZD medications, including 5-HT-selective drugs. Due to the possible delayed clinical response of these drugs, such investigations need to evaluate for the putative "anxiolytic" response with both acute and chronic administration of these drugs.

Finally, clinical studies of serotonergic function in patients with GAD are needed to advance our understanding of the underlying pathophysiology of this disorder. Such studies (e.g., behavioral and neuroendocrine responses to 5-HT precursors and agonists) are needed to further explore hypotheses concerning the underlying serotonergic state (e.g., 5-HT excess or deficiency) and possible hypersensitivity of postsynaptic 5-HT receptors (Kahn et al., 1988b) in GAD. In addition, studies of both the acute and chronic effects of 5-HT-selective drugs on 5-HT function are needed to further elucidate their underlying mechanisms of action. Investigations utilizing even more selective and specific 5-HT agonists and antagonists (as these become available) may also help to identify such mechanisms of action as well as further clarify the possible interactions between the different 5-HT receptor subtypes and their involvement in the etiology and modulation of anxiety.

REFERENCES

Amano, M., Goto, A., Sakai, A. et al. (1993). Comparison of the anticonflict effect of buspirone and its major metabolite 1-(2-pyrimidinyl)-piperazine (1-PP) in rats. Jpn. J. Pharmacol., 61(4), 311–317.

American Psychiatric Association (1980). Diagnostic and Statistical Manual of Mental Disorders, 3rd edn. American Psychiatric Association, Washington, DC.

American Psychiatric Association (1987). Diagnostic and Statistical Manual of Mental Disorders, 3rd edn, revised. American Psychiatric Association, Washington, DC.

American Psychiatric Association (1994). Diagnostic and Statistical Manual of Mental Disorders, 4th edn. American Psychiatric Association, Washington, DC.

Amsterdam, J. D. (1992). Gepirone, a selective serotonin (5HT1A) partial agonist in the treatment of major depression. Prog. Neuropsychopharmacol. Biol. Psychiatry, 16(3), 271–280.

Andrade, R. and Nicoll, R. A. (1987). Novel anxiolytics discriminate between postsynaptic serotonin receptors mediating different physiological responses on single neurons of the rat hippocampus. *Naunyn Schmiedebergs Arch. Pharmacol.*, **336**(1), 5–10.

Aprison, M. H. and Hingtgen, J. N. (1972). Serotonin and behavior: a brief summary. *Fed. Proc.*, **31**(1), 121–129.

Balster, R. L. (1990). Abuse potential of buspirone and related drugs. *J. Clin. Psychopharmacol.*, **10**, 31S–37S.

Barlow, D. H., Blanchard, E. B., Vermilyea, J. A. *et al.* (1986). Generalized anxiety and generalized anxiety disorder: description and reconceptualization. *Am. J. Psychiatry*, **143**, 40–44.

Barone, J. A., Bierman, R. H., Cornish, J. W. *et al.* (1986). Safety evaluation of ritanserin: an investigational serotonin antagonist. *Drug. Intell. Clin. Pharm.*, **20**(10), 770–775.

Batki, S. L. (1990). Buspirone in drug users with AIDS or AIDS-related complex. *J. Clin. Psychopharmacol.*, **10**, 111S–115S.

Baudrie, V., De Vry, J., Broqua, P. *et al.* (1993). Subchronic treatment with anxiolytic doses of the 5-HT1A receptor agonist ipsapirone does not affect 5-HT2 receptor sensitivity in the rat. *Eur. J. Pharmacol.*, **231**(3), 395–406.

Bill, D. J., Fletcher, A., Glenn, B. D. and Knight, M. (1992). Behavioural studies on WAY100289, a novel 5-HT3 receptor antagonist, in two animal models of anxiety. *Eur. J. Pharmacol.*, **218**(2–3), 327–334.

Blier, P. and de Montigny, C. (1987). Modification of 5-HT neuron properties by sustained administration of the 5-HT1A agonist gepirone: electrophysiological studies in the rat brain. *Synapse*, **1**(5), 470–480.

Bodnoff, S. R., Suranyi-Cadotte, B., Quirion, R. and Meaney, M. J. (1989). A comparison of the effects of diazepam versus several typical and atypical anti-depressant drugs in an animal model of anxiety. *Psychopharmacology*, **97**(2), 277–279.

Böhm, C., Placchi, M., Stallone, F. *et al.* (1990). A double-blind comparison of buspirone, clobazam, and placebo in patients with anxiety treated in a general practice setting. *J. Clin. Psychopharmacol.*, **10**(3 Suppl.), 38S–42S.

Borison, R. L., Albrecht, J. W. and Diamond, B. I. (1990). Efficacy and safety of a putative anxiolytic agent: ipsapirone. *Psychopharmacol. Bull.*, **26**(2), 207–210.

Bradley, P. B., Engel, G., Feniuk, W. *et al.* (1986). Proposals for the classification and nomenclature of functional receptors for 5-hydroxytryptamine. *Neuropharmacology*, **25**(6), 563–576.

Brawman-Mintzer, O., Lydiard, R. B., Emmanuel, N. *et al.* (1993). Psychiatric comorbidity in patients with generalized anxiety disorder. *Am. J. Psychiatry*, **150**, 1216–1218.

Bressa, G. M., Marini, S. and Gregori, S. (1987). Serotonin S2 receptors blockage and generalized anxiety disorders: a double-blind study on ritanserin and lorazepam. *Int. J. Clin. Pharmacol. Res.*, **7**(2), 111–119.

Brody, J. F., Jr (1970). Behavioral effects of serotonin depletion and of p-chlorophenylalanine (a serotonin depletor) in rats. *Psychopharmacologia*, **17**, 14–33.

Cameron, O. G., Thyer, B. A., Nesse, R. M. and Curtis, G. C. (1986). Symptom profiles of patients with DSM-III anxiety disorders. *Am. J. Psychiatry*, **143**, 1132–1137.

Carli, M., Prontera, C. and Samanin, R. (1989). Evidence that central 5-hydroxytryptaminergic neurones are involved in the anxiolytic activity of buspirone, *Br. J. Pharmacol.*, **96**(4), 829–836.

Ceulemans, D. L., Hoppenbrouwers, M. L., Gelders, Y. G. and Reyntjens, A. J. (1985). The influence of ritanserin, a serotonin antagonist, in anxiety disorders: a double-blind placebo-controlled study versus lorazepam, *Pharmacopsychiatry*, **18**(5), 303–305.

Chaput, Y., de Montigny, C. and Blier, P. (1986). Effects of a selective 5-HT reuptake blocker, citalopram, on the sensitivity of 5-HT autoreceptors: electrophysiological studies in the rat brain. *Naunyn Schmiedebergs Arch. Pharmacol.*, **333**, 342–345.

Charney, D. S., Woods, S. W., Goodman, W. K. and Heninger, G. R. (1987). Serotonin function in anxiety. II. Effects of the serotonin agonist MCPP in panic disorder patients and healthy subjects. *Psychopharmacology*, **92**, 14–24.

Charney, D. S., Woods, S. W., Krystal, J. H. and Heninger, G. R. (1990). Serotonin function and human anxiety disorders. *Ann. NY Acad. Sci.*, **600**, 558–572.

Chase, T. N., Katz, R. I. and Kopin, I. J. (1970). Effect of diazepam on fate of intracisternally injected serotonin C14. *Neuropharmacology*, **9**, 103–108.

Chouinard, G., Annable, L., Fontaine, R. and Solyom, L. (1982). Alprazolam in the treatment of generalized anxiety and panic disorders: a double-blind placebo-controlled study. *Psychopharmacology*, **77**, 229–233.

Cloez-Tayarani, I., Harel-Dupas, C. and Fillion, G. (1992). Inhibition of [3H] gamma-aminobutyric acid release from guinea-pig hippocampal synaptosomes by serotonergic agents. *Fundam. Clin. Pharmacol.*, **6**(8–9), 333–341.

Cloninger, C. R., Martin, R. L., Guze, S. B. and Clayton, P. J. (1990). The empirical structure of psychiatric comorbidity and its theoretical significance. In *Comorbidity of Mood and Anxiety Disorders* (eds J. D. Maser and C. R. Cloninger), pp. 439–462. American Psychiatric Press, Washington, DC.

Cohn, J. B. and Rickels, K. (1989). A pooled, double-blind comparison of the effects of buspirone, diazepam and placebo in women with chronic anxiety. *Curr. Med. Res. Opin.*, **11**(5), 304–320.

Collinge, J. and Pycock, C. (1982). Differential actions of diazepam on the release of [³H]-5-hydroxytryptamine from cortical and midbrain raphe slices in the rat. *Eur. J. Pharmacol.*, **85**, 9–14.

Commissaris, R. L. and Rech, R. H. (1982). Interactions of metergoline with diazepam, quipazine, and hallucinogenic drugs on a conflict behavior in the rat. *Psychopharmacology*, **76**, 282–285.

Costall, B. and Naylor, R. J. (1992). Astra Award Lecture. The psychopharmacology of 5-HT$_3$ receptors. *Pharmacol. Toxicol.*, **71**(6), 401–415.

Costall, B., Jones, B. J., Kelly, M. E. *et al.* (1989). The effects of ondansetron (GR38032F) in rats and mice treated subchronically with diazepam. *Pharmacol. Biochem. Behav.*, **34**(4), 769–778.

Costall, B., Domeney, A. M., Farre, A. J. *et al.* (1992). Profile of action of a novel 5-hydroxytryptamine1A receptor ligand E-4424 to inhibit aversive behavior in the mouse, rat and marmoset. *J. Pharmacol. Exp. Ther.*, **262**(1), 90–98.

Craft, R. M., Howard, J. L. and Pollard, G. T. (1988). Conditioned defensive burying as a model for identifying anxiolytics. *Pharmacol. Biochem. Behav.*, **30**(3), 775–780.

Critchley, M. A. and Handley, S. L. (1987). Effects in the X-maze anxiety model of agents acting at 5-HT1 and 5-HT2 receptors. *Psychopharmacology*, **93**(4), 502–506.

Csanalosi, I., Schweizer, E., Case, W. G. and Rickels, K. (1987). Gepirone in anxiety: a pilot study. *J. Clin. Psychopharmacol.*, **7**(1), 31–33.

Den Boer, J. A. and Westenberg, G. M. (1988). Effect of a serotonin and noradrenaline uptake inhibitor in panic disorder: a double-blind comparative study with flovoxamine and maprotiline. *Int. Clin. Psychopharmacol.*, **3**, 59–74.

Den Boer, J. A., Westenberg, H. K., Kamerbeek, W. D. *et al.* (1987). Effects of serotonin uptake inhibitors in anxiety disorders: a double-blind comparison of clomipramine and fluvoxamine. *Int. Clin. Psychopharmacol.*, **2**, 21–32.

Dominic, J. A., Sinha, A. K. and Barchas, J. D. (1975). Effect of benzodiazepine compounds on brain amine metabolism. *Eur. J. Pharmacol.*, **32**, 124–127.

Dourish, C. T., Hutson, P. H. and Curzon, G. (1986). Putative anxiolytics 8-OH-DPAT, buspirone and TVX Q 7821 are agonists at 5-HT$_{1A}$ autoreceptors in the raphé nuclei. *Trends Pharmacol. Sci.*, **7**, 212–214.

Dunner, D. L., Ishiki, I., Avery, D. H. *et al.* (1986). Effects of alprazolam and diazepam on anxiety and panic attacks in panic disorder: a controlled study. *J. Clin. Psychiatry*, **47**, 458–460.

Durcan, M. J., Lister, R. G., Eckardt, M. J. and Linnoila, M. (1988). Behavioral interactions of fluoxetine and other 5-hydroxytryptamine uptake inhibitors with ethanol in tests of anxiety, locomotion and exploration. *Psychopharmacology*, **96**(4), 528–533.

Eison, A. S. and Yocca, F. D. (1985). Reduction in cortical 5HT$_2$ receptor sensitivity after continuous gepirone treatment. *Eur. J. Pharmacol.*, **111**, 389–392.

Eison, A. S., Eison, M. S., Stanley, M. and Riblet. L. A. (1986). Serotonergic mechanisms in the behavioral effects of buspirone and gepirone. *Pharmacol. Biochem. Behav.*, **24**(3), 701–707.

Eison, M. S. (1990). Serotonin: a common neurobiologic substrate in anxiety and depression. *J. Clin. Psychopharmacol.*, **10**(3 Suppl.), 26S–30S.

Engel, J. A., Hjorth, S., Svensson, K. *et al.* (1984). Anticonflict effect of the putative serotonin receptor agonist 8-hydroxy-2-(di-n-propylamino)tetralin (8-OH-DPAT). *Eur. J. Pharmacol.*, **105**, 365–368.

Enkelmann, R. (1991). Alprazolam versus buspirone in the treatment of outpatients with generalized anxiety disorder. *Psychopharmacology*, **105**(3), 428–432.

Eriksson, E. and Humble, M. (1990). Serotonin in psychiatric pathophysiology: a review of data from experimental and clinical research. In *Progress in Basic and Clinical Pharmacology: The Biological Basis of Psychiatric Treatment* (eds R. Pohl and S. Gershon), pp. 66–119. Karger AG, Basel.

Feighner, J. P. (1987). Buspirone in the long-term treatment of generalized anxiety disorder. *J. Clin. Psychiatry*, **48**, 3–6.

Feighner, J. P. and Boyer, W. F. (1989). Serotonin-1A anxiolytics: an overview. *Psychopathology*, **1**, 21–26.

Feighner, J. P. and Cohn, J. B. (1989). Analysis of individual symptoms in generalized anxiety: a pooled, multistudy, double-blind evaluation of buspirone. *Neuropsychobiology*, **21**(3), 124–130.

Fernández-Guasti, A. and López-Rubalcava, C. (1990). Evidence for the involvement of the 5-HT1A receptor in the anxiolytic action of indorenate and ipsapirone. *Psychopharmacology*, **101**(3), 354–358.

File, S. E. and Andrews, N. (1993). Enhanced anxiolytic effect of zacopride enantiomers in diazepam-withdrawn rats. *Eur. J. Pharmacol.*, **237**(1), 127–130.

File, S. E. and Johnston, A. L. (1989). Lack of effects of 5HT3 receptor antagonists in the social interaction and elevated plus-maze tests of anxiety in the rat. *Psychopharmacology*, **99**(2), 248–251.

Filip, M., Baran, L., Siwanowicz, J. *et al.* (1992). The anxiolytic-like effects of 5-hydroxytryptamine3 (5-HT3) receptor antagonists. *Pol. J. Pharmacol. Pharm.*, **44**(3), 261–269.

Gandara, D. R., Harvey, W. H., Monaghan, G. G. *et al.* (1993). Delayed emesis following high-dose cisplatin: a double-blind randomised comparative trial of ondansetron (GR 38032F) versus placebo. *Eur. J. Cancer*, **1**(8), S35–S38.

Gardner, C. R. (1986). Recent developments in 5HT-related pharmacology of animal models of anxiety. *Pharmacol. Biochem. Behav.*, **24**, 1479–1485.

Geller, I. and Blum, K. (1970). The effects of 5-HTP on para-chlorophenylalanine (*p*-CPA) attentuation of "conflict" behavior. *Eur. J. Pharmacol.*, **9**, 319–324.

Geller, I., Hartmann, R. J., Croy, D. J. and Haber, B. (1974). Attenuation of conflict behavior with cinanserin, a serotonin antagonist: reversal of the effect with 5-hydroxytryptophan and α-methyltryptamine. *Res. Commun. Chem. Pathol. Pharmacol.*, **7**(1), 165–174.

Gillespie, D. D., Manier, D. H., Sanders-Bush, E. and Sulser, F. (1988). The serotonin/norepinephrine-link in brain. II. Role of serotonin in the regulation of beta adrenoceptors in the low agonist affinity conformation. *J. Pharmacol. Exp. Ther.*, **244**(1), 154–159.

Gleeson, S., Ahlers, S. T., Mansbach, R. S. *et al.* (1989). Behavioral studies with anxiolytic drugs. VI. Effects on punished responding of drugs interacting with serotonin receptor subtypes. *J. Pharmacol. Exp. Ther.*, **250**(3), 809–817.

Glitz, D. A. and Pohl, R. (1991). 5-HT1A partial agonists: what is their future? *Drugs*, **41**(1), 11–18.

Godbout, R., Chaput, Y., Blier, P. and de Montigny, C. (1991). Tandospirone and its metabolite, 1-(2-pyrimidinyl)-piperazine. I. Effects of acute and long-term administration of tandospirone on serotonin neurotransmission. *Neuropharmacology*, **30**(7), 679–690.

Goldberg, H. L. (1984). Buspirone hydrochloride: a unique new anxiolytic agent. Pharmacokinetics, clinical pharmacology, abuse potential and clinical efficacy. *Pharmacotherapy*, **4**(6), 315–324.

Goodman, W. K., McDougle, C. J. and Price, L. H. (1992). Pharmacotherapy of obsessive compulsive disorder. *J. Clin. Psychiatry*, **53**, 29–37.

Gorea, E. and Adrien, J. (1988). Serotonergic regulation of noradrenergic coerulean neurons: electrophysiological evidence for the involvement of 5-HT$_2$ receptors. *Eur. J. Pharmacol.*, **154**, 285–291.

Gorman, J. M., Liebowitz, M. R., Fyer, A. J. *et al.* (1987). An open trial of fluoxetine in the treatment of panic attacks. *J. Clin. Psychopharmacol.*, **7**(5), 329–332.

Goudie, A. J. and Leathley, M. J. (1991). Evaluation of the dependence potential of the selective 5-H1A agonist ipsapirone in rats and of its effects on benzodiazepine withdrawal. *Psychopharmacology*, **103**(4), 529–537.

Green, J. A., Watkin, S. W., Hammond, P. *et al.* (1989). The efficacy and safety of GR38032F in the prophylaxis of ifosfamide-induced nausea and vomiting. *Cancer Chemother. Pharmacol.*, **24**(2), 137–139.

Grunberg, S. M., Lane, M., Lester, E. P. *et al.* (1993). Randomized double-blind comparison of three dose levels of intravenous ondansetron in the prevention of cisplatin-induced emesis. *Cancer Chemother. Pharmacol.*, **32**(4), 268–272.

Hart, R. P., Colenda, C. C. and Hamer, R. M. (1991). Effects of buspirone and alprazolam on the cognitive performance of normal elderly subjects. *Am. J. Psychiatry*, **148**(1), 73–77.

Harto, N. E., Branconnier, R. J., Spera, K. F. and Dessain, E. C. (1988). Clinical profile of gepirone, a nonbenzodiazepine anxiolytic. *Psychopharmacol. Bull.*, **24**(1), 154–160.

Heller, A. H., Beneke, M., Kuemmel, B. *et al.* (1990). Ipsapirone: evidence for efficacy in depression. *Psychopharmacol. Bull.*, **26**(2), 219–222.

Higgins, G. A., Bradbury, A. J., Jones, B. J. and Oakley, N. R. (1988). Behavioural and biochemical consequences following activation of 5HT1-like and GABA receptors in the dorsal raphe nucleus of the rat. *Neuropharmacology*, **27**(10), 993–1001.

Higgins, G. A., Nguyen, P., Joharchi, N. and Sellers, E. M. (1991). Effects of 5-HT3 receptor antagonists on behavioural measures of naloxone-precipitated opioid withdrawal. *Psychopharmacology*, **105**(3), 322–328.

Hingtgen, J. N., Fuller, R. W., Mason. N. R. and Aprison, M. H. (1985). Blockade of a 5-hydroxytryptophan-induced animal model of depression with a potent and selective 5-HT2 receptor antagonist (LY53857). *Biol. Psychiatry*, **20**(6), 592–597.

Hjorth, S. and Magnusson, T. (1988). The 5-HT$_{1A}$ receptor agonist, 8-OH-DPAT, preferentially activates cell body 5-HT autoreceptors in rat brain in vivo. *Naunyn Schmiedebergs Arch. Pharmacol.*, **338**, 463–471.

Hoehn-Saric, R., McLeod, D. R. and Hipsley, P. A. (1993). Effect of fluvoxamine on panic disorder. *J. Clin. Psychopharmacol.*, **13**(5), 321–326.

Idzikowski, C., Cowen, P. J., Nutt, D. and Mills, F. J. (1987). The effects of chronic ritanserin treatment on sleep and the neuroendocrine response to L-tryptophan. *Psychopharmacology*, **93**(4), 416–420.

Jann, M. W. (1988). Buspirone: an update on a unique anxiolytic agent. *Pharmacotherapy*, **8**(2), 100–116.

Jenkins, S. W., Robinson, D. S., Fabre, L., Jr *et al.*(1990). Gepirone in the treatment of major depression. *J. Clin. Psychopharmacol.*, **10**(3 Suppl.), 77S–85S.

Johnston, A. L. and File, S. E. (1986). 5-HT and anxiety: promises and pitfalls. *Pharmacol. Biochem. Behav.*, **24**, 1467–1470.

Jones, B. J., Costall, B., Domeney, A. M. *et al.* (1988). The potential anxiolytic activity of GR38032F, a 5-HT3-receptor antagonist. *Br. J. Pharmacol.*, **93**(4), 985–993.

Kahn, R. S. and Westenberg, H. G. (1985). L-5-Hydroxytryptophan in the treatment of anxiety disorders. *J. Affect. Disord.* **8**(2), 197–200.

Kahn, R. J., McNair, D. M., and Frankenthaler, L. M. (1987). Tricyclic treatment of general-ized anxiety disorder. *J. Affect. Disord.*, **13**(2), 145–151.

Kahn, R. S., Asnis, G. M., Wetzler, S. and van Praag, H. M. (1988a). Neuroendocrine evi-dence for serotonin receptor hypersensitivity in panic disorder. *Psychopharmacology*, **96**, 360–364.

Kahn, R. S., van Praag, H. M., Wetzler, S. *et al.* (1988b). Serotonin and anxiety revisited. *Biol. Psychiatry*, **23**, 189–208.

Kaltwasser, M. T. (1991). Acoustic startle induced ultrasonic vocalization in the rat: a novel animal model of anxiety? *Behav. Brain Res.*, **43**(2), 133–137.

Kamali, F., Stansfield, S. C., Ashton, C. H. *et al.* (1992). Absence of withdrawal effects of ritanserin following chronic dosing in healthy volunteers. *Psychopharmacology*, **108**(1–2), 213–217.

Katz, R. J., Landau, P. S., Lott, M. *et al.* (1993). Serotonergic (5-HT2) mediation of anxiety: therapeutic effects of serazepine in generalized anxiety disorder. *Biol. Psychiatry*, **34**, 41–44.

Kilts, C. D., Commissaris, R. L., Cordon, J. J. and Rech, R. H. (1982). Lack of central 5-hydroxytryptamine influence on the anticonflict activity of diazepam. *Psychopharmacology*, **78**, 156–164.

Klein, D. F. (1964). Delineation of two drug-responsive anxiety syndromes. *Psychopharmacologia*, **5**, 397–408.

Klein, D. F. (1980). Anxiety reconceptualized. *Compr. Psychiatry*, **21**, 411–427.

Kostowski, W., Dyr, W., Krzascik, P. *et al.* (1992). 5-Hydroxytryptamine 1A receptor ago-nists in animal models of depression and anxiety. *Pharmacol. Toxicol.*, **71**(1), 24–30.

Lakoski, J. M. and Aghajanian, G. K. (1985). Effects of ketanserin on neuronal responses to serotonin in the prefrontal cortex, lateral geniculate and dorsal raphe nucleus. *Neuropharmacology*, **24**(4), 265–273.

Laurent, J. P., Mangold, M., Humbel, U. and Haefely, W. (1983). Reduction by two benzodi-azepines and pentobarbitone of the multiunit activity in substantia nigra, hippocampus, nucleus locus coeruleus, and nucleus dorsal raphé dorsalis of *encéphale isolé* rats. *Neuropharmacology*, **22**(4), 501–511.

Laws, D., Ashford, J. S. and Austee, J. A. (1990). A multicenter double-blind comparative study of fluvoxamine versus lorazepam in mixed anxiety and depression treated in gener-al practice. *Arch. Gen. Psychiatry*, **81**, 185–189.

Leysen, J. E., Van Gompel, P., Gommeren, W. *et al.* (1986). Down regulation of serotonin-S2 receptor sites in rat brain by chronic treatment with the serotonin-S2 antagonists: ritanserin and setoperone. *Psychopharmacology*, **88**(4), 434–444.

Li, Q., Rittenhouse, P. A., Levy, A. D. *et al.* (1992). Neuroendocrine responses to the sero-tonin2 agonist DOI are differentially modified by three 5-HT1A agonists. *Neuropharmacology*, **31**(10), 983–989.

López-Rubalcava, C., Saldívar, A. and Fernández-Guasti, A. (1992). Interaction of GABA and serotonin in the anxiolytic action of diazepam and serotonergic anxiolytics. *Pharmacol. Biochem. Behav.* **43**(2), 433–440.

Martin, K. F. and Mason, R. (1987). Ipsapirone is a partial agonist at 5-hydroxytryptamine 1A (5-HT1A) receptors in the rat hippocampus: electrophysiological evidence. *Eur. J. Pharmacol.*, **141**(3), 479–483.

Marty, M., Droz, J. P., Pouillart, P. *et al.* (1989). GR38032F, a 5HT3 receptor antagonist, in the prophylaxis of acute cisplatin-induced nausea and vomiting. *Cancer Chemother. Pharmacol.*, **23**(6), 389–391.

Mendels, J. and Frazer, A. (1974). Brain biogenic amine depletion and mood. *Arch. Gen. Psychiatry*, **30**, 447–451.

Merikangas, K. R. (1990). Comorbidity for anxiety and depression: review of family and genetic studies. In *Comorbidity of Mood and Anxiety Disorders* (eds J. D. Maser and C. R. Cloninger), pp. 331–348. American Psychiatric Press, Washington, DC.

Miczek, K. A., Mos, J. and Olivier, B. (1989). Brain 5-HT and inhibition of aggressive behavior in animals: 5-HIAA and receptor subtypes. *Psychopharmacol. Bull.*, **25**(3), 399–403.

Monferini, E., Gaetani, P., Rodriguez y Baena, R. *et al.* (1993). Pharmacological characterization of the 5-hydroxytryptamine receptor coupled to adenylyl cyclase stimulation in human brain. *Life Sci.*, **52**(9), L61–L65.

Mos, J., Olivier, B., Poth, M. and van Aken, H. (1992). The effects of intraventricular administration of eltoprazine, 1-(3-trifluoromethylphenyl)piperazine hydrochloride and 8-hydroxy-2-(di-n-propylamino)tetralin on resident intruder aggression in the rat. *Eur. J. Pharmacol.*, **212**(2–3), 295–298.

Murphy, D. L., Pato, M. T. and Pigott, T. A. (1990). Obsessive-compulsive disorder: treatment with serotonin-selective uptake inhibitors, azapirones, and other agents. *J. Clin. Psychopharmacol.*, **10**(3 Suppl.), 91S–100S.

Murphy, S. M., Owen, R. and Tyrer, P. (1989). Comparative assessment of efficacy and withdrawal symptoms after 6 and 12 weeks' treatment with diazepam or buspirone. *Br. J. Psychiatry*, **154**, 529–534.

Olivier, B., Mos, J., van der Heyden, J. and Hartog, J. (1989). Serotonergic modulation of social interactions in isolated male mice. *Psychopharmacology*, **97**(2), 154–156.

Ortiz, A., Pohl, R. and Gershon, S. (1987). Azaspirodecanediones in generalized anxiety disorder: buspirone. *J. Affect. Disord.*, **13**(2), 131–143.

Pazos, A., Probst, A. and Palacios, J. M. (1987). Serotonin receptors in the human brain: III. Autoradiographic mapping of serotonin-1 receptors *Neuroscience,* **21**(1), 97–122.

Pecknold, J. C., Matas, M., Howarth, B. G. *et al.* (1989). Evaluation of buspirone as an antianxiety agent: buspirone and diazepam versus placebo, *Can. J. Psychiatry,* **34**(8), 766–771.

Peroutka, S. J. (1985). Selective interaction of novel anxiolytics with 5-hydroxytryptamine1A receptors. *Biol. Psychiatry,* **20**(9), 971–979.

Peroutka, S. J. and Snyder, S. H. (1979). Multiple serotonin receptors: differential binding of [^{3}H]5-hydroxytryptamine, [^{3}H]lysergic acid diethylamide, and [^{3}H]spiroperidol. *Mol. Pharmacol.*, **16**, 687–699.

Petracca, A., Nisita, C., McNair, D. *et al.* (1990). Treatment of generalized anxiety disorder: preliminary clinical experience with buspirone. *J. Clin. Psychiatry*, **51**, 31–39.

Prather, P. L., Rezazadeh, S. M., Lane, J. D. *et al.* (1993). Conflicting evidence regarding the efficacy of ondansetron in benzodiazepine withdrawal. *J. Pharmacol. Exp. Ther.*, **264**(2), 622–630.

Pratt, J., Jenner, P., Reynolds, E. H. and Marsden, C. D. (1979). Clonazepam induces decreased serotonergic activity in the mouse brain. *Neuropharmacology*, **18**, 791–799.

Pratt, J. A., Jenner, P. and Marsden, C. D. (1985). Comparison of the effects of benzodiazepines and other anticonvulsant drugs on synthesis and utilization of 5-HT in mouse brain. *Neuropharmacology*, **24**, 59–68.

Raiteri, M., Paudice, P. and Vallebuona, F. (1993). Inhibition by 5-HT$_3$ receptor antagonists of release of cholecystokinin-like immunoreactivity from the frontal cortex of freely moving rats. *Naunyn Schmiedebergs Arch. Pharmacol.*, **347**(1), 111–114.

Rakel, R. E. (1990). Long-term buspirone therapy for chronic anxiety: a multicenter international study to determine safety. *South. Med. J.*, **83**(2), 194–198.

Rasmussen, K. and Aghajanian, G. K. (1986). Effect of hallucinogens on spontaneous and sensory-evoked locus coeruleus unit activity in the rat: reversal by selective 5-HT$_2$ antagonists. *Brain Res.*, **385**(2), 395–400.

Rausch, J. L., Ruegg, R. and Moeller, F. G. (1990). Gepirone as a 5-HT1A agonist in the treatment of major depression. *Psychopharmacol. Bull.*, **26**(2), 169–171.

Rickels, K. (1987). Antianxiety therapy: potential value of long-term treatment. *J. Clin. Psychiatry*, **48**, 7–11.

Rickels, K. and Schweizer, E. (1993). The treatment of generalized anxiety disorder in patients with depressive symptomatology. *J. Clin. Psychiatry*, **54**, 20–23.

Rickels, K., Schweizer, E., Csanalosi, I. *et al.* (1988). Long-term treatment of anxiety and risk of withdrawal: prospective comparison of clorazepate and buspirone. *Arch. Gen. Psychiatry*, **45**(5), 444–450.

Robinson, D., Napoliello, M. J. and Schenk, J. (1988). The safety and usefulness of buspirone as an anxiolytic drug in elderly versus young patients. *Clin. Ther.*, **10**(6), 740–746.

Robinson, D. S., Alms, D. R., Shrotriya, R. C. *et al.* (1989). Serotonergic anxiolytics and treatment of depression. *Psychopathology*, **1**, 27–36.

Rowan, M. J. and Anwyl, R. (1986). Neurophysiological effects of buspirone and ipsapirone in the hippocampus: comparison with 5-hydroxytryptamine. *Eur. J. Pharmacol.*, **132**(1), 93–96.

Sanger, D. J., Joly, D. and Zivkovic, B. (1984). Behavioral effects of nonbenzodiazepine anxiolytic drugs: a comparison of CGS 9896 and zopiclone with chlordiazepoxide. *J. Pharmacol. Exp. Ther.*, **232**(3), 831–837.

Sanghera, M. K., McMillen, B. A. and German, D. C. (1983). Buspirone, a non-benzodiazepine anxiolytic, increases locus coeruleus noradrenergic neuronal activity. *Eur. J. Pharmacol.*, **86**, 107–110.

Sannerud, C. A., Ator, N. A. and Griffiths, R. R. (1993). Behavioral pharmacology of tandospirone in baboons: chronic administration and withdrawal, self-injection and drug discrimination. *Drug Alcohol Depend.*, **32**(3), 195–208.

Schefke, D. M., Fontana, D. J. and Commissaris, R. L. (1989). Anti-conflict efficacy of buspirone following acute versus chronic treatment. *Psychopharmacology*, **99**(3), 427–429.

Scheibe, G., Grohmann, R. and Buchheim, P. (1990). Pilot study on the therapeutic efficacy, clinical safety, and dosage finding of enciprazine in out-patients with anxious and anxious-depressive syndromes. *Arzneimittelforschung*, **40**(6), 644–646.

Schneier, F. R., Liebowitz, M. R., Davies, S. O. *et al.* (1990). Fluoxetine in panic disorder. *J. Clin. Psychopharmacol.*, **10**(2), 119–121.

Schuckit, M. A. (1984). Clinical studies of buspirone. *Psychopathology*, **3**, 61–68.

Schweizer, E., Rickels, K., Csanalosi, I. *et al.* (1990). A placebo-controlled study of enciprazine in the treatment of generalized anxiety disorder: a preliminary report. *Psychopharmacol. Bull.*, **26**(2), 215–217.

Sharp, T., Bramwell, S. R. and Grahame-Smith, D. G. (1989). 5-HT1 agonists reduce 5-hydroxytryptamine release in rat hippocampus in vivo as determined by brain microdialysis. *Br. J. Pharmacol.*, **96**(2), 283–290.

Shimizu, H., Kumasaka, Y., Tanaka, H. *et al.* (1992a). Anticonflict action of tandospirone in a modified Geller–Seifter conflict test in rats. *Jpn. J. Pharmacol.*, **58**(3), 283–289.

Shimizu, H., Tatsuno, T., Tanaka, H. *et al.* (1992b). Serotonergic mechanisms in anxiolytic effect of tandospirone in the Vogel conflict test. *Jpn. J. Pharmacol.*, **59**(1), 105–112.

Söderpalm, B., Hjorth, S. and Engel, J. A. (1989). Effects of 5-HT$_{1A}$ receptor agonists and L-5-HTP in Montgomery's conflict test. *Pharmacol. Biochem. Behav.*, **32**, 259–265.

Soubrie, P. (1986). [Serotonergic neurons and behavior] (English abstract only). *J. Pharmacol.*, **17**(2), 107–112.

Sprouse, J. S. and Aghajanian, G. K. (1988). Responses of hippocampal pyramidal cells to putative serotonin 5-HT$_{1A}$ and 5-HT$_{1B}$ agonists: a comparative study with dorsal raphe neurons. *Neuropharmacology*, **27**(7), 707–715.

Sramek, J. J., Cutler, N. R., Costa, J. F. *et al.* (1993). Depression in the course of treatment of generalized anxiety disorder with lorazepam, ipsapirone, and placebo: results from a multicenter trial. *Depression*, **1**, 172–176.

Stahl, P. C. and Aitken, C. A. (1993). A double-blind comparison of paroxetine and amitriptyline in community patients with depression and associated anxiety. 146th American Psychiatric Association Annual Meeting, unpublished poster, San Francisco, May 22–27.

Stefanski, R., Palejko, W., Kostowski, W. and Plaznik, A. (1992). The comparison of benzodiazepine derivatives and serotonergic agonists and antagonists in two animal models of anxiety. *Neuropharmacology*, **31**(12), 1251–1258.

Strand, M., Hetta, J., Rosen, A. *et al.* (1990). A double-blind, controlled trial in primary care patients with generalized anxiety: a comparison between buspirone and oxazepam. *J. Clin. Psychiatry*, **51**, 40–45.

Task Force on DSM-IV (1991). *DSM-IV Options Book*. American Psychiatric Association, Washington, DC.

Task Force on DSM-IV (1993). *DSM-IV Draft Criteria*. American Psychiatric Association, Washington, DC.

Taylor, D. P., Riblet, L. A., Stanton, H. C. *et al.* (1982). Dopamine and antianxiety activity. *Pharmacol. Biochem. Behav.*, **1**, 25–35.

Temple, D. L., Jr, Yevich, J. P. and New, J. S. (1982). Buspirone: chemical profile of a new class of anxioselective agents. *J. Clin. Psychiatry*, **43**(12 Pt 2), 4–10.

Tompkins, E. C., Clemento, A. J., Taylor, D. P. and Perhach, J. L., Jr (1980). Inhibition of aggressive behaviour in rhesus monkeys by buspirone. *Res. Commun. Psychol. Psychiatr. Behav.*, **5**(4), 337–352.

Trulson, M. E., Preussler, D. W., Howell, G. A. and Frederickson, C. J. (1982). Raphe unit activity in freely moving cats: effects of benzodiazepines. *Neuropharmacology*, **21**, 1045–1050.

Tye, N. C., Everitt, B. J. and Iversen, S. D. (1977). 5-Hydroxytryptamine and punishment. *Nature*, **268**, 741–743.

Verge, D., Daval, G., Patey, A. *et al.* (1985). Presynaptic 5-HT autoreceptors on serotonergic cell bodies and/or dendrites but not terminals are of the $5-HT_{1A}$ subtype. *Eur. J. Pharmacol.*, **113**, 463–464.

Wang, W. H. and Lovick, T. A. (1992). Inhibitory serotonergic effects on rostral ventrolateral medullary neurons. *Pflugers Arch.*, **422**(2), 93–97.

Weissman, M. M. (1990). Evidence for comorbidity of anxiety and depression: family and genetic studies. In *Comorbidity of Mood and Anxiety Disorders* (eds J. D. Maser and C. R. Cloninger), pp. 349–365. American Psychiatric Press, Washington, DC.

Westenberg, H. G. and Den Boer, J. A. (1989). Serotonin-influencing drugs in the treatment of panic disorder. *Psychopathology*, **1**, 68–77.

Wettstein, J. G. (1988). Behavioral effects of acute and chronic buspirone. *Eur. J. Pharmacol.*, **151**(2), 341–344.

White, S. M., Kucharik, R. F. and Moyer, J. A. (1991). Effects of serotonergic agents on isolation-induced aggression. *Pharmacol. Biochem. Behav.*, **39**(3), 729–736.

Wieland, S., Fischette, C. T. and Lucki, I. (1993). Effect of chronic treatments with tandospirone and imipramine on serotonin-mediated behavioral responses and monoamine receptors. *Neuropharmacology*, **32**(6), 561–573.

Wise, C. D., Berger, B. D. and Stein, L. (1972). Benzodiazepines: anxiety-reducing activity by reduction of serotonin turnover in the brain. *Science*, **177**, 180–183.

Wright, I. K., Heaton, M., Upton, N. and Marsden, C. A. (1992). Comparison of acute and chronic treatment of various serotonergic agents with those of diazepam and idazoxan in the rat elevated X-maze. *Psychopharmacology*, **107**(2–3), 405–414.

Yocca, F. D. (1990). Neurochemistry and neurophysiology of buspirone and gepirone: interactions at presynaptic and postsynaptic 5-HT1A receptors. *J. Clin. Psychopharmacol.*, **10**(3 Suppl.). 6S–12S.

Yocca, F. D., Eison, A. S., Hyslop, D. K. *et al.* (1991). Unique modulation of central 5-HT2 receptor binding sites and 5-HT2 receptor-mediated behavior by continuous gepirone treatment. *Life Sci.*, **49**(24), 1777–1785.

Part V

POST-TRAUMATIC
STRESS DISORDER

16 The Body Keeps the Score: The Evolving Psychobiology of Post-traumatic Stress

BESSEL A. VAN DER KOLK

Trauma Clinic, Harvard Medical School, Boston, Massachusetts, USA

BACKGROUND

For more than a century, ever since people's responses to overwhelming experiences were first systematically explored, it has been noted that the psychological effects of trauma are stored in somatic memory and expressed as changes in the biological stress response. In 1889, Pierre Janet postulated that intense emotional reactions make events traumatic by interfering with the integration of the experience into existing memory schemes. Intense emotions, Janet thought, cause memories of particular events to be dissociated from consciousness, and to be stored, instead, as visceral sensations (anxiety and panic), or as visual images (nightmares and flashbacks). Janet also observed that traumatized patients seemed to react to reminders of the trauma with emergency responses that had been relevant to the original threat, but that had no bearing on current experience. He noted that victims had trouble learning from experience: unable to put the trauma behind them, their energies were absorbed by keeping their emotions under control at the expense of paying attention to current exigencies. They became fixated to the past, in some cases by being obsessed with the trauma, but more often by behaving and feeling like they were traumatized over and over again without being able to locate the origins of these feelings (van der Kolk and van der Hart, 1989, 1991).

Freud also thought that the tendency to stay fixated on the trauma is biologically based: "After severe shock . . . the dream life continually takes the patient back to the situation of his disaster from which he awakens with renewed terror . . . the patient has undergone a physical fixation to the trauma" (Freud, 1919/1954). Pavlov's investigations continued the tradition of explaining the effects of trauma as the result of lasting physiological alterations. He, and others employing his paradigm, coined the term "defensive reaction" for a cluster of innate reflexive responses to environmental threat (Pavlov, 1926). Many studies

Advances in the Neurobiology of Anxiety Disorders. Edited by H. G. M. Westenberg, J. A. Den Boer and D. L. Murphy
©1996 John Wiley & Sons Ltd

have shown how the response to potent environmental stimuli (unconditional stimuli, US) becomes a conditioned reaction. After repeated aversive stimulation, intrinsically non-threatening cues associated with the trauma (conditional stimuli, CS) become capable of eliciting the defensive reaction by themselves (conditional response, CR). A rape victim may respond to conditioned stimuli, such as the approach by an unknown man, as if she were about to be raped again, and experience panic. Pavlov also pointed out that individual differences in temperament accounted for the diversity of long-term adaptations to trauma.

Abraham Kardiner (1941), who first systematically defined post-traumatic stress for American audiences, noted that sufferers from "traumatic neuroses" develop an enduring vigilance for and sensitivity to environmental threat, and stated that "the nucleus of the neurosis is a physioneurosis. This is present on the battlefield and during the entire process of organization; it outlives every intermediary accommodative device, and persists in the chronic forms. The traumatic syndrome is ever present and unchanged". In *Men under Stress*, Grinker and Spiegel (1945) catalog the physical symptoms of soldiers in acute post-traumatic states: flexor changes in posture, hyperkinesis, "violently propulsive gait", tremor at rest, mask-like facies, cogwheel rigidity, gastric distress, urinary incontinence, mutism, and a violent startle reflex. They noted the similarity between many of these symptoms and those of diseases of the extrapyramidal motor system. Today we can understand them as the result of stimulation of biological systems, particularly of ascending amine projections. Contemporary research on the biology of PTSD, generally uninformed by this earlier research, confirms that there are persistent and profound alterations in stress hormones secretion and memory processing in people with post-traumatic stress disorder (PTSD).

THE SYMPTOMATOLOGY OF PTSD

Starting with Kardiner (1941), and closely followed by Lindemann (1944), a vast literature on combat trauma, crimes, rape, kidnapping, natural disasters, accidents and imprisonment have shown that the trauma response is biphasic: hypermnesia, hyperreactivity to stimuli and traumatic re-experiencing coexist with psychic numbing, avoidance, amnesia and anhedonia (American Psychiatric Association, 1987, 1993; Horowitz, 1978; van der Kolk, 1987a). These responses to extreme experiences are so consistent across traumatic stimuli that this biphasic reaction appears to be the normative response to any overwhelming and uncontrollable experience. In many people who have undergone severe stress, the post-traumatic response fades over time, while it persists in others. Much work remains to be done to spell out issues of resilience and vulnerability, but magnitude of exposure, prior trauma, and social support appear to be the three most significant predictors for developing chronic PTSD (Kulka *et al.*, 1990; McFarlane, 1988).

In an apparent attempt to compensate for chronic hyperarousal, traumatized people seem to shut down: on a behavioral level, by avoiding stimuli reminiscent of the trauma; on a psychobiological level, by emotional numbing, which extends to both trauma-related, and everyday experience (Litz and Keane, 1989). Thus, people with chronic PTSD tend to suffer from numbing of responsiveness to the environment, punctuated by intermittent hyperarousal in response to conditional traumatic stimuli. However, as Pitman has pointed out (Pitman *et al.*, 1983), in PTSD, the stimuli that precipitate emergency responses may not be conditional enough: many triggers not directly related to the traumatic experience may precipitate extreme reactions. Thus, people with PTSD suffer both from generalized hyperarousal and from physiological emergency reactions to specific reminders (American Psychiatric Association, 1987, 1993).

The loss of affective modulation that is so central in PTSD may help explain the observation that traumatized people lose the capacity to utilize affect states as signals (Krystal, 1978). Instead of using feelings as cues to attend to incoming information, in people with PTSD arousal is likely to precipitate flight or fight reactions (Strian and Klicpera, 1978). Thus, they are prone to go immediately from stimulus to response without making the necessary psychological assessment of the meaning of what is going on. This makes them prone to freeze, or, alternatively, to overreact and intimidate others in response to minor provocations (van der Kolk, 1987a; van der Kolk and Ducey, 1989).

PSYCHOPHYSIOLOGY

Abnormal psychophysiological responses in PTSD have been demonstrated on two different levels: (1) in response to specific reminders of the trauma and (2) in response to intense, but neutral stimuli, such as acoustic startle. The first paradigm implies heightened physiological arousal to sounds, images, and thoughts related to specific traumatic incidents. A large number of studies have confirmed that traumatized individuals respond to such stimuli with significant conditioned autonomic reactions, such as heart rate, skin conductance and blood pressure (van der Kolk and Ducey, 1989; Dobbs and Wilson, 1960; Malloy *et al.*, 1983; Kolb and Multipassi, 1982; Blanchard *et al.*, 1986; Pitman *et al.*, 1987). The highly elevated physiological responses that accompany the recall of traumatic experiences that happened years, and sometimes decades before, illustrate the intensity and timelessness with which traumatic memories continue to affect current experience (van der Kolk and van der Hart, 1991; Pitman *et al.*, 1993). This phenomenon has generally been understood in the light of Peter Lang's work (Lang, 1979), which shows that emotionally laden imagery correlates with measurable autonomic responses. Lang has proposed that emotional memories are stored as "associative networks," which are activated when a person is confronted with situations that stimulate a sufficient number of elements that make up these networks. One significant measure of treatment outcome that has become widely accepted in recent years is a decrease in physiological arousal in response to imagery related to the trauma

(Keane and Kaloupek, 1982). However, Shalev et al. (1992a) have shown that desensitization to specific trauma-related mental images does not necessarily generalize to recollections of other traumatic events, as well.

Kolb (1987) was the first to propose that excessive stimulation of the central nervous system (CNS) at the time of the trauma may result in permanent neuronal changes that have a negative effect on learning, habituation, and stimulus discrimination. These neuronal changes would not depend on actual exposure to reminders of the trauma for expression. The abnormal startle response characteristic of PTSD (American Psychiatric Association, 1993) is a paradigm of such neuronal changes. Despite the fact that an abnormal acoustic startle response (ASR) has been seen as a cardinal feature of the trauma response for over half a century, systematic explorations of the ASR in PTSD have just begun. The ASR consists of a characteristic sequence of muscular and autonomic responses elicited by sudden and intense stimuli (Shalev and Rogel-Fuchs, 1993; Davis, 1984). The neuronal pathways involved consist of only a small number of mediating synapses between the receptor and effector and a large projection to brain areas responsible for CNS activation and stimulus evaluation (Davis, 1984). The ASR is mediated by excitatory amino acids such as glutamate and aspartate and is modulated by a variety of neurotransmitters and second messengers at both the spinal and supraspinal level (Davis, 1986). Habituation of the ASR in normals occurs after three to five presentations (Shalev and Rogel-Fuchs, 1993).

Several studies have demonstrated abnormalities in habituation to the ASR in PTSD (Shalev et al., 1993; Ornitz and Pynoos, 1989; Butler et al., 1990; Ross et al., 1989). Shalev et al. (1993) found a failure to habituate both to CNS and ANS-mediated responses to ASR in 93% of the PTSD group, compared with 22% of the control subjects. Interestingly, people who previously met criteria for PTSD, but no longer do so now, continue to show failure of habituation of the ASR (van der Kolk et al., unpublished data; Pitman et al., unpublished data), which raises the question whether abnormal habituation to acoustic startle is a marker of, or a vulnerability factor for, developing PTSD.

The failure to habituate to acoustic startle suggests that traumatized people have difficulty evaluating sensory stimuli, and mobilizing appropriate levels of physiological arousal (Shalev and Rogel-Fuchs, 1993). Thus, the inability of people with PTSD to properly integrate memories of the trauma and, instead, to get mired in a continuous reliving of the past, is mirrored physiologically in the misinterpretation of innocuous stimuli, such as the ASR, as potential threats.

THE HORMONAL STRESS RESPONSE AND THE PSYCHOBIOLOGY OF PTSD

Post-traumatic stress develops following exposure to events that are intensely distressing. Intense stress is accompanied by the release of endogenous, stress-responsive neurohormones, such as cortisol, epinephrine and norepinephrine

(NE), vasopressin, oxytocin and endogenous opioids. These stress hormones help the organism mobilize the required energy to deal with the stress, ranging from increased glucose release to enhanced immune function. In a well-functioning organism, stress produces rapid and pronounced hormonal responses. However, chronic and persistent stress inhibits the effectiveness of the stress response and induces desensitization (Axelrod and Neisine, 1984).

Much still remains to be learned about the specific roles of the different neurohormones in the stress response. NE is secreted by the locus coeruleus (LC) and distributed through much of the CNS, particularly the neocortex and the limbic system, where it plays a role in memory consolidation and helps initiate fight/flight behaviors. Adrenocorticotropin (ACTH) is released from the anterior pituitary, and activates a cascade of reactions, eventuating in release of glucocorticoids from the adrenals. The precise interrelation between hypothalamic–pituitary–adrenal (HPA) axis hormones and the catecholamines in the stress response is not entirely clear, but it is known that stressors that activate NE neurons also increase corticotropin-releasing factor (CRF) concentrations in the LC (Dunn and Berridge, 1987), while intracerebral ventricular infusion of CRF increases NE in the forebrain (Valentino and Foote, 1988). Glucocorticoids and catecholamines may modulate each other's effects: in acute stress, cortisol helps regulate stress hormone release via a negative feedback loop to the hippocampus, hypothalamus and pituitary (Munck et al., 1984) and there is evidence that corticosteroids normalize catecholamine-induced arousal in limbic midbrain structures in response to stress (Bohus and DeWied, 1978). Thus, the simultaneous activation of corticosteroids and catecholamines could stimulate active coping behaviors, while increased arousal in the presence of low glucocorticoid levels may promote undifferentiated fight or flight reactions (Yehuda et al., 1990).

While acute stress activates the HPA axis and increases glucocorticoid levels, organisms adapt to chronic stress by activating a negative feedback loop that results in (1) decreased resting glucocorticoid levels in chronically stressed organisms (Meaney et al., 1989) (2) decreased glucocorticoid secretion in response to subsequent stress (Yehuda et al., 1990) and (3) increased concentration of glucocorticoid receptors in the hippocampus (Sapolsky et al., 1984). Yehuda has suggested that increased concentration of glucocorticoid receptors could facilitate a stronger glucocorticoid negative feedback, resulting in a more sensitive HPA axis and a faster recovery from acute stress (Yehuda et al., 1991a).

Chronic exposure to stress affects both acute and chronic adaptation: it permanently alters how an organism deals with its environment on a day-to-day basis, and it interferes with how it copes with subsequent acute stress (Yehuda et al., 1991a).

NEUROENDOCRINE ABNORMALITIES IN PTSD

Since PTSD appears to involve a persistent activation of the biological stress response upon exposure to stimuli reminiscent of the trauma, research has focused on applying the lessons learned from the effects of chronic and severe stress on the biology of other species to people with PTSD (van der Kolk *et al.*, 1985; Krystal *et al.*, 1989).

CATECHOLAMINES

Neuroendocrine studies of Vietnam veterans with PTSD have found good evidence for chronically increased sympathetic nervous system activity in PTSD. One study (Kosten *et al.*, 1987) found elevated 24 h excretions of urinary NE and epinephrine in PTSD combat veterans compared with patients with other psychiatric diagnoses. While Pitman and Orr (1990b) did not replicate these findings in 20 veterans and 15 combat controls, the mean urinary NE excretion values in their combat controls (58.0 μg per day) were substantially higher than those previously reported in normal populations. The expected compensatory downregulation of adrenergic receptors in response to increased levels of NE was confirmed by a study that found decreased platelet α_2-adrenergic receptors in combat veterans with PTSD, compared with normal controls (Perry *et al.*, 1987). Another study also found an abnormally low α_2-adrenergic receptor-mediated adenylate cyclase signal transduction (Lerer *et al.*, 1987). In a recent study Southwick *et al.* (1993) used yohimbine injections (0.4 mg/kg), which activate noradrenergic neurons by blocking the α_2-autoreceptor, to study noradrenergic neuronal dysregulation in Vietnam veterans with PTSD. Yohimbine precipitated panic attacks in 70% of subjects and flashbacks in 40%. Subjects responded with larger increases in plasma 3-methoxy-4-hydroxyphenethylene-glycol (MHPG) than controls. Yohimbine precipitated significant increases in all PTSD symptoms.

CORTICOSTEROIDS

Two studies have shown that veterans with PTSD have low urinary cortisol excretion, even when they have comorbid major depressive disorder (Yehuda *et al.*, 1990; Mason *et al.*, 1988). One study failed to replicate this finding (Pitman and Orr, 1990b). In a series of studies, Yehuda *et al.* (1990, 1991b) found increased numbers of lymphocyte glucocorticoid receptors in Vietnam veterans with PTSD. Interestingly, the number of glucocorticoid receptors was proportional to the severity of PTSD symptoms. Yehuda *et al.* (1991b) has also reported the results of an unpublished study by Heidi Resnick, in which acute cortisol response to trauma was studied from blood samples from 20 acute rape victims. Three months later, a prior trauma history was taken, and the subjects were evaluated for the presence of PTSD. Victims with a prior history of sexual abuse were significantly more likely to have developed PTSD three months following the rape than rape victims who did not develop PTSD. Cortisol levels shortly after the rape were correlated with histories of prior assaults: the mean initial cortisol level of individuals with a prior assault history was 15 μg/dl compared to 30 μg/dl in individuals without. These findings can be interpreted to mean either that prior exposure to traumatic events result in a blunted cortisol response to subsequent trauma, or in a quicker return of cortisol to baseline following stress. The fact that Yehuda *et al.* (1991a) also found subjects with PTSD to be hyperresponsive to low doses of dexamethasone argues for an enhanced sensitivity of the HPA feedback in traumatized patients.

SEROTONIN

While the role of serotonin (5-HT) in PTSD has not been systematically investigated, both the fact that inescapably shocked animals develop decreased CNS 5-HT levels (Valzelli, 1982) and that 5-HT reuptake blockers are effective pharmacological agents in the treatment of PTSD, justify a brief consideration of the potential role of this neurotransmitter in PTSD. Decreased 5-HT in humans has repeatedly been correlated with impulsivity and aggression (Brown *et al.*, 1979; Mann, 1987; Coccaro *et al.*, 1989). The literature tends to readily assume that these relationships are based on genetic traits. However, studies of impulsive, aggressive and suicidal patients seem to find at least as robust an association between those behaviors and histories of childhood trauma (Green, 1978; van der Kolk *et al.*, 1991; Lewis, 1992). It is likely that both temperament and experience affect relative CNS 5-HT levels (van der Kolk, 1987a).

Low 5-HT in animals is also related to an inability to modulate arousal, as exemplified by an exaggerated startle (Gerson and Baldessarini, 1980; Dupue and Spoont, 1989), and increased arousal in response to novel stimuli, handling, or pain (Dupue and Spoont, 1989). The behavioral effects of 5-HT depletion on animals is characterized by hyperirritability, hyperexcitability, and hypersensitivity, and an "exaggerated emotional arousal and/or aggressive display, to relatively mild stimuli" (Dupue and Spoont, 1989). These behaviors bear a striking resemblance to the phenomenology of PTSD in humans. Finally, 5-HT abnormalities are thought to be central in obsessive thinking. 5-HT reuptake inhibitors have been found to be the most effective pharmacological treatment of both obsessive thinking in people with obsessive-compulsive disorder (OCD) (Jenike *et al.*, 1990), and of obsessive preoccupation with traumatic memories in people with PTSD (van der Kolk *et al.*, 1993; van der Kolk and Saporta, 1991).

ENDOGENOUS OPIOIDS

Stress-induced analgesia (SIA) has been described in experimental animals following a variety of inescapable stressors such as electric shock, fighting, starvation and cold-water swim (Akil *et al.*, 1983). In severely stressed animals, opiate withdrawal symptoms can be produced both by termination of the stressful stimulus or by naloxone injections. Stimulated by the findings that fear activates the secretion of endogenous opioid peptides, and that SIA can become conditioned to subsequent stressors and to previously neutral events associated with the noxious stimulus, we tested the hypothesis that in people with PTSD re-exposure to a stimulus resembling the original trauma will cause an endogenous opioid response that can be indirectly measured as naloxone-reversible analgesia (van der Kolk *et al.*, 1989; Pitman *et al.*, 1990). We found that two decades after the original trauma, people with PTSD developed opioid-mediated analgesia in response to a stimulus resembling the traumatic stressor, which we correlated with a secretion of endogenous opioids equivalent to 8 mg of morphine. Self-reports of emotional responses suggested that endogenous opioids were responsible for a relative blunting of the emotional response to the traumatic stimulus.

PAIN, NUMBING, AND DISSOCIATION

When young animals are isolated, and older ones attacked, they respond initially with aggression (hyperarousal–fight–protest), and, if that does not produce the required results, with withdrawal (numbing–flight–despair). Fear-induced attack or protest patterns in the young serve to attract protection, and in mature animals to prevent or counteract the predator's activity. During external attacks pain inhibition is a useful defensive capacity, because attention to pain would interfere with effective defense: grooming or licking wounds would attract the opponent and stimulate further attack (Siegfried *et al.*, 1990). Thus defensive and pain-motivated behaviors are mutually inhibitory. Stress-induced analgesia protects organisms against feeling pain while engaged in defensive activities. As early as 1949, Beecher (1946), after observing that wounded soldiers required less morphine, speculated that "strong emotions can block pain." Today, we can reasonably assume that this is due to the release of endogenous opioids (van der Kolk *et al.*, 1989; Pitman *et al.*, 1990).

Endogenous opioids, which inhibit pain and reduce panic, are secreted after prolonged exposure to severe stress. Siegfried *et al.* (1990) have observed that memory is impaired in animals when they can no longer actively influence the outcome of a threatening situation. They showed that both the freeze response and panic interfere with effective memory processing: excessive endogenous opioids and NE both interfere with the storage of experience in explicit memory. Freeze/numbing responses may serve the function of allowing organisms to not "consciously experience" or to remember situations of overwhelming stress (and which thus will also keep them from learning from experience). We have proposed that the dissociative reactions in people in response to trauma may be analogous to this complex of behaviors that occur in animals after prolonged exposure to severe uncontrollable stress (van der Kolk *et al.*, 1989).

DEVELOPMENTAL LEVEL AFFECTS THE PSYCHOBIOLOGICAL EFFECTS OF TRAUMA

While most studies on PTSD have been done on adults, particularly on war veterans, in recent years a small prospective literature is emerging that documents the differential effects of trauma at various age levels. Anxiety disorders, chronic hyperarousal, and behavioral disturbances have been described with some regularity in traumatized children (Bowlby, 1969; Cicchetti, 1985; Terr, 1991). In addition to the reactions to discrete, one-time, traumatic incidents documented in these studies, intrafamilial abuse is increasingly recognized to produce complex post-traumatic syndromes (Cole and Putnam, 1991). This recognition opens up the boundaries between the current concept of PTSD and a spectrum of trauma-related disorders (van der Kolk *et al.*, 1988; Herman, 1992), which has started to be explored in the Field Trials for DSM-IV under the rubric of Disorders of Extreme Stress (van der Kolk *et al.*, 1992).

While current research on traumatized children is outside the scope of this review, it is important to recognize that a range of neurobiological abnormalities are beginning to be identified in this population. Research in the last decade has shown that many children who have been victims of intrafamilial abuse have chronic problems with affect modulation, ranging from extremes in hyper-reactivity to psychic numbing (Green, 1978; Lewis, 1992; Cicchetti, 1985; van der Kolk *et al.*, 1992). Frank Putnam's prospective, but as yet unpublished, studies are showing major neuroendocrine disturbances in sexually abused girls compared with normals. Research on the psychobiology of childhood trauma can be profitably informed by the vast literature on the psychobiological effects of trauma and deprivation in non-human primates (van der Kolk, 1987a; Reite and Fields, 1985).

TRAUMA AND MEMORY

THE FLEXIBILITY OF MEMORY AND THE ENGRAVING OF TRAUMA

One hundred years ago, Pierre Janet (1889) suggested that the most fundamental of mental activities is the storage and categorization of incoming sensations into memory, and the retrieval of those memories under appropriate circumstances. He, like contemporary memory researchers, understood that memory is an active and constructive process and that remembering depends on existing mental schemata (Freud, 1919/1954; Calvin, 1990). In general, once an event or a particular bit of information is integrated into existing mental schemes, it will no longer be accessible as a separate, immutable entity, but be distorted both by prior experience, and by the emotional state at the time of recall (Freud, 1919/1954). Trauma, per definition, is accompanied by memory disturbances, consisting of both hypermnesias and amnesias (American Psychiatric Association, 1987, 1993). There is now enough information available about the biology of memory storage and retrieval to start building coherent hypotheses regarding the underlying psychobiological processes involved in these memory disturbances (Freud, 1919/1954; Pitman and Orr, 1990a; Pitman *et al.*, 1987, 1993).

In the beginning of this century Janet already noted that: "certain happenings . . . leave indelible and distressing memories—memories to which the sufferer continually returns, and by which he is tormented by day and by night" (Janet, 1919/1925). Clinicians and researchers dealing with traumatized patients have repeatedly made the observation that the sensory experiences and visual images related to the trauma seem not to fade over time, and appear to be less subject to distortion than ordinary experiences (Janet, 1889; Pitman and Orr, 1990b; van der Kolk *et al.*, 1984). When people are traumatized, they are said to experience "speechless terror": the emotional impact of the event may interfere with the capacity to capture the experience in words or symbols. Piaget (1962) thought that under such circumstances failure of semantic memory leads to the organization of memory on a somatosensory or iconic level (such as somatic sensations, behavioral enactments, nightmares and flashbacks). He pointed out: "It is precisely because there is no immediate accommodation that there is complete dissociation of the inner activity from the external world. As the external world is solely represented by images, it is assimilated without resistance (i.e. unattached to other memories) to the unconscious ego."

TRAUMATIC MEMORIES ARE STATE DEPENDENT

Research has shown that, under ordinary conditions, many traumatized people, including rape victims (Kilpatrick *et al.*, 1985), battered women (Hilberman and Munson, 1978) and abused children (Green, 1980) have a fairly good psychosocial adjustment. However, they do not respond to stress the way other people do. Under pressure, they may feel or act as if they were traumatized all over again. Thus, high states of arousal seem to selectively promote retrieval of traumatic memories, sensory information, or behaviors associated with prior traumatic experiences (American Psychiatric Association, 1987, 1993). The tendency of traumatized organisms to revert to irrelevant emergency behaviors in response to minor stress has been well documented in animals, as well. Studies at the Wisconsin primate laboratory have shown that rhesus monkeys with histories of severe early maternal deprivation display marked withdrawal or aggression in response to emotional or physical stimuli (such as exposure to loud noises, or the administration of amphetamines), even after a long period of good social adjustment (Kraemer, 1985). In experiments in mice, Mitchell and his colleagues (1985) found that the relative degree of arousal interacts with prior exposure to high stress to determine how an animal will react to novel stimuli. In a state of low arousal, animals tend to be curious and seek novelty. During high arousal, they are frightened, avoid novelty, and perseverate in familiar behavior, regardless of the outcome. Under ordinary circumstances, an animal will choose the most pleasant of two alternatives. When hyperaroused, it will seek whatever is familiar, regardless of the intrinsic rewards. Thus, animals who have been locked in a box in which they were exposed to electric shocks and then released return to those boxes when they are subsequently stressed.

Mitchell concluded that this perseveration is non-associative, i.e. uncoupled from the usual reward systems.

In people, analogous phenomena have been documented: memories (somatic or symbolic) related to the trauma are elicited by heightened arousal (Solomon *et al.*, 1985). Information acquired in an aroused or otherwise altered state of mind is retrieved more readily when people are brought back to that particular state of mind (Phillips and LePiane, 1980; Rawlins, 1980). State-dependent memory retrieval may also be involved in dissociative phenomena in which traumatized persons may be wholly or partially amnestic for memories or behaviors enacted while in altered states of mind (van der Kolk and van der Hart, 1989, 1991; Putnam, 1989).

Contemporary biological researchers have shown that medications that stimulate autonomic arousal may precipitate visual images and affect states associated with prior traumatic experiences in people with PTSD, but not in controls. In patients with PTSD the injection of drugs such as lactate (Rainey *et al.*, 1987) and yohimbine (Southwick *et al.*, 1993) tends to precipitate panic attacks, flashbacks (exact reliving experiences) of earlier trauma, or both. In our own laboratory, approximately 20% of PTSD subjects responded with a flashback of a traumatic experience when they were presented with acoustic startle stimuli.

TRAUMA, NEUROHORMONES AND MEMORY CONSOLIDATION

When people are under severe stress, they secrete endogenous stress hormones that affect the strength of memory consolidation. Based on animal models it has been widely assumed (van der Kolk and van der Hart, 1991; van der Kolk *et al.*, 1985; Charney *et al.*, 1993) that massive secretion of neurohormones at the time of the trauma plays a role in the long-term potentiation (LTP) (and thus, the overconsolidation) of traumatic memories. Mammals seem equipped with memory storage mechanisms that ordinarily modulate the strength of memory consolidation according to the strength of the accompanying hormonal stimulation (McGaugh, 1989). This capacity helps the organism evaluate the importance of subsequent sensory input according to the relative strength of associated memory traces. This phenomenon appears to be largely mediated by NE input to the amygdala (LeDoux, 1990; Adamec, 1978). In traumatized organisms, the capacity to access relevant memories appears to have gone awry: they become overconditioned to access memory traces of the trauma and to "remember" the trauma whenever aroused. While NE seems to be the principal hormone involved in producing LTP, other neurohormones secreted under particular stressful circumstances, such as endorphins and oxytocin, actually inhibit memory consolidation (Zager and Black, 1985).

The role of NE in memory consolidation has been shown to have an inverted U-shaped function (McGaugh, 1989): both very low and very high levels of CNS NE activity interfere with memory storage. Excessive NE release at the time of the trauma, as well as the release of other neurohormones, such as endogenous opioids, oxytocin and vasopressin, are likely to play a role in creating the hypermnesias and the amnesias that are a quintessential part of PTSD (American Psychiatric Association, 1987, 1993). It is of interest that childbirth, which can be extraordinarily stressful, almost never seems to result in post-traumatic problems (Moleman et al., 1992). Oxytocin may play a protective role that prevents the overconsolidation of memories surrounding childbirth.

Physiological arousal in general can trigger trauma-related memories, while, conversely, trauma-related memories precipitate generalized physiological arousal. It is likely that the frequent reliving of a traumatic event in flashbacks or nightmares cause a re-release of stress hormones which further kindle the strength of the memory trace (van der Kolk et al., 1985). Such a positive feedback loop could cause subclinical PTSD to escalate into clinical PTSD (Pitman et al., 1993), in which the strength of the memories appears so deeply engraved that Pitman and Orr (1990a) have called it "the Black Hole" in the mental life of the PTSD patient, that attracts all associations to it, and saps current life of its significance.

MEMORY, TRAUMA AND THE LIMBIC SYSTEM

The limbic system is thought to be the part of the CNS that maintains and guides the emotions and behavior necessary for self-preservation and survival of the species (MacLean, 1985), and that is critically involved in the storage and retrieval of memory. During both waking and sleeping states signals from the sensory organs continuously travel to the thalamus whence they are distributed to the cortex (setting up a "stream of thought"), to the basal ganglia (setting up a "stream of movement") and to the limbic system where they set up a "stream of emotions" (Papez, 1937), which determines the emotional significance of the sensory input. It appears that most processing of sensory input occurs outside of conscious awareness, and only novel, significant or threatening information is selectively passed on to the neocortex for further attention. Since people with PTSD appear to overinterpret sensory input as a recurrence of past trauma and since recent studies have suggested limbic system abnormalities in brain imaging studies of traumatized patients (Saxe et al., 1992; Bremner et al., 1992), a review of the psychobiology of trauma would be incomplete without considering the role of the limbic system in PTSD (see also Teicher et al., 1993). Two particular areas of the limbic system have been implicated in the processing of emotionally charged memories: the amygdala and the hippocampus.

The amygdala

Of all areas in the CNS, the amygdala is most clearly implicated in the evaluation of the emotional meaning of incoming stimuli (LeDoux, 1986). Several investigators have proposed that the amygdala assigns free-floating feelings of significance to sensory input, which the neocortex then further elaborates and imbues with personal meaning (MacLean, 1985; LeDoux, 1986; Adamec, 1991; O'Keefe and Bouma, 1969). Moreover, it is thought to integrate internal representations of the external world in the form of memory images with emotional experiences associated with those memories (Calvin, 1990). After assigning meaning to sensory information, the amygdala guides emotional behavior by projections to the hypothalamus, hippocampus and basal forebrain (LeDoux, 1986; Adamec, 1991; Squire and Zola-Morgan, 1991).

The septohippocampal system

This system, which anatomically is adjacent to the amygdala, is thought to record in memory the spatial and temporal dimensions of experience and to play an important role in the categorization and storage of incoming stimuli in memory. Proper functioning of the hippocampus is necessary for explicit or declarative memory (Squire and Zola-Morgan, 1991). The hippocampus is thought to be involved in the evaluation of spatially and temporally unrelated events, comparing them with previously stored information and determining whether and how they are associated with each other, with reward, punishment, novelty or non-reward (Adamec, 1991; Gray, 1982). The hippocampus is also implicated in playing a role in the inhibition of exploratory behavior and in obsessional thinking, while hippocampal damage is associated with hyper-responsiveness to environmental stimuli (Altman *et al.*, 1973; O'Keefe and Nadel, 1978).

The slow maturation of the hippocampus, which is not fully myelinated till after the third or fourth year of life, is seen as the cause of infantile amnesia (Jacobs and Nadel, 1985; Schacter and Moscovitch, 1982). In contrast, it is thought that the memory system that subserves the affective quality of experience (roughly speaking procedural, or "taxon" memory) matures earlier and is less subject to disruption by stress (O'Keefe and Nadel, 1978). As the CNS matures, memory storage shifts from primarily sensorimotor (motoric action) and perceptual representations (iconic), to symbolic and linguistic modes of organization of mental experience (Piaget, 1962). With maturation, there is an increasing ability to categorize experience, and link it with existing mental schemes. However, even as the organism matures, this capacity, and with it, the hippocampal localization system, remains vulnerable to disruption (Yehuda *et al.*, 1991a; Adamec, 1991; Gray, 1982; Nadel and Zola-Morgan, 1984; Sapolsky *et al.*, 1990). A variety of external and internal stimuli, such as stress-induced corticosterone production (Pfaff *et al.*, 1971), decreases hippocampal activity. However, even when stress interferes with hippocampally mediated memory storage and categorization, it is likely that some mental representation of the experience is laid down by means of a system that records affective experience, but that has no capacity for symbolic processing and placement in space and time.

Decreased hippocampal functioning causes behavioral disinhibition, possibly by stimulating incoming stimuli to be interpreted in the direction of "emergency" (fight/flight) responses. The neurotransmitter 5-HT plays a crucial role in the capacity of the septohippocampal system to activate inhibitory pathways that prevent the initiation of emergency responses until it is clear that they will be of use (Gray, 1982). This observation made us very interested in a possible role for serotonergic agents in the treatment of PTSD.

"EMOTIONAL MEMORIES ARE FOREVER"

In animals, high-level stimulation of the amygdala interferes with hippocampal functioning (Adamec, 1991; Squire and Zola-Morgan, 1991). This implies that intense affect may inhibit proper evaluation and categorization of experience. In mature animals one-time intense stimulation of the amygdala will produce lasting changes in neuronal excitability and enduring behavioral changes in the direction of either fight or flight (LeDoux et al., 1991). In kindling experiments with animals, Adamec et al. (1980) have shown that, following growth in amplitude of amygdala and hippocampal seizure activity, permanent changes in limbic physiology cause lasting changes in defensiveness and in predatory aggression. Pre-existing "personality" played a significant role in the behavioral effects of amygdala stimulation in cats: animals that are temperamentally insensitive to threat and prone to attack tend to become more aggressive, while in highly defensive animals different pathways were activated, increasing behavioral inhibition (Adamec et al., 1980).

In a series of experiments, LeDoux has utilized repeated electrical stimulation of the amygdala to produce conditioned fear responses. He found that cortical lesions prevent their extinction. This led him to conclude that, once formed, the subcortical traces of the conditioned fear response are indelible, and that "emotional memory may be forever" (LeDoux et al., 1991). In 1987, Lawrence Kolb postulated that patients with PTSD suffer from impaired cortical control over subcortical areas responsible for learning, habituation, and stimulus discrimination. The concept of indelible subcortical emotional responses, held in check to varying degrees by cortical and septohippocampal activity, has led to the speculation that delayed-onset PTSD may be the expression of subcortically mediated emotional responses that escape cortical, and possibly hippocampal, inhibitory control (van der Kolk and van der Hart, 1991; Pitman et al., 1993; Charney et al., 1993; Nijenhuis, 1991; Shalev et al., 1992b).

Decreased inhibitory control may occur under a variety of circumstances: under the influence of drugs and alcohol, during sleep (as nightmares), with aging, and after exposure to strong reminders of the traumatic past. It is conceivable that traumatic memories then could emerge, not in the distorted fashion of ordinary recall, but as affect states, somatic sensations or as visual images (nightmares (Janet, 1919/1925) or flashbacks (Southwick et al., 1993)) that are timeless and unmodified by further experience.

PSYCHOPHARMACOLOGICAL TREATMENT

The goal of treatment of PTSD is to help people live in the present, without feeling or behaving according to irrelevant demands belonging to the past. Psychologically, this means that traumatic experiences need to be located in time and place and distinguished from current reality. However, hyperarousal, intrusive reliving, numbing and dissociation get in the way of separating current reality from past trauma. Hence, medications that affect these PTSD symptoms are often essential for patients to begin to achieve a sense of safety and perspective from which to approach their tasks. While numerous articles have been written about the drug treatment of PTSD, to date only 134 people with PTSD have been enrolled in published double-blind studies. Most of these have been Vietnam combat veterans. Unfortunately, up until recently, only medications which seem to be of limited therapeutic usefulness have been the subject of adequate scientific scrutiny. While the only published double-blind studies of medications in the treatment of PTSD have been tricyclic antidepressants and monoamine oxidase inhibitors (Frank *et al.*, 1988; Bleich *et al.*, 1987; Davidson and Nemeroff, 1989). It is sometimes assumed that they therefore also are the most effective. Three double-blind trials of tricyclic antidepressants have been published (Frank *et al.*, 1988; Davidson and Nemeroff, 1989; Reist *et al.*, 1989), two of which demonstrated modest improvement in PTSD symptoms. While positive results have been claimed for numerous other medications in case reports and open studies, at the present time there are no data about which patient and which PTSD symptom will predictably respond to any of them.

Success has been claimed for just about every class of psychoactive medication, including benzodiazepines (van der Kolk, 1987b), tricyclic antidepressants (Frank *et al.*, 1988; Reist *et al.*, 1989), monamine oxidase inhibitors (Frank *et al.*, 1988; Hogben and Cornfield, 1981), lithium carbonate (van der Kolk, 1987b), β-adrenergic blockers and clonidine (Kolb *et al.*, 1984), carbamezapine (Lipper *et al.*, 1986) and antipsychotic agents. The accumulated clinical experience seems to indicate that understanding the basic neurobiology of arousal and appraisal is the most useful guide in selecting medications for people with PTSD (Davidson and Nemeroff, 1989; Reist *et al.*, 1989). Autonomic arousal can be reduced at different levels in the CNS: through inhibition of LC noradrenergic activity with clonidine and the β-adrenergic blockers (Kolb *et al.*, 1984; Famularo *et al.*, 1988), or by increasing the inhibitory effect of the γ-aminobutyric acid (GABA)-ergic system with GABA-ergic agonists (the benzodiazepines). During the past two years a number of case reports and open clinical trials of fluoxetine were followed by our double-blind study of 64 PTSD subjects with fluoxetine (van der Kolk *et al.*, 1993). Unlike the tricyclic antidepressants, which were effective on either the intrusive (imipramine) or numbing (amitryptiline) symptoms of PTSD, fluoxetine proved to be effective for the whole spectrum of PTSD symptoms. It also acted more rapidly than the tricyclics. The fact that fluoxetine has proven to be such an effective treatment for PTSD supports a larger role of the serotonergic system in PTSD (van der Kolk and Saporta, 1991). Double-blind Rorschach tests revealed that subjects on fluoxetine became able to take distance from the emotional impact of incoming stimuli and to become able to utilize cognition to harness the emotional responses to unstructured visual stimuli (van der Kolk *et al.*, unpublished).

While the subjects improved clinically, their startle habituation got worse (van der Kolk, Orr, Fisler and Michaels, unpublished). The 5-HT$_{1A}$ agonist buspirone shows some promise to be able to facilitate habituation to startle (Giral *et al.*, 1988) and thus may play a useful adjunctive role in the pharmacotherapy of PTSD. Even newer research has suggested abnormalities of the MNDA receptor and of glutamate in PTSD (Krystal, 1993), opening up potential new avenues for the psychopharmacological treatment of PTSD.

SUMMARY

Ever since people's responses to overwhelming experiences have been systematically explored, it has been noted that the trauma is stored in somatic memory and expressed as changes in the biological stress response. Intense emotions at the time of the trauma initiate the long-term conditional responses to reminders of the trauma, and are responsible for the amnesias and hypermnesias characteristic of PTSD. Continued physiological hyperarousal and altered stress hormone secretion affect the ongoing evaluation of sensory stimuli.

While memory ordinarily is an active and constructive process, in PTSD failure of semantic memory may lead to the organization of experience on somatosensory or iconic levels that are relatively impervious to change. The inability of people with PTSD to integrate traumatic experiences and, instead, to continuously relive the past, is mirrored physiologically and hormonally in the misinterpretation of innocuous stimuli as potential threats.

Animal research suggests that intense emotional memories are stored outside of the localization system and are difficult to extinguish. Cortical and septohippocampal activity can inhibit the expression of these subcortically based emotional memories. The effectiveness of this inhibition is, in part, dependent on physiological arousal and neurohormone activity. This formulation has implications for both the psychotherapy and pharmacotherapy of PTSD.

ACKNOWLEDGMENT

The author wishes to thank Rita Fisher Ed.M. for her editorial assistance.

REFERENCES

Adamec, R. E. (1978). Normal and abnormal limbic system mechanisms of emotive biasing. In *Limbic Mechanisms* (eds K. E. Livingston and O. Hornykiewicz). Plenum Press, New York.

Adamec, R. E. (1991). Partial kindling of the ventral hippocampus: identification of changes in limbic physiology which accompany changes in feline aggression and defense. *Physiol. Behav.*, **49**, 443–454.

Adamec, R. E., Stark-Adamec, C. and Livingston, K. E. (1980). The development of predatory aggression and defense in the domestic cat. *Neural Biol.*, **30**, 389–447.

Akil, H., Watson, S. J. and Young, E. (1983). Endogenous opioids: biology and function. *Annu. Rev. Neurosci.*, **7**, 223–255.

Altman, J., Brunner, R. L. and Bayer, S. A. (1973). The hippocampus and behavioral maturation. *Behav. Biol.*, **8**, 557–596.

American Psychiatric Association (1987). *Diagnostic and Statistical Manual of Mental Disorders*, 3rd edn, revised. American Psychiatric Association, Washington, DC.

American Psychiatric Association (1993). *Diagnostic and Statistical Manual of Mental Disorders*, 4th edn. American Psychiatric Association, Washington, DC.

Axelrod, J. and Neisine, (1984). Stress hormones, their interaction and regulation. *Science*, **224**, 452–459.

Beecher, H. K. (1946). Pain in men wounded in battle. *Ann. Surg.*, **123**, 96–105.

Blanchard, E. B., Kolb, L. C. and Gerardi, R. J. (1986). Cardiac response to relevant stimuli as an adjunctive tool for diagnosing post traumatic stress disorder in Vietnam veterans. *Behav. Ther.*, **17**, 592–606.

Bleich, A., Siegel, B., Garb, B. *et al.* (1987). PTSD following combat exposure: clinical features and pharmacological management. *Br. J. Psychiatry*, **149**, 365–369.

Bohus, B. and DeWied, D. (1978). Pituitary–adrenal system hormones and adaptive behavior. In *General, Comparative, and Clinical Endocrinology of the Adrenal Cortex*, Vol. 3. (eds I. Chester-Jones and I. W. Henderson). Academic Press, New York.

Bowlby, J. (1969). *Attachment and Loss*, Vol. 1. Basic Books, New York.

Bremner, J. D., Seibyl, J. P., Scott, T. M. (1992). Depressed hippocampal volume in post-traumatic stress disorder (New Research Abstract 155). *Proceedings of the 145th annual meeting of the American Psychiatric Association*, Washington, DC, May 1992.

Brown, G. L., Ballenger, J. C., Minichiello, M. D. and Goodwin, F. K. (1979). Human aggression and its relationship to cerebrospinal fluid 5-hydroxy-indolacetic acid, 3-methoxy-4-hydroxy-phenyl-glycol, and homovannilic acid. In *Psychopharmacology of Aggression* (ed. M. Sandler). Raven Press, New York.

Butler, R. W., Braff, D. L. and Rausch, J. L. (1990). Physiological evidence of exaggerated startle response in a subgroup of Vietnam veterans with combat-related PTSD. *Am. J. Psychiat.*, 1308–1322.

Calvin, W. H. (1990). *The Cerebral Symphony*. Bantam, New York.

Charney, D. S., Deutch, A. Y., Krystal, J. H. *et al.* (1993). Psychobiologic mechanisms of post traumatic stress disorder. *Arch. Gen. Psychiatry*, **50**, 294–305.

Cicchetti, D. (1985). The emergence of developmental psychopathology. *Child Dev.*, **55**, 1–7.

Coccaro, E. F., Siever, L. J., Klar, H. M. and Maurer, P. (1989). Serotonergic studies in patients with affective and personality disorders. *Arch. Gen. Psychiatry*, **46**, 587–598.

Cole, P. M. and Putnam, F. W. (1991). Effect of incest on self and social functioning: a developmental psychopathology perspective. *J. Consult. Clin. Psychol.*, **60**, 174–184.

Davidson, J. R. T. and Nemeroff, C. B. (1989). Pharmacotherapy in PTSD: historical and clinical considerations and future directions. *Psychopharmacol. Bull.*, **25**, 422–425.

Davidson, J., Kudler, H. and Smith, R. (1990). Treatment of post-traumatic stress disorder with amitriptyline and placebo. *Arch. Gen. Psychiatry*, **47**, 259–266.

Davis, M. (1984). The mammalian startle response. In *Neural Mechanisms of Startle Behavior* (ed. R. C. Eaton). Plenum Press, New York.

Davis, M. (1986). Pharmacological and anatomical analysis of fear conditioning using the fear-potentiated startle paradigm. *Behav. Neurosci.*, **100**, 814–824.

Dobbs, D. and Wilson, W. P. (1960). Observations on the persistence of traumatic war neurosis. *J. Ment. Nerv. Dis.*, **21**, 40–46.

Dunn, A. J. and Berridge, C. W. (1987). Corticotropin-releasing factor administration elicits stresslike activation of cerebral catecholamine systems. *Pharmacol. Biochem. Behav.*, **27**, 685–691.

Dupue, R. A. and Spoont, M. R. (1989). Conceptualizing a serotonin trait: a behavioral model of constraint. *Ann. NY Acad. Sci.*, **12**, 47–62.

Falcon, S., Ryan, C. and Chamberlain, K. (1985). Tricyclics: possible treatment for posttraumatic stress disorder. *J. Clin. Psychiatry*, **46**, 385–389.

Famularo, R., Kinscherff, R. and Fenton, T. (1988). The Propranolol treatment for childhood posttraumatic stress disorder, acute type: a pilot study. *Am. J. Dis. Child.*, **142**, 1244–1247.

Frank, J. B., Kosten, T. R., Giller, E. L. and Dan, E. (1988). A randomized clinical trial of phenelzine and imipramine in PTSD. *Am. J. Psychiatry*, **145**, 1289–1291.

Freud, S. (1919/1954). *Introduction to Psychoanalysis and the War Neuroses. Standard Edition*, Vol. 17 (ed. and trans. Strachey), pp. 207–210. Hogarth Press, London.

Gerson, S. C. and Baldessarini, R. J. (1980). Motor effects of serotonin in the central nervous system. *Life Sci.*, **27**, 1435–1451.

Giral, P., Martin, P. and Soubrie, P. (1988). Reversal of helpless behavior in rats by putative 5-HT1A agonists. *Biol. Psychiatry*, **23**: 237–242.

Gray, J. (1982). *The Neuropsychology of Anxiety: An Inquiry into the Functions of the Septo-hippocampal System*. Oxford University Press, Oxford.

Green, A. H. (1978). Self-destructive behavior in battered children. *Am. J. Psychiatry*, **135**, 579–582.

Green, A. (1980) *Child Maltreatment*. Aronson, New York.

Grinker, R. R. and Spiegel, J. J. (1945). *Men Under Stress*. McGraw-Hill, New York.

Herman, J. L. (1992). Complex PTSD: a syndrome in survivors of prolonged and repeated trauma. *J. Traum. Stress*, **5**, 377–391.

Hilberman, E. and Munson, M. (1978). Sixty battered women. *Victimology*, **2**, 460–461.

Hogben, G. L. and Cornfield, R. B. (1981). Treatment of traumatic war neurosis with phenalzine. *Arch. Gen. Psychiatry*, **38**, 440–445.

Horowitz, M. (1978). *Stress Response Syndromes*, 2nd edn. Jason Aronson, New York.

Jacobs, W. J. and Nadel, L. (1985). Stress-induced recovery of fears and phobias. *Psychol. Rev.*, **92**, 512–531.

Janet, P. (1889). *L'Automatisme Psychologique*. Alcan, Paris.

Janet, P. (1919/1925). *Les Medications Psychologiques* (three volumes). Felix Alcan, Paris.

Jenike, M. A., Baer, L., Summergrad, P. *et al.* (1990). Sertroline in obsessive-compulsive disorder: a double blind study. *Am. J. Psychiatry*, **147**, 923–928.

Kardiner, A. (1941) *The Traumatic Neuroses of War*. Hoeber, New York.

Keane, T. M. and Kaloupek, D. G. (1982). Imaginal flooding in the treatment of post-traumatic stress disorder. *J. Consult. Clin. Psychol.*, **50**, 138–140.

Kilpatrick, D. G., Veronen, L. J. and Best, C. L. (1985). Factors predicting psychological distress in rape victims. In *Trauma and its Wake* (ed. C. Figley). Brunner/Mazel, New York.

Kolb, L. C. (1987). Neurophysiological hypothesis explaining posttraumatic stress disorder. *Am. J. Psychiatry*, **144**, 989–995.

Kolb, L. C. and Multipassi, L. R. (1982). The conditioned emotional response: a subclass of chronic and delayed post traumatic stress disorder. *Psychiatr. Ann.*, **12**, 979–987.

Kolb, L. C., Burris, B. C. and Griffiths, S. (1984). Propranolol and clonidine in the treatment of post traumatic stress disorders of war. In *Post Traumatic Stress Disorder: Psychological and Biological Sequelae* (ed. B. A. van der Kolk). American Psychiatric Press, Washington, DC.

Kosten, T. R., Mason, J. W., Giller, E. L. *et al.* (1987). Sustained urinary norepinephrine and epinephrine elevation in PTSD. *Psychoneuroendocrinology*, **12**, 13–20.

Kraemer, G. W. (1985). Effects of differences in early social experiences on primate neuro-biological–behavioral development. In *The Psychobiology of Attachment and Separation* (eds Reite *et al.*). Academic Press, Orlando, FL.

Krystal, H. (1978). Trauma and affects. *Psychoanal. Study Child*, **33**, 81–116.

Krystal, J. (1993). Neurobiological mechanisms of dissociation. Paper presented at the American Psychiatric Association Meeting, San Francisco, May 1993.

Krystal, J. H., Kosten, T. R., Southwick, S. *et al.* (1989). Neurobiological aspects of PTSD: review of clinical and preclinical studies. *Behav. Ther.*, **20**, 177–198.

Kulka, R. A., Schlenger, W. E., Fairbank, J. A. *et al.* (1990). *Trauma and the Vietnam War Generation: Report of Findings from the National Vietnam Veterans' Readjustment Study.* Brunner Mazel, New York.

Lang, P. J. (1979). A bio-informational theory of emotional imagery. *Psychophysiology*, **16**, 495–512.

LeDoux, J. (1986). *Mind and Brain: Dialogues in Cognitive Neuroscience.* Cambridge University Press, New York.

LeDoux, J. E. (1990). Information flow from sensation to emotion: plasticity of the neural computation of stimulus value. In *Learning Computational Neuroscience: Foundations of Adaptive Networks* (eds M. Gabriel and J. Morre). MIT Press, Cambridge, MA.

LeDoux, J. E., Romanski, L. and Xagoraris, A. (1991). Indelibility of subcortical emotional memories. *J. Cogn. Neurosci.*, **1**, 238–243.

Lerer, B., Bleich, A. and Kotler, M. (1987). Post traumatic stress disorder in Israeli combat veterans: effect of phenylzine treatment. *Arch. Gen. Psychiatry*, **44**, 976–981.

Lewis, D. O. (1992). From abuse to violence: psychophysiological consequences of maltreatment. *J. Am. Acad. Child Adolesc. Psychiatry*, **31**, 383–391.

Lindemann, E. (1944). Symptomatology and management of acute grief. *Am. J. Psychiatry*, **101**, 141–148.

Lipper, S., Davidson, J. R. T., Grady, T. A. *et al.* (1986). Preliminary study of carbamezapine in post-traumatic stress disorder. *Psychosomatics*, **27**, 8479–854.

Litz, B. T. and Keane, T. M. (1989). Information processing in anxiety disorders: application to the understanding of post-traumatic stress disorder. *Clin. Psychol. Rev.*, **9**, 243–257.

MacLean, P. D. (1985). Brain evolution relating to family, play, and the separation call. *Arch. Gen. Psychiatry*, **42**, 505–417.

Malloy, P. F., Fairbank, J. A. and Keane, T. M. (1983). Validation of a multimethod assessment of post traumatic stress disorders in Vietnam veterans. *J. Consult. Clin. Psychol.*, **51**, 4–21.

Mann, J. D. (1987). Psychobiologic predictors of suicide. *J. Clin. Psychiatry*, **48**, 39–43.

Mason, J., Giller, E. L. and Kosten, T. R. (1988). Elevated norepinephrine/cortisol ratio in PTSD. *J. Ment. Nerv. Dis.*, **176**, 498–502.

McFarlane, A. C. (1988). The longitudinal course of posttraumatic morbidity: the range of outcomes and their predictors. *J. Nerv. Ment. Dis.*, **176**, 30–39.

McGaugh, J. L. (1989). Involvement of hormonal and neuromodulatory systems in the regulation of memory storage. *Annu. Rev. Neurosci.*, **2**, 255–287.

Meaney, M. J., Aitken, D. H., Viau, V. *et al.* (1989). Neonatal handling alters adrenocortical negative feedback sensitivity and hippocampal type II glucocorticoid binding in the rat. *Neuroendocrinology*, **50**, 597–604.

Mitchell, D., Osborne, E. W. and O'Boyle, M. W. (1985). Habituation under stress: shocked mice show non-associative learning in a T-maze. *Behav. Neurobiol.*, **43**, 212–217.

Moleman, N., van der Hart, O. and van der Kolk, B. A. (1992). The partus stress reaction: a neglected etiological factor in post-partum psychiatric disorders. *J. Nerv. Ment. Dis.*, **180**, 271–272.

Munck, A., Guyre, P. M. and Holbrook, N. J. (1984). Physiological functions of glucocorticoids in stress and their relation to pharmacological actions. *Endocr. Rev.*, **93**, 9779–9783.

Nadel, L. and Zola-Morgan, S. (1984). Infantile amnesia: a neurobiological perspective. In *Infant Memory* (ed. M. Moscovitch). Plenum Press, New York.

Nijenhuis, F. (1991). Multiple personality disorder, hormones, and memory. Paper presented at the International Conference on Multiple Personality Disorder, Chicago.

O'Keefe, J. and Bouma, H. (1969). Complex sensory properties of certain amygdala units in the freely moving cat. *Exp. Neurol.*, **23**, 384–398.

O'Keefe, J. and Nadel, L. (1978). *The Hippocampus as a Cognitive Map*. Clarendon Press, Oxford.

Ornitz, E. M. and Pynoos, R. S. (1989). Startle modulation in children with post traumatic stress disorder. *Am. J. Psychiatry*, **146**, 866–870.

Papez, J. W. (1937). A proposed mechanism of emotion. *Arch. Neurol. Psychiatry*, **38**, 725–743.

Pavlov, I. P. (1926). *Conditioned reflexes: An Investigation of the Physiological Activity of the Cerebral Cortex* (ed. and trans. G. V. Anrep). Dover Publications, New York.

Perry, B. D., Giller, E. L. and Southwick, S. M. (1987). Altered plasma alpha-2 adrenergic receptor affinity states in PTSD. *Am. J. Psychiatry*, **144**, 1511–1512.

Pfaff, D. W., Silva, M. T. and Weiss, J. M. (1971). Telemetered recording of hormone effects on hippocampal neurons. *Science*, **172**, 394–395.

Phillips, A. G. and LePiane, F. G. (1980). Disruption of conditioned taste aversion in the rat by stimulation of amygdala: a conditioning effect, not amnesia. *J. Comp. Physiol. Psychol.*, **94**, 664–674.

Piaget, J. (1962). *Play, Dreams, and Imitation in Childhood*. W. W. Norton, New York.

Pitman, R. and Orr, S. (1990a). *The Black Hole of Trauma. Biol, Psychiatry*, **26**, 221–223.

Pitman, R. K. and Orr, S. P. (1990b). Twenty-four hour urinary cortisol and cathecholamine excretion in combat-related post-traumatic stress disorder. *Biol. Psychiatry*, **27**, 245–247.

Pitman, R. K., Orr, S. P., Forgue, D. F. *et al.* (1987). Psychophysiologic assessment of post-traumatic stress disorder imagery in Vietnam combat veterans. *Arch. Gen. Psychiatry*, **44**, 970–975.

Pitman, R. K., van der Kolk, B. A., Orr, S. P. and Greenberg, M. S. (1990). Naloxone reversible stress induced analgesia in post traumatic stress disorder. *Arch. Gen. Psychiatry*, **47**, 541–547.

Pitman, R., Orr, S. and Shalev, A. (1993). Once bitten twice shy: beyond the conditioning model of PTSD. *Biol. Psychiatry*, **33**, 145–146.

Putnam, F. W. (1989). *Diagnosis and Treatment of Multiple Personality Disorder*. Guilford Press, New York.

Rainey, J. M., Aleem, A., Ortiz, A. *et al.* (1987). Laboratory procedure for the inducement of flashbacks. *Am. J. Psychiatry*, **144**, 1317–1319.

Rawlins, J. N. P. (1980). Associative and non-associative mechanisms in the development of tolerance for stress: the problem of state dependent learning. In *Coping and Health* (eds S. Levine and H. Ursin). Plenum Press, New York.

Reist, C., Kauffman, C. D. and Haier, R. J. (1989). A controlled trial of desipramine in 18 men with post-traumatic stress disorder. *Am. J. Psychiatry*, **146**, 513–516.

Reite, M. and Fields, F. (eds) (1985). *The Psychobiology of Attachment and Separation*. Academic Press, Orlando, FL.

Ross, R. J., Ball, W. A. and Cohen, M. E. (1989). Habituation of the startle response in post traumatic stress disorder. *J. Neuropsychiatry*, **1**, 305–307.

Sapolsky, R., Krey, L. and McEwen, B. S. (1984). Stress down-regulates corticosterone receptors in a site specific manner in the brain. *Endocrinology*, **114**, 287–292.

Sapolsky, R. M., Uno Hideo, Rebert, C. S. and Finch, C. E. (1990). Hippocampal damage associated with prolonged glucocorticoid exposure in primates. *J. Neurosci.*, **10**, 2897–2902.

Saxe, G. N., Vasile, R. G., Hill, T. C. *et al.* (1992). SPECT imaging and multiple personality disorder. *J. Nerv. Ment. Dis.*, **180**, 662–663.

Schacter, D. L. and Moscovitch, M. (1982). Infants, amnesics, and dissociable memory systems. In *Infant Memory* (ed. M. Moscovitch). Plenum Press, New York.

Shalev, A. Y. and Rogel-Fuchs, Y. (1993). Psychophysiology of PTSD: from sulfur fumes to behavioral genetics. *J. Ment. Nerv. Dis.* (in press).

Shalev, A. Y., Orr, S. P., Peri, T. *et al.* (1992a). Physiologic responses to loud tones in Israeli patients with post-traumatic stress disorder. *Arch. Gen. Psychiatry*, **49**, 870–875.

Shalev, A., Rogel-Fuchs, Y. and Pitman, R. (1992b). Conditioned fear and psychological trauma. *Biol. Psychiatry*, **31**, 863–865.

Shalev, A. Y., Orr, S. P., Peri, T. *et al.* (1993). Physiologic responses to loud tones in Israeli patients with post traumatic stress disorder. *Arch. Gen. Psychiatry*, **49**, 870–875.

Siegfried, B., Frischknecht, H. R. and Nunez de Souza, R. (1990). An ethological model for the study of activation and interaction of pain, memory, and defensive systems in the attacked mouse: role of endogenous opoids. *Neurosci. Biobehav. Rev.*, **14**, 481–490.

Solomon, Z., Garb, R., Bleich, A. and Grupper, D. (1985) Reactivation of combat-related post-traumatic stress disorder. *Am. J. Psychiatry*, **144**, 51–55.

Southwick, S. M., Krystal, J. H., Morgan, A. *et al.* (1993). Abnormal noradrenergic function in post traumatic stress disorder. *Arch. Gen. Psychiatry*, **50**, 266–274.

Squire, L. R. and Zola-Morgan, S. (1991). The medial temporal lobe memory system. *Science*, **253**, 2380–2386.

Strian, F. and Klicpera, C. (1978). Die Bedeutung psychoautonomische Reaktionen im Entstehung und Persistenz von Angstzustanden. *Nervenarzt*, **49**, 576–583.

Teicher, M. H., Glod, C. A., Surrey, J. and Swett, C. (1993). Early childhood abuse and limbic system ratings in adult psychiatric outpatients. *J. Neuropsychiatr. Clin. Neurosci.* (in press).

Terr, L. C. (1991). Childhood traumas: an outline and overview. *Am. J. Psychiatry*, **148**, 10–20.

Valentino, R. J. and Foote, S. L. (1988). Corticotropin releasing hormone increases tonic, but not sensory-evoked activity of noradrenergic locus coeruleus in unanesthetized rats. *J. Neurosci.*, **8**, 1016–1025.

Valzelli, L. (1982). Serotonergic inhibitory control of experimental aggression. *Psychopharmacol. Res. Commun.*, **12**, 1–13.

van der Kolk, B. A. (1987a). *Psychological Trauma*. American Psychiatric Press, Washington, DC.

van der Kolk, B. A. (1987b). Drug treatment of post traumatic stress disorder. *J. Affect. Disorders*, **13**, 203–213.

van der Kolk, B. A. (1988). The trauma spectrum: the interaction of biological and social events in the genesis of the trauma response. *J. Traum. Stress*, **1**, 273–290.

van der Kolk, B. A. and Ducey, C. P. (1989). The psychological processing of traumatic experience: Rorschach patterns in PTSD. *J. Traum. Stress*, **2**, 259–274.

van der Kolk, B. A. and Saporta, J. (1991). The biological response to psychic trauma: mechanisms and treatment of intrusion and numbing. *Anxiety Res.*, **4**, 199–212.

van der Kolk, B. A. and van der Hart, O. (1989). Pierre Janet and the breakdown of adaptation in psychological trauma. *Am. J. Psychiatry*, **146**, 1530–1540.

van der Kolk, B. A. and van der Hart, O. (1991). The intrusive past: the flexibility of memory and the engraving of trauma. *Am. Imago*, **48**, 425–454.

van der Kolk, B. A., Blitz, R., Burr, W. and Hartmann, E. (1984). Nightmares and trauma. *Am. J. Psychiatry*, **141**, 187–190.

van der Kolk, B. A., Greenberg, M. S., Boyd, H. and Krystal, J. H. (1985). Inescapable shock, neurotransmitters and addiction to trauma: towards a psychobiology of post traumatic stress. *Biol. Psychiatry*, **20**, 314–325.

van der Kolk, B. A., Greenberg, M. S., Orr, S. P. and Pitman, R. K. (1989). Endogenous opioids and stress induced analgesia in post traumatic stress disorder. *Psychopharmacol. Bull.*, **25**, 108–112.

van der Kolk, B. A., Perry, J. C. and Herman, J. L. (1991). Childhood origins of self-destructive behavior. *Am. J. Psychiatry*, **148**, 1665–1671.

van der Kolk, B. A., Roth, S. and Pelcovitz, D. (1992). *Field Trials for DSM IV, Post Traumatic Stress Disorder. II: Disorders of Extreme Stress*. American Psychiatric Association, Washington, DC.

van der Kolk, B. A., Dreyfuss, D., Michaels, M. *et al.* (1993). Fluoxetine in post traumatic stress disorder. *J. Clin. Psychiatry* (in press).

Yehuda, R., Southwick, S. M. *et al.* (1990). Interactions of the hypothalamic–pituitary adrenal axis and the catecholaminergic system in posttraumatic stress disorder. In *Biological Assessment and Treatment of PTSD* (ed. E. L. Giller). American Psychiatric Press, Washington, DC.

Yehuda, R., Giller, E. L., Southwick, S. M. *et al.* (1991a). Hypothalamic–pituitary–adrenal dysfunction in posttraumatic stress disorder. *Biol. Psychiatry*, **30**, 1031–1048.

Yehuda, R., Lowy, M. T. and Southwick, S. M. (1991b). Lymphocyte glucortoid receptor number in posttraumatic stress disorder. *Am. J. Psychiatry*, **148**, 499–504.

Zager, E. L. and Black, P. M. (1985). Neuropeptides in human memory and learning processes. *Neurosurgery*, **17**, 355–369.

17 Peptidergic Alterations in Stress: Focus on Corticotropin-releasing Factor

[1,2]JOHN W. KASCKOW AND [3]CHARLES B. NEMEROFF
[1]Department of Psychiatry, University of Cincinnati College of Medicine, Cincinnati, Ohio, USA, [2]Cincinnati VA Medical Center, Psychiatry Service, Cincinnati, Ohio, USA, [3]Department of Psychiatry and Behavioral Sciences, Emory University School of Medicine, Atlanta, Georgia, USA

Corticotropin-releasing factor (CRF) is a 41 amino acid-containing peptide found in the central nervous system (CNS) and in certain peripheral tissues as well. In its role as a hypothalamic hypophysiotropic hormone, CRF is the major physiologic regulator of the secretion of adrenocorticotropic hormone (ACTH), β-endorphin, and other pro-opiomelanocortin (POMC)-derived peptides from the anterior pituitary gland. CRF is believed to orchestrate the mammalian stress response, at least partly by activation of the hypothalamic–pituitary–adrenal (HPA) axis. In addition to mediating the endocrine response to stress, CRF also appears to integrate the autonomic, immunologic and behavioral responses to stress. Indeed, there is considerable data which has accumulated to support this widespread role for CRF. In this chapter, we will initially discuss the basic neurobiology of CRF and then describe the evidence implicating a role for CRF as the major neuroregulator mediating the stress response. The discussion of the latter will focus on how the concentration of CRF in extracellular fluid may change after exposure to stress and moreover will review the evidence that CRF injected directly into various brain regions leads to behaviors observed following exposure to stress. Finally, the clinical database relevant to CRF will be described.

The amino acid composition of CRF has been highly conserved throughout evolution. It is found in mammals and birds, and closely related structural homologs can be found in amphibians and fish which mediate their respective stress responses. Evolutionarily it appears that CRF-like compounds first functioned to mobilize sources of energy in animals; however, its role in higher animals has become more complex.

Vale et al. (1981) isolated and characterized ovine CRF as a 41 amino acid-containing peptide from ovine hypothalamus. Aguilera et al. (1982) determined that the bioactivity of the peptide resides in the C-terminal 27 amino acid

Advances in the Neurobiology of Anxiety Disorders. Edited by H. G. M. Westenberg, J. A. Den Boer and D. L. Murphy
©1996 John Wiley & Sons Ltd

residues. In 1983, Numa's group (Furutani *et al.*, 1983; Shibahara *et al.*, 1983) structurally characterized the gene encoding ovine and human CRF. The CRF gene was found to contain two exons, the latter encoding the functional protein (Thompson *et al.*, 1987). In addition, a large intronic sequence was found whose function remains obscure.

In the CNS, the most widely studied localization of CRF is in the paraventricular nucleus (PVN) of the hypothalamus (Bloom *et al.*, 1982). The PVN CRF-containing cell bodies project nerve terminals to the median eminence. In the median eminence, CRF is released into the primary plexus of the hypothalamo-hypophysial portal system. Some CRF fibers from the PVN also project to other hypothalamic nuclei and other extrahypothalamic brain sites. CRF-containing perikarya are also present in the supraoptic, suprachiasmatic, preoptic, premamillary, periventricular and arcuate nuclei as well as in magnocellular PVN neurons (Kawata *et al.*, 1982; Antoni *et al.*, 1983, Daikoku *et al.*, 1984; Piekut and Joseph, 1985).

CRF neurons have also been identified in the cerebral cortex, limbic system and in brain stem nuclei associated with regulation of the autonomic nervous system (Swanson *et al.*, 1983) (see Figure 1). Within these regions, the highest density of CRF-containing cells are located in the amygdala, bed nucleus of the stria terminalis, lateral hypothalamus, central gray area, dorsal tegmentum, locus coeruleus, parabrachial nucleus, dorsal vagal complex and inferior olive.

In addition to the studies demonstrating localization of CRF peptides to the above regions by immunohistochemistry and radioimmunoassay, DeSouza

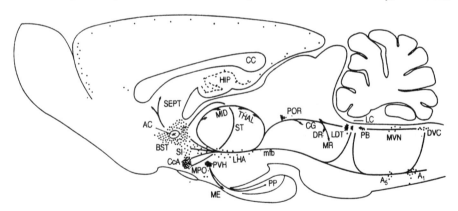

Figure 1 Major CRF-stained cell groups (dots) and fiber systems in the rat brain. CC, corpus callosum; HIP, hippocampus; SEPT, septal region; AC, anterior commissure; BST, bed nucleus of the stria terminalis; SI, substantia innominata; CcA, central nucleus of the amygdala; MPO, medial preoptic area; PVH, PVN of hypothalamus; ME, median eminence; PP, posterior pituitary; LHA, lateral hypothalamic area; mfb, medial forebrain bundle; MID THAL, midline thalamic nuclei; ST, stria terminalis; POR, perioculomotor nucleus; CG, central gray; DR, dorsal raphe; MR, median raphe; LDT, laterodorsal tegmental nucleus; LC, locus coeruleus; PB, parabrachial nucleus; MVN, medial vestibular nucleus; DVC, dorsal vagal complex; A_5, A_1, noradrenergic cell groups (Reprinted by permission of S. Karger AG, Basel from Swanson *et al.*, 1983)

(1987) described the heterogeneous distribution of CRF receptors in the anterior pituitary and in the CNS; high densities of CRF receptors in the CNS include the olfactory bulb, cerebellum, cerebral cortex and several limbic system structures. It is of interest that CRF is strategically placed to influence the activity of the major monoamine-containing neuronal systems in the CNS.

The structure of the CRF receptor has now been elucidated. Binding of various ligands to the CRF receptor is increased by divalent cations and decreased by guanyl nucleotides (Perrin *et al.*, 1986). Signal transduction studies involving the CRF receptor indicate that its activation is coupled to the cyclic AMP second messenger system (Battaglia *et al.*, 1987). Although there is limited evidence implicating other signal transduction systems in the receptor-mediated actions of CRF (Owens and Nemeroff, 1991), there is ample evidence that cyclic AMP appears to regulate transcription of the CRF gene (Spengler *et al.*, 1992). However, very little work has been performed to identify other pathways involved in transcriptional regulation. Analysis of the CRF promoter reveals cyclic AMP regulatory regions as well as other regulatory sites involving transcription factors CTF/NPI and CPI (Vamvakopoulos *et al.*, 1990).

As noted above, CRF is clearly the major physiologic regulator of the HPA axis, the major endocrine axis activated by stress. Stress as defined by Selye (1936) is a non-specific response to any demand, frequently noxious, upon the body. Stress responses involve overactivation of the body's normal activational processes (Hennessey and Levine, 1979). Psychological stress is important, especially in combination with physical stressors in activating the HPA axis (Mason, 1971). Indeed, Burchfield (1979) redefined stress as "anything which causes an alteration of psychological homeostatic processes." Examples of psychological stressors include defeat/frustration, conflict or fear whereas typical physical stressors include exposure to pain, heat, cold and toxins.

When the HPA axis is activated, CRF acts on the anterior pituitary corticotrophs to release ACTH, which in turn acts on the adrenal cortex to release glucocorticoids, e.g., corticosterone in the rat, cortisol in primates. Soon after the isolation and characterization of CRF, the role of CRF in activation of the HPA axis was firmly established. Rivier *et al.* (1982) demonstrated that almost complete blockade of pituitary–adrenal responsiveness occurs following administration of a CRF antiserum, which neutralizes the actions of endogenous CRF.

CRF perikarya in the PVN are innervated by a myriad of neurons which modulate the activity of the CRF cells and therefore modify HPA activity. These include serotonergic (Liposits and Paul, 1987), dopaminergic (Liposits and Paul, 1989), and γ-aminobutyric acid (GABA)-ergic inputs (Meister *et al.*, 1988). Serotonergic inputs are stimulatory (Nakagama *et al.*, 1986). GABA-ergic/benzodiazepine agonists have been reported to inhibit CRF neuronal activity (Kalogeras *et al.*, 1990) whereas cholinergic and noradrenergic inputs are believed to be stimulatory (Suda *et al.*, 1985; Plotsky *et al.*, 1989). There is also evidence for a role for opioids modulating CRF secretion (Buckingman, 1986; Buckingman and Cooper, 1987; Tsagarakis *et al.*, 1989).

In addition, glucocorticoids, of course, act via negative feedback on the hypothalamus to regulate CRF release. Thus glucocorticoids decrease CRF immunoreactivity in the hypothalamus (Suda *et al.*, 1984). Conversely, Sawchenko (1987) reported that loss of glucocorticoids following adrenalectomy is associated with increased CRF immunostaining in the PVN; this is abolished by glucocorticoid replacement. Adrenalectomy also increases PVN c-fos immunoreactivity (Jacobsen *et al.*, 1990) and increases in CRF PVN mRNA as determined by *in situ* hybridization (Beyer *et al.*, 1988), the latter response inhibited by dexamethasone treatment (Kovacs and Mezey, 1987).

In modulating the HPA axis, glucocorticoids act at extrahypothalamic sites including the anterior pituitary and the hippocampus in addition to the hypothalamus. Glucocorticoids diminish anterior pituitary ACTH release (Giguere *et al.*, 1982). Adrenalectomy leads to a reducton in anterior pituitary CRF receptor concentration, presumably due to CRF hypersecretion, and this can be reversed by glucocorticoid supplementation, presumably due to inhibition of CRF release (Wynn *et al.*, 1983, 1985). Similarly, chronic corticosterone treatment leads to decreases in anterior pituitary CRF receptor number (Hauger *et al.*, 1987). Sapolsky *et al.* (1989) reported that fornix transection, which disrupts hippocampal input to the hypothalamus, renders the normally glucocorticoid-sensitive releases of CRF resistant. Hippocampectomy or destruction of the dorsal hippocampus results in a four-fold increase in PVN CRF mRNA production (Herman *et al.*, 1989).

Most importantly to the theme of this chapter, stress is known to alter regional rat brain CRF concentrations. Our group (Chappell *et al.*, 1986) exposed rats to acute 3 h cold immobilization stress or a 14-day regimen of daily stressors. Both acute and chronic stress paradigms led to a 50% decrease in median eminence CRF concentrations. Murakami *et al.* (1989) studied earlier time points and reported increases in CRF content in the median eminence 2.5 but not 5 min after ether stress. These early changes are thought to reflect changes in processing or packaging of CRF in granules; already at 2.5 min, ACTH levels had risen and CRF was already secreted.

Moldow *et al.* (1987) reported restraint stress-associated decreases in hypothalamic CRF concentrations 15 min after the initiation of stress. If the animals were treated with cycloheximide, this effect was abolished indicating that the increases observed were likely indicative of new protein synthesis. Similarly, Haas and George (1988) demonstrated increases in median eminence CRF content 24 h after a single 5 min footshock. Anisomycin, an inhibitor of protein synthesis, abolished this increase, and produced decreases in hypothalamic CRF concentrations.

Physical and behavioral stresses that activate the HPA axis and alter CRF tissue concentrations also alter CRF gene expression. These stressors include intraperitoneal hypertonic saline, naloxone-induced opiate withdrawal, swimming and restraint stress. CRF mRNA changes are seen as early as 4 h and last as long as 24 h after exposure to stress (Harbuz and Lightman, 1989). Herman *et al.* (1992) utilized intronic CRF probes to study changes in CRF mRNA expression following metyrapone administration, a drug that blocks adrenal steroid formation. Probes directed against the CRF exon indicated CRF mRNA levels were elevated 60 min after metyrapone treatment. Heteronuclear RNA increases, as detected by a CRF intronic probe, were seen as early as 15–30 min following metyrapone treatment. It would be interesting to determine how quickly heteronuclear CRF RNA rises in stress paradigms in comparison to the studies above which have measured total mRNA.

CRF, administered directly into the CNS, produces behaviors similar to those observed following exposure to stress. Structures that comprise the limbic system and the locus coereleus (LC) appear to be some of the neural substrates involved in activating the neuroendocrine stress responses. Intracerebroventricular (i.c.v.), but not peripheral, CRF produced dose-dependent increases in locomotor activity in a familiar environment and in the open field (Veldhuis and deWied, 1984; Eaves et al., 1985; Berridge and Dunn, 1986; Sherman and Kalin, 1987).

Moreover, the CRF antagonist, α-helical CRF_{9-41}, blocks the actions of centrally applied CRF (K. T. Britton et al., 1986b) whereas dexamethasone is ineffective in this regard; this suggests that pituitary–adrenal activation is not mediating the CNS effects of CRF (D. R. Britton et al., 1986b; K. T. Britton et al., 1986a). Britton and Indyk (1990) reported that ganglionic blocking drugs partially attenuate the locomotor activation of i.c.v. CRF, implying that the observed behaviors are secondary to increased sympathetic tone. Furthermore, CRF-induced locomotor activation is not reduced by destruction of dopaminergic nerve terminals (Swerdlow and Koob, 1985) or by treatment with opiate antagonists (Koob et al., 1984).

CRF has been shown to alter appetitive behaviors. CRF i.c.v. inhibits feeding in rats and sheep in different experimental paradigms (Britton et al., 1982; Gosnell et al., 1983). Decreases in food consumption after CRF administration have been observed even after administration of agents known to stimulate food intake such as muscimol, norepinephrine, neuropeptide Y, dynorphin, ethylketocyclazocine, and insulin (Levine et al., 1983; Morley et al., 1985; Heinrichs et al., 1992b). CRF will even prevent intake of familiar food seen in nutritionally deficient rats (Heinrichs and Koob, 1992). The available evidence suggests that CRF acts on the paraventricular nucleus to inhibit feeding because microinjection of CRF into this region is effective in this regard. In contrast, CRF was not effective following microinjection into the lateral hypothalamus, ventromedial hypothalamus, globus pallidus or caudate (Krahn et al., 1988).

Central CRF administration inhibits sexual behavior in male and female rats, an effect similar to that observed in animals exposed to stress (Sirinathsinghji et al., 1989). Microinjection of CRF into the arcuate–ventromedial area of the hypothalamus or the mesencephalic central gray area also suppressed sexual receptivity in female rats (Sirinathsinghji, 1986, Sirinathsinghji, 1987).

CRF injected centrally produces an anxiogenic and fear response, quite similar to what is observed after exposure to a stress. Britton et al. (1982) reported that i.c.v. CRF in rats increases the frequency of behaviors normally observed when animals are exposed to a novel environment. Increases in grooming and freezing behaviors were seen; decreases in rearing and the number of approaches to a food pellet were also seen. In mice, reduced time was spent in contact with novel stimuli; this resembled behaviors observed following periods of restraint stress. The CRF receptor antagonist, α-helical CRF$_{9-41}$ blocked this response when administered i.c.v. (Berridge and Dunn, 1986; Berridge and Dunn, 1987).

In the conflict test, an animal model used to reveal anxiogenic and anxiolytic properties of drugs, CRF has been shown to produce suppression of punished and non-punished responding, an effect characteristic of anxiety-provoking substances. This is not mediated by HPA axis activation (D. R. Britton et al., 1986). In addition, GABA-ergic mechanisms are implicated because ethanol (Britton and Koob, 1986) and chlordiazepoxide (Britton et al., 1985) block this CRF effect.

There are other stress-related behaviors produced by CRF. Central CRF administration potentiates acoustic startle in rats, an effect which can be blocked by the CRF receptor antagonist α-helical CRF (Swerdlow et al. 1989). This effect can also be blocked by chlordiazepoxide (Swerdlow et al., 1986). CRF produces an anxiogenic effect in a social interaction test. It decreases social interaction without altering locomotion and is reversed by the CRF receptor antagonist (Dunn and File, 1987). CRF facilitates stress-induced fighting induced by inescapable footshock (Tazi et al., 1987). The CRF receptor antagonist blocks this effect as well as stress-induced fighting behavior and also blocks anxiety observed in rats following exposure to odors associated with fear-induced urination and defecation from a different set of rats (Takahashi et al., 1990).

CRF i.c.v. increases stress-induced freezing behaviors elicited by mild electric footshock (Sherman and Kalin, 1988). The CRF receptor antagonist blocks the effects of both CRF-induced and shock-induced "freezing" when given 20 min prior to footshock. (Kalin et al., 1988; Kalin and Takahshi, 1990). Cole et al. (1990) showed that prior restraint stress enhances locomotor responses to saline injections and the intensity of stereotypic behaviors to amphetamine in rats. These sensitizing effects of stress can be attenuated by i.c.v. injections of the CRF receptor antagonist at the time of the initial stressor.

CRF also produces both taste and place aversions (Heinrichs et al., 1991). As highlighted above, psychological stress is an important factor in activating the HPA axis. Heinrichs et al. (1992b) recently reported that α-helical CRF$_{9-41}$ reverses the decreases in exploration in the elevated plus-maze induced by social defeat. Similar effects are observed with other stresses, including restraint stress and ethanol withdrawal (Baldwin et al. 1991). The CRF receptor antagonist will also reduce restraint stress-induced decreases in food intake (Krahn et al., 1986).

Kalin et al. (1989) studied the effects of i.c.v. CRF on non-human primate infants. Infant rhesus monkeys emit frequent distress vocalizations and alter activity levels when transiently separated from their mothers. CRF, at doses greater than 10 ng i.c.v., inhibited the increases in activity levels without affecting distress vocalizations. Large doses of CRF i.c.v. produce behavioral despair similar to that observed after long-term maternal separation (Kalin *et al.*, 1983; Kalin, 1990).

One of the neural substrates where CRF acts appears to be the LC (Valentino *et al.*, 1983). When administered i.c.v. or directly into the LC, CRF activates LC neurons as assessed electrophysiologically (Valentino *et al.*, 1983) and neurochemically (Butler *et al.*, 1990). Valentino and Wehby (1988) reported that the CRF receptor antagonist, when injected directly into the LC, reverses activation of the LC produced by hemodynamic stress. Butler *et al.* (1990) provided evidence for the LC to be the site mediating CRF-induced anxiogenesis. Bilateral infusions of CRF (1–100 ng) into the LC of rats produced a dose-dependent increase in the time spent in the darkened compartment and decreased time spent exploring the outside of the compartment, measures of increased anxiety. The investigators also showed that the concentration of 3,4-dihydroxyphenylglycol, a metabolite of norepinephrine, in forebrain projection areas was elevated, suggesting that CRF increased LC noradrenergic neuronal turnover. Moreover, Cole and Koob (1988) reported that propranolol, a β-adrenergic receptor antagonist, blocked the reduction in punished responding produced by i.c.v. CRF administration in the conflict test, thus also implicating noradrenergic neural mechanisms in the effects of CRF. GABA-ergic mechanisms appear also to be important in interacting with LC CRF activity. Owens and Nemeroff (1991) demonstrated that a triazolobenzodiazepine, alprazolam, produces effects in the LC opposite to that of acute or chronic stress, i.e. that acute and chronic alprazolam administration decreases LC CRF concentrations (see Figure 2).

The amygdala has also been strongly implicated in the behavioral actions of CRF. Heinrichs *et al.* (1992a) reported that behavioral exploration is suppressed by doses of CRF 100-fold lower, after microinjections into the amygdala than when injected i.c.v. The same is true for rats exposed to social defeat followed by 30 min of prolonged threat and then placed on the elevated plus-maze. Rats in this paradigm spend less time than controls on the open arms but this reduction can be reversed by the bilateral injection of 250 ng α-helical CRF_{9-41} directly into the central nucleus of the amygdala. Lee and Tsai (1989) and Liang and Lee (1988) showed that CRF injections into the central nucleus of the amygdala produce locomotor stimulation in mice, facilitate inhibitory avoidance learning and reduce exploratory behaviors in rats.

Davis (1992) has recently reported that lesions of the central nucleus of the amygdala abolish fear-potentiated startle. Low-level stimulation of this region enhances acoustic startle amplitude. CRF has been found to be contained in many of the central amygdala neurons which project to the PVN, preoptic region and bed nucleus of the stria terminalis.

Gray (1990) concludes that amygdalofugal CRF pathways participate in the autonomic, endocrine and behavioral stress response. In fact, when the central nucleus of the amygdala is stimulated, there are increases in respiration, cardiac

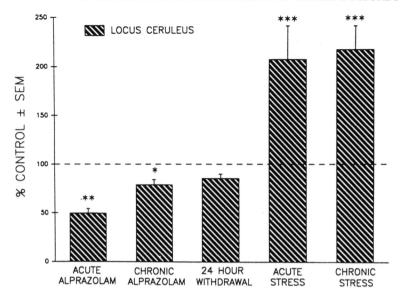

Figure 2 Effects of alprazolam and stress on CRF concentrations in the locus coeruleus. The anxiolytic/antidepressant triazolobenzodiazepine, alprazolam, produces effects in the locus coeruleus opposite to those of acute or chronic stress but not alprazolam withdrawal. $p < 0.05$, $^{**}p < 0.01$, $^{***}p < 0.001$ compared with controls (Reprinted by permission from Owens *et al.*, 1991)

output and emotional responses. In addition, lesions to the central nucleus of the amygdala block the rise in plasma ACTH concentration observed after immobilization stress (Beaulieu *et al.*, 1986). Lesions of the central nucleus of the amygdala also block corticosterone secretion following psychological stressors (Van der Kar *et al.*, 1991). More studies are needed to determine precisely which type of stressors activate the amygdala and exactly which neuroanatomical pathways are implicated (Koob *et al.*, 1993).

Not only are more studies needed to better understand exactly how CRF mediates the stress response, but we need to more closely scrutinize the potential roles for CRF in the pathophysiology of a variety of devastating psychiatric disorders. Psychosocial stressors are known to play a pre-eminent role in the pathogenesis of affective disorders (Kendler *et al.*, 1993; Brown and Harris, 1989) and various investigators have provided evidence which links HPA axis hyperactivity with affective and perhaps anxiety disorders. Included in these studies are findings which support a role for CRF hypersecretion in major depression (Nemeroff, 1988). It has long been known that patients with major depression frequently exhibit dexamethasone non-suppression (Carroll *et al.*, 1981) and other evidence of adrenocortical hyperactivity. Later, depressed patients were shown to exhibit a blunted ACTH response following CRF administration (Gold *et al.*, 1984; Holsboer *et al.*, 1984). Krishnan *et al.* (1993) reported that blunted ACTH response to CRF occurs in dexamethasone non-suppressors.

Nemeroff *et al.* (1984) originally reported that CRF-like immunoreactivity was increased in the cerebrospinal fluid (CSF) of patients with major depression. This has been confirmed in subsequent studies (Arato *et al.*, 1989; Banki *et al.*, 1987; France *et al.*, 1988) (see Figure 3). In panic disorder, Roy-Byrne *et al.* (1986) reported blunted ACTH responses to CRF, suggesting that CRF dysregulation plays a role in this anxiety disorder. However, CSF CRF concentrations are not elevated in patients with panic disorder (Jolkkonen *et al.*, 1993). Smith *et al.* (1989) reported a reduced ACTH response to CRF in patients with post-traumatic stress disorder, one-half of whom also fulfilled the DSM-III cri-

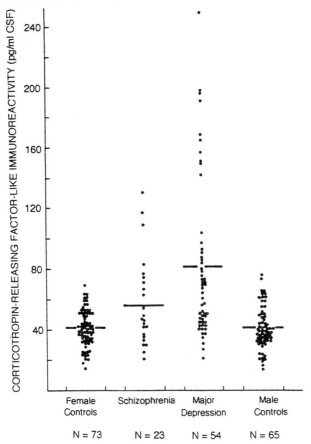

Figure 3 CSF CRF-like immunoreactivity in patients with schizophrenia (as defined in *Diagnostic and Statistical Manual of Mental Disorders*, 3rd edn (DSM-III), patients with DSM-III major depression, and control subjects with various peripheral neurologic diseases. Patients with DSM-III major depression exhibited a markedly higher (almost two-fold) CSF CRF concentration than the control subjects (Newman–Keuls test, $p < 0.001$). The mean CSF CRF concentrations in the depressed group was also significantly higher than that of the schizophrenic group (Newman–Keuls test, $p < 0.05$). Six (26%) of the 23 schizophrenic patients and 24 (44%) of the 54 depressed patients had higher CSF CRF concentrations than the highest value among the sex-matched control subjects (from Banki *et al.*, *Am. J. Psychiatry*, **144**, 873–877, 1987, the American Psychiatric Association. Reprinted by permission)

teria for major depression. Further study of CRF regulation in various anxiety disorders is of interest as well as in mixed depression–anxiety states. Lipophilic CRF receptor antagonists may represent a novel class of antidepressants and/or anxiolytic agents.

An area which clearly also warrants more extensive exploration is the study of CRF gene regulation. As described above, only cyclic AMP-mediated effects have been well explored and other signal transduction pathways implicated in CRF transcription need to be elucidated. It is possible that dysregulation of the CRF gene at the level of transcriptional control could play a significant role in certain disease processes.

CRF was isolated slightly over a decade ago, yet a remarkable literature about it has accrued. We expect the knowledge of this peptide to continue to expand rapidly in the next decade. We hope to better understand its precise role in stress and in clinical syndromes exacerbated by stress.

ACKNOWLEDGMENTS

Supported by NIMH MH-42088 and the John D. and Catherine T. MacArthur Foundation (C.B.N.). J.W.K. is the recipient of a Pfizer Fellowship and a NARSAD Young Investigator's Award.

REFERENCES

Aguilera, G., Harwood, J. P., Wilson, J. X. *et al.* (1986). Receptor-mediated actions of corticotropin-releasing factor in pituitary gland and nervous system. *Neuroendocrinology*, **43**, 79–88.

Antoni, F. A., Palkovits, M., Makara, G. B. *et al.* (1983). Immunoreactive corticotropin-releasing hormone in the hypothalamoinfundibular tract. *Neuroendocrinology*, **36**, 415–423.

Arato, M., Banki, C. M., Bissette, G. and Nemeroff, C. B. (1986). Elevated cerebrospinal corticotropin-releasing factor in suicide victims. *Biol. Psychiatry*, **25**, 355–359.

Baldwin, H. A., Rassnick, S., Rivier, J. *et al.* (1991). CRF antagonist reverses the "anxiogenic" response to ethanol withdrawal in the rat. *Psychopharmacology*, **103**, 227–232.

Banki, C. M., Bissette, G., Arato, M. *et al.* (1987). Cerebrospinal fluid corticotropin-releasing factor like immunoreactivity in depression and schizophrenia. *Am. J. Psychiatry*, **144**, 873–877.

Battaglia, G., Webster, E. L. and DeSouza, E. B. (1987). Characterization of corticotropin releasing factor receptor-mediated adenylate cyclase activity in the rat central nervous system. *Synapse*, **1**, 572–581.

Beaulieu, S., Di Paolo, T. and Barden, N. (1986). Control of ACTH secretion by the central nucleus of the amygdala: implications of the serotonergic system and its relevance to glucocorticoid delayed negative feedback mechanism. *Neuroendocrinology*, **44**, 247–254.

Berridge, C. W. and Dunn, A. J. (1987). A corticotropin-releasing factor antagonist reverses the stress-induced changes of exploratory behavior in mice. *Horm. Behav.*, **21**, 393–401.

Beyer, H. S., Matta, S. G. and Sharp, B. M. (1988). Regulation of the messenger RNA for corticotropin-releasing factor in the paraventricular nucleus and other brain sites of the rat. *Endocrinology*, **123**, 2117–2123.

Bloom, F. E., Battenberg, E. L. F., Rivier, J. and Vale, W. (1982). Corticotropin releasing factor (CRF) immunoreactive neurons and fibers in rat hypothalamus. *Regul. Pept.*, **4**, 43–48.

Britton, D. R. and Indyk, E. (1990). Central effects of corticotropin-releasing factor(CRF): evidence for similar interactions with environmental novelty and with caffeine. *Psychopharmacology*, **101**, 366–370.

Britton, D. R., Koob, G. F., Rivier, J. and Vale, W. (1982). Intraventricular corticotropin-releasing factor enhances behavioral effects of novelty. *Life Sci.*, **31**, 363–367.

Britton, D. R., Varela, M., Garcia, A. and Rosenthal, M. (1986). Dexemethasone suppresses pituitary–adrenal but not behavioral effects of centrally administered CRF. *Life Sci.*, **38**, 211–216.

Britton, K. T. and Koob, G. F. (1986). Alcohol reverses the proconflict effect of corti-cotropin-releasing factor. *Regul. Pept.*, **16**, 315–320.

Britton, K. T., Morgan, J., Rivier, J. *et al.* (1985). Chlordiazepoxide attenuates response suppression induced by corticotropin-releasing factor in the conflict test. *Psychopharmacology*, **86**, 170–174.

Britton, K. T., Lee, G., Dana, R. *et al.* (1986a). Activating and "anxiogenic" effects of corti-cotropin-releasing factor are not inhibited by blockade of the pituitary–adrenal system with dexamethasone. *Life Sci.*, **39**, 1281–1286.

Brown, G. W. and Harris, T. O. (1989). *Life Events and Illness*. Guilford Press, New York.

Buckingham, J. C. (1986). Stimulation and inhibition of corticotropin-releasing factor secretion by beta-endorphin. *Neuroendocrinology*, **42**, 148–152.

Buckingham, J. C. and Cooper, T. A. (1987). Interrelationships of opioidergic and adrenergic mechanisms controlling the secretion of corticotropin-releasing factor in the rat. *Neuroendocrinology*, **46**, 199–206.

Burchfield, S. (1979). The stress response: a new perspective. *Psychosom. Med.*, **41**, 661–671.

Butler, P. D., Weiss, J. M., Stout, J. C. and Nemeroff, C. B. (1990). Corticotropin-releasing factor produces fear-enhancing and behavioral activating effects following infusion into the locus coeruleus. *J. Neurosci.*, **10**, 176–183.

Carroll, B. J., Feinberg, M., Greden, J. R. *et al.* (1981). A specific laboratory test for the diagnosis of melancholia. *Arch. Gen. Psychiatry*, **38**, 15–22.

Chappell, P. B., Smith, M. A., Kilts, C. D. *et al.* (1986). Alterations in corticotropin-releasing factor-like immunoreactivity in discrete rat brain regions after acute and chronic stress. *J. Neurosci.*, **6**, 2908–2914.

Cole, B. J. and Koob, G. F. (1988). Propranolol antagonizes the enhanced conditioned fear produced by corticotropin-releasing factor. *J. Pharmacol. Exp. Ther.*, **247**, 902–910.

Cole, B. J., Cador, M., Stinus, L. *et al.* (1990). Central administration of CRF antagonist blocks the development of stress-induced behavioral sensitization. *Brain Res.*, **512**, 343–346.

Daikoku, S., Okamura, Y., Kawano, H. *et al.* (1984). CRF-containing neurons of the rat hypothalamus. *Cell Tissue Res.*, **238**, 539–544.

Davis, M. (1992). The Role of the amygdala in fear-potentiated startle: implications for animal models of anxiety. *Trends Pharmacol. Sci.*, **13**, 35–41.

DeSouza, E. B. (1987). Corticotropin-releasing factor receptors in the rat central nervous system: characterization and regional distribution. *J. Neurosci.*, **7**, 88–100.

Dunn, A. J. and File, S. E. (1987). Corticotropin-releasing factor has an anxiogenic action in the social interaction test. *Horm. Behav.*, **21**, 193–202.

Eaves, M., Britton, K. T., Rivier, J. *et al.* (1985). Effects of corticotropin-releasing factor on locomotor activity in hypophysectomized rats. *Peptides*, **4**, 923–926.

France, R. D., Urban, B., Krishnan, K. R. R. *et al.* (1988). Cerebrospinal fluid corticotropin-releasing factor-like immunoreactivity in chronic pain patients with and without major depression. *Biol. Psychiatry*, **23**, 86–88.

Furutani, Y., Morimoto, Y., Shibahara, S. *et al.* (1983). Cloning and sequence analysis of cDNA for ovine corticotropin-releasing factor precursor. *Nature (Lond.)*, **301**, 537–540.

Giguere, V., Labrie, F., Cote, J. *et al.* (1982). Stimulation of cyclic AMP accumulation and corticotropin release by synthetic ovine corticotopin-releasing factor in rat anterior pituitary cells: site of glucocorticoid action. *Proc. Natl Acad. Sci. USA*, **79**, 3466–3469.

Gold, P. W., Chrousos, G., Kellner, C. *et al.* (1984). Psychiatric implications of basic and clinical studies with corticotropin-releasing factor. *Am. J. Psychiatry*, **141**, 619–627.

Gosnell, B. A., Morley, J. E. and Levine, A. S. (1983) A comparison of the effects of corticotropin-releasing factor and sauvagine on food intake. *Pharmacol. Biochem. Behav.*, **19**, 771–775.

Gray, T. S. (1990). The organization and possible function of amygdaloid corticotropin-releasing factor pathways. In *Corticotropin Releasing Factor: Basic and Clinical Studies of a Neuropeptide* (eds E. D. Desouza and C. B. Nemeroff), pp. 53–68. CRC Press, Boca Raton, FL.

Haas, D. A. and George, S. (1988). Single or repeated mild stress increases synthesis and release of hypothalamic corticotropin-releasing factor. *Brain Res.*, **461**, 230–237.

Harbuz, M. S. and Lightman, S. L. (1989). Glucocorticoid inhibition of stress-induced changes in hypothalamic corticotropin-releasing factor mRNA and proenkephalin A messenger RNA. *Neuropeptides*, **14**, 17–20.

Heinrichs, S. C. and Koob, G. F. (1992). Corticotropin-releasing factor modulates dietary preference in nutritionally and physically stressed rats. *Psychopharmacology*, **109**, 177–184.

Heinrichs, S. C., Britton, K. T. and Koob, G. F. (1991). Both conditioned taste preference and aversion induced by corticotropin-releasing factor. *Pharmacol. Biochem. Behav.*, **40**, 717–721.

Heinrichs, S. C., Cole, B. J., Pich, E. M. *et al.* (1992a). Brain corticotropin-releasing factor attenuates feeding induced by neuropeptide Y or a tail-pinch stressor. *Peptides*, **13**, 879–884.

Heinrichs, S. C., Pich, E. M., Miczek, K. *et al.* (1992b). Corticotropin-releasing factor antagonist reduces emotionality in socially defeated rats via direct neurotropic action. *Brain Res.*, **581**, 190–197.

Hennessey, J. W. and Levine, S. (1979). Stress, arousal and the pituitary adrenal system: a psychoendocrine hypothesis. In *Progress in Psychobiology and Physiological Psychology*, 8th edn (eds J. M. Sprague and A. N. Epstein), pp. 133–178. Academic Press, New York.

Herman, J. P., Schafer, M. K. H., Young, E. A. *et al.* (1989). Evidence for hippocampal regulation of neuroendocrine neurons of the hypothalamo-pituitary–adrenocortical axis. *J. Neurosci.*, **9**, 3072–2082.

Herman, J. P., Schafer, M. K. H., Thompson, R. C. and Watson, S. J. (1992). Rapid regulation of corticotropin-releasing hormone gene transcription *in vivo. Mol. Endocrinol.*, **6**, 1061–1069.

Holsboer, F., Von Bardeleben, U., Gerken, A. *et al.* (1984). Blunted corticotropin and normal cortisol response to human corticotropin-releasing factor in depression. *N. Engl. J. Med.*, **311**, 1127.

Jacobson, L., Sharp, F. R. and Dallman, M. F. (1990). Induction of fos-like immunoreactivity in hypothalamic corticotropin-releasing factor neurons after adrenalectomy in the rat. *Endocrinology*, **126**, 1709–1719.

Jolkkonen, J., Lepola, U., Bissette, G. and Nemeroff, C. B. (1993). Cerebrospinal fluid corticotropin-releasing factor is not affected in panic disorder. *Biol. Psychiatry*, **33**, 136–138.

Kalin, N. H. (1990). Behavioral and endocrine studies of corticotropin-releasing hormone in primates. In *Corticotropin-releasing Factor: Basic and Clinical Studies of a Neuropeptide* (eds E. B. DeSouza and C. B. Nemeroff), pp. 275–289. CRC Press, Boca Raton, FL.

Kalin, N. H. and Takahashi, L. K. (1990). Fear-motivated behavior induced by prior shock experience is mediated by corticotropin-releasing hormone systems. *Brain Res.*, **509**, 80–84.

Kalin, N. H., Shelton, S. E., Kraemer, G. and McKinney, W. (1983). Corticotropin-releasing factor administered intracerebroventricularly to rhesus monkeys. *Peptides*, **4**, 217–220.

Kalin, N. H., Sherman, J. E. and Takahashi, L. K. (1988). Antagonism of endogenous CRH systems attenuates stress-induced freezing behavior in rats. *Brain Res.*, **457**, 130–135.

Kalin, N. H., Shelton, S. E. and Barksdale, C. M. (1989). Behavioral and physiologic effects of CRH administered to infant primates undergoing maternal separation. *Neuropsychopharmacology*, **2**, 97–104.

Kalogeras, K. T., Calogero, A. E., Kuribayashi, T. *et al.* (1990). *In vitro* and *in vivo* effects of the triazolobenzodiazepine alprazolam on hypothalamic–pituitary–adrenal function: pharmacological and clinical implications. *J. Clin. Endocrinol. Metab.*, **70**, 1462–1471.

Kawata, M., Hashimoto, K., Takahara, J. and Sano, Y. (1982). Immunohistochemical demonstration of the localization of corticotropin-releasing factor containing neurons of the hypothalamus of mammals including primates. *Anat. Embryol.*, **165**, 303–313.

Kendler, K. S., Kessler, R. C., Neale, M. C. *et al.* (1993). The prediction of major depression in women: toward an integrated etiologic model. *Am. J. Psychiatry*, **150**, 1139–1148.

Koob, G. F., Swerdlow, N., Seeligson, M. *et al.* (1984). Effects of alphafluphenthixol and naloxone on CRF-induced locomotor activation. *Neuroendocrinology*, **39**, 459–464.

Koob, G. F., Heinrichs, S. C., Pich, E. M. *et al.* (1993). The role of corticotropin-releasing factor in behavioral responses to stress. In *Corticotropin-releasing Factor: Ciba Foundation Symposium 172*, pp. 277–295. Wiley, Chichester.

Kovacs, K. J. and Mezey, E. (1987). Dexamethasone inhibits corticotropin-releasing factor gene expression in the rat paraventricular nucleus. *Neuroendocrinology*, **46**, 365–368.

Krahn, D. D., Gosnell, B. A., Grace, M. and Levine, A. S. (1986). CRF antagonist partially reverses CRF and stress-induced effects on feeding. *Brain Res. Bull.*, **17**, 285–289.

Krahn, D. D., Gosnell, B. A., Levine, A. S. and Morley, J. E. (1988). Behavioral effects of corticotropin-releasing factor: localization and characterization of central effects. *Brain Res.*, **443**, 63–69.

Krishnan, K. R. R., Ritchie, J. C., Reed, D. *et al.* (1993). The corticotropin-releasing factor stimulation test in patients with major depression: relationship to dexamethasone test results. *Depression*, **1**, 133–136.

Lee, E. H. Y. and Tsai, M. J. (1989). The hippocampus and amygdala mediate the locomotor stimulating effects of corticotropin-releasing factor in mice. *Behav. Neurol. Biol.*, **51**, 412–423.

Levine, A. S., Rogers, B., Kneip, J. *et al.* (1983). Effect of centrally administered corticotropin-releasing factor (CRF) on multiple feeding paradigms. *Neuropharmacology*, **22**, 337–339.

Liang, K. C. and Lee, E. H. Y. (1988). Intra-amygdala injections of corticotropin-releasing factor facilitate inhibitory avoidance learning and reduce exploratory behavior in rats. *Psychopharmacology*, **96**, 232–236.

Liposits, Z. P. C. and Paul, W. K. (1987). Synaptic interaction of serotonergic actions and corticotropin-releasing factor (CRF) synthesizing neurons in the hypothalamic paraventricular nucleus of the rat. *Histochemistry*, **86**, 541–549.

Liposits, Z. P. C. and Paul, W. K. (1989). Association of dopaminergic fibers with corticotropin-releasing hormone (CRH)-synthesizing neurons in the paraventricular nucleus of the rat hypothalamus. *Histochemistry*, **93**, 119–127.

Mason, J. W. (1971). A re-evaluation of the concept of "non-specificity" in stress specificity theory. *J. Psychiatr. Res.*, **8**, 323–333.

Meister, B., Hokfelt, T., Geffard, M. and Oertel, W. (1988). Glutamic acid decarboxylase- and γ-aminobutyric acid-like immuno-reactivities in corticotopin-releasing factor-containing parvocellular neurons of the hypothalamic paraventricular nucleus. *Neuroendocrinology*, **48**, 516–526.

Moldow, R. W., Kastin, A. J., Graf, M. and Fischman, A. J. (1987). Stress mediated changes in hypothalamic corticotropin-releasing factor-like immunoreactivity. *Life Sci.*, **40**, 413–418.

Morley, J. E., Levine, A. S., Gosnell, B. A. and Krahn, D. D. (1985). Peptides as central regulators of feeding. *Brain Res. Bull.*, **14**, 511–519.

Murakami, K., Akana, S., Dallman, M. F. and Ganong, W. F. (1989). Correlation between the stress-induced transient increase in corticotropin-releasing hormone content of the median eminence of the hypothalamus and adrenocorticotropic hormone secretion. *Neuroendocrinology*, **49**, 233–241.

Nakagama, Y., Suda, T., Yajima, F. *et al.* (1986). Effects of serotonin, cyproheptadine and reserpine on corticotropin-releasing factor release from the rat hypothalamus *in vitro*. *Brain Res.*, **386**, 232–239.

Nemeroff, C. B., Widerlow, E., Bissette, G. *et al.* (1984). Elevated concentrations of corticotropin-releasing factor-like immunoreactivity in depressed patients. *Science*, **226**, 1342.

Owens, M. J., Bissette, G. and Nemeroff, C. B. (1989). Acute effects of alprazolam and adinazolam on the concentrations of corticotropin-releasing factor in rat brain. *Synapse*, **4**, 196–202.

Owens, M. J. and Nemeroff, C. B. (1991). Physiology and pharmacology of corticotropin-releasing factor. *Pharmacol. Rev.*, **43**, 425–473.

Owens, M. J., Vargas, M. A., Knight, D. L., Nemeroff, C. B. (1991). The effects of alprazolam on corticotropin-releasing factor neurons in the rat brain: acute time course, chronic treatment and abrupt withdrawal. *J. Pharmacol. Exp. Ther.*, **258**, 349–356.

Perrin, M. H., Haas, Y., Rivier, J. E. and Vale, W. W. (1986). Corticotropin releasing factor binding to the anterior pituitary receptor is modulated by divalent cations and guanyl nucleotides. *Endocrinology*, **118**, 1171–1179.

Piekut, D. T. and Joseph, S. A. (1985). Relationship of CRF-immunostained cells and magnocellular neurons in the paraventricular nucleus of rat hypothalamus. *Peptides*, **6**, 873–882.

Plotsky, P. M., Cunningham, E. T., Jr and Widmaier, E. P. (1989). Catecholaminergic modulation of corticotropin-releasing factor and adrenocorticotropin secretion. *Endocr. Rev.*, **10**, 437–458.

Rivier, C., Rivier, J. and Vale, W. (1982). Inhibition of adrenocorticotropic hormone secretion in the rat by immunoneutralization of corticotropin-releasing factor. *Science*, **218**, 377–379.

Roy-Byrne, P. P., Olde, T., Post, R. *et al.* (1986). The corticotropin-releasing factor stimulation test in patients with panic disorder. *Am. J. Psychiatry*, **143**, 896–899.

Sawchenko, P. E. (1987). Adrenalectomy-induced enhancement of CRF and vasopressin immunoreactivity in parvocellular neurosecretory neurons: anatomic, peptide and steroid specificity. *J. Neurosci.*, **7**, 1093–1106.

Seyle, H. (1936), A syndrome produced by diverse noxious agents. *Nature*, **32**, 138.

Sherman, J. E. and Kalin, N. H. (1987). The effects of ICV-CRH on novelty-induced behavior. *Pharmacol. Biochem. Behav.*, **26**, 699–703.

Sherman, J. E. and Kalin, N. H. (1988). ICV-CRH alters stress-induced freezing behavior without affecting pain sensitivity. *Pharmacol. Biochem. Behav.*, **30**, 801–807.

Sirinathsinghi, D. J. S. (1986). Regulation of lordosis behavior in the female rat by corticotropin-releasing factor, b-endorphin/cortocotropin and leutinizing hormone-releasing hormone neuronal systems in the medial preoptic area. *Brain Res.*, **375**, 49–56.

Sirinathsinghi, D. J. S. (1987). Inhibitory influence of corticotropin-releasing factor on components of sexual behavior in the rat male., *Brain Res.*, **407**, 185–190.

Sirinathsinghi, D., Rees, L. H., Rivier, J. and Vale, W. (1989). Corticotropin-releasing factor is a potent inhibitor of sexual receptivity in the female rat. *Nature*, **305**, 232–235.

Smith, M. A., Davidson, J., Ritchie, J. *et al.* (1989). The corticotropin-releasing hormone test in patients with post traumatic stress disorder. *Biol. Psychiatry*, **26**, 349–355.

Spengler, D., Rupprecht, R., Van, L. P. and Hoelsboer, F. (1992). Identification and characterization of a 3′, 5′-cyclic adenosine monophosphate-responsive element in the human CRF gene promoter. *Mol. Endocrinol.*, **6**, 1931–1941.

Suda, T., Tomori, N., Tozawa, F. *et al.* (1984). Effect of dexamethasone on immunoreactive corticotropin-releasing factor in the rat median eminence and intermediate-posterior pituitary. *Endocrinology*, **114**, 851–854.

Suda, T., Yajima, F., Tomori, N. *et al.* (1985). *In vitro* study of immunoreactive corticotropin-releasing factor release from the rat hypothalamus. *Life Sci.*, **37**, 1499–1504.

Swanson, L. W., Sawchenko, P. E., Rivier, J. and Vale, W. W. (1983). Organization of ovine corticotropin-releasing factor immunoreactive cells and fibers in the rat brain: an immunohistochemical study. *Neuroendocrinology*, **36**, 165–186.

Swerdlow, N. R. and Koob, G. F. (1985). Separate neural substrates of the locomotor activating properties of amphetamine, heroin, caffeine and corticotropin-releasing factor (CRF) in the rat. *Pharmacol. Biochem. Behav.*, **23**, 303–307.

Swerdlow, N. R., Geyer, M. A., Vale, W. W. and Koob, G. F. (1986). Corticotropin-releasing factor potentiates acoustic startle in rats: blockade by chlordiazepoxide. *Psychopharmacology*, **88**, 147–152.

Swerdlow, N. R., Britton, K. T. and Koob, G. F. (1989). Potentiation of acoustic startle by corticotropin-releasing factor (CRF) and fear are both reversed by α-helical CRF (9–41). *Neuropsychopharmacology*, **2**, 285–292.

Takahashi, L. K., Kalin, N. H. and Baker, E. W. (1990). Corticotropin-releasing factor antagonist attenuates defensive-withdrawal behavior elicited by odors of stressed conspecifics. *Behav. Neurosci.*, **104**, 386–389.

Tazi, A., Dantzer, R., LeMoal, M. *et al.* (1987). Corticotropin-releasing factor antagonist blocks stress-induced fighting in rats. *Regul. Pept.*, **18**, 37–42.

Thompson, R. C., Seasholtz, A. F. and Herbert, E. (1987). Rat corticotropin-releasing hormone gene: sequence and tissue specific expression. *Mol. Endocrinol.*, **1**, 363–368.

Tsagarakis, S., Navarra, P., Rees, L. H. *et al.* (1989). Morphine directly modulates the release of corticotropin-releasing factor-41 from the rat hypothalamus *in vitro*. *Neuroendocrinology*, **49**, 98–101.

Vale, W., Speiss, J. and Rivier, J. (1981). Characterization of a 41-residue ovine hypothalamic peptide that stimulates secretion of corticotropin and β-endorphin. *Science*, **213**, 1394–1397.

Valentino, R. J. and Wehby, R. G. (1988). Corticotropin-releasing factor: evidence for a neurotransmitter role in the locus ceruleus during hemodynamic stress. *Neuroendocrinology*, **48**, 674–677.

Valentino, R. J., Foote, S. L. and Aston-Jones, G. (1983). Corticotropin-releasing factor activates noradrenergic neurons of the locus coeruleus. *Brain Res.*, **270**, 363–367.

Vamvakopoulos, N. C., Kaul, M., Mayol, V. *et al.* (1990). Structural analysis of the regulatory region of the human corticotropin-releasing hormone gene. *FEBS Lett.*, **267**, 1–5.

Van der Kar, L. D., Peichowski, R. A., Rittenhouse, P. A. and Gray, T. S. (1991). Amygdaloid lesions: differential effect of conditioned stress and immobilization-induced increases in corticosterone and renin secretion. *Neuroendocrinology*, **54**, 89–95.

Veldhuis, H. D. and deWied, D. (1984). Differential behavioral actions of corticotropin-releasing factor (CRF). *Pharmacol. Biochem. Behav.*, **21**, 707–713.

Wynn, P. C., Aguilera, G., Norell, J. and Catt, K. J. (1983). Properties and regulation of high-affinity pituitary receptors for corticotropin-releasing factor. *Biochem. Biophys. Res. Commun.*, **110**, 602–208.

Wynn, P. C., Harwood, J. P., Catt, K. J. and Aguilera, G. (1985). Regulation of corticotropin-releasing factor (CRF) receptors in the rat pituitary gland: effects of adrenalectomy on CRF receptors and corticotroph responses. *Endocrinology*, **116**, 1653–1659.

Part VI

SOCIAL PHOBIA

18 Advances in the Psychopharmacology of Social Phobia

JOHAN A. DEN BOER, IRENE M. VAN VLIET AND HERMAN G. M. WESTENBERG
Department of Psychiatry, Academic Hospital, Utrecht, The Netherlands

INTRODUCTION

Anxiety in social situations, e.g. during public speaking, has been recognized throughout the ages as a severe and incapacitating experience. Already many centuries ago bodily as well as psychological symptoms, including anticipatory anxiety, were recognized.

> It confounds voice and memory, as Lucian wittingly brings in Jupiter Tragoedus so much afraid of his auditory, when he was to make a speech to the rest of the gods, that he could not utter a ready word . . . Many men are so amazed and astonished with fear, they know not where they are, what they say, what they do, and that which is worst, it tortures them many days before with continual affrights and suspicion (Burton, 1621 [reprint 1977], p. 261)

According to DSM-III-R criteria, social phobics are afraid of, and avoid situations in which the individual is exposed to the scrutiny of other people because of fear of acting in an embarrassing way (American Psychiatric Association, 1987). In these situations such patients experience both subjective and somatic symptoms of anxiety, including trembling, blushing and sweating.

Epidemiological studies have suggested that this disorder is equally common in males and females (Marks and Gelder, 1966; Solyom *et al.*, 1986; Amies *et al.*, 1983), and the lifetime prevalence is estimated at 2.8% (Regier *et al.*, 1988). The age of onset is usually in late adolescence (Marks and Gelder, 1966; Amies *et al.*, 1983; Solyom *et al.* 1986). In spite of the fact that together with panic disorder and obsessive-compulsive disorder, social phobia has a high descriptive validity, a high degree of comorbidity has been described. Disorders with the highest rate of co-occurrence are agoraphobia, simple phobia, major depression and obsessive-compulsive disorder (Schneier *et al.*, 1992).

A variety of theories, most of them not of a biological nature, have been proposed to explain the origins of social phobia. Traditionally the treatment of

Advances in the Neurobiology of Anxiety Disorders. Edited by H. G. M. Westenberg, J. A. Den Boer and D. L. Murphy
©1996 John Wiley & Sons Ltd

social phobia has been the domain of psychotherapists: psychoanalytic psychotherapy or behavioral therapy (Emmelkamp, 1982; Leary, 1983; Nichols, 1974). Advances in cognitive-behavioral therapy have effectively reduced incapacitating and maladaptive social anxiety (Heimburg and Barlow, 1991).

From a sociological perspective De Swaan has attributed the rise of agoraphobia at the end of the nineteenth century to societal transformations during the initial phase of industrialization (de Swaan, 1981). Due to the fact that the social distance between the *petite bourgeoisie* and the working class became more difficult to maintain, he asserted that the public appearance of bourgeois women was increasingly dangerous. Because of these changes in society, de Swaan suggested that "the urban market place had become a threatened space, the scene of roughness, violent menace and erotic seduction". In spite of the appealing nature of this viewpoint, the evidence for this hypothesis is meager. Two points of criticism are relevant. First of all agoraphobia had already been described centuries ago, and thus before the onset of the societal transformations for which he postulates a causal relationship with the rise of agoraphobia. Secondly, transcultural studies suggest that the same clinical picture is present in totally different cultures like the eskimo's, who may suffer from "kayak angst", a clinical picture very similar to panic attacks resulting in avoidance behavior (Murphy, 1982). In a similar vein, a recent sociological study tried to explain the increased occurrence of social phobia, by assuming that social phobics reproduce the expressions of social distinction that were taken for granted one or two generations ago, but unfortunately empirical testing was unable to confirm this hypothesis (Gomperts, 1992).

SUBTYPES OF SOCIAL PHOBIA

In most studies different reliabilities for the different anxiety disorders have been reported. The kappa value of generalized anxiety disorder is generally found to be relatively low in most studies (Riskind *et al.*, 1987), whereas the reliability of other anxiety disorders such as simple phobia, panic disorder and obsessive-compulsive disorder was found to be higher (Barlow, 1985; Riskind *et al.*, 1987). In a recent reliability study in which DSM-III-R criteria were used throughout the study, DiNardo *et al.* (1993) reported a kappa value of 0.79 for social phobia as a principal diagnosis, although no distinction was made between specific and generalized subtypes of social phobia.

The latter distinction has become a focus of recent investigation since these subtypes were included in the DSM-III-R. Patients can be classified as suffering from the generalized subtype if the phobic situation includes most social situations. The specific subtype according the DSM-III-R requires fear for only specific situations (e.g. public speaking).

Investigations of the validity of this social phobia subtype distinction revealed that these subtypes show significant differences in severity in social phobia and social anxiety as well as in the level of general distress (Turner *et al.*, 1992). In general, patients with specific social phobia were less impaired in terms of social anxiety and showed lower levels of general distress than patients with the generalized subtype. There is circumstantial evidence that familial contribution may play a role in the development of social phobia. In a recent study in relatives of social phobia probands it was found that social phobia (DSM-III-R), occurring in the absence of other lifetime anxiety disorder diagnoses, was associated with an increased risk (16%) for social phobia, but not for other anxiety disorders (Fyer *et al.*, 1993).

GENERALIZED SOCIAL PHOBIA AND AVOIDANT PERSONALITY DISORDER

Three recent studies have addressed the overlap between avoidant personality disorder and generalized social phobia (Herbert *et al.*, 1992; Turner *et al.*, 1992; Holt *et al.*, 1992). Across the three studies the findings were largely consistent in that hardly any cases of avoidant personality disorder could be delineated, who did not also fulfill the criteria for generalized social phobia. A recent study in which children with social phobia were compared to avoidant disorder and avoidant disorder plus social phobia, it was found that there was a striking similarity between the three groups (Francis *et al.*, 1992). These findings question the validity of avoidant personality disorder and generalized social phobia as distinct disorders. A solution of this problem could be to radically abdicate from the categorical distinctions between axis I anxiety disorders and personality, and classify a patient on the degree to which he or she suffers from social avoidance, as suggested by Widiger (1992).

PSYCHOPHARMACOLOGY OF SOCIAL PHOBIA

It is only during the last decade that the psychopharmacology of social phobia has been subject to consistent investigation. The early experiences with β-blocking drugs and irreversible non-selective monoamine oxidase inhibitors (MAOIs) provided sufficient evidence to suggest that pharmacotherapy could play a major role in the treatment of social phobia.

BENZODIAZEPINES

Successful treatment of generalized anxiety disorder and panic disorder with the triazolobenzodiazepine alprazolam has prompted investigations into the efficacy of this compound in social phobia. In two open studies, alprazolam was found to be effective in reducing severity of social anxiety and avoidance behavior (Reich *et al.*, 1988; Lydiard *et al.*, 1988). However, the efficacy of MAOIs appeared to be superior to alprazolam (Gelernter *et al.*, 1991).

In two small controlled studies positive effects of clonazepam were reported (Munjack *et al.*, 1991a; Reiter *et al.*, 1990). In the largest study thus far, Davidson *et al.* (1991) reported that 22 out of 26 social phobics (84.6%) showed good improvement with clonazepam. A major limitation of the latter study is that only the Clinical Global Impression scale was used, thus no specific information on social phobic anxiety or avoidance could be deduced from their study.

It is important to note that benzodiazepines have strong sedative properties and thus it is not known whether the reductions in social anxiety and avoidance are due to this sedative effect or whether there is a specific anxiolytic effect leading to diminished social avoidance.

β-ADRENERGIC BLOCKERS

The majority of studies with β-blockers have been performed in patients with a subtype of social anxiety, i.e. performance anxiety.

In several controlled studies in a variety of performing arts and sports, the use of β-blockers has appeared to be useful in reducing autonomic symptoms, such as palpitations and tremors (Brantigan *et al.*, 1982; Hartley *et al.*, 1983; Gates *et al.*, 1985; James and Savage, 1984). As a secondary effect anxiety reduction is achieved. Since not all β-blockers (e.g. atenolol) cross the blood–brain barrier, it is argued that the efficacy of β-blockers in performance anxiety is related to a attenuation of autonomic symptoms and not by a central reduction in anxiety.

In social phobia only a small number of studies using β-blockers have been published. Propranolol was found to be ineffective in the treatment of social phobia (Falloon *et al.*, 1981). In contrast Gorman and coworkers (1985) reported a good treatment response in social phobics with atenolol. In subsequent double–blind studies with MAOIs the limited efficacy of β-blockers in the treatment of generalized social phobia was further corroborated. In these studies no significant differences were found between placebo and atenolol (Liebowitz *et al.*, 1991, 1992). In other anxiety disorders, e.g. panic disorder, β-blockers appear to have only limited therapeutic value (Hayes and Schulz, 1987).

MONOAMINE OXIDASE INHIBITORS

In several studies beneficial effects of MAOIs in the treatment of social phobia have been reported. In most studies with the non-selective and irreversible MAOI phenelzine a reduction in social anxiety has been reported (Kelly *et al.*, 1970; Solyom *et al.*, 1973, 1981; Tyrer *et al.*, 1973; Tyrer and Steinberg, 1975; Mountjoy *et al.*, 1977; Liebowitz *et al.*, 1985).

There are, however, a number of methodological flaws with regard to the older studies with MAOIs. Firstly, in most studies mixed patient groups of agoraphobic, simple phobic and social phobic patients were used. Secondly, only small numbers of patients were studied. Thirdly, in the early studies vague diagnostic criteria were used (e.g. "phobic anxiety states"), and, moreover, low dosages were used as compared with those used in depressed patients (Tyrer et al., 1973; Solyom et al., 1973; Mountjoy et al., 1977; Solyom et al., 1981). It is thus impossible to determine whether the patients with social phobia as a separate group actually improved by treatment with phenelzine (see Table 1).

More recent studies revealed that tranylcypromine led to a marked improvement in 60% of social phobia patients (Versiani et al., 1988). Phenelzine has also recently been investigated in well-designed studies. In the study by Gelernter et al. (1991) four treatment conditions were compared: alprazolam (plus instructions for exposure: IE), phenelzine (plus IE), placebo (plus IE) and cognitive-behavioral therapy. Results showed that 63% of the phenelzine-treated patients were responders, whereas the response rate was only 39% in the alprazolam-treated group, 24% in the cognitive-behavioral group and 20% in the placebo group. The number of patients per group was too small to detect possible differences in treatment outcome, therefore it was concluded that all four treatment conditions were effective in reducing social anxiety and distress. An important limitation of this study is the fact that the therapeutic gains might have been related to increased exposure which was combined with all pharmacotherapeutic treatments.

In a study by Liebowitz et al. (1992) it was reported that phenelzine led to marked improvement in two-thirds of patients with social phobia, whereas atenolol could not be distinguished from placebo.

A major risk of the use of the conventional and irreversible MAOIs has been the development of hypertensive crises, due to potentiation of the tyramine pressor effect ("cheese effect"). The monoamine neurotransmitters, such as serotonin (5-hydroxytryptamine, 5-HT) and norepinephrine (NE), are preferentially deaminated by MAO-A, whereas other amines, such as phenylethylamine are endogenous substrates for MAO-B (Robinson and Kurtz, 1987). Tyramine, which was held responsible for the serious side effects of MAOIs, and dopamine are substrates for both types of enzymes. MAOIs leaving the B-form of MAO intact allow this isoenzyme to deaminate tyramine and thus no dietary measures are required during treatment with selective MAO-A inhibitors.

RECENT FINDINGS WITH SELECTIVE MAO-A INHIBITORS

So far the experiences with selective MAO-A inhibitors has been limited. Versiani et al. (1992) studied the effects of moclobemide and phenelzine in a double-blind parallel-group, placebo-controlled flexible dose study. Moclobemide is the prototype of the new generation of selective and reversible MAO-A inhibitors. It increases the content of 5-HT, NE and dopamine in the brain (review: Haefely et al. 1992). Seventy-eight patients with social phobia, 26 on moclobemide (mean dose 580±55 mg per day), 26 on phenelzine (67±15 mg per day), and 26 on placebo were included. It was found that on the social

Table 1. Controlled studies of MAOIs in social phobia

Study	Patients (N)	Design	Dose (mg)	Duration	Results
Tyrer et al. (1973)	Ag/SP (N=32)	Phenelzine Placebo	to 90	8 weeks	Phenelzine > placebo
Solyom et al. (1973)	Ag/SP (N=30)	Flooding Phenelzine Placebo	to 45	3 months	Flooding+ phenelzine effective
Mountjoy et al. (1977)	Anx. neur. (N=36) SP/Ag (N=22)	Phenelzine Diazepam Placebo	to 75 15	4 weeks	Phenelzine+ diazepam placebo in SP
Solyom et al. (1981)	Ag/SP (N=40)	2×2 Phenelzine placebo; exposure vs no exposure	to 45	6 weeks	Phenelzine > placebo on anxiety in exposure. No significant difference between exposure and phenelzine
Gelernter et al. (1991)	SP (N=65)	Phenelzine+IE Alprazolam+IE Placebo+IE Cogn. Behav.	to 90 to 7.3	12 weeks	All treatments effective. Phenelzine > alprazolam
Liebowitz et al. (1992)	SP (N=74) DSM–III-R	Phenelzine Atanolol Placebo	60 100	8 weeks	Phenelzine >atenolol Atenolol > placebo (NS)
Van Vliet et al. (1992)	SP (N=30) DSM-III-R	Brofaromine Placebo	150	12 weeks	Significant effect of brofaromine (> placebo) on social anxiety and avoidance
Versiani et al. (1992)	SP N=78 (DSM–III-R)	Moclobemide Phenelzine Placebo	to 600 90	16 weeks	Both moclobemide and phenelzine led to improvement of SP symptoms. After 16 weeks: 82% of moclobemide; 91% of phenelzine-treated patients asymptomatic

Ag, agoraphobia; Cogn. behav., cognitive-behavioral therapy; IE, instructions for exposure; SP, social phobia; Anx, neur., anxiety neurosis; NS, not significant.

phobia scale both phenelzine and moclobemide were significantly superior to placebo.

In our center we investigated the efficacy of brofaromine in a double-blind placebo-controlled design (Van Vliet et al. 1992). Similar to moclobemide, brofaromine selectively and competitively inhibits MAO-A, the enzyme responsible for the deamination of biogenic amines. In animal studies brofaromine has been shown to increase levels of NE, dopamine and 5-HT dose-dependently in rat brain (Waldmeier and Baumann, 1983). In addition to these effects brofaromine displayed weak 5-HT uptake inhibitory properties in synaptosomal preparations at doses about 30 times higher than those that inhibited MAO-A (Waldmeier and Stocklin, 1989).

Twenty-one females and nine males who fulfilled DSM-III-R criteria for social phobia were included. Patients were studied for 12 weeks in a double-blind, placebo-controlled design. If patients judged themselves to be improved they could continue their medication under double-blind conditions in a follow-up period which lasted another 12 weeks.

The dose of brofaromine was gradually increased from 50 to 150 mg daily (75 mg b.i.d.) in three weeks.

Efficacy of the treatment was assessed using the Social Phobia Scale (SPS; Liebowitz, 1987), the Spielberger State–Trait Anxiety Inventory (STAI; Van der Ploeg *et al.,* 1981), the Hamilton Anxiety Scale (Hamilton, 1967), and the Symptom Checklist 90-items (SCL-90).

Plasma levels of brofaromine and 3-methoxy-4-hydroxyphenylglycol (MHPG) were assessed at baseline and at week 4, 8 and 12. Plasma levels of 5-hydroxyindoleacetic acid (5-HIAA), melatonin and homovanillic acid (HVA) were measured on admission and week 12.

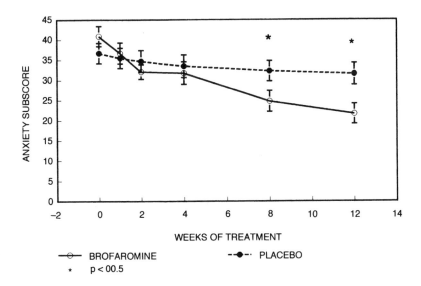

Figure 1 Mean ($\pm$ SEM) score on the anxiety subscale of the Social Phobia Scale in patients with social phobia treated with brofaromine (n=15) or placebo (n=14). Brofaromine was found to be superior to placebo from week 8.

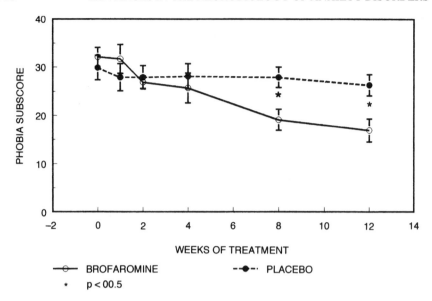

Figure 2 Mean (±SEM) score on the avoidance subscale of the Social Phobia Scale in patients with social phobia treated with brofaromine (*n*=15) or placebo (*n*=14). Brofaromine showed a statistically different treatment response from week 8 (Reprinted from Van Vliet *et al.*, Psychopharmacological treatment of social phobia, *Eur. Neuropsychopharmacol*, **12**, 1992, with kind permission from Elsevier Science–NL, Sara Burgerhartstraat 25, 1055 KV Amsterdam, The Netherlands).

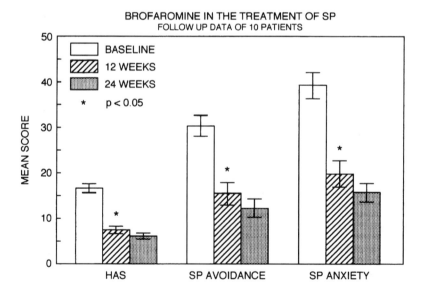

Figure 3 Mean (±SEM) score on the HAS, and the avoidance and anxiety subscales of the Social Phobia Scale during the follow-up period (Reprinted from Van Vliet *et al.*, Psychopharmacological treatment of social phobia, *Eur. Neuropsychopharmacol*, **12**, 1992, with kind permission from Elsevier Science–NL, Sara Burgerhartstraat 25, 1055 KV Amsterdam, The Netherlands).

CLINICAL RESULTS

Most notably we found a reduction in anxiety in social situations, as well as a decrease in social avoidance as measured using the social phobia scale (Figures 1 and 2). The SCL-90 revealed a reduction in interpersonal sensitivity and in the subscore anxiety and phobic avoidance. Ten patients who continued their treatment during the follow-up period continued to benefit from treatment with brofaromine (Figure 3).

Our results are similar to those obtained in previous studies in which (non-selective and irreversible) MAOIs were studied, and are in accordance with the results obtained with moclobemide. It should, however, be noted that the sample size is small and thus larger numbers of patients need to be studied before firm conclusions about efficacy can be drawn. In keeping with the pharmacological profile of brofaromine, we found a decrease in plasma MHPG, 5-HIAA and HVA. Biochemical and neuroendocrine results are discussed in detail elsewhere (Van Vliet et al., 1992).

A comprehensive biological theory of social phobia is lacking. During normal social anxiety, like public speaking, a two- to three-fold increase in plasma adrenaline was found (Liebowitz et al., 1985). During an adrenaline challenge study in 11 social phobics, however, only three patients experienced anxiety (Liebowitz, 1987). In addition, there is evidence indicating that a simple increase in plasma levels of adrenaline alone is inadequate to cause social anxiety (Papp et al., 1988).

It is not clear whether dopamine is involved in the pathogenesis of social phobia. Such a "dopaminergic theory" of social phobia is supported by the fact that MAOIs which have greater dopamine agonistic effects than tricyclic antidepressants (TCAs) are more effective in treating school phobias (Gittleman-Klein and Klein, 1972, 1973). Further support was suggested by a study from King and coworkers (1986), who reported a positive correlation of cerebrospinal fluid dopamine levels and self-reported extraversion in 16 social phobics. In addition, there is one case study reporting efficacy of the dopamine agonist bupropion in social phobia (Emmanuel et al., 1991).

It is unlikely that treatment studies with MAO-A inhibitors will shed more light on underlying biological mechanisms involved in social phobia, as these drugs lead to increases in several monoaminergic systems.

RECENT FINDINGS WITH SEROTONERGIC AGENTS IN SOCIAL PHOBIA

There is only circumstantial evidence that antidepressants like clomipramine and imipramine are effective in the treatment of social phobia (Gungras, 1977; Beaumont, 1977; Pecknold et al., 1982; Benca et al., 1986). Virtually no information is available on the effects of selective serotonergic drugs in the treatment of social phobia. Two open studies have reported the successful use of the 5-HT$_{1A}$ agonist buspirone in social phobia, albeit the scales used in these studies were not especially designed to measure social anxiety or avoidance, therefore they remain inconclusive (Schneier et al., 1990; Munjack et al. 1991). There are some case reports which have documented the efficacy of fluoxetine in social phobia (Sternbach, 1990; Schneier et al., 1992). Recently two open studies were published reporting efficacy of fluoxetine in patients with social phobia (Black et al., 1992; Van Ameringen et al., 1993), but well-designed studies are lacking.

In view of the fact that treatment with MAOIs affects two monoamine systems, no specific information can be derived from these studies with respect to the involvement of serotonergic or noradrenergic neuronal systems in social phobia.

With respect to other anxiety disorders there is abundant data suggesting involvement of 5-HT, particularly in panic disorder and obsessive-compulsive disorder (Den Boer and Westenberg, 1988, 1990, 1991; Westenberg and Den Boer, 1994).

In order to shed more light on this serotonergic theory, we performed a study with the selective serotonin reuptake inhibitor (SSRI) fluvoxamine in which 30 outpatients (17 females, 13 males) suffering from social phobia according to the DSM-III-R were enrolled in a double-blind placebo-controlled 12-week study. Patients with other anxiety disorders or with a major affective disorder were excluded. A score of 15 or higher on the Hamilton Depression Scale was an exclusion criterion. The dosage of fluvoxamine used was 150 mg, gradually increasing from 50 mg in the first week. Treatment efficacy was assessed by means of the Social Phobia Scale (anxiety and phobic avoidance subscales), the

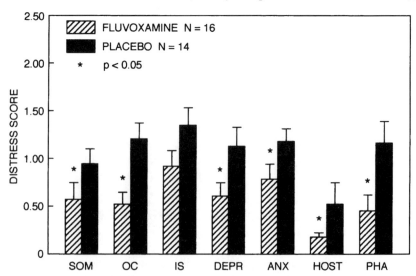

Figure 4 Factor scores of the Symptom Checklist 90 in patients with social phobia treated with fluvoxamine or placebo at the end of the treatment period. Fluvoxamine was superior to placebo on the factors SOM, OC, DEPR, ANX, HOST, PHA. SOM, somatization; OC, obsessive-compulsive; IS, interpersonal sensitivity; DEPR, depression; ANX, anxiety; HOST, hostility; PHA, phobic anxiety. (Reprinted from Van Vliet et al., A novel psychopharmacological approach to social phobia, *Psychopharmacology*, 1993, with kind permission of Elsevier Science–NL, Sara Burgerhartstraat 25, 1055 KV Amsterdam, The Netherlands).

SCL-90, Hamilton Anxiety Scale (HAS) and the State Anxiety Inventory. There were two drop-outs in the placebo group, due to lack of efficacy. If patients judged themselves to be improved they could continue their medication in a follow-up period which lasted another 12 weeks. Fifteen patients in the fluvoxamine group continued and none in the placebo group.

Fluvoxamine was found to be superior to placebo on virtually all psychometric scales. Social anxiety as measured with the Social Phobia Scale showed a statistically significant decrease compared with baseline in the fluvoxamine but not in the placebo group. Social phobic avoidance was reduced in both groups but there was a trend to greater improvement in the fluvoxamine group.

The score of all symptom factors of the SCL-90 (except the symptom factor Interpersonal Sensitivity) showed a statistically significant difference in favor of fluvoxamine. The results of the SCL-90 after treatment are depicted in Figure 4.

During the follow-up period of 12 weeks a further improvement was found in patients treated with fluvoxamine. General anxiety, social anxiety and social phobic avoidance declined further.

In conclusion: the SSRI fluvoxamine reduces general anxiety as measured with the HAS and has beneficial effects on social anxiety and social phobic avoidance as assessed using the Social Phobia Scale in patients suffering from social phobia. The effects appear to require a longer treatment period, probably similar to the treatment period in depressed patients or patients with panic disorder. This study supports the notion that serotonergic neural systems may be implicated in the pathophysiology of social phobia (Van Vliet et al., 1993).

It is difficult to explain why different anxiety disorders like panic disorder and social phobia might respond to the same pharmacological treatment. There is a large body of evidence suggesting that SSRIs as well as MAOIs are effective in the treatment of panic disorder (Den Boer and Westenberg, 1988, 1990). A parsimonious explanation as to why two different anxiety disorders respond to the same pharmacological treatment might be the fact that two subtypes of social phobia exist: generalized social phobia and discrete social phobia. The first type might show the greatest overlap with panic disorder patients and respond well to antidepressants and MAOIs. The second type, discrete social phobia, which is characterized by surges of autonomic activation, should respond to β-adrenergic blockers.

Another explanation could be that certain symptom profiles and behavioral dimensions within different diagnostic entities respond to SSRIs and MAOIs, irrespective of nosological diagnosis (Van Praag et al., 1987). It is well known that several psychiatric disorders like boulimia, panic disorder, obsessive-compulsive disorder and depressive disorders can be successfully treated with 5-HT uptake inhibitors. In depressive subtypes there is preliminary evidence that symptoms related to anxiety and aggression are the first ones to disappear with antidepressant treatment (Van Praag, 1992). It is conceivable, although at the present state of knowledge still speculative, that the same reasoning could be applied to generalized social phobia. If the effect of fluvoxamine or other specific 5-HT uptake inhibitors is confirmed in other studies, then one should look at common symptom profiles among patients suffering from, for example, panic disorder, obsessive-compulsive disorder and social phobia, which respond to 5-HT uptake inhibitors.

PRELIMINARY FINDINGS WITH PEPTIDES IN THE TREATMENT OF SOCIAL PHOBIA

Several neuropeptides have been implicated in the pathogenesis of anxiety, but clinical research is still in its infancy. Animal models have suggested anxiogenic effects for corticotropin-releasing hormone (CRH; Thatcher-Britton et al., 1985). In patients with panic disorder, two studies reported a blunted (adrenocorticotrophic hormone (ACTH) response to CRH (Roy-Byrne et al., 1986; Holsboer et al., 1987).

Neuropeptide Y (NPY), a peptide which is found in the gastrointestinal tract and in the central nervous systems (CNS), has also been implicated in anxiety. NPY is colocalized with NE in noradrenergic neurons in the brain stem and with γ-aminobutyric acid (GABA) in the cortex (Hendry et al., 1984). Considering these associations with monoaminergic systems a role in the pathogenesis of different anxiety disorder is probable. Moreover, in animal models "anxiolytic" effects of NPY have been reported (Heilig et al., 1988).

A third peptide which has been postulated to be involved in anxiety is cholecystokinin (CCK), a peptide which is abundant in the CNS. Preclinical and clinical studies have suggested a role in anxiety, most notably panic disorder, but it is likely that also in other anxiety disorders this peptide plays an important role in the regulation of anxiety (Van Megen et al., 1993; Bradwejn et al., 1994).

It has been suggested that peptides related to the pituitary ACTH, including the ACTH(4–9) analog Org 2766, increase the motivational value of environmental stimuli, by inducing a state of arousal in limbic structures of the midbrain. ACTH and related peptides may also be involved in behavior related to fear in animals. In the social interaction model of anxiety, ACTH(1–24) and ACTH(4–10) have been shown to reduce active social contact in rats, which has been interpreted as an anxiogenic effect (File, 1979). The social interaction model is an example of a new animal model of anxiety, which is based on manipulation of novelty and uncertainty. It has been shown that the amount of time rats engage in active social interaction can be manipulated by varying the familiarity of the environment as well as the level of illumination. In this model a reduction of social interaction between pairs of male rats is observed, when placed in a novel, well-lit environment (File and Hyde, 1978; File, 1980). This reduction in social interaction could be reversed by subacute administration of benzodiazepines (File and Velluci, 1978). Interestingly, the MSH/ACTH(4–9) analog Org 2766 has similar effects to benzodiazepines in this model, in that this peptide increases social interaction. Increased social interaction has been related to anxiolytic activity (File, 1981; File and Hyde, 1978) because chronic treatment with benzodiazepines, which have been shown to possess anxiolytic activity in humans, increase social interaction in rats (review: Gardner and Guy, 1984). Thus, based upon the effects in this animal model, Org 2766 may have anxiolytic activity in humans.

In some clinical studies a reduced anxiety level has been described, e.g. in demented elderly patients following oral treatment with this peptide (Ferris *et al.*, 1981; for review see Pigache and Rigter, 1981). Most clinical studies however, have studied the link between ACTH/MSH peptides and mood or cognition. In none of these studies was convincing evidence obtained for an antidementia or antidepressive efficacy, although decreases in feelings of tiredness and increases in alertness were reported (Gaillard, 1981; Tinklenberg and Thornton, 1983; Heuser *et al.*, 1993).

Table 2. Assessment results of Org 2766 in social phobia

	Org 2766		Placebo	
	Baseline	Week 6	Baseline	Week 6
HAM-A	15.5 ± 2.7	11.7 ± 4.8	15.2 ± 1.2	12.5 ± 4.4
HAM-D total	7.3 ± 2.2	6.8 ± 1.7	6.7 ± 1.0	5.3 ± 2.3
SDS/ZUNG	44.3 ± 10.4	38.5 ± 13.8	38.5 ± 6.9	35.5 ± 9.7
STAI	47.7 ± 16.7	35.2 ± 16.8	41.0 ± 6.1	32.8 ± 9.5
GSI	1.2 ± 1.0	0.5 ± 0.4	0.7 ± 0.3	0.4 ± 0.3

HAM-A, Hamilton Rating Scale for Anxiety; HAM-D, Hamilton Rating Scale for Depression; SDS/ZUNG, Zung's Self Rating Depression Scale; STAI, State–Trait Anxiety Inventory; GSI, General Symptom Index of the 90-item Symptom Checklist.

In the present studies we explored the clinical efficacy of Org 2766 in a double-blind placebo-controlled design in patients with anxiety disorders. Three groups of patients were investigated, suffering from panic disorder, generalized anxiety disorder or social phobia, all according to DSM-III-R criteria (Den Boer *et al.*, 1992).

The results reported herein will be confined to patients (n=12) with social phobia. Treatment with Org 2766 and placebo resulted in a small decrease in both the "anxiety" and the "avoidance" subscales of the social phobia scale. The mean ($\pm$SD) anxiety score in the Org 2766 group was 41.3 ± 12.3 before and 35.0 ± 13.9 after treatment. In the placebo group the mean baseline anxiety score was 27.8 ± 13.0 and was 22.0 ± 8.1 at the end of treatment. The mean avoidance score in the Org 2766 group was 29.0 ± 16.1 and 29.2 ± 17.0 before and after treatment, respectively. In the placebo group the mean avoidance score was 17.8 ± 7.3 and 18.3 ± 8.5, respectively. Statistical analysis did not reveal significant differences. Other psychometric assessments are summarized in Table 2. No significant effects were present on any of the psychometric assessments. No side effects were reported.

In social phobia patients, Org 2766 did not result in a significant decrease in anxiety experienced in social situations, nor in a reduction in social avoidance. The social interaction model has been used as a model predicting anxiolytic activity of benzodiazepines and other experimental compounds. The predictive value of the social interaction test for newer compounds can only be critically assessed after clinical evaluation.

In the present study, however, no clear anxiolytic activity for Org 2766 could be observed, thus casting doubt on the predictive value of the social interaction test as a predictor for anxiolytic activity in patients with anxiety disorders.

SUMMARY AND CONCLUSIONS

There is increasing evidence that the new generation of reversible and selective MAO-A inhibitors like moclobemide and brofaromine are of therapeutic value in the treatment of social phobic complaints, whereas β-blockers appear to be only of limited value. Only one study has been published in which anxiolytic effects of the MSH/ACTH(4–9) analog Org 2766 has been investigated. The results indicate that there is no evidence for anxiolytic effects of this experimental compound. There is one controlled study indicating that social anxiety is reduced during treatment with the selective 5-HT uptake inhibitor fluvoxamine, although the effects on social avoidance were limited. Furthermore a relatively long treatment period was required to reach the observed anxiolytic effect. In numerous clinical studies it has been established that MAO-A inhibitors as well as 5-HT uptake inhibitors are therapeutic in patients with depression and panic disorder. Recently it has been shown that 5-HT uptake inhibitors such as clomipramine, fluvoxamine and fluoxetine are effective in treating patients with obsessive-compulsive disorder. These findings may argue for a common underlying mechanism, at least for those symptoms within different diagnostic categories, related to anxiety. The findings also provide empirical evidence suggesting that MAO-A inhibitors and 5-HT uptake inhibitors can be appropriate treatments for different disorders with overlapping symptom clusters.

REFERENCES

American Psychiatric Association on Nomenclature and Statistics (1987). *Diagnostic and Statistical Manual of Mental Disorders*, 3rd edn, revised. American Psychiatric Association, Washington, DC.

Amies, P. L., Gelder, M. G. and Shaw, P. M. (1983). Social phobia: a comparative clinical study. *Br. J. Psychiatry*, **142**, 174–179.

Barlow, D. H. (1985). The dimension of anxiety disorders. In *Anxiety and the Anxiety Disorders* (eds A. H. Tuma and J. D. Maser), pp. 479–500. Erlbaum, Hillsdale, NJ.

Beaumont, G. (1977). A large open multicentre trial of clomipramine in the management of phobic disorders. *J. Int. Med. Res.*, **5**, 116–123.

Benca, R., Matuzas, W. and Al-Sadir, J. (1986). Social phobia, MVP and response to imipramine (letters to the editors). *J. Clin. Psychopharmacol.*, **6**, 50–51.

Black, B., Uhde, T. W. and Tancer, M. E. (1982). Fluoxetine for the treatment of social phobia. *J. Clin. Psychopharmacol.*, **82**(4), 293–295.
Bradwejn, J., Koszycki, D., van Megen, H. *et al.* (1994). The panicogenic effects of CCK-tetrapeptide are antagonized by L-365,260, a central CCK receptor antagonist in patients with panic disorder. *Arch. Gen. Psychiatry*, **51**, 486–493.
Brantigan, C. O., Brantigan, T. A. and Joseph, N. (1982). Effect of a beta-blockade and beta-stimulation on stage fright. *Am. J. Med.*, **72**, 88–94.
Burton, R. (1621). *The Anatomy of Melancholy* (reprinted 1977). Dent, London.
Davidson, J. R. T., Ford, S. M., Smith, R. D. and Potts, N. L. S. (1991). Long-term treatment of social phobia with clonazepam. *J. Clin. Psychiatry*, **52** (11, Suppl.), 16–20.
Deltito, J. A. and Stam, M. (1990). Psychopharmacology treatment of avoidant personality disorder. *Compr. Psychiatry*, **30**, 498–509.
Den Boer, J. A. and Westenberg, H. G. M. (1988). Effects of a serotonin and noradrenaline uptake inhibitor in panic disorder: a double blind comparative study with fluvoxamine and maprotiline. *Int. Clin. Psychopharmacol.*, **3**, 59–74.
Den Boer, J. A. and Westenberg, H. G. M. (1990). Serotonin function in panic disorders: a double blind placebo controlled study with fluvoxamine and ritanserine. *Psychopharmacology*, **102**, 85–94.
Den Boer, J. A. and Westenberg, H. G. M. (1991). Do panic attacks reflect an abnormality in serotonin receptor subtypes? *Hum. Psychopharmacol.*, **6**, 25–30.
Den Boer, J. A., Westenberg, H. G. M. and De Vries, H. (1992). The MSH/ACTH analog ORG 2766 in anxiety disorders. *Peptides*, **13**, 109–112.
DiNardo, P. A., Moras, K., Barlow, D. H. *et al.* (1993). Reliability of DSM-III-R anxiety disorder categories. *Arch. Gen. Psychiatry*, **50**, 251–256.
Emmanuel, N. P., Lydiard, R. B. and Ballenger, J. C. (1991). Treatment of social phobia with bupropion. *J. Clin. Psychopharmacol.*, **11**(4), 276–277.
Emmelkamp, P. M. C. (1982). *Phobic and Obsessive Compulsive Disorder: Theory, Research and Practice*. Plenum Press, New York.
Falloon, I. R., Lloyd, G. G. and Harpin, R. (1981). The treatment of social phobia. *J. Nerv. Ment. Dis.*, **169**, 180–184.
Ferris, S. H., Reisberg, B. and Gershon, S. (1981). Neuropeptide modulation of cognition and memory in humans. In *Aging in the 1980s: Selected Contemporary Issues in the Psychology of Aging* (ed. L. Poon), pp. 212–220. American Psychological Association, Washington, DC.
File, S. E. (1979). Effects of ACTH 4–10 in the social interaction test of anxiety. *Brain Res.*, **171**, 157–160.
File, S. E. (1980). The use of social interaction as a method for detecting anxiolytic activity of chlordiazepoxide-like drugs. *J. Neurosci. Methods*, **2**, 219–238.
File, S. E. (1981). Contrasting effects of Org 2766 and alpha-MSH on social and exploratory behavior in the rat. *Peptides*, **2**, 255–260.
File, S. E. and Hyde, J. R. G. (1978). Can social interaction be used to measure anxiety? *Br. J. Pharmacol.*, **62**, 19–24.
File, S. E. and Velluci S. V. (1978). Studies on the role of ACTH and 5-HT in anxiety, using an animal model. *J. Pharm. Pharmacol.*, **30**, 105–110.
Francis, G., Last, C. G. and Strauss, C. C. (1992). Avoidant disorder and social phobia in children and adolescents. *J. Acad. Child Adolesc. Psychol.*, **31**(6), 1086–1089.
Fyer, A. J., Mannuzza, S., Chapman, T. F. *et al.* (1993). A direct interview family study of social phobia. *Arch. Gen. Psychiatry*, **50**, 286–293.
Gaillard, A. W. K. (1981). ACTH analogs and human performance. In *Endogenous Peptides and Learning and Memory Processes* (eds J. L. Martinez, R. A. Jensen, R. B. Messing *et al.*, pp. 181–196. Academic Press, New York.
Gardner, C. R. and Guy, A. P. (1984). A social interaction model of anxiety sensitive to acutely administered benzodiazepines. *Drug Rev. Res.*, **4**, 207–216.

Gates, G. A., Saegert, P., Wilson, N. *et al.* (1985). Effects of beta blockade on singing performance. *Ann. Otol. Rhinol. Laryngol.*, **94**, 570–574.

Gelernter, C. S., Uhde, T. W., Cimbolic, P. *et al.* (1991). Cognitive-behavioral and pharmacological treatments of social phobia. *Arch. Gen. Psychiatry*, **48**, 938–945.

Gittleman-Klein, R. and Klein, D. (1972). Controlled imipramine treatment in school phobia. *Arch. Gen. Psychiatry*, **25**, 204–207.

Gittleman-Klein, R. and Klein, D. (1973). School Phobia: diagnostic considerations in the light of imipramine effects. *J. Nerv. Ment. Dis.*, **156**, 193–215.

Gomperts, W. (1992). *De opkomst van de sociale fobie (The Rise of Social Phobia)*. Bert Bakker, Amsterdam.

Gorman, J. M. and Gorman, L. K. (1987). Drug treatment of social phobia. *J. Affect. Disord.*, **13**, 183–192.

Gorman, J. M., Liebowitz, M. R., Fyer, A. J. *et al.* (1985). Treatment of social phobia with atenolol. *J. Clin. Psychopharmacol.*, **5**, 669–677.

Gungras, M. (1977). An uncontrolled trial of clomipramine in the treatment of phobic and obsessional states in general practice. *J. Int. Med. Psychol.*, **32**, 50–55.

Haefely, W., Burkard, W. P., Cesura, A. M. *et al.* (1992). Biochemistry and pharmacology of moclobemide, a prototype RIMA. *Psychopharmacology*, **118**, S6–S14

Hamilton, M. (1967). Development of a rating scale for primary depressive illness. *Br. J. Clin. Psychol.*, **6**, 50–55.

Hartley, L. R., Ungapen, S., Davie, I. and Spencer, D. J. (1983). The effect of beta blocking drugs on speaker's performance and memory. *Br. J. Psychiatry*, **142**, 512–517.

Hayes, P. E. and Schulz, S. C. (1987). BDZ, beta-blockers in anxiety disorders. *J. Affect. Disord.*, **13**, 119–130.

Heilig, M., Söderpalm, B., Engel, J. A. and Widerlöv, E. (1988). Centrally administered neuropeptide-Y (NPY) produces anxiolytic effects in animal anxiety models. *Psychopharmacology*, **98**, 524–529.

Heimburg, R. G. and Barlow, D. H. (1991). New developments in cognitive-behavioral therapy for social phobia. *J. Clin. Psychiatry*, **52**, 21–29.

Hendry, S. H. C., Jones, E. G., Felipe, J. *et al.* (1984). Neuropeptide containing neurons of the cerebral cortex are also GABA-ergic. *Proc. Natl. Acad. Sci., USA*, **1**, 6526–6530.

Herbert, J. D., Hope, D. A. and Bellack, A. S. (1992). Validity of the distinction between generalized social phobia and avoidant personality disorder. *J. Abnorm. Psychol.*, **101**, 332–229.

Heuser, I., Heuser-Link, M., Gotthardt, U. *et al.* (1993). Behavioral effects of a synthetic corticotropin 4–9 analog in patients with depression and patients with alzheimer's disease. *J. Clin. Psychopharmacol.*, **13**, 171–174.

Holsboer, F., Bardeleben, U. van, Heuser, I. and Steiger, A. (1987). Corticotropin releasing hormone in patients with depression, alcoholism and panic disorder. *Horm. Metab. Res.*, **16**, 80–88.

Holt, C. S., Heimberg, R. G. and Hope, D. A. (1992). Avoidant personality disorder and the generalized subtype in social phobia. *J. Abnorm. Psychol.*, **101**, 318–325.

James, I. M. and Savage, I. (1984). Beneficial effects of nadolol on anxiety-induced disturbances of performance in musicians: a comparison with diazepam and placebo. *Am. Heart J.*, **108**, 1150–1155.

Kelly, D., Guirguis, W., Frommer, E. *et al.* (1970). Treatment of phobic states with antidepressants: a retrospective study of 246 patients. *Br. J. Psychiatry*, **116**, 387–398.

King, R. J., Mefford, I. N., Wang, C. *et al.* (1986). CSF dopamine levels correlate with extraversion in depressed patients. *Psychiatr. Res.*, **19**, 305.

Leary, M. (1983). *Understanding Social Anxiety: Social, Personality and Clinical Perspectives*. Sage, Beverly Hills, CA.

Liebowitz, M. R. (1987). Social phobia. *Mod. Probl. Pharmacopsychiatry*, **22**, 141–173.

Liebowitz, M. R., Gorman, J. H., Fyer, A. J. and Klein, D. F. (1985). Social phobia. *Arch. Gen. Psychiatry*, **42**, 729–736.

Liebowitz, M. R., Schneier, F. R., Hollander, E. *et al.* (1991). Treatment of social phobia with drugs other than benzodiazepines. *J. Clin. Psychiatry*, **52** (11, Suppl.), 10–15.

Liebowitz, M. R., Schneier, F., Campeas, R. *et al.* (1992). Phenelzine vs atenolol in social phobia. *Arch. Gen. Psychiatry*, **49**, 290–300.

Lydiard, R. B., Laraia, M. T., Howell, E. F. and Ballenger, J. C. (1988). Alprazolam in the treatment of social phobia. *J. Clin. Psychiatry*, **49** (1), 17–19.

Marks, M. and Gelder, M. G. (1966). Different ages of onset in varieties of phobia. *Am. J. Psychiatry*, **123**, 218–221.

Mountjoy, C. Q., Roth, M., Garside, R. F. and Leitch, I. M. (1977). A clinical trial of phenelzine in anxiety depressive and phobic neurosis. *Br. J. Psychiatry*, **131**, 486–492.

Munjack, D. J., Baltazar, P. L., Bohn, P. B. *et al.* (1991a). Clonazepam for the treatment of social phobia: a pilot study. *J. Clin. Psychiatry*, **51** (5, suppl.), 35–40.

Munjack, D. J., Bruns, J., Baltazar, P. L. *et al.* (1991b). A pilot study of buspirone in the treatment of social phobia. *J. Anxiety Disord.*, **5**, 87–98.

Murphy, H. B. M. (1982). *Comparative Psychiatry: The International and Intercultural Distribution of Mental Illness.* Springer-Verlag, New York.

Nichols, K. A. (1974). Severe social anxiety. *Br. J. Med. Psychol.*, **47**, 301–306.

Papp, L. A., Gorman, J. M., Liebowitz, M. R. *et al.* (1988). Epinephrine infusions in patients with social phobia. *Am. J. Psychiatry*, **145**(6), 733–736.

Pecknold, J. C., McClure, D. J., Appeltauer, L. *et al.* (1982). Does tryptophan potentiate clomipramine in the treatment of agoraphobic and social phobia patients? *Br. J. Psychiatry*, **140**, 484–490.

Pigache, R. M. and Rigter, H. (1981). Effects of peptides related to ACTH on mood and vigilance in man. *Front. Horm. Res.*, **8**, 193–207.

Regier, D. A., Boyd, J. H., Burke, J. D., Jr *et al.* (1988). One month prevalence of mental disorders in the United States: based on five epidemiologic catchment area sites. *Arch. Gen. Psychiatry*, **45**, 977–986.

Reich, J., Yates, W. and Tes, W. (1988). A pilot study of treatment of social phobia with alprazolam. *Am. J. Psychiatry*, **145**(5), 590–594.

Reiter, S. R., Pollack, M. H., Rosenbaum, J. F. and Cohen, L. S. (1990). Clonazepam for the treatment of social phobia. *J. Clin. Psychiatry*, **51**, 470–472.

Riskind, J. H., Beck, A. T., Berchik, R. J. *et al.* (1987). Reliability of DSM-IIR diagnoses for major depression and generalized anxiety disorder using the structured clinical interview for DSM-IIIR. *Arch. Gen. Psychiatry*, **44**, 817–820.

Robinson, D. S. and Kurtz, N. M. (1987). Monoamine oxidase inhibiting drugs: pharmacological and therapeutic issues. In *Psychopharmacology, The Third Generation in Progress* (ed. H. Y. Meltzer), pp. 777–783. Raven Press, New York.

Roy-Byrne, P. P., Uhde, T. W., Post, R. M. *et al.*, (1986). The corticotropin hormone stimulation test in patients with panic disorder. *Am. J. Psychiatry*, **143**, 896–899.

Schneier, F. R., Johnson, J., Hornig, C. D. *et al.* (1992a). Social phobia; comorbidity and morbidity in an epidemiological sample. *Arch. Gen. Psychiatry*, **49**, 282–288.

Schneier, F. R., Chin, S. J., Hollander, E. and Liebowitz, M. R. (1992b). Fluoxetine in social phobia (letter to the editor). *J. Clin. Psychopharmacol.*, **12**, 62–63.

Schneier, F., Campeas, R. and Fallon, B. (1990). Buspirone in social phobia (abstract). Presentation at the 17th Congress of Collegium Internationale Neuro Psychopharmacologicum, Kyoto, Japan.

Solyom, L., Heseltine, G. F. D., McClure, D. J. *et al.* (1973). Behaviour therapy vs drug therapy in the treatment of phobic neurosis. *Can. J. Psychiatry*, **18**, 25–31.

Solyom, C., Solyom, L., La Pierre, Y. *et al.* (1981). Phenelzine and exposure in the treatment of phobias. *Biol. Psychiatry*, **16**, 239–247.

Solyom, L., Ledwidge, B. and Solyom, C. (1986). Delineating social phobia. *Br. J. Psychiatry*, **149**, 464–470.

Sternack, H. (1990). Fluoxetine treatment of social phobia. *J. Clin. Psychopharmacol.*, **10**, 230.

Swaan, A. de (1981). The politics of agoraphobia: on changes in emotional and relational management. *Theory and Society*, **10**, 359–185.

Thatcher-Britton, K., Morgan, J., Rivier, J. *et al.* (1985). Chlordiazepoxide attenuates response suppression induced by corticotropin releasing factor in the conflict test. *Psychopharmacology*, **86**, 170–174.

Tinklenberg, J. R. and Thornton, J. E. (1983). Neuropeptides in geriatric psychopharmacology. *Psychopharmacol. Bull.*, **19**, 198–211.

Turner, S. M., Beidel, D. C. and Townsley, R. M. (1992). Social phobia: a comparison of specific and generalized subtypes and avoidant personality disorder. *J. Abnorm Psychol.*, **101**(2), 326–331.

Tyrer, P. and Steinberg, D. (1975). Symptomatic treatment of agoraphobia and social phobics: a follow-up study. *Br. J. Psychiatry*, **127**, 163–168.

Tyrer, P., Candy, J. and Kelly, D. (1973). A study of the clinical effects of phenelzine and placebo in the treatment of phobic anxiety. *Psychopharmacology*, **2**, 237–254.

Van Ameringen, M., Mancini, C. and Streiner, D. L. (1993). Fluoxetine efficacy in social phobia. *J. Clin. Psychiatry*, **54**(1), 27–32.

Van der Ploeg, H. M., Delfares, P. B. and Spielberger, C. D. (1981). *Handleiding bij de zelfbeoordelingsvragenlijst.* Swets and Zeitlinger, Lisse.

Van Megen, H. J. G. M., Den Boer, J. A. and Westenberg, H. G. M. (1994). On the significance of cholecystokinin receptors in panic disorder. In *Progress in Neuropsychopharmacology and Biological Psychiatry*, **18**, 1235–1246.

Van Praag H. M. (1992). About the centrality of mood lowering in mood disorders. *Eur. Neuropsychopharmacol.*, **2**, 393–404.

Van Praag, H. M., Kahn, R. J., Asnis, G. M. *et al.* (1987). Denosologisation of biological psychiatry or the specificity of 5-HT disturbances in psychiatric disorders. *J. Affect. Disord.*, **13**, 1–8.

Van Vliet, I. M., Den Boer, J. A. and Westenberg, H. G. M. (1992). Psychopharmacological treatment of social phobia: clinical and biochemical effects of brofaromine, a selective MAO-A inhibitor. *Eur. Neuropsychopharmacol.*, **12**, 21–29.

Van Vliet, I. M., Den Boer, J. A. and Westenberg, H. G. M. (1993). A novel psychopharmacological approach to social phobia; a double blind placebo controlled study with fluvoxamine. *Psychopharmacology* (in press).

Versiani, M., Mundinn, F. D., Wardi, A. E. and Liebowitz, M. R. (1988). Tranylcypromine in social phobia. *J. Clin. Psychopharmacol.*, **8**, 279–283.

Versiani, M., Nardi, A. E., Mindim, F. D. *et al.* (1992). Pharmacotherapy of social phobia: a controlled study with moclobemide and phenelzine. *Br. J. Psychiatry*, **161**, 353–360.

Waldmeier, P. C. and Baumann, P. A. (1983). A new reversible and selective inhibitor of MAO-A, on biogenic amine levels and metabolism in rat brain. *Naunyn Schiedebergs Arch. Pharmacol.*, **324**, 20–26.

Waldmeier, P. C. and Stocklin, L. (1989). The reversible MAO inhibitor, brofaromine, inhibits serotonin uptake in vivo. *Eur. J. Pharmacol.*, **169**, 197–204.

Westenberg, H. G. M. and Den Boer, J. A. (1994). The neuropharmacology of anxiety: a review on the role of serotonin. In *Handbook of Depression and Anxiety* (eds J. A. Den Boer and J. M. A. Sitsen, pp. 405–446. Marcel Dekker, New York.

Widiger, Th.A. (1992). Generalized social phobia versus avoidant personality disorder: a commentary on three studies. *J. Abnorm. Psychol.*, **101**, 340–343.

Part VII

INTEGRATIVE VIEW

19 Serotonin-related, Anxiety/Aggression-driven, Stressor-precipitated Depression: A Psychobiological Hypothesis

H. M. VAN PRAAG
Academic Psychiatric Center, University of Limburg, Maastricht, The Netherlands

HYPOTHESIS

The hypothesis I will submit in this paper is composed of three components. First, a subgroup of depression exists in which serotonergic (serotonin = 5-hydroxytryptamine = 5-HT) dysfunctions play a pathogenetic role. Second, in those so-called 5-HT-related depressions, dysregulation of anxiety and/or aggression are the primary symptoms while mood-lowering is a derivative phenomenon. Third, the 5-HT-related anxiety/aggression-driven depressions are precipitated by stressors, in individuals that are susceptible to the psychologically disrupting effects of (certain types) of psychotraumatic events. The evidence in favor of these three components I will discuss separately.

5-HT-RELATED DEPRESSION

5-HT DISTURBANCES

In a subgroup of depression disturbances in central serotonergic systems have been ascertained. The most significant of them are lowering of baseline and post-probenecid levels of 5-hydroxyindoleacetic acid (5-HIAA), the major metabolite of 5-HT. These phenomena can be considered as an indication of diminished metabolism of 5-HT in (certain parts of) the central nervous system (CNS) (Van Praag et al., 1970; Van Praag and Korf, 1971; Meltzer and Lowy, 1987; Westenberg and Verhoeven, 1988).

Receptor studies with challenge tests using more or less specific 5-HT agonists revealed changes in 5 HT receptor sensitivity (Caldecott-Hazard et al., 1991; Siever et al., 1991; Cowen and Wood, 1991; Cowen, 1993), while single-

Advances in the Neurobiology of Anxiety Disorders. Edited by H. G. M. Westenberg, J. A. Den Boer and D. L. Murphy
©1996 John Wiley & Sons Ltd

photon emission computed tomography (SPECT) studies indicated an increase of 5-HT$_2$ receptor density in the frontal cortex of some depressed patients (D'haenen *et al.*, 1992). Increased numbers of 5-HT$_2$ receptors have also been found in the frontal cortex of suicide victims (Arango *et al.*, 1990) and on blood platelets in depression (Arora and Meltzer, 1989) in particular suicidal depressions (Pandey *et al.*, 1990). It is unknown whether low cerebrospinal fluid (CSF) 5-HIAA, 5-HT challenge test disturbances and signs of increased 5-HT$_2$ receptor density intercorrelate.

The changes in 5-HT receptor status could be primary and the diminution of 5-HT metabolism secondary, i.e. compensatory; or, vice versa, the changes in 5-HT metabolism could be primary with adaptive alterations in 5-HT receptor density and/or sensitivity as a consequence. The latter hypothesis seems at present more likely than the former (Cowen, 1993).

SPECIFICITY

Lowering of CSF 5-HIAA appeared not to be·correlated with type of depressive syndrome, type of mood disorder or severity of the depression (Van Praag, 1992a). The changes in 5-HT metabolism were, instead, linked to components of the depression, in particular with heightened anxiety (Figure 1) and aggression dysregulation, both inwardly and outwardly directed (Figure 2) (Kahn *et al.*, 1988a, 1988b; Asberg *et al.*, 1986, 1987; Eison and Eison, 1994).

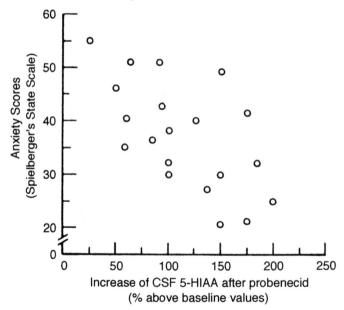

Figure 1 Concentration of 5-HIAA in CSF in relation to the degree of trait anxiety in patients with major depression, melancholic type (endogenous depression; vital depression). (Reprinted from Van Praag, 1988, by permission of Oxford University Press.)

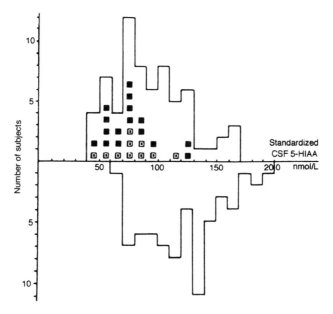

Figure 2 Standardized concentration of CSF 5-HIAA in patients who have attempted suicide (upward) and healthy volunteer control subjects (downward). Black boxes indicate suicide attempts by a violent method (any method other than drug overdose, taken by mouth, or a single wrist cut). "D" indicates a subject who subsequently died from suicide, in all cases but one within one year after the lumbar puncture (Asberg *et al.*, 1986)

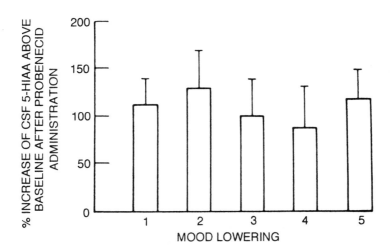

Figure 3 Concentration of 5-HIAA in CSF in relation to the degree of mood lowering as assessed by the treating physician on a five-point scale in untreated patients with major depression, melancholic type (Van Praag, 1992a)

Interestingly, no correlation could be established between lowering of CSF 5-HIAA and mood-lowering (Van Praag, 1992a) (Figure 3).

The correlation between 5-HT disturbances on the one hand, and dysregulated anxiety- and aggression-regulation on the other, is not restricted to depression but was found in non-depressive psychiatric disorders as well (Van Praag et al., 1987, 1990; Traskman Bendz et al., 1993; Winchel and Stanley, 1991; Deakin and Graeff, 1991; Brain and Haug, 1992; Coccaro, 1992; Nutt and Lawson, 1992; Simeon et al., 1992; Pratt, 1992; Handley and McBlane, 1993; Benkert et al., 1993). Thus, 5-HT disturbances in depression appear to be what I have called functionally specific, rather than syndromally or nosologically specific. They occur across diagnoses (Van Praag et al., 1975, 1987, 1990).

PATHOGENETIC RELEVANCE

In most depressed patients the 5-HT disturbances, as manifested in the lowering of CSF 5-HIAA, persist in times of remission (Van Praag, 1977, 1992a; Traskman et al., 1981; Asberg et al., 1987). Maintenance treatment of recurrent unipolar depression with 5-hydroxytryptophan (5-HTP), in combination with a peripheral decarboxylase inhibitor, normalizes the CSF 5-HIAA level and reduces the relapse frequency of depression (Van Praag and Haan, 1979, 1980a, 1980b). 5-HTP is a 5-HT precursor that is centrally readily transformed into 5-HT. It could thus be expected to eliminate the alleged deficit in 5-HT synthesis in certain forms of depression.

The observation that additional supply of 5-HT exercises a prophylactic effect in recurrent unipolar depression we considered to be an indication that the 5-HT disturbances in certain types of depression are part of the pathophysiology of those conditions, and not just secondary phenomena, marginal with respect to the pathogenetic process.

ANXIETY AND/OR AGGRESSION-DRIVEN DEPRESSION

In a subgroup of depressive patients, a depressive episode is heralded by increased anxiety, and/or signs of dysregulated outward directed aggression (irritability, crankiness, bursts of anger). Mood-lowering in those cases comes later (Fava and Kellner, 1991; Van Praag, 1992a, 1992b) (Table 1). In addition, in some depressive patients, the first symptoms to respond to antidepressants are anxiety and aggression, while mood elevation appears to be a latecomer (Katz et al., 1991).

The two subgroups—the one in which anxiety/aggression heralds the depres-

Table 1. First manifestation of depression in 50 patients with major depression and 50 with dysthymia and the occurrence of those features in a normal control group (Van Praag, 1992)

	Major depression		Dysthymic depression		Controls (n = 50)
	Symptoms pronounced	Symptoms mild or absent	Symptoms pronounced	Symptoms mild or absent	
Low spirits	11	39	42	8	2
Anxiety	41	9	24	26	3
Irritability	38	12	21	29	4
Inability to enjoy	16	34	7	43	1
Lack of drive	18	32	11	39	2
Diminished concentration	21	29	17	33	2
Difficulties thinking through	12	38	8	42	1
Fatigue	9	41	29	21	6
Disturbed sleep	24	26	24	26	3
Diminished appetite	14	36	6	44	2

Table 2. Correlation between anxiety and aggression in acute psychiatric patients from different diagnostic categories. (Reprinted from Apter *et al.*, Interrelations among anxiety, aggression, impulsivity and mood, *Psychiatry Research*, **32**, 191–199, 1990, with kind permission from Elsevier Science Ireland Ltd, Bay ISK, Shannon Industrial Estate, Co. Clare, Ireland)

	Suicide risk	Violent risk	Impulsivity	State anxiety	Trait anxiety
Suicide risk	0.53*	0.50*	0.47*	0.67*	
Violent risk		0.39**	0.33**	0.48*	
Impulsivity			0.33**	0.48*	

$*p < 0.001$; $**p < 0.01$.

sion and the other in which anxiety/aggression is first to respond to antidepressants—coincide to a large extent. Fifty-nine percent of depressed patients in whom anxiety/aggression appeared as precursor symptoms showed an early response of anxiety and aggression to antidepressants. In the group of patients with early symptoms of a different nature this percentage was 29.

Anxiety and aggression, finally, are not independent phenomena but occur highly intercorrelated, across diagnoses (Apter *et al.*, 1990; Katon and Roy-Byrne, 1991; Coryell *et al.*, 1992) (Table 2).

Based on these data we formulated the hypothesis of an anxiety/aggression-driven depression, i.e. a subtype of depression in which dysregulated aggression and/or anxiety are the primordial symptoms, while mood-lowering is a derivative.

DO THE SUBGROUP OF 5-HT-RELATED DEPRESSION AND THE SUBGROUP OF ANXIETY/AGGRESSION-DRIVEN DEPRESSION COINCIDE?

LINKAGE OF 5-HT DISTURBANCES AND ANXIETY/AGGRESSION

The 5-HT disturbances observed in a subgroup of depression supposedly carry pathogenetic significance. Moreover they are strongly linked to the anxiety and aggression dimensions of the depressive syndrome.

If a subgroup of anxiety/aggression-driven depression does indeed exist, one would expect patients with anxiety/aggression as precursor symptoms of depression to be overrepresented in the group of 5-HT-related depression, i.e. the patients with lowered CSF 5-HIAA. This could indeed be shown. In the low-CSF 5-HIAA group, 62% of patients mentioned anxiety/aggression, not mood-lowering, as the first manifestations of depression. In the normoserotonergic group this percentage amounted to 30.

In other words, dysfunctional serotonergic status and the occurrence of anxiety/aggression as early symptoms of depression are clearly coupled. Anxiety- and aggression-dysregulation are the first symptoms to occur and hence are probably primordial and "driving", i.e. driving the patient into a full-blown state of depression. Moreover in the hyposerotonergic patients a successful treatment with antidepressants is often inaugurated by amelioration of anxiety- and aggression-dysregulation. Mood elevation occurs later, supposedly because the driving mechanisms have first to be switched off.

Parkinson's disease is frequently accompanied by depression (Gothan et al., 1986), a complication possibly related to destruction of serotonergic neurons (Mayeux et al. 1988). Interestingly, anxiety is a prominent feature of Parkinson depression that frequently precedes the onset of the depression (Henderson et al., 1992). Parkinson depression possibly belongs to the group of 5-HT-related, anxiety/aggression-driven depressions (Van Praag, 1993).

THERAPEUTIC EXPECTATIONS

If a 5-HT-related subgroup of depression existed in which anxiety and aggression are the driving forces, one would expect that those depressions would preferentially respond tᴏ compounds that diminish anxiety and/or aggression via regulation of the serotonergic system. So far some findings suggest that at least part of this prediction is being fulfilled.

Members of the azapirone class of compounds have been successfully used as anxiolytics. These compounds are partial agonists of $5-HT_{1A}$ receptors (e.g. buspirone and ipsapirone). Anxiolytic activity has also been reported of flesinoxan, a non-azapirone, full $5-HT_{1A}$ agonist. The anxiolytic potential of these compounds is contingent on regulation of serotonergic circuits (Lopez-Ibor, 1988; Eison and Eison, 1993; Deakin, 1993). Increasing evidence indicates that such compounds, *in addition*, possess antidepressant properties (Ansseau *et al.*, 1993; Rickels *et al.*, 1990; Heller *et al*, 1990; Stahl *et al*, 1992; Deakin, 1993). Unknown is whether the group of 5-HT-related, anxiety- and/or aggression-driven depressions respond preferentially.

Eltoprazine is a rather selective agonist of 5-HT_{1B} receptors and exhibits in animals a strong and selective aggression-reducing action. Human data, though very scarce, show a similar action (Verhoeven *et al.*, 1992). In addition some, admittedly very preliminary, findings suggest an additional antidepressive component. Data on a possible preferential effect in 5-HT-related, anxiety- and/or aggression-driven depression are not available.

LIFE EVENTS AND 5-HT-RELATED ANXIETY/AGGRESSION-DRIVEN DEPRESSION

LIFE EVENTS AND 5-HT-RELATED DEPRESSION

The 5-HT disturbances in depression—at least the lowering of the CSF 5-HIAA level—are permanent. Depression frequently takes a recurrent rather than a chronic course. Assuming that the 5-HT disturbances have pathogenetic significance, we hypothesized that the 5-HT disturbances could possibly be conceived as vulnerability factors, decreasing coping ability, and increasing the risk of depression in case of mounting stress (Van Praag and Haan, 1980a).

In order to get an impression of the stress level prior to the onset of depression we used the life event scale developed by Paykel *et al.* (1971). Based on data obtained from 213 psychiatric patients and 160 relatives of psychiatric patients, these authors rank-ordered 61 life events according to their psychotraumatic weight. We extended the "top five" events a score of 12, the subsequent five a score of 11, and so on, so that the last six events received a score of 1. If a patient mentioned more than one event the scores were averaged.

From a cohort of 203 patients with depression, of whom CSF 5-HIAA had been measured, we contrasted those 25 with the lowest CSF 5-HIAA concentrations with those with the highest CSF 5-HIAA values in terms of the seriousness, i.e. the "weight" of the life events that had occurred in the three months prior to the onset of the depression.

The average weight of life events that had occurred in that period was significantly less in the low-CSF 5-HIAA group than in the high-CSF 5-HIAA group (Figure 4). This observation permits two explanations. First, 5-HT-related depression arises in large measure autonomously, i.e. independent of psychotraumatic events. Second, in 5-HT-related depression the susceptibility for (certain) psychotraumatic events is increased, which is why ostensibly insignificant events still exercise a powerful decompensating effect. The probability of the second hypothesis is greater than that of the first, a conclusion which is based on considerations discussed in the next section.

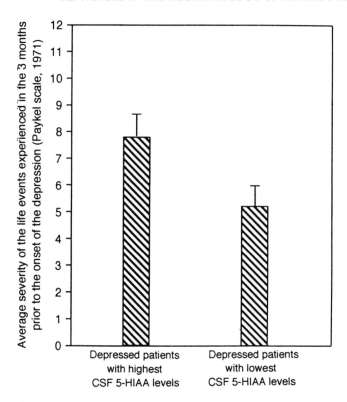

Figure 4 Average weight of the stressor(s) in 25 depressive patients with the lowest CSF 5-HIAA concentration and the 25 depressed patients with the highest CSF 5-HIAA values, sampled from a group of 203 patients suffering from various types of depression, in whom CSF 5-HIAA was measured

PERSONALITY AND 5-HT-RELATED DEPRESSION

In the group of low-CSF 5-HIAA depressives, manifestations of personality disorder were more prevalent than in the group of high-CSF 5-HIAA depressives. In this study we focused on egosyntonic as opposed to egodystonic symptoms. Egodystonic symptoms of personality disorder are experienced by the patient as pathological. Examples are excessive fears, outspoken moodinesss and perfectionism with difficultie⸗ to terminate, to a degree that task completion is interfered with. Egosyntonic symptoms, on the other hand, are experienced as part of one's self—"it is just the way I am, doctor"—though they may profoundly compromise the quality of and the satisfaction with one's life. Egosyntonic personality disorder corresponds with Freud's concept of character neurosis. The transition from egosyntonic to egodystonic personality disorder is gradual, but yet the distinction is important, because these "character neuroses" (mild forms of personality disorder, one could say) largely escape the present assessment instruments of personality disorders and thus remain a stepchild of experimental psychiatry.

To trace symptoms of egosyntonic personality disorder we did not rely on available questionnaires because they are largely geared towards the egodystonic counterparts. Instead we used structured interview techniques focusing on phenomenological phenomena in the sense of Jaspers (1948). That is, we concentrated on the individual's own experiences (Van Praag, 1989, 1992b). In this case we tried to explore whether the patient experienced his or her personality make-up as being neurotic, i.e. as a source of dissatisfaction and displeasure. We qualified a personality as (character-) neurotically disturbed if, in a structured interview, the following experiential qualities were thought to be present by at least two independently scoring clinicians:

1. Basic feelings of discontent with one's life situation and one's own psychological make-up. Feelings that life has treated one unfairly, in that it had blessed most others with more pleasure and satisfaction than oneself.
2. Unhappiness with one's personal relations, ranging from parental relations and school- and work-experiences, to marital relations and relations with one's children. The other is felt to be not forthcoming, distant, threatening, cold, abrasive or in any other way not meeting the individual's expectations and needs. As a consequence, a chronic feeling of loneliness and solitude has developed.
3. Emotional instability, in that the basic discontent ignites a range of emotions varying form mood-lowering to guilt, anger, despair and anxiety. These emotions are generally intense, vary abruptly and frequently, sometimes ignited by traceable events in the life situation, sometimes not clearly so.

Each of the three factors we scored on a five-point scale ranging from 4 to 0, so that a maximum score of 12 and a minimum score of 0 could be obtained. Interviews were done when the patients were in remission (Hirschfeld et al., 1983). The average score on the three items was 9.8 in the group of low-5-HIAA depressives and 6.1 in that of high-5-HIAA depressives. The former group thus held a larger proportion of (ostensibly) "asymptomatic" or "minor" personality disorder than the group of high-5-HIAA depressives.

Moreover, we explored in detailed free interviews the character of the life events occurring in the three months prior to the onset of the depression. In the low-5-HIAA group the majority ranked rather low on the Paykel scale. Rating them on a global impact scale ranging from 0 (unimportant) to 4 (severely disrupting) the patients themselves, however, considered them to be severe (mean rating 3.1), i.e. as serious blows to an already meagre sense of independence and self-appreciation. Examples are a derogatory remark of one's employer, a disappointing date, an expected invitation that had not been forthcoming. Due to personality imperfections these individuals were vulnerable for psychotraumatic events, particularly those that reinforced feelings of insecurity, loneliness, non-acceptance, and dependence.

In conclusion, in 5-HT-related depression the susceptibility for (certain) life events is increased, which is why seemingly insignificant events may exercise, psychologically, a powerful decompensating effect.

5-HT-RELATED, ANXIETY/AGGRESSION-DRIVEN, STRESSOR-PRECIPATED DEPRESSION

A mental state with which an individual cannot adequately cope generates, initially, feelings of discomfort and thereupon a conglomerate of physical and psychological symptoms carrying the name of stress syndrome. The traumatic events generating these conditions are called stressors (Seyle, 1980). The composition of the stress syndrome varies considerably between individuals, but two elements are almost universally present, i.e. anxiety and anger. Anger might be overt or suppressed and directed towards the instigators of the stress, or towards oneself for being unable to handle the stressful situation adequately. Stress syndrome-prone individuals—in short, stress-prone individuals—more readily than normals develop stress symptoms under burdensome conditions.

Patients with 5-HT-related depression can be considered to be stress-prone, first, because of a biological impairment, i.e. a trait-related 5-HT disturbance, linked to instability of anxiety- and aggression-regulation. That is why these individuals will readily respond with anxiety and/or anger in taxing conditions. Stress-proneness is further conditioned by debilitating personality traits and corresponding oversensitiveness for the unsettling effects of (particular) psychotraumatic life events.

The biological and psychological impairments converge, in making patients with 5-HT-related depression susceptible to the stress syndrome, the anxiety/aggression components of which serve as pacemakers for mood-lowering, driving the patient into a full-blown depression.

With this, a 5-HT-related, anxiety/aggression-driven, stressor-precipitated depression has been conceptualized: an as yet hypothetical construct I set out to define and to support.

SUMMARY

The concept of a 5-HT-related, anxiety- and/or aggression-driven, stressor-precipitated depression is formulated and discussed. It comprises the following elements:

1. The serotonergic disturbances found in some depressed individuals—particularly lowered CSF 5-HIAA—are linked to the anxiety and the aggression components of the depressive syndrome.
2. In this type of depression, called 5-HT-related depression, dysregulation of anxiety and/or aggression is primordial and mood-lowering is a derivative

phenomenon. In other words this is a group of anxiety/aggression-driven depressions.

3. The serotonergic impairment in certain types of depression is a trait phenomenon, i.e. persists during remission. This disturbance makes the individual susceptible to perturbation of anxiety- and aggression-regulation. Anxiety and (overt or suppressed) anger are core constituents of the stress syndrome. Thus, the serotonergic disturbance will induce a heightened sensitivity for stressful events, i.e. the latter will induce, more readily than normal, stress phenomena, among which are anxiety and anger. The latter psychological features induce lowering of mood and thus "drive" the patient into a full-blown depression.

Furthermore it is predicted that anxiolytics and serenics (i.e. antiaggressive drugs) that act via normalization of serotonergic circuits will exert an antidepressant effect in 5-HT-related depression, *in addition* to their therapeutic actions in anxiety disorders and states of increased aggressiveness, respectively.

The exact nature of the serotonergic impairment in 5-HT-related depression has yet to be elucidated.

REFERENCES

Ansseau, M., Pitchot, W., Moreno, A. G. *et al.* (1993). Pilot study of flesinoxan, a 5-HT1A agonist, in major depression: effects on sleep REM latency and body temperature. *Hum. Psychopharmacol.*, **8**, 279–283.

Apter, A., Praag van, H. M., Plutchik, R. *et al.* (1990). Interrelations among anxiety, aggression, impulsivity, and mood: a serotonergically linked cluster, *Psychiatr. Res.*, **32**, 191–199.

Arango, V., Ernsberger, *et al.* (1990). Autoradiographic demonstration of increased serotonin 5-HT$_2$ and β-adrenergic receptor binding sites in the brain of suicide victims. *Arch. Gen. Psychiatry*, **47**, 10380.

Arora, R. C. and Meltzer, H. Y. (1989). Increased serotonin$_2$ (5-HT$_2$) receptor binding as measured by ^{3}H-lysergic acid diethylamide (^{3}H-LSD) in the blood platelets of depressed patients. *Life Sci.*, **44**, 725.

Asberg, M., Norstrom, P. and Traskman-Bendz, L. (1986). Biological factors in suicide. In *Suicide* (ed. A. Roy). Williams & Wilkins, Baltimore.

Asberg, M., Schalling, D., Traskman-Bendz, L. and Wagner, A. (1987). Psychobiology of suicide, impulsivity, and related phenomena. In *Psychopharmacology: The Third Generation of Progress* (ed. H. Y. Meltzer). Raven Press, New York.

Benkert, O., Wetzel, H. and Szegedi, A. (1993). Serotonin dysfunctions syndromes: a functional common denominator for classification of depression, anxiety, and obsessive-compulsive disorder. *Int. Clin. Psychopharmacol.*, **8** (Suppl. 1), 3–14.

Brain, P. F. and Haug, M. (1992). Hormonal and neurochemical correlates of various forms of animal "aggression." *Psychoneuroendocrinology*, **17**, 537–551.

Caldecott-Hazard, S., Guze, B. H., Kling, M. A. *et al.* (1991). Clinical and biochemical aspects of depressive disorders: I. Introduction, classification, and research techniques. *Synapse*, **8**, 185–211.

Coccaro, E. F. (1992). Impulsive aggression and central serotonergic system function in humans: an example of a dimensional brain–behavior relationship. *Int. Clin. Psychopharmacol.*, **7**, 3–12.

Coryell, W., Endicott, J. and Winokur, G. (1992). Anxiety syndromes as epiphenomena of primary major depression: outcome and familial psychopathology. *Am. J. Psychiatry*, **149**, 100–107.

Cowen, P. J. (1993). Serotonin receptor subtypes in depression: evidence from studies in neuroendocrine regulation. *Clin. Neuropharmacol.*, **16** (Suppl. 3), S6–S18.

Cowen, P. J. and Wood, D. J. (1991). Biological markers of depression. *Psychol. Med.*, **21**, 831–836.

Deakin, J. F. W. (1993). A review of clinical efficacy of 5-HT$_{1A}$ agonists in anxiety and depression. *J. Psychopharmacol.*, **7**, 283–289.

Deakin, J. F. and Graeff, F. G. (1991). Critique, 5-HT and mechanisms of defence. *J. Psychopharmacol.*, **5**, 305–315.

D'haenen, H., Bossuyt, A., Mertens, J. *et al.* (1992). SPECT imaging of serotonin$_2$ receptors in depression. *Psychiatr. Res.*, **45**, 227–237.

Eison, A. S. and Eison, M. S. (1994). Serotonergic mechanisms in anxiety. *Prog. Neuropsychopharmacol. Biol. Psychiatry*, **18**, 47–62.

Fava, G. A. and Kellner, R. (1991). Prodromal symptoms in affective disorders. *Am. J. Psychiatry*, **148**, 823–830.

Gotham, A., Brown, R. G. and Marsen, C. D. (1986). Depression in Parkinson's disease: a quantitative and qualitative analysis. *J. Neurol. Neurosurg. Psychiatry*, **49**, 381–389.

Handley, S. L. and McBlane (1993). 5HT drugs in animal models of anxiety. *Psychopharmacology*, **112**, 13–20.

Heller, A. H., Beneke, M., Kuemmel, B. *et al.* (1990). Ipsapirone: evidence for efficacy in depression. *Psychopharmacol. Bull.*, **26**, 219–222.

Henderson, R., Jurlan, R., Kersun, J. M. and Como, P. (1992). Preliminary examination of the comorbidity of anxiety and depression in Parkinson's disease. *J. Neuropsychiatry*, **4**, 257–264.

Hirschfeld, R., Klerman, G. L., Clayton, P. J. *et al.* (1983). Assessing personality: effects of the depressive state on trait measurement. *Am. J. Psychiatry*, **140**, 695–699.

Jaspers, K. (1948). *Allgemeine Psychopathologie*, Springer, Berlin.

Kahn, R. S., Wetzler, S., Van Praag, H. M. and Asnis, G. M. (1988a). Behavioral indications for serotonin receptor hypersensitivity in panic disorder. *Psychiatr. Res.*, **25**, 101–104.

Kahn, R. S., Wetzler, S., Van Praag, H. M. and Asnis, G. M. (1988b). Neuroendocrine evidence for 5-HT receptor hypersensitivity in patients with panic disorder. *Psychopharmacology*, **96**, 360–364.

Katon, W. and Roy-Byrne, P. P. (1991). Mixed anxiety and depression. *J. Abnorm. Psychol.*, **100**, 337–345.

Katz, M. M., Koslow, S., Maas, J. *et al.* (1991). Identifying the specific clinical actions of amitriptyline: irrelationships of behavior, affect, and plasma levels in depression. *Psychol. Med.*, **21**, 599–611.

Lopez-Ibor, J. J. (1988). The involvement of serotonin in psychiatric disorders and behavior. *Br. J. Psychiatry*, **153**, 26–39.

Mayeux, R., Stern, Y., Sano, M. *et al.* (1988). The relationship of serotonin to depression in Parkinson's disease, *Mov. Disord.*, **3**, 237–244.

Meltzer, H. J. and Lowy, M. T. (1987). The serotonin hypothesis of depression. In *Psychopharmacology: The Third Generation of Progress* (ed. H. J. Meltzer). Raven Press, New York.

Nutt, D. and Lawson, C. (1992). Panic attacks: a neurochemical overview of models and mechanisms. *Br. J. Psychiatry*, **160**, 165–178.

Pandey, G. N., Pandey, S. C., Janicak P. G. *et al.* (1990). Platelet serotonin-2 receptor binding sites in depression and suicide. *Biol. Psychiatry*, **28**, 215.

Paykel, E. G., Prusoff, B. A. and Uhlenhuth, E. H. (1971). Scaling of life events. *Arch. Gen. Psychiatry*, **24**, 340–347.

Pratt, J. A. (1992). The neuroanatomical basis of anxiety. *Pharmacol. Ther.*, **55**, 149–181.

Rickels, K., Amsterdam, J., Clary, C. *et al.* (1990). Buspirone in depressed outpatients: a controlled study. *Psychopharmacol. Bull.*, **26**, 163–167.

Selye, H. (ed.) (1980). *Selye's Guide to Stress Research*, Vol. 1. Van Nostrand Reinhold, New York.

Siever, L. J., Kahn, R. S., Lawlor, B. A. *et al.* (1991). II. Critical issues in defining the role of serotonin in psychiatric disorders. *Pharmacol. Rev.*, **43**, 509–525.

Simeon, D., Stanley, B., Frances, A. *et al.* (1992). Self-mutilation in personality disorders: psychological and biological correlates. *Am. J. Psychiatry*, **149**, 221–226.

Stahl, S. M., Gastpar, M., Keppel Hesselink, J. M. and Traber, J. (eds) (1992). *Serotonin 1A receptors*. Raven Press, New York.

Traskman, L., Asberg, M., Bertilsson, L. and Sjostrand, L. (1981). Monoamine metabolites in CSF and suicidal behavior. *Arch. Gen. Psychiatry*, **38**, 633–636.

Traskman-Bendz, L., Alling, C., Alsén, M. *et al.* (1993). The role of monoamines in suicidal behavior. *Acta Psychiatr. Scand.* (Suppl. 371), 45–47.

Van Praag, H. M. (1977). Significance of biochemical parameters in the diagnosis, treatment and prevention of depressive disorders. *Biol. Psychiatry*, **12**, 101–131.

Van Praag, H. M. (1988). Serotonergic mechanisms and suicidal behavior. *Psychiatr. Psychobiol.*, **3**, 335–346.

Van Praag, H. M. (1989). Diagnosing depression: looking backward into the future, *Psychiatr. Dev.*, **4**, 375–394.

Van Praag, H. M. (1992a). About the centrality of mood lowering in mood disorders. *Eur Neuropsychopharmacol.*, **2**, 393–404.

Van Praag, H. M. (1992b). *Make Believes in Psychiatry or the Perils of Progress*. Brunner Mazel, New York.

Van Praag, H. M. (1993). Serotonin and affective psychopathology in Parkinson's disease: a psychobiological hypothesis with therapeutic consequences. In *Mental Dysfunction in Parkinson's Disease* (eds E. C. Wolters and P. Scheltens), pp. 325–348. VU Amsterdam.

Van Praag, H. M. and Haan de, S. (1979). Central serotonin metabolism and frequency of depression. *Psychiatr. Res.*, **1**, 219–224.

Van Praag, H. M. and Haan de, S. (1980a). Depression vulnerability and 5-hydroxytryptophan prophylaxis. *Psychiatr. Res.*, **3**, 75–83.

Van Praag, H. M. and Haan de, S. (1980b). Central serotonin deficiency: a factor which increases depression vulnerability? *Acta Psychiatr. Scand. Suppl.*, **61**, 89–95.

Van Praag, H. M. and Korf, J, (1971). Endogenous depressions with and without disturbances in the 5-hydroxytryptamine metabolism: a biochemical classification? *Psychopharmacology*, **19**, 148–152.

Van Praag, H. M., Korf, J. and Puite, J. (1970). 5-Hydroxyindoleacetic acid levels in the cerebrospinal fluid of depressive patients treated with probenecid. *Nature*, **225**, 1259–1260.

Van Praag, H. M., Korf, J., Lakke, J. P. W. F. and Schut, T. (1975). Dopamine metabolism in depression, psychoses and Parkinson's disease: the problem of the specificity of biological variables in behaviour disorders. *Psychol. Med.*, **5**, 138–146.

Van Praag, H. M., Kahn, R. S., Asnis, G. M. *et al.* (1987). Denosologization of biological psychiatry or the specificity of 5-HT disturbances in psychiatric disorders. *J. Affect. Disord.*, **13**, 1–8.

Van Praag, H. M., Asnis, G. M., Kahn, R. S. *et al.* (1990). Monoamines and abnormal behavior: a multi-aminergic perspective. *Br. J. Psychiatry*, **157**, 723–734.

Verhoeven, W. M. A., Tuinier, S., Sijben, N. A. S., Berg van den, Y. W. H. M., Witte de, E. P. P. M., Pepplinkhuizen, L., and Nieuwenhuizen van, O. (1992). Eltoprazine in mentally retarded self-injuring patients, *Lancet*, 340, 1037–1038.

Westenberg, H. G. M., Verhoeven, W. M. A. (1988). CSF monoamine metabolites in patients and controls: support for a bimodal distribution in major affective disorders. *Acta Psychiatr. Scand.*, 478, 541–749.

Winchel, R. M., and Stanley, M. (1991). Self-injurious behavior; a review of the behavior and biology of self-mutilation, *Am. J. Psychiatry*, 148, 306–317.

Index

Note: Page numbers in *italic* refer to figures and/or tables

Index compiled by Caroline S. Sheard